Audrey –

In appreciation of your support and friendship. My best wishes to you and Steve for continued success in your academic careers.

– Paul

OUTPATIENT ANESTHESIA

Edited by

Paul F. White, M.D., Ph.D.

Professor and Assistant to the Chairman
Director, Division of Clinical Research
Department of Anesthesiology
Washington University School of Medicine
St. Louis, Missouri

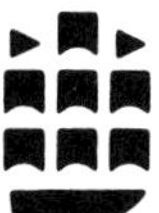

Churchill Livingstone
New York, Edinburgh, London, Melbourne

Library of Congress Cataloging-in-Publication Data

Outpatient anesthesia / edited by Paul F. White.
p. cm.
Includes bibliographical references.
ISBN 0-443-08437-8
1. Anesthesia. 2. Surgery, Outpatient. I. White, Paul F., date.
[DNLM: 1. Ambulatory Care. 2. Ambulatory Surgery. 3. Anesthesia. WO 200 094]
RD82.088 1990
617.9′6—dc20
DNLM/DLC
for Library of Congress 90-1556
CIP

Distributed in the United Kingdom by Churchill Livingstone, Robert Stevenson House, 1–3 Baxter's Place, Leith Walk, Edinburgh EH1 3AF, and by associated companies, branches, and representatives throughout the world.

Accurate indications, adverse reactions, and dosage schedules for drugs are provided in this book, but it is possible that they may change. The reader is urged to review the package information data of the manufacturers of the medications mentioned.

The Publishers have made every effort to trace the copyright holders for borrowed material. If they have inadvertently overlooked any, they will be pleased to make the necessary arrangements at the first opportunity.

Acquisitions Editor: *Toni M. Tracy*
Assistant Editor: *Nancy Terry*
Copy Editor: *Kathleen P. Lyons*
Production Designer: *Angela Cirnigliaro*
Production Supervisor: *Sharon Tuder*

Printed in the United States of America

First published in 1990

To my loving parents,
Paul and Kathryn White

Contributors

Jeffrey L. Apfelbaum, M.D.
Associate Professor, Department of Anesthesia and Critical Care, University of Chicago Division of Biological Sciences Pritzker School of Medicine; Director of Outpatient Surgery, University of Chicago Hospitals and Clinics, Chicago, Illinois

Frederic A. Berry, M.D.
Professor of Anesthesiology and Pediatrics, Department of Anesthesiology, University of Virginia School of Medicine, Charlottesville, Virginia

Casey D. Blitt, M.D.
Old Pueblo Anesthesiology, Ltd.; Chairman, Department of Anesthesiology, Tucson Medical Center; Former Professor, Department of Anesthesiology, University of Arizona College of Medicine, Tucson, Arizona

Burton S. Epstein, M.D.
Seymour Alpert Professor and Chairman, Department of Anesthesiology, The George Washington University School of Medicine and Health Sciences, Washington, DC

Robert J. Fragen, M.D.
Professor of Clinical Anesthesia, Department of Anesthesia, Northwestern University Medical School, Chicago, Illinois

Gareth W. Jones, B.Sc., M.B., B.S., M.R.C.P.
Instructor, Department of Anesthesiology, Virginia Commonwealth University Medical College of Virginia School of Medicine, Richmond, Virginia

Surinder K. Kallar, M.D.
Professor, and Director of Ambulatory Anesthesia, Department of Anesthesiology, Virginia Commonwealth University Medical College of Virginia School of Medicine, Richmond, Virginia

Laura L. Katz, J.D.
Associate and Health Care Specialist, Ober, Kaler, Grimes and Shriver, Attorneys at Law, Baltimore, Maryland

Kari Korttila, M.D., Ph.D.
Associate Professor, Department of Anaesthesia, Women's Hospital, University of Helsinki, Helsinki, Finland

J. Lance Lichtor, M.D.
Associate Professor, Department of Anesthesia and Critical Care, University of Chicago Division of Biological Sciences Pritzker School of Medicine, Chicago, Illinois

Michael A. Marschall, M.D.
Assistant Professor, Division of Plastic Surgery, Department of Surgery, University of Illinois College of Medicine at Chicago; Attending Plastic Surgeon, Cook County Hospital, Chicago, Illinois

Helen McKebery, R.N., R.M.
Charge Nurse, Day Surgery Unit, Box Hill Hospital, Melbourne, Australia

Charles H. McLeskey, M.D.
Associate Professor, and Director of Academic Affairs, Department of Anesthesiology, University of Colorado School of Medicine, Denver, Colorado

Michael F. Mulroy, M.D.
Staff Anesthesiologist, Department of Anesthesiology, Virginia Mason Clinic, Seattle, Washington

David M. Nibel, B.A.
University of Colorado School of Medicine, Denver, Colorado

Frederick K. Orkin, M.D.
Associate Professor, Department of Anesthesia, University of California, San Francisco, School of Medicine; Anesthesiologist, UCSF Surgery Center, Medical Center of the University of California, San Francisco, California

Beverly K. Philip, M.D.
Assistant Professor, Department of Anaesthesia, Harvard Medical School; Director, Day Surgery Unit, Brigham and Women's Hospital, Boston, Massachusetts

S. Mark Poler, M.D.
Assistant Professor, Department of Anesthesiology, Washington University School of Medicine; Medical Director of Outpatient Surgery, Barnes Hospital at Washington University Medical Center, St. Louis, Missouri

Michael F. Roizen, M.D.
Professor and Chairman, Department of Anesthesia and Critical Care, and Professor, Department of Medicine, University of Chicago Division of Biological Sciences Pritzker School of Medicine, Chicago, Illinois

Gita Rupani, M.D.
Assistant Professor, Department of Anesthesia and Critical Care, University of Chicago Division of Biological Sciences Pritzker School of Medicine, Chicago, Illinois

Bruce D. Schreider, M.D., Ph.D.
Clinical Associate Professor, and Vice Chairman, Division of Clinical Affairs, Department of Anesthesia and Critical Care, University of Chicago Division of Biological Sciences Pritzker School of Medicine, Chicago, Illinois

Richard C. Schultz, M.D.
Professor, Division of Plastic Surgery, Department of Surgery, University of Illinois College of Medicine at Chicago, Chicago, Illinois

David J. Steward, M.B.
Professor, Department of Anaesthesiology, University of British Columbia Faculty of Medicine; Anaesthetist-in-Chief, British Columbia's Children's Hospital, Vancouver, British Columbia, Canada

Robert K. Stoelting, M.D.
Professor and Chairman, Department of Anesthesia, Indiana University School of Medicine, Indianapolis, Indiana

Linda Dickey White, R.N., M.S., C.N.O.R.
Director, Operating Rooms and Postanesthesia Care Unit, Barnes Hospital at Washington University Medical Center, St. Louis, Missouri

Paul F. White, M.D., Ph.D.
Professor and Assistant to the Chairman, and Director, Division of Clinical Research, Department of Anesthesiology, Washington University School of Medicine, St. Louis, Missouri

James B. Wieland, J.D.
McGuire and Wieland, Attorneys at Law, San Mateo, California

John Zelcer, M.B., B.S., B.Med.Sc.(Hons)
Clinical Instructor, Department of Anaesthesia, St. Vincent's Hospital, University of Melbourne, Melbourne, Victoria, Australia

Foreword

The 1980s was a time of remarkable change in clinical medicine, but no aspect has proved to be more profound, pervasive, and influential in the delivery of health care than the development of outpatient anesthesia and surgery. Today, virtually all minor surgery and a substantial portion of major surgery have been shifted from almost exclusively hospital-based, inpatient procedures to a diversity of outpatient procedures in freestanding and hospital affiliated units.

While surgical procedures are much the same whether performed in the inpatient or outpatient setting, anesthesia and nursing care required for these procedures are different. Patients coming to an outpatient facility the day of surgery and going home the same day present a myriad of new and unique problems with which anesthesiologists and nurses must cope. Initially, anesthesiologists attempted to adapt their care of outpatients to the traditional, standard anesthetic techniques used for many years with inpatients. This approach was fraught with problems. Gradually, through clinical trial and error, they learned what worked and adjusted the anesthetic technique to the outpatient setting. What has emerged is a new discipline, making outpatient anesthesia the most rapidly growing area in clinical anesthesia.

Throughout the developmental period of outpatient anesthesia, there has been an inadequate scientific foundation upon which to base clinical decisions and choices. Recognizing the need to develop sound research programs to investigate the issues unique to outpatient anesthesia, several anesthesiologists have focused all of their substantial research and clinical talents on this new subspecialty. Foremost among these is Paul F. White, M.D., Ph.D., the editor of *Outpatient Anesthesia*. No one in the field of anesthesia has contributed more to the scientific development of outpatient anesthesia than Paul. He is ideally suited to edit this text since he has dealt personally with all the critical issues in his research, teaching, and clinical care. He brings the breadth and depth of expertise that are seldom obtainable in an editor. In addition, he has assembled a group of contributors, all of whom are well-known and knowledgeable in their assigned area. This coalition of exceptional skill and experience has resulted in a text that is concise, comprehensive, authoritative, and readable. It offers its readers alternatives in care based on research analysis as well as clinical experience, and, where appropriate, the best solutions to patient management are offered and justified.

C. Philip Larson, Jr., M.D.
Professor, Departments of
Anesthesia and Surgery
Division of Neurosurgery
Stanford University
School of Medicine
Stanford, California

Preface

Over the past two decades, outpatient (ambulatory) surgery has become a widely accepted form of health care for millions of Americans. In the 1980s, 600 freestanding outpatient surgery centers were performing over one million operations each year. At the present time, outpatient procedures performed in hospital-affiliated centers account for over 40 percent of all operations performed in the hospital setting. Similar growth patterns are being reported in Europe, Canada, and Australia. With the explosive growth in outpatient surgery, both practitioners and medical organizations have recognized the need for improved care of this increasing patient population. *Outpatient Anesthesia* focuses on the perioperative care of outpatients undergoing elective surgery. The book is intended as a resource for anesthesiologists, both in practice and training, as well as other physicians, nurses, and health care professionals involved in ambulatory surgery care.

The contributors, acknowledged authorities in their respective fields, explore a variety of important issues in outpatient anesthesia and surgery, including preoperative assessment, choice of anesthesia, intraoperative monitoring, pain management, and postoperative complications, as well as outpatient facility and personnel, regulatory issues, and medicolegal considerations. All of these aspects of anesthesia care are presented to give the reader a comprehensive analysis of this vital area of surgical care. Chapters focusing on pediatric and geriatric patients outline the special problems that need to be addressed for these patient populations.

Duplication of specific issues is inevitable in a multiauthored text and may result in a variety of opposing opinions. As editor, I feel these differences of opinion illustrate for the reader the dynamics of this advancing field of medicine. With this in mind, Dr. Burton Epstein, one of the pioneers in modern outpatient anesthesia, discusses some of these major controversies in the field and comments on the varying opinions presented in the text.

I am hopeful that the work gathered here will prove useful to all health care professionals involved in the care of patients undergoing ambulatory surgery. If it succeeds in this, the book will have accomplished its intention.

The efforts of all the contributing authors are graciously acknowledged. Finally, I would like to thank my anesthesia, nursing, and surgery colleagues at the University of California, San Francisco, Stanford University, and Washington University for their helpful discussions and insights regarding the management of outpatients. Thanks are also owed my publisher, Churchill Livingstone. Without the dedication and invaluable assistance of Ms. Nancy Terry and the superb copy editing of Ms. Kathleen Lyons, as well as the encouragement of Ms. Toni Tracy, this book would not have been completed. Finally, I would like to express my sincere appreciation to my family—Linda, Kristine, and Lisa—and friends for their support and encouragement during this project.

Paul F. White, M.D., Ph.D.

Contents

1

Outpatient Anesthesia—An Overview

Paul F. White

Outpatient (ambulatory) surgery is widely practiced in the United States and is increasing in popularity throughout the world. The practice of ambulatory surgery was first described in the early 1900s by Drs. J. H. Nicoll at the Glasgow Royal Hospital for Sick Children and R. M. Waters at the "Down-Town" Anesthesia Clinic in Sioux City, Iowa.[1,2] However, it was not until the 1960s that the first hospital-based ambulatory surgery facilities were established at the University of California in Los Angeles and George Washington University in Washington, DC.[3,4] In 1970, the first successful freestanding outpatient facility was established in Phoenix, Arizona (Surgicenter) by Drs. W. A. Reed and J. L. Ford.[5] However, the concept of outpatient surgery was not readily accepted by surgeons and anesthesiologists because of concerns about postoperative complications and follow-up care.

In 1974, an organization for the advancement of freestanding ambulatory surgical centers was established to improve the quality of outpatient care. Currently, this organization is known as the Federated Ambulatory Surgery Association (FASA). However, it was not until 1984 that outpatient anesthesia was formally recognized as an anesthesia subspecialty with the establishment of the Society for Ambulatory Anesthesia (SAMBA). The SAMBA organization was granted representation in the American Society of Anesthesiologists (ASA) in 1989. A copy of the ASA Guidelines for Ambulatory Surgical Facilities can be found in Appendix 1-1. In the 1980s, ambulatory surgery continued to grow, with over 600 freestanding outpatient surgery centers performing more than one million operations per year. These figures should continue to increase with the expected growth in office-based surgery units.[6] At present, hospital-affiliated outpatient surgery procedures currently account for over 40 percent of all operations performed in the hospital setting.

In providing the optimal care for this large surgical population, cooperation is required between physicians, nurses, and other ancillary health care providers, such as administrators, receptionists, lab technicians, and orderlies. In this textbook, experts with diverse experiences in the care of outpatients undergoing elective ambulatory surgical procedures have contributed chapters concerning important issues facing this specialty area. In this introductory chapter, I will review a broad range of topics, including patient selection, preoperative preparation, use of premedication, selection of an anesthetic technique, and discharge criteria. Although these topics will be discussed in greater detail by the contributing authors, the objective of this introductory chapter is to provide an overview of the material contained in this textbook.

The rapid growth and development of the subspecialty of outpatient anesthesia has created a new role for the anesthesiologist as a specialist with clinical, administrative, and communicative skills. An understanding of nursing and surgical considerations for the outpatient undergoing ambulatory surgery is important in order to provide optimal anesthetic care for this patient population (see Ch. 4 through 6). Although the ability to "give a good anesthetic" is essential in the outpatient setting, it is also important for anesthesiologists specializing in this surgical area to have a sound rational basis for choice of pharmacologic agents, procedures, and monitoring and to be knowledgeable in both the preoperative and postoperative management of outpatients undergoing ambulatory surgery.

RATIONALE FOR OUTPATIENT ANESTHESIA

When Ralph Waters first described his outpatient anesthesia clinic in Iowa, he made the prediction that "the future for such a venture is bright."[2] Indeed, seven decades later, we are seeing a dramatic increase in the demand for outpatient surgery. During the last 10 years, the American Hospital Association has reported a significant increase in outpatient procedures each year, while inpatient procedures have continued to decline. Perrin et al reported a 30 percent decrease in pediatric inpatient surgical procedures as a result of shifting cases to the outpatient setting.[7] Hospitalization for many procedures (e.g., cataract extraction) is now considered "inappropriate."[8] In fact, it has become more difficult to convince insurance and health care agencies that there are indeed some patients who benefit from overnight hospitalization prior to their "minor" operative procedure.

In providing care for a diverse surgical population, it is important to have a well-organized facility and well-trained personnel (see Ch. 2). Although gynecologic surgery is still the most common type of outpatient procedure, nearly all surgical subspecialties are contributing to the increasing number of operations performed on an outpatient basis (Table 1-1). Current estimates are that 40 to 60 percent of all surgical procedures could be performed in outpatient surgery centers. Thus, outpatient surgery has progressed from the practice of performing simple procedures in a physician's office to the total care of a broad spectrum of surgical patients in freestanding ambulatory surgery centers. The ability to perform more extensive operations on an outpatient basis has focused increasing interest on outpatient anesthesia.

As discussed in Chapter 3, several factors have contributed to the explosive growth in ambulatory surgery. First, hospital costs are decreased 25 to 75 percent for many operations performed in the outpatient setting.[9–14] For any given procedure, fewer laboratory tests are ordered and fewer pharmacy items are prescribed for outpatients (versus inpatients).[6,15] Unfortunately, many of the articles purporting to show that outpatient care is less costly are anecdotal reports.[16] Procedures requiring specialized postoperative care (such as physical therapy) may actually be more costly when performed on an outpatient basis.[14] Second, for many patients, ambulatory surgery is less disruptive to their personal lives because it decreases separation from their familiar home environments. Third, pediatric and immunocompromised cancer and transplant patients may also benefit as a result of the decreased risk of hospital-acquired infections.[17] Finally, there are preliminary data that suggest that the incidence of respiratory complications (e.g., pulmonary embolus and pneumonia) may also be decreased.[18]

The ability to provide high-quality and

Table 1-1. Operative Procedures Routinely Performed on an Outpatient Basis

Surgical specialty	Types of procedures
Dental	Extraction, restoration
Dermatology	Excise skin lesion
Ear, nose, and throat	Adenoidectomy, antrostomy, microlaryngoscopy, myringotomy, nasal polypectomy, tonsillectomy
Eye	Cataract extraction, chalazion excision, exam under anesthesia, nasolacrimal duct probing, ptosis repair, strabismus correction, tonometry
General	Biopsy, endoscopy, excisions of masses (e.g., lipomas, lymph nodes), fissurectomy, hemorrhoidectomy, herniorrhaphy, incision and drainage of abscesses, varicose vein stripping
Gynecology	Biopsy, dilatation and curettage/extraction, marsupialization of Bartholin's cyst, laparoscopy
Medicine	Bronchoscopy, endoscopy, sigmoidoscopy
Orthopaedic	Carpal tunnel decompression, exostectomy, ganglionectomy, hand/foot procedure, manipulation under anesthesia
Pain	Chemical sympathectomy, intrathecal/epidural injection, nerve block
Pediatric	Biopsy, circumcision, endoscopy, herniorrhaphy, release of adhesions, suture removal
Plastic	Cosmetic procedure (e.g., scar removal, blepharoplasty, otoplasty), septorhinoplasty
Urology	Circumcision, cystoscopy, frenulectomy, meatotomy, orchiopexy, vasectomy

(Adapted from McTaggart RA: Selection of patients for day care surgery. Can Anaesth Soc J 30:543, 1983 as appears in White PF: Outpatient anesthesia. p. 1895. In Miller RD (ed): Anesthesia. 2nd Ed. New York, Churchill Livingstone, 1986, with permission.)

cost-effective care has made outpatient surgery one of the fastest growing areas in our health care delivery system. However, some health care providers have questioned whether we and our patients really need ambulatory surgery.[19] In one study,[20] 30 percent of patients undergoing laparoscopy on an ambulatory basis stated that they would prefer to be admitted overnight for a similar procedure in the future because of postoperative fatigue and discomfort. While concluding that "we can expect an increasing proportion of surgical patients to be cared for in a day-care surgery facility," Hatch makes the valid point that "empty beds do not cost zero dollars to maintain but 80 percent of the cost of a bed being utilized for patient care."[19] Although costs of hospitalized care may increase, the more widespread availability of outpatient surgery should allow the community to obtain more health care for its money. In addition, the expanded availability of outpatient surgery could decrease waiting lists in many countries.[21]

PREOPERATIVE ASSESSMENT

If ambulatory surgery is to be successful, outpatients must be properly selected and prepared for surgery (see Chs. 7 and 9). Although the majority of patients seen in outpatient facilities are classified as ASA physical status I or II, medically stable ASA III and IV patients are now considered acceptable candidates for outpatient surgery. A prospective study by Natof involving nearly 18,000 patients found no increase in the incidence of perioperative complications in patients with pre-existing disease.[22] He attributes success in managing this higher risk population to prudent patient selection involving thorough preoperative evaluation and close communication between surgeon, anesthesiologist, and primary care physician.[22] However, a more recent multicenter study found an increased risk of perioperative complications in patients who had pre-existing cardiovascular diseases (Table 1-2).[18] It was noted that the risk associated with this condition, or any

Table 1-2. Factors Predisposing to Complications During and After Outpatient Anesthesia

Factors	Incidence
Preexisting disease	
None (ASA physical status I)	1/156
Diabetes mellitus	1/149
Asthma	1/139
Chronic pulmonary disease	1/112
Hypertension (diuretic therapy)	1/87 (1/64)[a]
Heart disease	1/74[a]
Type of anesthesia	
Local only	1/268
Regional only	1/277
Local/regional with sedation	1/106[a]
General (combination techniques)	1/120[a]
Duration of anesthesia	
Less than 1 hr	1/155
1 to 2 hr	1/84
2 to 3 hr	1/54[a]
Greater than 3 hr	1/35[a]

[a] Significantly different from initial value for the group, $P < .05$.

(Data from Federated Ambulatory Surgery Association.[18])

other pre-existing disease, was reduced when symptoms were under good control for at least 3 months prior to the operation. Interestingly, the pre-existing disease had a causal relationship to the complication experienced less than one percent of the time.

The acceptability of patients at the extremes of age (e.g., less than 6 months and greater than 70 years) has been questioned at some ambulatory centers; however, age alone should not be considered a deterrent in the selection of patients (see Ch. 7 and 16). It is difficult to evaluate the effect of aging on recovery because of age-related differences in the mix of surgical procedures and anesthetic techniques,[23] yet most studies have failed to demonstrate an age-related increase in discharge times or incidence of complications following outpatient anesthesia. However, recovery of fine motor skills and cognitive function after general anesthesia (or local anesthesia with sedation) is slower in older outpatients.[24–26]

At the other extreme, ex-preterm infants (less than 48 weeks postconceptual age) appear to be at increased risk for the development of postoperative respiratory complications (apnea and periodic breathing, for example).[27–30] Infants at increased risk of developing postoperative respiratory complications (e.g., history of prematurity, bronchopulmonary dysplasia, apnea, or irregular respirations during induction) should be admitted to the hospital for 12 to 24 hours and carefully observed during the early recovery period. Recently, Welborn et al. reported that the use of caffeine, 10 mg/kg IV, can minimize the possibility of prolonged postoperative apneic episodes in high-risk infants.[31] Full-term infants under 6 months of age undergoing minor surgery, (such as inguinal hernia repairs, minor plastic surgery, myringotomies, and examination under anesthesia), can be successfully managed as outpatients, tolerating a 3 to 6 hour fast without difficulty.[32] Nevertheless, a recent case report described postoperative apnea in a full-term infant.[33] Although a history of recent upper respiratory tract infection does not increase the risk of respiratory complications during the perioperative period in otherwise healthy children,[34] a higher incidence of desaturation ($SaO_2 \leq 90$ percent) has been reported in these children during transfer to the recovery room.[35] The available data emphasize the importance of judging the suitability of patients for ambulatory surgery on a case-by-case basis.

While the importance of preoperative assessment is obvious, evaluation of the surgical outpatient can present some logistic problems for the anesthesiologist. In the chapters discussing the preoperative assessment of pediatric (Ch. 7), adult (Ch. 9), and geriatric outpatients (Ch. 16), the authors describe several alternative approaches to dealing with this difficult problem. A visit with the anesthesiologist prior to the day of surgery is desirable because it minimizes cancellations and improves overall efficiency of the surgical facility. Unfortunately, this practice is not possible in many busy outpatient centers. In contrast to the inpatient setting,[36,37] a preoperative interview by an anesthesiologist does not necessarily decrease anxiety in outpatients.[38]

Anesthesiologists vary with respect to the means by which they judge a patient's fitness for a surgical procedure.[39] An alternative approach to evaluating outpatients is to use a preanesthetic screening questionnaire to obtain information about the patient's medical problems, previous operations, drug history, and family history, and to provide a general review of systems (Fig. 1-1). Based on a careful history and physical examination, it is possible to minimize unnecessary laboratory testing (Table 1-3). A computerized questionnaire can be more accurate in listing positive and negative historic information than a physician interview and can be used to predict the need for preoperative laboratory testing (see Ch. 9).[40,41] This type of screening mechanism may allow for more appropriate and cost-effective laboratory testing in the future.[42,43] Ideally, this would be supplemented with a letter of consent containing essential information (e.g., preoperative laboratory tests, NPO status, arrival time, discharge requirements) that should be read and signed by the patient (or legal guardian). Additionally, it is important to identify the individual who will be responsible for taking the patient home. When outpatients are given both verbal and printed instructions that they are required to read and sign, compliance improves significantly.[44,45] Hence, surgeons must understand the preoperative requirements for anesthesia and be capable of communicating this information to their patients.

As discussed in Chapter 2, a wide variety of surgical procedures are being performed on an outpatient basis (Table 1-1). Even angioplastic and angiographic procedures are now commonly performed on an outpatient basis.[46,47] In the past, procedures expected to require more than 60 to 90 minutes of anesthesia were not scheduled on an outpatient basis because it was assumed that these patients would require a prolonged recovery period. However, cases lasting 2 to 4 hours (oral surgery or plastic surgery, for example) are currently being performed successfully at many outpatient facilities. In a retrospective analysis, Meridy[23] found no obvious correlation between the duration of anesthesia and the recovery time. However, for gynecologic procedures, Kitz et al.[48] found a direct relationship between the length of the operation (and anesthesia) and the duration of the recovery room stay. Furthermore, the incidence of postoperative complications would appear to be related to the length of the operative procedure.[18,49] The FASA special study found that operations lasting less than 1 hour were associated with a complication rate of one in 155 patients, while operations requiring more than 2 hours of anesthesia were associated with a complication rate of one in 48 patients.

Procedures in which postoperative surgical complications are likely to occur should be performed on an inpatient basis (see Ch. 5 and 18). While autologous blood transfusions are being administered during some outpatient operations (e.g., reduction mammoplasty, liposuction), procedures associated with excessive fluid shifts are more appropriately handled in the hospital setting. Similarly, operative procedures requiring prolonged immobilization and parenteral analgesic therapy are not ideally suited to the outpatient model. The availability of newer analgesic therapies, such as ambulatory PCA, may alter the latter recommendation in the near future (see Ch. 19). Although injection of a long-acting local anesthetic at the site of the surgical incision can decrease the postoperative analgesic requirement, postoperative pain should be controllable with oral analgesics (e.g., acetaminophen with codeine). If the patient has to travel a long distance following discharge, careful consideration must be given to the potential for airway problems, the

OUTPATIENT PREANESTHESIA QUESTIONNAIRE

This questionnaire is designed to assist the doctors who will be taking care of you (or your child). It will help us to learn more about your health (or the health of your child). Please fill it out as completely as possible and return it to the reception desk.

Name:____________________________ Age:____ Sex:____
Height:________ Weight:_____ Occupation:________________
Home address:________________________ Home phone: _________
________________________ Local phone: _________

Referring physician (surgeon): ____________________
Reason (type of operation): ____________________
Date of operation: ____________________

How would you rate your overall health? (Please circle)

excellent good fair poor

Has there been a recent change in your health?

Yes _____ No _____ Comment ____________________

How physically active are you? (Please circle)

very active (no restrictions)	somewhat active (walk up stairs)	not active (unable to walk)

Previous Hospitalizations:

Date (month/year)	Hospital	Problem(s)	Type of operation	Type of anesthesia
1.				
2.				
3.				
4.				
5.				

Do you have or have you ever had any of these problems? (Please circle)

1. Heart attack or heart failure
2. Stroke
3. Kidney or bladder problems
4. Liver problems or hepatitis
5. High blood pressure
6. Diabetes
7. Bleeding problems
8. Cancer
9. Seizure or epilepsy
10. Rheumatic fever
11. Arthritis
12. Lung problems, (e.g., pneumonia, emphysema, bronchitis, asthma)
13. Other ____________

Please name any medicine that you are presently taking: include all prescription and non-prescription drugs (even aspirin):

1. ____________________
2. ____________________
3. ____________________
4. ____________________
5. ____________________

Fig. 1-1. Preoperative questionnaire used to obtain pertinent medical history prior to ambulatory surgery. (*Figure continues.*)

Are you allergic to, or have you had unusual reactions following the use of adhesive tapes, medicine, or drugs? Please list the items and the type of reaction you experienced:

____

____

Have you ever taken steroids such as prednisone or cortisone? Yes _____ No _____
If so, when were they last used? ____________________

Do you have any of the following: (Please circle)
false teeth, capped teeth, loose teeth,
or teeth that need dental care, specify ____________________

Have you or any of your close relatives encountered problems or complications with anesthesia? Yes _____ No _____ If so, what? ____________________

At the present time, do you have? (please check appropriate boxes):

- [ ] chest pain or tightness with exercise
- [ ] blackouts or dizziness (light-headedness)
- [ ] palpitations or irregular heart beats
- [ ] pain in your legs with exercise
- [ ] ankle or leg swelling
- [ ] shortness of breath at night
- [ ] shortness of breath with exercise
- [ ] chronic cough or sputum (phlegm)
- [ ] blood in your sputum
- [ ] black or tarry stools, diarrhea
- [ ] frequent nausea and vomiting
- [ ] temporary loss or blurring of vision
- [ ] temporary weakness or numbness of one or more limbs
- [ ] facial weakness, numbness or difficulty speaking
- [ ] burning with urination or frequent urination
- [ ] arthritis or joint pains
- [ ] back or neck pain
- [ ] excessive bleeding following minor cuts or dental surgery
- [ ] recent weight loss
- [ ] difficulty walking
- [ ] pregnancy

Have you had any recent problems with : (Please circle)
a "cold", "flu", bronchitis, laryngitis, sore throat, fever

Do you smoke? Yes _____ No _____ How many years? _____ Packs per day _____
Do you drink alcoholic beverages? Yes _____ No _____ Drinks per day _____
Do you use any other "recreational" drugs? Yes _____ No _____ Type __________
Do you wish to discuss the possible complications of anesthesia? Yes _____ No _____

<u>Questions for the anesthesiologist:</u>

1. ____
2. ____
3. ____

Thank you for your assistance.

Fig. 1-1. (*Continued*).

Table 1-3. Guidelines for Preoperative Studies in Healthy Outpatients Undergoing Superficial Surgical Procedures

	Men (age range)[b]			Women (age range)[b]		
	<50	50 to 70	>70	<50	50 to 70	>70
Complete blood cell count/hematocrit		√	√	√	√	√
Electrolyte panel[a]			√			√
Human chorionic gonadotropin				(√)		
Chest x-ray			√			√
Electrocardiogram[a]		√	√		√	√

√ Situations in which tests should be ordered.

[a] Electrolyte panel and electrocardiogram are recommended for patients chronically receiving cardiovascular drugs.

[b] Platelets, prothrombin time/partial thromboplastin time, and bleeding time are only recommended for patients with known or suspected bleeding disorders or coagulopathies.

likelihood of hemorrhage, and postoperative pain management. Indeed, the recent FASA multicenter study showed that 69 percent of all perioperative complications occurred after discharge from the ambulatory surgery center. This finding emphasizes the importance of providing clearly understood discharge instructions and ensuring that a responsible adult is available to monitor the patient at home, and suggests that out-of-town patients should spend their first postoperative night within a reasonable distance of the outpatient facility.

In the recovery room, anesthesia appears to be a contributing factor in over 60 percent of the reported side effects (see Ch. 18). Of the anesthetic-related causes for unexpected hospitalization after ambulatory surgery (15 to 30 percent of all cases), intractable nausea and vomiting, airway problems (e.g., stridor, bronchospasm), inability to void, dizziness, and delayed emergence are the most common.[23,50] In pediatric outpatients, protracted vomiting accounted for 33 percent of the unanticipated admissions after ambulatory surgery.[51] Common surgically related problems necessitating admission to the hospital (30 to 50 percent of all cases) include intractable pain, excessive bleeding, surgical misadventures (bowel burn or perforation and uterine perforation, for example), errors in diagnosis, and parenteral drug therapy (e.g., antibiotics).[23,50,51] Other causes of unanticipated admissions after ambulatory surgery include the need for more intensive monitoring and social factors such as a lack of appropriate transportation or a responsible escort. In many cases, both surgery and anesthesia contributed to the occurrence of side effects after ambulatory surgery.[18] For example, laparoscopy is associated with a high incidence of postoperative morbidity, including nausea, vomiting, and myalgias, as well as abdominal or shoulder pain. Some studies indicate that only 33 to 57 percent of outpatients undergoing laparoscopy are able to resume normal activities within 48 hours, and that the majority of these patients require 2 to 5 days to completely recover from this operation.[52,53] Thus, it is important to have an efficient mechanism for admitting outpatients to the hospital should the need arise.

Most well-organized outpatient facilities have an overall hospitalization rate of less than 1 percent.[18,54] However, the transfer rate will be higher in ambulatory centers with a larger proportion of neonate, elderly patients, and ASA physical status III-IV outpatients.[54] The incidence of emergency hospitalizations for life-threatening complications was one in 12,500 patients in the recent multicenter study.[18] Yet, even allegedly minor procedures (e.g., midtrimester abortions) can be associated with serious life-threatening complications, such as disseminated intravascular coagulation.[55]

Close cooperation between surgeons and anesthetists regarding patient selection, preoperative assessment and preparation, and types of operations performed in the outpatient setting will minimize the number of unexpected hospitalizations.

PREMEDICATION

The use of premedication in the outpatient setting has been a subject of considerable interest and debate (see Ch. 7, 10, and 16). Primary indications for preoperative medication include anxiolysis, sedation (especially for pediatric patients), analgesia, amnesia, vagolysis, and prophylaxis against postoperative emesis and aspiration pneumonia. Despite these recognized indications, premedication is not routinely used in most ambulatory surgery facilities in the United States. An important concern in outpatient anesthesia is prompt recovery, and many anesthesiologists avoid using centrally active depressant premedicants because they believe these drugs could prolong the recovery period.[54,56]

Interestingly, most clinical studies involving the use of sedative-anxiolytic and analgesic drugs have not found a prolonged recovery following the use of premedication in the outpatient setting.[57–62] In a retrospective study, Meridy concluded that premedication with diazepam or hydroxyzine did not prolong recovery times.[23] In a prospective study, Jakobsen et al.[58] demonstrated that diazepam, 0.25 mg/kg PO, was superior to placebo in decreasing preoperative apprehension without delaying discharge. Similarly, intramuscular midazolam produced sedation, amnesia, and anxiolysis without prolonged recovery in both children[59,60] and adults.[61,62] In those situations in which it is not feasible to administer intramuscular premedication (e.g., lack of holding area, insufficient time), small bolus doses of midazolam, 1 to 2 mg IV, do not appear to adversely affect recovery after outpatient anesthesia.[63,64] Although larger doses are required because of first-pass metabolism, oral midazolam has been reported to be highly effective in both adults[65] and children.[66] Other benzodiazepines (temazepam and triazolam, for example) are also effective following oral administration.[65,67–70] Alternative means of administration include intranasal and rectal routes.[71,72] Even though these premedicants can impair coordinative and reactive skills for 5 to 12 hours,[73] some studies have found a decrease in recovery times when analgesic or antiemetic premedication is given immediately prior to induction of outpatient anesthesia.[74,75] Furthermore, premedication with sedative and/or analgesic drugs does not appear to increase the percentage of outpatients at risk of developing aspiration pneumonitis.[76] Hence, the judicious use of preoperative medication can be extremely beneficial to outpatients without increasing postoperative morbidity.

The routine use of narcotic analgesics for premedication has been criticized, with the exception of cases in which the patient is experiencing acute or chronic pain. The traditional opioid premedicant combinations, such as morphine-scopolamine and atropine-papaveretum, increase the incidence of postoperative nausea and vomiting in outpatients.[59,61,77] Although the agonist-antagonist analgesic nalbuphine produced sedation and decreased side effects during induction, its use was also associated with an increased incidence of postoperative nausea and vomiting.[78] Investigators have also reported that the use of small doses of the potent opioid analgesics (e.g., fentanyl, 1 to 3 μg/kg, alfentanil, 5 to 15 μg/kg, and sufentanil, 0.1 to 0.3 μg/kg) prior to the induction of general anesthesia can decrease anxiety and facilitate early recovery as a result of the analgesic's ability to decrease the anesthetic requirement and to provide postoperative analgesia.[74,79–83] However, the use of these potent, rapid-acting opioids also contributes to an increased incidence of post-anesthetic nausea and vomiting.[62,79–82] Oral transmucosal fentanyl (in the form of a lollipop) can provide effective preoperative sedation and analgesia.[84] Other studies suggest that transmucosal opioid administration also increases the incidence of pruritis and emetic sequelae.[85] Interestingly, when oral meperidine was combined with diazepam and atropine, there was no apparent increase in the incidence of nausea and vomiting.[86]

Postoperative nausea and vomiting is a common problem after general anesthesia and, because it can delay discharge and may result in unexpected hospital admissions, it is particularly disturbing to outpatients.[23,75,79,87,88] Factors that have been alleged to increase the incidence of postoperative nausea and vomiting include the patient's body habitus and medical condition, the type of surgery performed (laparoscopy, orchiopexy, strabismus surgery, therapeutic abortions), assisted ventilation using a facemask, and anesthetic and analgesic medications (fentanyl, etomidate, isoflurane, or N_2O).[89]

Many different pharmacologic and nonpharmacologic regimens have also been evaluated to reduce emesis, including acupuncture and acupressure.[90–92] Outpatient studies involving both children and adults indicate that droperidol, 5 to 75 μg/kg IV, can be a highly effective prophylactic antiemetic.[87,93–102] To minimize its side effects, including sedation and dysphoria, the lowest effective dose is recommended. Metoclopramide, a gastrokinetic agent that facilitates gastric and small bowel motility, is another useful antiemetic. Although somewhat controversial,[100–110] investigators have reported that both orally and parenterally administered metoclopramide possesses antiemetic properties. The variable responses may be partly related to the dosage, route, and timing of the drug's administration.[111] The combination of metoclopramide, 10 to 20 mg IV, and low-dose droperidol, 0.5 to 1.0 mg IV, appears to be more effective than droperidol alone.[75] Transdermal scopolamine can also be effective in decreasing emetic sequelae after outpatient procedures.[112–115] However, transdermal scopolamine's onset of action is slow, its effectiveness is highly variable, and its side effects (e.g., dry mouth, visual disturbances, dysphoria) can be troublesome. Hence, transdermal scopolamine should be restricted to outpatients at high risk (e.g., history of motion sickness) who are undergoing procedures frequently associated with postoperative nausea and vomiting, such as laparoscopy. The antihistaminic drug hydroxyzine and the antiarrhythmic drug lidocaine have also been reported to be effective in decreasing emetic sequelae.[116,117] Several newer drugs (e.g., domperidone, clebopride, ondansetron), which are alleged to possess antiemetic activity, are under active clinical investigation.

Another controversial aspect of premedication in outpatients relates to the need for prophylactic medication to decrease the risk of pulmonary injury from aspiration of gastric contents (see Chs. 10 and 18). Since some outpatients may have a large residual gastric volume (Fig. 1-2),[118] and 40 to 60 percent of outpatients could be defined as "at risk" of aspiration pneumonitis (i.e., gastric volume > 25 ml with pH < 2.5) despite overnight fasting,[76,119–122] a variety of premedication regimens has been evaluated to reduce this risk (Table 1-4). However, the incidence of pulmonary aspiration appears to be low (less than one per 35,000) in elective surgical patients without specific risk factors.[127] The H_2-receptor antagonists cimetidine and ranitidine are both effective in decreasing the percentage of patients at risk for pulmonary aspiration injury.[123,128,129] Some experts recommend the routine of an H_2-blocker whenever a facemask technique is used during outpatient anesthesia.[130]

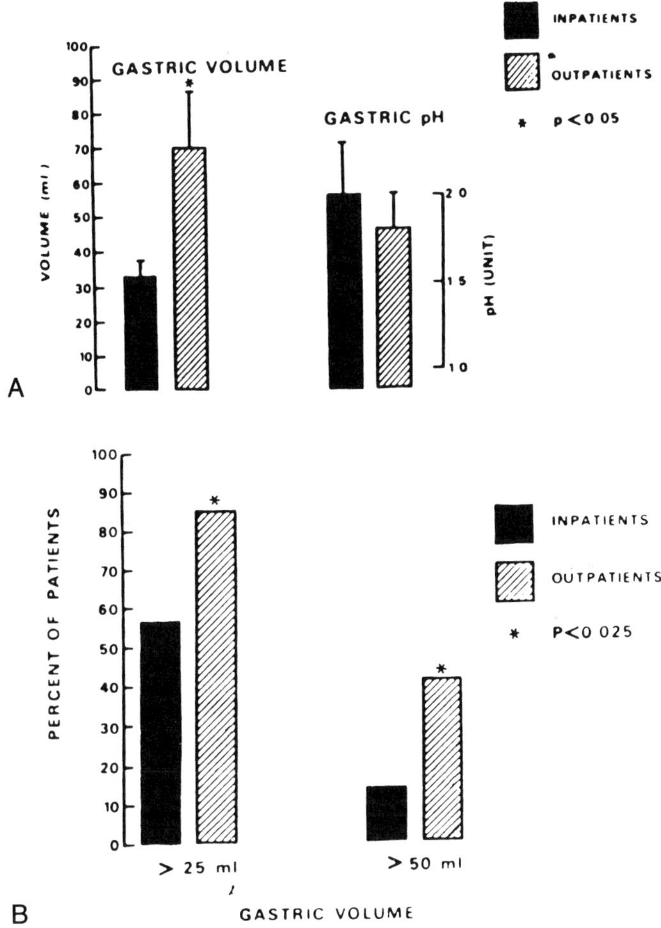

Fig. 1-2. (**A**) Comparison of mean gastric volume and pH values at the time of induction in outpatients and inpatients. (**B**) Relative frequencies of large gastric volumes among outpatients compared with inpatients. (From Ong et al,[118] with permission.)

Since prolonged fasting does not guarantee an empty stomach at the time of induction, several investigators have questioned the value of even a 4- to 5-hour fast prior to elective surgery.[122,131] Sutherland et al. found that 50 and 44 percent of outpatients complained of moderate-to-severe hunger and thirst, respectively, after an overnight fast.[132] These investigators postulated that hunger and thirst contributed significantly to preoperative anxiety. More important, 14 percent of young female outpatients presenting to the operating room in the afternoon after an overnight fast had a serum glucose concentration of less than 45 μg/dl.[133] Maltby et al. reported that ingestion of 150 ml of water as late as 2 hours prior to surgery significantly decreased the severity of thirst without increasing gastric volume in fasted outpatients.[122] More recently, these investigators reported that ingestion of either coffee or orange juice (150 ml) 2 to 3 hours before induction of anesthesia had no significant effect on re-

Table 1-4. Prophylactic Regimens Used to Decrease the Risk of Aspiration Pneumonitis in Outpatients

Medication/dose	Dosing interval (min)[a]	Gastric volume (ml)[a]	Gastric pH[a]	Patients with pH <2.5 and volume >25 ml (%)	Untreated "controls" with pH <2.5 and volume >25 ml (%)[b]	References
Ranitidine 1.5 mg/kg IV	83 (± 6.4)	11 (± 2)	6.8 (± 18)	0	36	Manchikanti and Roush[120]
Ranitidine 150 mg PO	113 (± 8.4)	1 (± 2)	5.2 (± 0.3)	0	35	Sutherland et al[121]
	154 (± 13)	10 (± 2)	6.4 (± 0.41)	5	60	Manchikanti et al[123]
with 150 ml water	144 (± 17)	8 (± 7)	5.5 (± 1.8)	0	46	Maltby et al[122]
with 150 ml water	159 (± 37)	10 (± 13)	6.2 (± 1.5)	0	48	Maltby et al[124]
with 150 ml coffee	160 (± 34)	14 (± 15)	5.7 (± 2.1)	6	38	Maltby et al[124]
with 150 ml juice	142 (± 37)	15 (± 17)	5.4 (± 2.1)	8	42	Maltby et al[124]
Cimetidine 300 mg PO	146 (± 9.9)	13 (± 2)	5.0 (± 0.44)	4	48	Manchikanti and Roush[119]
Bicitra 15 ml PO and metoclopramide 10 mg IV	50 (± 3.5)	22 (± 4)	3.4 (± 0.29)	4	36	Manchikanti et al[125]
Bicitra 30 ml PO and metoclopramide 10 mg IV	50 (± 3.6)	26 (± 6)	3.7 (± 0.30)	8	36	Manchikanti et al[125]
Bicitra 15 ml PO	45 (± 3.5)	32 (± 6)	3.2 (± 0.21)	12	36	Manchikanti et al[125]
Bicitra 30 ml PO	46 (± 3.5)	58 (± 9)	3.7 (± 0.17)	12	36	Manchikanti et al[125]
Cimetidine 400 mg PO	105 (± 6.1)	13 (± 2)	5.0 (± 0.4)	12	35	Stock and Sutherland[126]

[a] Mean values ± SD.
[b] Average duration of fasting, 12 to 14 hours.

sidual gastric volume or pH in adults.[134] Compared with fasted outpatients, patients who received coffee or orange juice with oral ranitidine 2 to 3 hours prior to induction of anesthesia had lower residual gastric volumes, higher pH values, and a decreased incidence of moderate or severe thirst.[124] Similarly, preoperative administration of apple juice (3 to 5 ml/kg), with or without ranitidine (2 mg/kg), decreased gastric volume, thirst, and hunger in children.[135,136] Yet, other studies suggest that decreasing the traditional fasting period and giving oral premedication before general anesthesia may increase gastric volume in pediatric outpatients.[137] While arbitrary restrictions (e.g., NPO after midnight) on when outpatients may ingest fluids prior to an elective operation appear to be unwarranted, further studies are clearly needed.

Use of metoclopramide in combination with an H_2-blocking drug has been advocated by some investigators to decrease postoperative emesis and further reduce the risk of aspiration.[138] However, other studies have failed to demonstrate a significant advantage of this drug combination over an H_2-receptor antagonist alone.[108,120] When a rapid change in gastric pH and volume is necessary, a combination of sodium citrate and metoclopramide is a useful alternative to the H_2 blockers.[125,139] Although pharmacologic manipulation of gastric contents[126] and/or gastroesophageal sphincter tone[140] does not prevent aspiration and cannot substitute for careful airway management and vigilance, these drugs offer a simple, inexpensive, safe, and effective way of reducing the risk of aspiration pneumonitis in certain "high-risk" patient populations (e.g., morbidly obese, diabetic, and pregnant outpatients). Other important issues related to the use of preoperative medication, including chronic drugs and prophylactic antibiotics, are discussed in Chapter 10.

OUTPATIENT ANESTHETIC TECHNIQUES

What are the primary considerations in choosing an anesthetic technique for outpatient surgery? Since both quality and efficiency are important, the ideal anesthetic for outpatients would produce a smooth onset of action, intraoperative amnesia and analgesia, good surgical conditions, and a short recovery period, with no side effects.[141] Each procedure presents unique challenges for the anesthesiologist (see Ch. 4). For example, the potential for intraoperative problems during laparoscopy, such as perforation of a viscus or a major blood vessel or electric injury to the bowel, exists whether the procedure is performed under local, regional, or general anesthesia.

If the patient is to receive general anesthesia for a laparoscopic procedure, is it necessary to "secure" the airway with an endotracheal tube? The practice in most centers has been to intubate *all* patients undergoing laparoscopy because of concerns about adequacy of ventilation (e.g., Trendelenberg position, pneumoperitoneum) and the possibility of passive regurgitation and aspiration. However, in situations in which the laparoscopy can be performed expeditiously, some anesthesiologists have chosen not to intubate the patient. By avoiding laryngoscopy and intubation, the amount of anesthetic drug administered would be decreased, and a faster recovery with fewer postoperative side effects (sore throat, for example) could be anticipated.[20,142] In addition, Kenefick et al. reported that spontaneous ventilation via a facemask did not result in significant hypercarbia or acidosis.[142] Thus, brief laparoscopic procedures can be safely performed on healthy, fasted, non-obese patients under general anesthesia without endotracheal intubation.

Although most outpatient procedures are

performed under general (or local) anesthesia, regional techniques can be extremely useful for a wide variety of urologic, gynecologic, and orthopaedic procedures (see Ch. 14). Finally, sedative-analgesic drugs can be valuable supplements to local anesthetic techniques during monitored anesthesia care (see Chs. 12 and 13).

General Anesthesia

The ability to deliver a safe and effective general anesthetic with minimal side effects and rapid recovery is critical in a busy outpatient surgery unit (see Ch. 15). General anesthesia remains the most widely used anesthetic technique for managing ambulatory surgery patients because of its popularity with patients, surgeons, and anesthesiologists.[143] Outpatients require the same basic equipment as inpatients for delivery of anesthetic drugs, monitoring, and resuscitation (see Ch. 11).[144] Routine intraoperative monitoring equipment for outpatient operations include a precordial stethoscope, an electrocardiogram, and a blood pressure cuff. In addition, a pulse oximeter and a capnograph are both extremely valuable monitors. The major risk factors for hypoxemia during outpatient general anesthesia include obesity, age (older than 35 years), lithotomy position, manual ventilation, and arousal.[145] Temperature monitoring is also recommended for young adults, adolescents, and children undergoing general anesthesia with known triggering agents for malignant hyperthermia.

The question of whether to start an intravenous line in outpatients arises frequently in pediatric patients undergoing brief surgical procedures. For procedures lasting less than 15 minutes that do not require intravenous administration of drugs or fluid (e.g., myringotomies, eye examinations under anesthesia), intravenous access is not essential. Preoperative fasting for periods of 10 to 15 hours does not result in hypoglycemia in healthy outpatients younger than 5 years of age.[32,146–148] However, for longer cases or for situations in which the patient has been without oral intake for an excessive period of time (more than 15 hours), an intravenous line is useful for the maintenance of fluid balance and glucose homeostasis,[32,133] as well as for facilitating administration of drugs during the perioperative period. Use of heated humidifiers will decrease fluid losses and conserve heat during longer outpatient procedures.[149] To facilitate access to important patient data during the perioperative period, many outpatient centers have adopted simplified anesthesia record systems that combine preoperative, intraoperative, and postoperative information (see Appendix 1-2).

Induction of Anesthesia

Induction of general anesthesia is usually accomplished with a rapid-acting intravenous anesthetic (see Ch. 15). Thiopental, the prototypic induction agent, is associated with a rapid induction of anesthesia without significant side effects.[150] Methohexital appears to be associated with slightly shorter awakening and recovery times than thiopental.[150–153] Nevertheless, full recovery of fine motor skills requires 6 to 8 hours after an induction dose of methohexital.[154] Newer intravenous agents (e.g., propofol) appear to offer advantages over the more traditional agents in the outpatient setting.

Etomidate has also been used for both induction and maintenance of general anesthesia during short outpatient procedures.[150,151] Although its use is associated with excellent hemodynamics and respiratory stability,[80,81,155] common adverse effects include pain on injection, postoperative nausea and vomiting, myoclonic movements, and transient suppression of adrenal steroidogenesis.[150,156,157] Because of its side effects, the use of etomidate is usually restricted to those clinical situations in which it offers an advantage over other available induction agents, such as for outpatients with coronary artery or cerebrovascular disease. Ketamine also compares unfavorably with the barbiturates for routine clinical use because of its prominent psychomimetic effects during the early postoperative period.[158,159] When its cardiostimulatory and bronchodilatory properties are advantageous, premedication with a benzodiazepine will decrease the incidence of ketamine-induced emergence reactions.[63,160] When the water-soluble benzodiazepine midazolam is used as the sole agent for induction in outpatients, its onset of action is slower and its recovery is prolonged compared with the barbiturate compounds.[161–163] However, small doses of midazolam, 1 to 3 mg IV, can be extremely effective in decreasing anxiety prior to induction of anesthesia.[63,64] Furthermore, flumazenil (Ro 15-1788), a specific benzodiazepine antagonist, can be administered at the end of surgery to reverse residual midazolam-induced sedation and amnesia and to facilitate the recovery process.[164] Compared with the newest intravenous induction agent (propofol), recovery after flumazenil antagonism of midazolam anesthesia is still significantly slow.[165] Recovery following induction of anesthesia with propofol appears to be more rapid than with the commonly used barbiturate compounds[166–170] (Fig. 1-3). Although propofol produces a greater degree of cardiovascular depression and pain on injection than the barbiturates, its use is associated with fewer postoperative side effects. While many anesthesiologists would consider propofol to be the intravenous induction agent of choice for outpatient anesthesia,[171] it appears to offer less advantages when anesthesia is maintained with inhaled agents.[172,173] For short outpatient procedures, induction and maintenance with a variable-rate infusion of propofol and nitrous oxide (N_2O) results in recovery times that compare favorably with both standard intravenous and inhaled anesthetic techniques[174–176] (Fig. 1-4). As part of a

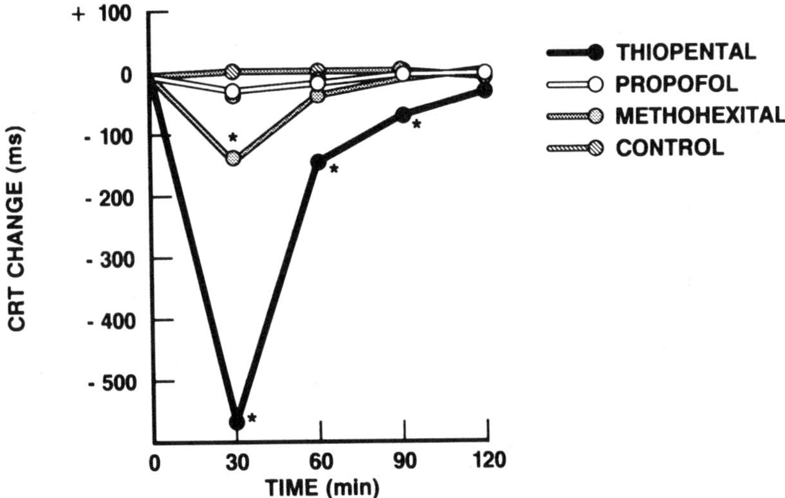

Fig. 1-3. Comparison of mean changes in choice reaction time (CRT) during the early postoperative period in untreated controls and outpatients who received either thiopental, methohexital, or propofol for induction of anesthesia. Astericks indicate values significantly different from control ($P < .05$). (From MacKenzie and Grant,[166] with permission.)

total intravenous anesthetic technique for gynecologic and urologic procedures,[177–179] propofol offers advantages over other commonly used anesthetic drugs. Recently, Marais et al. suggested that there were substantial potential benefits associated with propofol in improving the quality of outpatient care and reducing recovery room costs.[180] Nevertheless, complete recovery of psychomotor function may require up to 3 hours after induction and maintenance of outpatient anesthesia with propofol.[181]

In children, an inhalation induction is a useful alternative to the standard intravenous induction techniques (see Ch. 8). When an intravenous drug is used for induction followed by an inhalation agent during brief outpatient procedures, initial recovery may be prolonged compared with the use of a volatile agent alone[151] (Fig. 1-5). Although its use is associated with a higher incidence of arrhythmias,[182,183] halothane remains the drug of choice for inhalation induction in pediatric patients as it is associated with shorter induction times and fewer respiratory problems than either isoflurane or enflurane.[184–187] Unfortunately, inhalation inductions are frequently more time-consuming, and many patients object to the facemask as well as the pungent smell of inhaled agents. In cooperative patients, these complaints can be minimized by the use of the so-called "single breath" induction technique.[188] In unruly, frightened, or mentally retarded children, larger doses of intravenous anesthetics can be administered either intramuscularly (e.g., ketamine, 2 to 4 mg/kg) or rectally (e.g., methohexital, 20 to 30 mg/kg, etomidate, 3 to 6 mg/kg, ketamine, 25 to 50 mg/kg) prior to taking the patient to the operating room.[189–193] Use of the minimally effective dose will decrease recovery times and adverse reactions.[194] An alternative nonpharmacologic approach involves the use of play-oriented preoperative teaching to minimize the fear and discomfort during the induction period. Allowing parents to support their child during the induction of anesthesia can also be effective in relieving the child's anxiety and in producing a smooth induction of anesthesia.[195] When

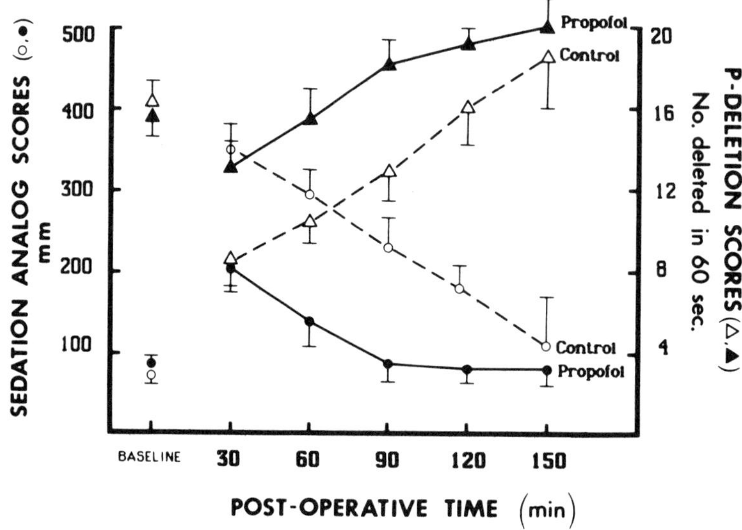

Fig. 1-4. Comparison of sedation scores and ability to perform the p-deletion test in healthy outpatients anesthetized with propofol-N_2O (solid lines) or a combination of thiopental-isoflurane-N_2O (control) (dotted lines). (Adapted from Doze et al.,[176] with permission.)

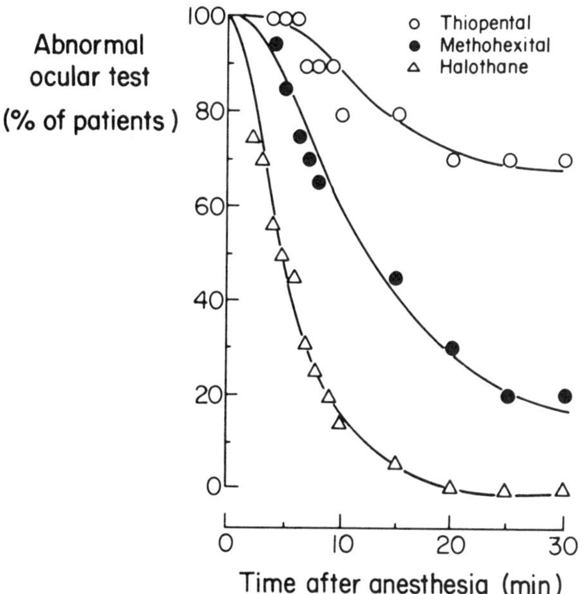

Fig. 1-5. Percentage of patients with abnormal Maddox wing readings (extraocular muscle balance) at various times after completion of surgery. Recovery curves demonstrate the effect of various induction agents. (From Hannington-Kiff,[152] with permission.)

administered 60 to 90 minutes prior to induction of anesthesia, a topical (dermally applied) cream containing a mixture of lidocaine and prilocaine (EMLA) can decrease pain at the intravenous injection site, thereby facilitating the use of conventional induction techniques in children.[196]

Maintenance of Anesthesia

Use of a volatile agent in combination with nitrous oxide (N_2O), 60 to 70 percent in oxygen, is the most popular technique for maintenance of anesthesia. The extremely low solubility of N_2O contributes to the rapid onset and recovery from its central nervous system effects, making it a valuable adjunct to most outpatient general anesthetics. Although some investigators have suggested that there is an association between the use of N_2O and postoperative nausea and/or vomiting,[197–200] recent studies question the role of N_2O in producing this side effect.[201–203] However, when N_2O is combined with opioid analgesics as part of a "balanced" anesthetic technique, the increase of emetic sequelae will be significantly higher.[197]

Volatile anesthetics are generally considered to be superior to intravenous anesthetics for maintenance during outpatient surgery because they are "more controllable," that is, changes in the depth of anesthesia can be made more rapidly because of the rapid uptake or elimination of volatile agents from the lungs. The more rapidly eliminated anesthetic vapors would theoretically provide faster recovery and earlier discharge of the patients from the outpatient facility. A similar spectrum of pharmacologic activity is produced by the three commonly used volatile agents (halothane, enflurane, and isoflurane). Several investigators have compared the times of recovery after anesthesia with these three agents. Although pediatric outpatients

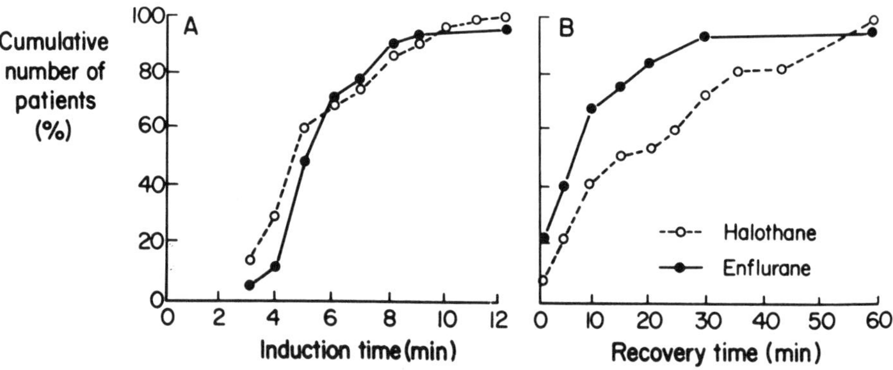

Fig. 1-6. (**A**) Induction times (from application of facemask until loss of consciousness) for pediatric outpatients. (**B**) Recovery times (from the end of anesthesia until return of consciousness) in pediatric outpatients. (Adapted from Davidson,[204] with permission.)

may experience a more rapid awakening after enflurane (versus halothane) anesthesia[184,204] (Fig. 1-6), most have reported that halothane is associated with the lowest incidence of perioperative complications and has not been found to significantly prolong recovery times.[184–187]

Studies involving adult outpatients undergoing brief procedures have shown no significant differences in recovery times between the three potent inhalational agents (Table 1-5).[152,205,206] However, some investigators have reported that enflurane is associated with a more rapid recovery than halothane or isoflurane.[207,208] For procedures lasting longer than 90 minutes, Valanne and Korttila found faster recovery times after isoflurane when compared with enflurane.[209] However, Tracey et al. reported that adult outpatients receiving isoflurane during gynecologic surgery had a higher incidence of postoperative complications (Table 1-6).[205] For brief outpatient anesthetic problems, enflurane has become the inhalation agent of choice for maintenance of anesthesia at many centers. However, delayed convulsions have been reported after enflurane anesthesia.[210]

Because of their decreased blood solubility, newer inhaled anesthetic agents should allow for a more rapid recovery after outpatient surgery compared with the currently available inhaled anesthetics.[211] The two new inhaled anesthetics of greatest interest to anesthesiologists are sevoflurane (a methyl-isopropyl ether) and desflurane (I-653, a fluorinated methyl-ethyl ether). Although sevoflurane is subject to breakdown by soda lime (at temperatures higher than 40°C), desflurane appears to be extremely stable, with minimal (if any) metabolic breakdown.[212] The solubility of desflurane

Table 1-5. Recovery Times Following Outpatient Anesthesia When Volatile Anesthetics Were Used as Adjuvants to Nitrous Oxide[a]

	Halothane (n = 20)	Enflurane (n = 20)	Isoflurane (n = 20)
Opens eyes (min)	5.5 (± 0.6)	5.1 (± 0.3)	6.2 (± 0.6)
Gives correct birth date (min)	6.4 (± 0.6)	5.8 (± 0.4)	7.4 (± 0.5)[b]
Completes postbox test	34.2 (± 3.2)	33.8 (± 3.1)	40.2 (± 4.2)

[a] Mean values ± SEM.
[b] Significantly different from enflurane group, $P < .05$.
(Modified from Carter et al.,[206] with permission.)

Table 1-6. Morbidity Following the Use of Halothane, Enflurane, or Isoflurane for Outpatient Gynecologic Surgery

Postoperative symptoms	Incidence (%)		
	Halothane	Enflurane	Isoflurane
Sore throat	68	64	64
Pain (analgesics)	52(0)	68(12)	54(20)
Malaise	28	44	44
Cough	16	40	44[a]
Dizziness	16	28	52[a]
Drowsiness	16	36	40
Myalgias	16	28	20
Smell anesthetic	28	12	40[a]
Headache	20	12	44[a]
Nausea	8	12	32[a]
Vomiting	4	4	12

[a] Significantly different from halothane or enflurane groups, $p < 0.05$.
(From Tracey et al.,[205] with permission.)

(0.42) is even lower than nitrous oxide (0.46), and preliminary studies suggest that awakening and recovery of psychomotor function occurs rapidly following discontinuation of this agent.[213] Clinical evaluations of both desflurane and sevoflurane are presently in progress. These two new inhalational agents may prove to be extremely useful in the outpatient setting.

In those situations in which inhaled anesthetics should be avoided (e.g., midtrimester abortions, severe pulmonary disease),[150,214] infusions of intravenous drugs will allow the anesthetist to improve the titration of the rapid and short-acting intravenous anesthetics and analgesics. With intravenous infusion (versus intermittent bolus) techniques, the amount of drug administered is less and recovery times are shorter.[215] Anesthetic and analgesic infusions can be administered in a manner analogous to conventional inhalational agents. For brief outpatient gynecologic procedures, barbiturate infusions, such as thiopental, 10 to 20 mg/min, and methohexital, 3 to 7 mg/min, are useful adjuvants to nitrous oxide, 70 percent in oxygen.[150] The use of a variable-rate infusion of propofol (4 to 12 mg/min) has been shown to be highly effective in outpatient surgery, and was associated with fewer side effects and earlier ambulation and discharge compared with barbiturate or inhalation-based anesthetic techniques.[174,176] Even though outpatients may be clinically fit for discharge 1 hour after surgery when short-acting intravenous anesthetics and analgesics are used, memory and cognitive functioning may require 2 to 3 hours to return to normal.[216]

Narcotic (opioid) analgesics are frequently administered as adjuvants during the immediate preinduction period. Narcotics can reduce the requirement for sedative-hypnotic drugs and inhalation agents, thereby decreasing recovery times and postoperative pain (Table 1-7).[74,80,217] Although morphine (and its derivatives) and meperidine can be used in outpatient anesthesia,[62,74] they are not as popular as the more potent, rapid, and shorter-acting narcotic analgesics (e.g., fentanyl, sufentanil, and alfentanil).[217–220] Small doses of these potent analgesics can effectively attenuate the cardiostimulatory response to laryngoscopy and intubation, and they are also useful supplements to the intravenous and inhaled anesthetics during the maintenance period.[221–223] Alfentanil's extremely rapid onset of action and short duration of effect make it particularly useful in the outpatient setting.[224–229] When administered by continuous infusion,[228,229] the anesthetist can more precisely titrate the alfentanil dose to

Table 1-7. Effect of Fentanyl Premedication on Hypnotic Requirements, Recovery Times, and Side Effects Following Induction and Maintenance of Anesthesia With Either Thiopental or Etomidate

Treatment group	Premedication	Hypnotic dose (mg)[a]	Recovery times (min)[a]			Side effects (%)			
			Awake	Oriented	Cognitive	Pain	Myoclonus	Nausea	Vomiting
Thiopental	None	618 ± 67	17 ± 4	24 ± 7	106 ± 9	0	0	9	9
	Fentanyl	398 ± 60	4 ± 1	8 ± 2	97 ± 13	0	0	22	22
Etomidate	None	67 ± 7	8 ± 2	13 ± 3	93 ± 9	55	66	44	33
	Fentanyl	44 ± 8	4 ± 1	8 ± 2	75 ± 10	36	45	36	36

[a] Mean values ± SEM.
(From Horrigan et al.,[80] with permission.)

produce the desired clinical effect. Most investigators have reported significantly more rapid emergence after an alfentanil-based (versus fentanyl-based) anesthetic technique (Fig. 1-7).[225–228] The addition of alfentanil improved anesthetic conditions and decreased postoperative morbidity after both propofol and thiopental-enflurane anesthesia.[175] Use of alfentanil as an adjunct to methohexital or propofol can produce general anesthesia without the need for inhaled agents (i.e., total intravenous anesthesia).[177,229]

Most investigators have demonstrated a more rapid initial recovery from anesthesia when fentanyl or one of its newer analogs was administered as part of a nitrous oxide–narcotic-relaxant ("balanced") technique (Table 1-8).[208,230–235] Furthermore, use of a balanced technique as an alternative to an inhaled agent may decrease the requirement for postoperative analgesics and contribute to a shorter recovery room stay.[236] However, recovery of cognitive function and reaction time 3 to 6 hours after surgery with an inhalation technique compared favorably with a narcotic-based technique (Fig. 1-8).[234,235,237–239] Since outpatient studies have consistently reported a higher incidence of postoperative nausea and/or vomiting when fentanyl, sufentanil, or alfentanil was used as an alternative to the volatile agents,[234,235,238–240] antiemetic prophylaxis or treatment will be required more frequently when a narcotic-based technique is used. Prophylactic techniques are preferred because the postoperative administration of centrally active antiemetics (e.g., droperidol) can contribute to a delayed recovery of psychomotor function after outpatient surgery. Use of the agonist-antagonist analgesic drugs, such as nalbuphine and butorphanol, as alternatives to the potent opioid agonists appears to result in an even higher incidence of postoperative side effects.[241–243] If antagonist drugs (naloxone, anticholinesterases, and anticholinergics, for example) are required when using a balanced technique, the potential for adverse drug interactions and side effects in the early recovery period would be increased compared with an inhalational technique. Of the side effects occurring during the early postoperative period after outpatient anesthesia, headaches are more frequent with volatile anesthetics while nausea and vomiting are more common after nitrous-narcotic-relaxant techniques (Table 1-9).[233,238,239,244,245]

The use of muscle relaxants may be required in outpatient anesthesia to facilitate endotracheal intubation and to optimize the surgical conditions. In addition, their use can decrease the anesthetic requirement and recovery time (Fig. 1-9).[246] Prior to the introduction of the intermediate-acting nondepolarizing muscle relaxants, succinylcholine infusion (0.1 to 0.2 percent) was the most frequently used muscle relaxant during outpatient anesthesia. Unfortunately, administration of succinylcholine may be associated with muscle pain lasting up to 4

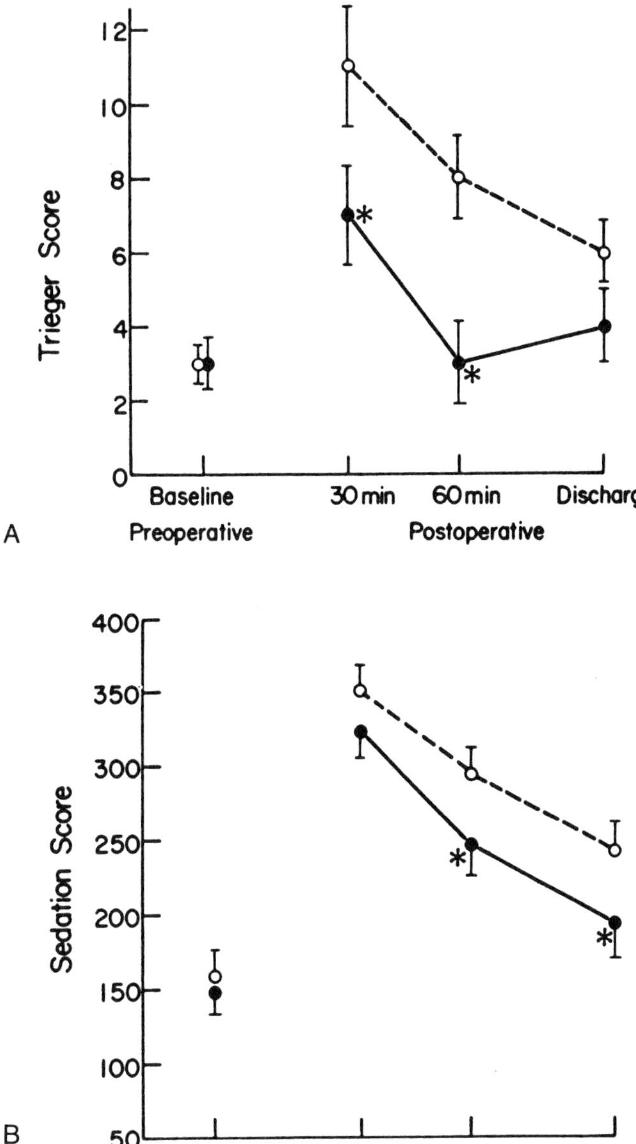

Fig. 1-7. (**A**) Change in Trieger scores (number of dots missed) as a function of time after awakening from anesthesia (mean values ± SEM). (**B**) Change in sedation analog scores (sum of five 100-mm analog scales, with 0 [no sedation] to 100 [maximal sedation] for each scale) as a function of time after awakening from anesthesia. Asterisk indicates significant differences ($P < 0.05$) between fentanyl (○- - - -○) and alfentanil (●———●) infusion groups at the indicated time intervals. (From White et al.,[228] with permission.)

days after the operation.[247,248] With the availability of shorter-acting nondepolarizing muscle relaxants (e.g., atracurium, 0.3 to 0.5 mg/kg, vecuronium, 0.06 to 0.08 mg/kg), prompt reversal of neuromuscular blockade can be achieved even after brief surgical procedures.[249–253] Although still controversial, it would appear that the use

Table 1-8. Comparative Recovery Times Following Outpatient Anesthesia with Enflurane, Isoflurane, or a "Balanced" Technique

Primary anesthetic	Awakening time[a] (min)	Arousal scores[b] at 20 min	Arousal scores[b] at 40 min
Enflurane	8.8 ± 2.4	2.0 ± 0.4	2.7 ± 0.5
Isoflurane	9.4 ± 4.8	2.0 ± 0.7	2.7 ± 0.4
Fentanyl	3.6 ± 2.6[c]	2.4 ± 0.5[c]	2.9 ± 0.3

[a] Time to first response (mean ± SD).
[b] Arousal state on a scale from 0 to 3 (mean ± SD).
[c] Fentanyl group significantly different from either enflurane or isoflurane, $P < .05$.
(From Azar et al.,[208] with permission.)

of nondepolarizing muscle relaxants may contribute to a decreased incidence of postoperative myalgias.[254,255] Factors other than succinylcholine also contribute to the occurrence of myalgias after outpatient surgery. In fact, Zahl and Apfelbaum demonstrated that the use of vecuronium (versus succinylcholine) did not lower the incidence or severity of muscle pain after laparoscopy.[256] When mivacurium (BW 1090U), a shorter-acting derivative of atracurium, is approved for clinical use, it should further

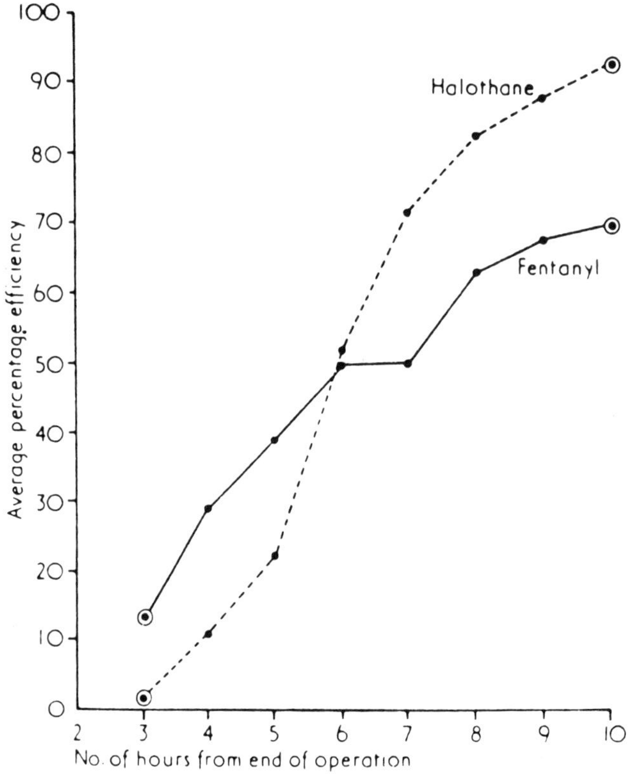

Fig. 1-8. Recovery of cognitive function in patients administered either halothane-nitrous oxide (●- - - -●) or fentanyl-pancuronium-nitrous oxide (●———●) for maintenance of anesthesia. (From Simpson et al.,[237] with permission.)

Table 1-9. Comparative Morbidity After Three Different Outpatient Anesthetic Techniques for Laparoscopy

	Primary Anesthetics		
Side Effects	Halothane/N_2O	Enflurane/N_2O	Fentanyl/N_2O
at Discharge			
Drowsy	68	50	57
Dizzy	45	39	43
Headache	20	6	14
Weak	90	64	64
Nausea	28	22	43
at 24 hr			
Drowsy	83	75	64
Dizzy	50	44	36
Headache	40	25	7
Weak	83	83	71
Nausea	10	11	29
Myalgias	80	72	57
at 48 hr			
Drowsy	33	33	21
Dizzy	23	28	14
Headache	30	25	14
Weak	55	3	43
Nausea	13		0
Myalgias	70	83	42

(From Dhamee et al.,[245] with permission.)

decrease the need for reversal agents in outpatient anesthesia. Although its onset of action is slower than succinylcholine,[257,258] mivacurium's rate of spontaneous recovery appears to be more rapid than the intermediate-acting nondepolarizing drugs.[259] When antagonism of nondepolarizing muscle relaxants is required, edrophonium (0.5 mg/kg) may offer an advantage in the outpatient setting because its onset of action appears to be faster than either neostigmine or pyridostigmine.[260] Furthermore, a recent study suggests that there is a relationship between postoperative emetic symptoms and the antagonism of neuromuscular blockade by neostigmine and atropine.[261]

Any comparison of general anesthetic techniques is complicated because of the many factors that can influence both early and late recovery after outpatient surgery. The incidence of postoperative symptoms after outpatient surgery is high irrespective of the anesthetic technique used (Table 1-9),[245] and is dependent on a multiplicity of factors, including gender (female), previous exposure to general anesthesia, endotracheal intubation, and the duration of the operative procedure.[49] Endotracheal intubation results in a higher incidence of airway-related complaints (e.g., sore throat, croup, hoarseness) and greater morbidity when assessed 4 hours after surgery.[20]

Given the high incidence of side effects after general anesthesia,[262] it can be difficult to determine when it is safe to discharge a patient following ambulatory surgery (see Ch. 17). Although a variety of tests have been devised to assess psychomotor recovery after general anesthesia (e.g., Aldrete score, Trieger dot test, electroencephalogram, stabilometry),[263–265] there are still no standardized discharge criteria. Complications and side effects after general anesthesia that commonly delay discharge include excessive bleeding, intolerable pain, prolonged emergence, dizziness, inability to urinate, and intractable nausea and vomiting.[49–53] Simple maneuvers can be used to decrease the incidence of some of these side effects. For example, infiltration of the mesosalpinx with bupivacaine 0.5 percent decreases postoperative pain after laparos-

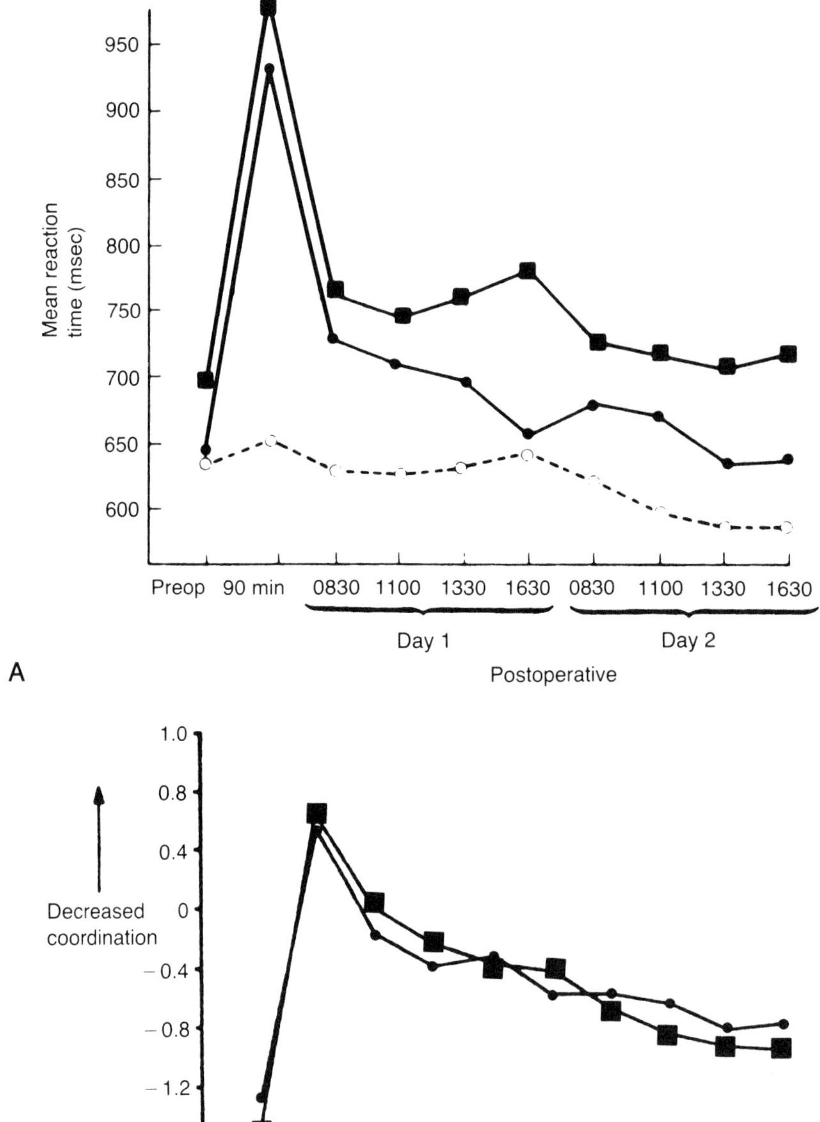

Fig. 1-9. (**A**) Effect of anesthesia on mean reaction time in three groups of patients: (○– – – –○) unanesthetized controls, (■———■) patients receiving halothane-N_2O with spontaneous ventilation, and (●———●) patients receiving thiopental-N_2O-relaxant with controlled ventilation. (**B**) Effect of anesthesia on coordination scores derived from visual analogue scales: (■———■) patients receiving halothane-N_2O with spontaneous ventilation, and (●———●) patients receiving thiopental halothane-N_2O-relaxant with controlled ventilation. (From Herbert et al.,[246] with permission.)

copic tubal sterilization under general anesthesia.[266] Although controversial,[267] use of airway heating may decrease postoperative shivering and recovery times after longer outpatient procedures.[149] Some anesthesiologists have even administered central stimulants such as doxapram in an effort to hasten arousal after outpatient general anesthesia.[268] There is no "ideal" general anesthetic agent or technique for outpatients; however, there is a vast array of pharmacologically active drugs that, when combined in a rational manner and carefully titrated, can produce the desired anesthetic conditions with an acceptable recovery profile.

Regional Anesthesia

Regional anesthesia can offer many advantages over general anesthesia for the ambulatory patient (see Ch. 14). In addition to limiting the anesthetized area to the surgical site, common side effects of general anesthesia are avoided (e.g., nausea, vomiting, dizziness, lethargy), the risks of aspiration pneumonitis and the side effects of endotracheal intubation are minimized, postanesthesia nursing care and patient recovery time may be decreased, and improved analgesia is provided in the early postoperative period.[269,270] Although some studies indicate that the incidence of postoperative complications may be lower and recovery time shorter in patients receiving regional anesthesia,[271] there is still debate as to whether it is truly "safer" than general anesthesia. Proper patient selection along with the skill and enthusiasm of the surgical and anesthesia teams would allow a wide variety of procedures to be performed with regional anesthetic techniques (Table 1-10).[269]

Central neural blockade using a spinal or epidural technique is the most widely used form of regional anesthesia. Spinal anesthesia is useful for lower extremity, urologic, and herniorrhaphy procedures in the ambulatory setting. Outpatients should be allowed to recover full sensory and motor function prior to discharge. Once the sensory deficits have resolved, residual sympathetic blockade and orthostatic hypotension are rarely problems on ambulation.[272] Concern over the effect of ambulation on postlumbar puncture headache may be unwarranted.[273] Nevertheless, many clinicians limit the use of subarachnoid blocks to patients over 60 years of age because the incidence of headache can be very high in younger outpatients.[274] The use of smaller needles (26 guage) and/or Quincke-type points may decrease the incidence of this potentially disturbing side effect.[275] The prophylactic use of analgesics or an epidural blood patch are ineffective in outpatients.[276,277] If a postlumbar puncture headache occurs and does not respond to hydration and oral analgesic medication, treatment with an epidural blood patch on an outpatient basis can be highly effective.[278,279] Cohen instructs patients to rest quietly for 1 hour after injection of 10 ml of blood before being discharged home.[279] The patient should avoid straining and maintain good oral fluid intake at home.

Epidural (and caudal) anesthesia has been advocated for outpatient lower extremity procedures, herniorrhaphy, and extracorporeal shock wave lithotripsy.[280–283] Short- and intermediate-acting local anesthetic drugs are sufficient for most outpatient procedures (e.g., 2-chloroprocaine, lidocaine, mepivacaine). Proper selection of the local anesthetic agent and the use of epinephrine should make the use of an epidural catheter unnecessary for most ambulatory procedures. Caudal blockade is a useful technique for anorectal surgery as well as for dilatation and curettage.[284] These procedures can also be performed with perianal infiltration or paracervical blocks, respectively.[285]

For brief superficial surgical procedures limited to a single extremity, the intrave-

Table 1-10. Summary of Regional Anesthetic Techniques for Outpatient Surgical Procedures

Nerve blocks of the head and neck	Blocks for superficial procedures on the abdominal wall (intercostal or field block)
Jaw wiring—mandibular block	Umbilical herniorrhaphy
Cervical node biopsy—cervical block	Excision of lipoma
Excision of mass in neck—cervical block	Removal of abdominal scar, stitch granuloma
Revision of lip scar—infraorbital block	Inguinal herniorrhaphy
Blepharoplasty—infraorbital and supraorbital block	
Dermabrasion of chin—mental block	Blocks for procedures involving the lower abdomen or perineum
Suture of scalp lacerations—scalp block	Spinal
	Fulguration, vaginal carcinoma
Blocks for superficial thorax procedures (intercostal block)	Fulguration, rectal carcinoma
Breast biopsy	Prostrate biopsy
Excision of axillary node	Caudal
Removal of sternal suture granuloma	Dilatation and curettage
Removal of lipoma from back	Cervical polypectomy
Excision of sternal sinus tract	Modified Shirodkar suture
	Incision and drainage of Bartholin cyst
Blocks of the upper extremity	Lumbar epidural
Interscalene (Winnie) or supraclavicular block	Incision and drainage of pilonidal cyst
Reduction of a dislocated shoulder	Diagnostic laparoscopy
Closed reduction of Colles fracture	Tubal ligation
Excision of bone cyst of hand	Inguinal herniorrhaphy
Excision of masses	
Debridement of osteo tracts	Blocks of the leg (sciatic and femoral nerve blocks)
Epicondylar stripping	Exostosectomy of the foot
Axillary or intravenous (Bier) block	Removal of screw from leg
Arthrodesis of finger joints	Bunionectomy
Repair of lacerated tendons	Foreign body removal from leg
Carpal tunnel syndrome	Excision of neuroma of foot
Removal of K wires	Correction of hammertoe
Excision of osteoma	Reduction of dislocated hip (lidocaine spinal)
Repair of digital nerves	
Excision of tumor	
Lipoma of forearm	

(From Bridenbaugh,[269] with permission.)

nous regional block is a simple and reliable technique.[286] This procedure can be used for either upper or lower extremity surgery, and use of a double tourniquet can decrease the incidence of tourniquet pain. If more profound and prolonged anesthesia of the upper extremity is required, a regional block of the brachial plexus can be used, such as an axillary block or interscalene block. Peripheral nerve blocks are also useful for surgery of the leg. Patel et al. found the "3 in 1" block (femoral, obturator, and lateral femoral cutaneous nerves using a perivascular technique) to be useful for outpatient knee arthroscopy, with excellent postoperative analgesia and a high degree of patient acceptance.[287] Nerve block at the ankle is also simple and effective for surgery of the foot.[288]

In pediatric outpatients, a regional block performed immediately after induction of general anesthesia can reduce the anesthetic requirement and provide profound postoperative analgesia and an earlier return to the child's usual bright and alert state after surgery.[289] Caudal anesthesia is a highly effective technique in children undergoing lower abnominal, perineal, and lower extremity procedures (see Chs. 8 and 14). Other useful techniques include blockade of the ilioinguinal and iliohypogastric nerves with bupivacaine to minimize postherniorrhaphy pain,[290] and the use of either a caudal, dorsal penile nerve block, subcutaneous ring block, or topical lidocaine ointment for postcircumcision pain.[291–296] Interestingly, simple wound infiltration with a local anesthetic solution or topical application of a local anesthetic gel were reported to be as effective as a caudal block or an ilioinguinal nerve block.[297–299]

Local Anesthesia

Of all the anesthetic techniques suitable for outpatients, local infiltration of the operative site with dilute solutions of local anesthetics may be the simplest and safest (see Ch. 13). As mentioned earlier, outpatient urologic procedures (e.g., vasovasotomy, orchiopexy, hydrocele and spermatocele repairs) under local anesthesia can significantly decrease the overall cost compared with inpatient procedures.[10,11] Even transurethral resection of the prostate has been performed under local anesthesia.[300] Outpatient knee arthroscopy is commonly performed under local anesthesia, bupivacaine 0.5 percent, 30 ml, for example.[143] Inguinal herniorrhaphy has also been performed under local anesthesia, with excellent patient acceptance and minimal postoperative complications.[301] Use of a retrobulbar block technique (versus general anesthesia) can decrease the incidence of postoperative emesis after ophthalmologic surgery.[302] Malhora et al. described a local anesthetic technique for lithotripsy that involved a combination of local infiltration and intercostal nerve blocks.[303] Unfortunately, only a limited number of operations can be performed with local infiltration or "field blocks." Yet, local anesthetic supplementation (e.g., infiltration with bupivacaine 0.25 to 0.5 percent) will decrease incisional pain in the recovery room. The use of topical local anesthetic techniques, including lidocaine creams, gels, and aerosols, can also provide effective analgesia in the early postoperative period.[299,304]

How does local anesthesia compare with general anesthesia with respect to recovery time and incidence of postoperative morbidity after outpatient surgery? The retrospective analysis by Meridy revealed that patients receiving local anesthesia had significantly shorter recovery time.[23] In contrast, Muir et al. found relatively minor differences in postoperative morbidity when comparing local and general anesthesia in young patients undergoing oral surgery.[305] As expected, patients receiving local anesthesia had greater difficulty eating on the day of the operation because of the residual neural blockade, while drowsiness and nausea were more common in the general anesthesia group. Surprisingly, 65 percent of those who had local anesthesia felt "unfit" to return to work or school on the day following their operation compared with only 28 percent in the group receiving general anesthesia.

Since the injection of local anesthetics can be associated with significant discomfort, the use of intravenous sedative and analgesic drugs (i.e., so-called conscious sedation techniques) during local anesthetic injections has been popularized by both oral and plastic surgeons.[306–308] This practice must be taken into consideration when assessing the safety of "local" anesthesia and monitored anesthesia care (see Ch. 12). The FASA study found the incidence of perioperative complications to be lowest in those patients receiving local anesthesia (Table 1-11).[18] In contrast, the incidence of complications was significantly higher in patients receiving local anesthesia with sedation. Overall, morbidity following the use of intravenous sedation is higher in women than men.[308] To understand the relationship between the sedation technique and perioperative morbidity, carefully controlled studies are needed.

Sedation During Local and Regional Anesthesia

Sedation during local anesthesia is often desirable to minimize the stress associated with the busy operating room environment (see Chs. 12 and 13). In addition, many patients are concerned about recall of intraoperative events. In a crossover study eval-

Table 1-11. Relationship of Anesthetic Technique to the Incidence of Postoperative Complications After Outpatient Surgery

Technique	No. of patients	No. of complications	Incidence
Local anesthesia only	10,169	38	1/268
Local anesthesia with sedation	10,229	96	1/106
General anesthesia	61,299	513	1/120
Regional block	1,936	7	1/277

(Data from Federated Ambulatory Surgery Association.[18])

uating the use of sedation in outpatient oral surgery,[309] 85 percent of the patients preferred surgery under local anesthesia with sedation to local anesthesia alone. Regardless of the route of administration, patient satisfaction was reported to be higher in the presence of more profound sedation.[310] Effective sedation-analgesia techniques can be used as alternatives to general (and regional) anesthesia in the outpatient setting.[311] However, the ever-present risk of ventilatory depression necessitates the use of effective respiratory monitors (e.g., precordial or pretracheal stethoscope, pulse oximeter, capnograph) and supplemental oxygen (e.g., nasal prongs). In a recent study, over 40 percent of patients who did not receive supplemental oxygen during local anesthesia with sedation experienced clinically significant oxygen desaturation.[312] Interestingly, hypoxia also occurred in some patients receiving only local anesthesia.

In 1966, Shane described an "intravenous amnesia" technique involving the use of small incremental doses of barbiturates, opioids, anticholinergics, and ataractics.[313] At present, the term "conscious sedation" implies the use of intravenous anesthetics and analgesics to supplement local or regional anesthesia. According to the American Dental Association,[314] conscious sedation is "a minimally depressed level of consciousness that retains the patient's ability to independently and continuously maintain an airway and respond appropriately to physical stimulation and verbal command, produced by a pharmacologic or non-pharmacologic method." Since the drugs commonly used to produce this altered state of consciousness produce dose-dependent central nervous system depression, conscious sedation lies on a continuum leading from minimal sedation (i.e., awake, relaxed state) to profound sedation (i.e., unconscious hypnotic state). The primary objectives of conscious sedation include adequate sedation with "minimal risk," relief of anxiety, amnesia, and relief from pain and other noxious stimuli.[315] Achieving an optimal balance between patient comfort and safety requires careful titration of sedative and analgesic drugs, appropriate monitoring of the cardiovascular, respiratory, and central nervous systems, and, most importantly, good communication with the patient and surgeon. A wide variety of intravenous drugs and techniques are currently used for producing conscious sedation (see Chs. 12 and 13).

The most popular techniques for conscious sedation involve the use of combinations of benzodiazepines (e.g., diazepam, midazolam) and opioid analgesics (e.g., fentanyl, sufentanil). Careful titration of sedative and analgesic drugs is required to minimize the potential for severe (life-threatening) respiratory depression. Although the most widely used technique involves a combination of midazolam and fentanyl, techniques that have a lower risk of ventilatory depression (i.e., midazolam-ketamine, midazolam-nalbuphine, or butorphanol) are becoming increasingly popular. In addition, with the availability of very rapid and short-acting sedative (propofol) and analgesic (alfentanil) drugs, it is possible to more precisely titrate these drugs to achieve the desired clinical endpoint without side effects or prolonged recovery times. For anesthesiologists to achieve an optimal outcome when using conscious sedation techniques, their clinical skills as "communicators" will be challenged as will their knowledge of basic pharmacology and physiology.

Several recent studies have compared midazolam and diazepam for sedation during local and regional techniques.[316–321] Midazolam is two to four times more potent that diazepam with respect to its sedative-amnestic properties.[317] When used as an intravenous adjuvant to topical (local) anesthesia, most investigators report a faster onset of action, more effective amnesia, and higher patient acceptance with midazolam than diazepam. In patients undergoing regional anesthesia with benzodiazepine-induced sedation, 80 percent of the patients receiving midazolam were wide awake 2 hours after the procedure, compared with 67 percent of those receiving diazepam.[319] In addition, 50 percent of patients in the midazolam group were completely amnestic for their surgery compared with only 18 percent in the diazepam group. McClure et al.[320] also compared these two drugs during spinal anesthesia, and reported that patients receiving midazolam experienced a higher incidence of intraoperative amnesia and less postoperative sedation. Use of oral midazolam (versus intravenous diazepam) was associated with greater patient and physician acceptance when used for conscious sedation in outpatients undergoing minor procedures.[321] A new sublingual lormetazepam formulation also appears to be an effective alternative to parenteral benzodiazepines for conscious sedation.[322] With the availability of flumazenil, it will be possible to reverse the residual sedative and amnestic effects of benzodiazepines prior to discharge (Fig. 1-10).[323–325] However, the short halflife of flumazenil (1 to 2 hours) might contribute to the recurrence of sedation after discharge from the outpatient facility.

While benzodiazepines are highly effective sedative-anxiolytic drugs, the addition of an opioid analgesic will significantly improve patient comfort during local anesthesia.[326] However, concurrent administration of opioid and benzodiazepine compounds will result in significant ventilatory depression and a higher incidence of apnea.[327,328] The apparent synergism between the benzodiazepines and opioid analgesics with respect to ventilatory depression may result from their ability to decrease hypoxic and hypercapnic respiratory drive, respectively. Use of an agonist-antagonist (e.g., butorphanol, nalbuphine) as an alternative to fentanyl will decrease the possibility of severe ventilatory depression. Preliminary studies suggest that these combinations (e.g., nalbuphine-diazepam) can be highly effective for sedation during local anesthesia.[329] When more profound sedation is required, a nalbuphine-methohexital combination was found to be effective.[330] Alternatively, use of a carefully titrated continuous intravenous infusion of the sedative-analgesic alfentanil can provide more profound analgesia than the agonist-antagonist analgesics and less ventilatory depression than the benzodiazepine-opioid combinations. Recently, alfentanil was reported to provide effective analgesia during gallstone lithotripsy.[331]

The combination of a benzodiazepine and ketamine is another useful alternative to the benzodiazepine-opioid techniques for intravenous sedation and analgesia.[317,332] When ketamine was used alone for sedation during intercostal nerve block procedures, physician and patient acceptance scores were higher than those associated with diazepam alone or with a droperidol-fentanyl combination.[333] However, if the patient is not adequately sedated with a benzodiazepine prior to administration of ketamine,

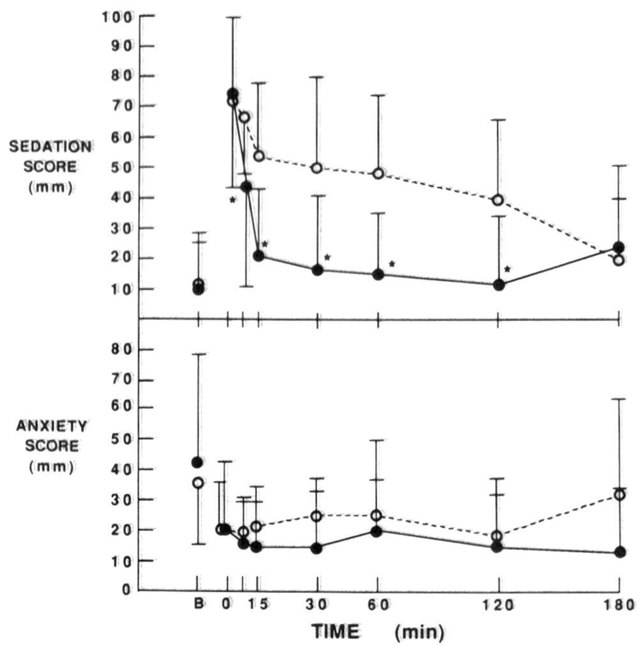

Fig. 1-10. Levels of sedation and anxiety immediately before (**B**) and at the conclusion of (●) midazolam sedation, and as a function of time following treatment with either saline (control, ○- - - -○) or flumazenil (●——●). Data represents mean values ± SD. Asterisks indicate significant differences between the two treatment groups, P < .05. (From White et al.,[323] with permission.)

marked cardiovascular stimulation can occur, and patients may experience unpleasant psychomimetic emergence reactions. When either midazolam or diazepam were administered as adjuvants to low-dose ketamine during plastic surgery procedures, midazolam was found to produce more profound intraoperative sedation, anxiolysis, and amnesia, less pain and venoirritation, and higher overall patient acceptance than diazepam.[317] The safety and efficacy of the midazolam-ketamine combination when used to supplement local anesthesia for outpatient dermatologic surgery has recently been confirmed.[334] However, amnesia after midazolam sedation can persist into the postoperative period.[317,335]

Barbiturates and etomidate have also been administered by infusion techniques to produce sedation during local anesthesia.[336] Care must be taken to titrate these drugs to avoid respiratory and hemodynamic depression. Although the newer intravenous sedative-hypnotic propofol is associated with slightly greater hemodynamic depression than methohexital, a propofol infusion is highly effective in producing rapid, smooth, and controllable sedation.[337,338] Compared with a midazolam infusion, use of a propofol infusion during local anesthesia results in a more rapid recovery of cognitive function.[339]

Inhalational analgesia with nitrous oxide, 30 to 50 percent, or enflurane, 0.5 percent, can also be used to supplement ambulatory procedures under regional anesthesia.[340,341] Care must be taken to avoid general anesthesia and its potential complications of excitement, respiratory depression, and aspiration. Frequent side effects (e.g., nausea, confusion), concern over operating room pollution, and the availability of improved medications for intravenous sedation limit the clinical usefulness of these inhalational analgesia techniques.

DISCHARGE CRITERIA

Accurate assessment of recovery of cognitive and psychomotor function is important in determining the appropriate time for discharge after ambulatory surgery (see Ch. 17).[342] The recovery room nurse, the surgeon, and the anesthesiologist, as well as the patient and the patient's responsible escort, all play important roles in determining when a "home ready" state has been achieved. According to the Joint Commission for the Accreditation of Hospitals guidelines, the ultimate decision to discharge a patient after an outpatient procedure rests with a "licensed, independent practioner with appropriate privileges who is familiar with the patient." Although the physician need not be physically present at the time of discharge, specific discharge criteria (that have been approved by the medical staff) must be rigorously applied when the nursing staff makes decisions regarding discharge from an ambulatory surgery unit (see Appendix 1-3). Thus, it is no longer necessary for a physician to examine a patient immediately prior to discharge from the facility. Nevertheless, from a medicolegal perspective (see Ch. 20), the physician as well as the nurse will be held responsible if an outpatient is prematurely discharged from an ambulatory facility.

A wide variety of psychomotor tests have been used to assess recovery following outpatient anesthesia.[343,344] Tests of cognitive function, such as processing (mental arithmetic, reaction time), integration (critical flicker fusion test), memory (digit span), and learning (word lists), have been used to assess recovery after outpatient anesthesia (Table 1-12). Tests of sensory (e.g., stimulus detection, auditing perception, Maddox Wing test, vigilance) and psychomotor function (e.g., choice reaction time, postbox test, Trieger dot test, tracking test) have also been used to determine home readiness (Fig. 1-11). Although these cognitive, sensory, and psychomotor tests provide information that can be used in developing practical discharge criteria, most of these tests are too complex and time-consuming to use in a busy clinical setting.[345] Simple tests of memory and sensorimotor coordination appear to be the most useful indices of recovery.[344] The Bender Gestalt Track Tracer Test is a reliable, valid, objective, noninvasive, inexpensive test which can be easily performed by outpatients (in less than 60 seconds).[346]

In general, discharge from an ambulatory facility requires that patients satisfy specific

Table 1-12. Assessing Recovery of Psychomotor and Cognitive Function After Outpatient Anesthesia

	Tests
Home readiness	Paper and pencil tests (e.g., Trieger) Maddox wing (extraocular muscle balance) Single reaction time Coordination and attention tests
Street fitness	Flicker fusion Psychomotor tests Electroencephalogram
Complete recovery	Reaction timing and coordinative skills Driving stimulation tests

(Adapted from Korttila,[343] with permission.)

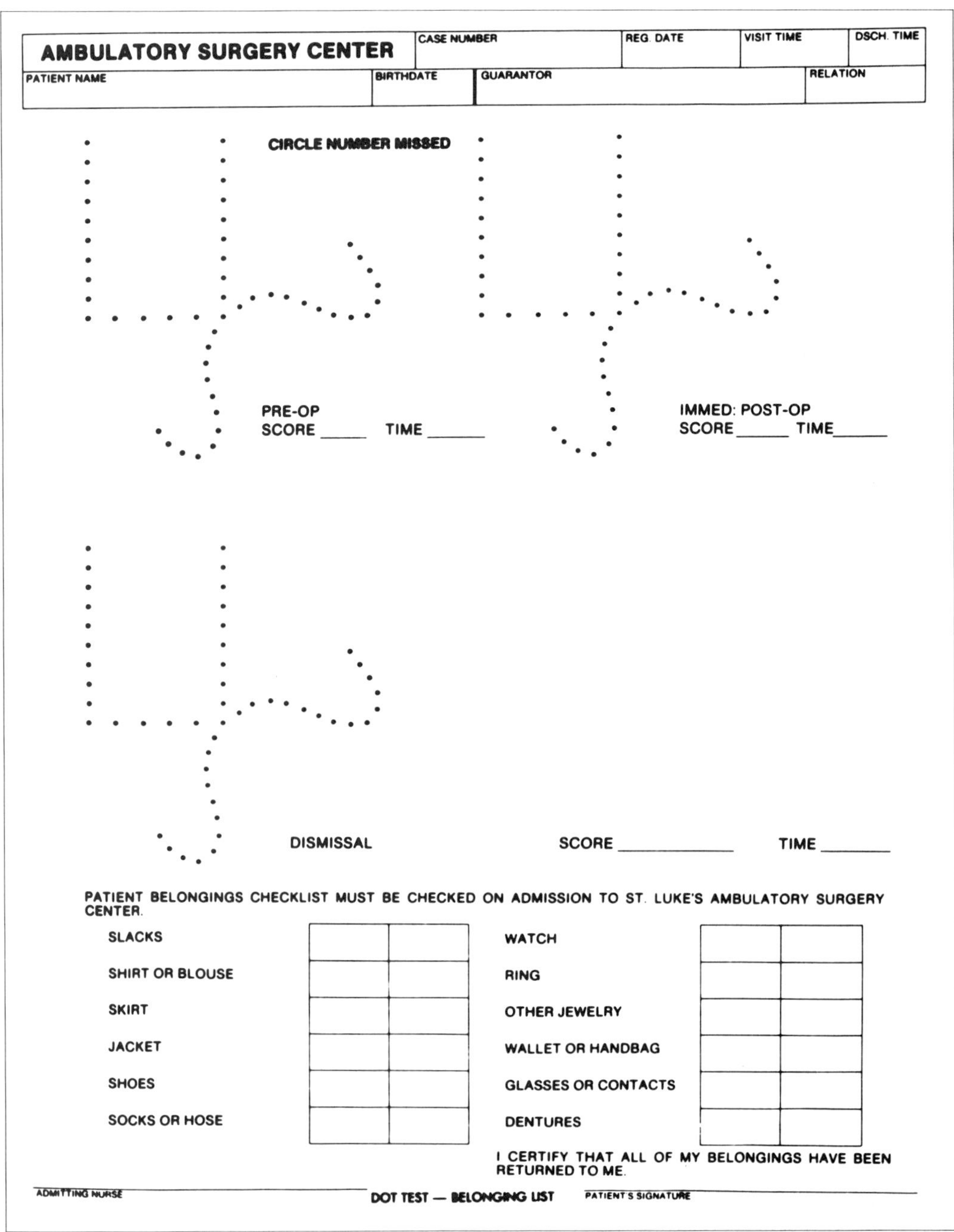

AMBULATORY SURGERY CENTER

CASE NUMBER	REG. DATE	VISIT TIME	DSCH. TIME

PATIENT NAME	BIRTHDATE	GUARANTOR	RELATION

CIRCLE NUMBER MISSED

PRE-OP
SCORE _____ TIME ______

IMMED: POST-OP
SCORE ______ TIME______

DISMISSAL SCORE ____________ TIME _______

PATIENT BELONGINGS CHECKLIST MUST BE CHECKED ON ADMISSION TO ST. LUKE'S AMBULATORY SURGERY CENTER.

SLACKS			WATCH		
SHIRT OR BLOUSE			RING		
SKIRT			OTHER JEWELRY		
JACKET			WALLET OR HANDBAG		
SHOES			GLASSES OR CONTACTS		
SOCKS OR HOSE			DENTURES		

I CERTIFY THAT ALL OF MY BELONGINGS HAVE BEEN RETURNED TO ME.

ADMITTING NURSE ______ DOT TEST — BELONGING LIST PATIENT'S SIGNATURE ______

Fig. 1-11. Use of Trieger dot test to assess recovery following outpatient anesthesia. (Courtesy of Dr. E. E. Fibuch, St. Luke's Hospital, Kansas City, Missouri.)

Discharge Criteria Used for Assessing Recovery After General Anesthesia

Stable vital signs for 30 minutes or more.

No new signs or symptoms after the operation.

No active bleeding or oozing.

Minimal nausea or emesis for 30 minutes or more.

Intact neurocirculatory function without evidence of swelling or impaired circulation after extremity surgery.

Ability to void (clear) urine after cystoscopic examination and herniorrhapy.

Orientation to person, time, and place.

Minimal dizziness after changing clothes and sitting for 10 minutes or more.

Pain controllable with oral analgesics.

Presence of responsible escort.

criteria which can be summarized on simplified checklists. Additional criteria must be applied when patients undergo regional anesthesia. With spinal or epidural anesthesia, it is generally accepted that motor and sensory functions return before sympathetic nerve function. However, several studies have reported recovery of sympathetic activity before complete regression of the subarachnoid block.[272,347,348] In fact, Alexander et al. suggested that patients can be safely discharged when they have two successive orthostatic blood pressure decreases of 10 percent or less after a spinal anesthetic.[349] Prior to ambulation, patients should have normal perianal ($S_{4\text{-}5}$) sensation, be able to plantar flex the foot, and have proprioception of the great toe.[272] Intact functioning of the sympathetic nerve supply to the bladder and urethra is necessary for urination. Thus, discharge criteria after spinal and epidural anesthesia should include return of normal sensation, muscle strength, and proprioception, as well as sympathetic nervous function.

Pain control is one of the most important factors in determining when a patient can be discharged from an outpatient facility.[350] Excessive postoperative pain is the most common surgical-related cause of unexpected hospital admissions after ambulatory surgery. Pain must be treated rapidly and effectively in order to minimize postoperative symptoms which can delay ambulation. In postoperative patients experiencing both pain and nausea, adequate treatment of their postoperative pain was often accompanied by resolution of their emetic symptoms.[351] As described in Chapter 19, pain management for outpatient surgery includes three essential components: use of potent, rapid-acting intravenous opioid analgesics to decrease the intraoperative anesthetic requirement and provide effective analgesia in the early recovery period, use of regional and local anesthetic techniques for analgesia during the perioperative period, and use of oral analgesics for controlling pain after discharge.

While local anesthetics are excellent adjuvants to other analgesic techniques, controversy surrounds their use in the outpatient setting. In a placebo-controlled study, Milligan et al. found that intra-articular bupivacaine provided no significant analgesic effect after outpatient arthroscopy.[352] While wound infiltration with bupivacaine usually decreases the severity of pain in the recovery room, these patients may complain of more severe pain after discharge (Sung Y-F, personal communications, 1989). Opioid compounds are the most effective in controlling early incisional pain (less than 24 hours after the operation), while nonsteroidal anti-inflammatory drugs are more effective in treating the pain associated with tissue edema and inflammation which occurs 24 to 72 hours after the operation. Intravenous diclofenac, a prostaglandin synthesis inhibitor, significantly decreased postoperative morbidity after outpatient oral surgery.[353]

Prior to leaving the outpatient facility, patients should have their dressings checked and be given both verbal and written instructions regarding their postoperative care. Most anesthetic-related postoperative side effects (e.g., pain, nausea and vomiting, dizziness, headache, myalgias) resolve within 24 hours.[49] However, if these symptoms persist, the patient should be encouraged to contact the facility regarding appropriate follow-up care. All patients must leave in the company of a responsible adult, and need to be aware of the recommendations regarding acceptable activities after discharge. The nursing staff should determine whether or not the escort is a responsible person (i.e., an adult who is both physically and intellectually capable of caring for the patient at home). Although patients are typically warned not to operate machinery or to make important decisions for 24 hours after anesthesia, studies evaluating the effect of halothane on reaction time after short outpatient anesthetics suggest that a patient's activity should be restricted for at least 2 days after receiving this general anesthetic (Fig. 1-9).[247]

As part of the discharge plan, the patient and the patient's escort should clearly understand how to access an emergency facility should a complication arise after the ambulatory center closes. Finally, all outpatient facilities should develop a follow-up plan after the patient has been discharged (Appendix 1-3). Nursing staff members at many outpatient facilities telephone the patient the day after surgery to assess their recovery from surgery and anesthesia. Other facilities rely on postcards or questionnaires for their postoperative follow-up.

SUMMARY

It is obvious that there is still much to learn about anesthesia for ambulatory surgery.[141] In reviewing the early experiences with outpatient anesthesia,[354] it is obvious that many of the same problems still exist. Indeed, recovery times are still too long and the incidences of common side effects remain too high. There is increasing evidence that arbitrary limits placed on the type of surgery, age of the patient, duration of the operation, preoperative fasting period, and use of premedication may be unwarranted. Yet, many controversies remain unresolved (see Ch. 21). Nevertheless, with proper perioperative assessment and care, ambulatory surgery can be safe, economic, and highly acceptable to patients and their families.[355] At present, the ability to provide adequate pain relief after outpatient anesthesia is the major limiting factor in determining the types of operative procedures that can be performed in this setting. Thus, the availability of high-quality home health care services will be critically important in the future expansion of outpatient surgery.

Irrespective of the definition one chooses to describe ambulatory surgery,[356,357] it is clear that the number of operations performed in the outpatient setting will continue to increase as we enter the 21st century. As originally described,[358] the basic principles of ambulatory surgery were applied to healthy children and adults undergoing "minor surgery." Over the last decade, increasing numbers of "high-risk" patients are presenting for surgical procedures on an outpatient basis. The proper selection and evaluation of patients for ambulatory surgery has assumed increased importance. Yet, very little is known about the optimal (anesthetic) techniques for managing outpatients with pre-existing diseases or those at the extremes of age.

In conclusion, the rational use of available combinations of anesthetic drugs and techniques can provide for a rapid and smooth induction, excellent intraoperative conditions, and a rapid recovery with minimal side effects. The incidences of anesthetic-related side effects (e.g., drowsiness, headache, nausea, myalgias, and dizziness) may be altered depending on the premedication, the anesthetic technique, and the skill of the anesthetist. Further studies are needed to determine the etiology of these adverse effects and the optimal therapeutic modalities. With the availability of more rapid and shorter-acting anesthetics, analgesics, and muscle relaxants, as well as improved techniques for administering these drugs, the care we provide to our expanding outpatient population should continue to improve in the future.

REFERENCES

1. Nicoll JM: The surgery of infancy. Br Med J 2:753, 1909
2. Waters RM: The "Down-Town" anesthesia clinic. Am J Surg 33:71, 1919
3. Cohen DO, Dillon JB: Anesthesia for outpatient surgery. JAMA 196:1114, 1966
4. Levy M-L, Coakley CS: Survey of in and out surgery—first year. South Med J 61:995, 1968
5. Ford JL, Reed WA: The Surgicenter™—an innovation in the delivery and cost of medical care. Ariz Med 26:804, 1969
6. Porterfield HW, Franklin LT: The use of general anesthesia in the office surgery facility. Clin Plast Surg 10:289, 1983
7. Perrin JM, Valvona J, Sloan FA: Changing patterns of hospitalization for children requiring surgery. Pediatrics 77:587, 1986
8. Siu AI, Sonnenberg FA, Manning WG, et al: Inappropriate use of hospitals in a randomized trial of health insurance plans. N Engl J Med 315:1259, 1986
9. Doberneck RC: Breast biopsy—a study of cost-effectiveness. Ann Surg 192:152, 1980
10. Caldamone AA, Rabinowitz R: Outpatient orchiopexy. J Urol 127:286, 1982
11. Kaye KW, Clayman RV, Lange PH: Outpatient hydrocele and spermatocele repair under local anesthesia. J Urol 130:269, 1983
12. Smith LE: Ambulatory surgery for anorectal diseases—an update. South Med J 79:163, 1986
13. Steckler RM: Outpatient thyroidectomy—a feasibility study. Am J Surg 152:417, 1986
14. Pineault R, Contandriopoulos A-P: Randomized clinical trial of one-day surgery—patient satisfaction, clinical outcomes, and costs. Med Care 23:171, 1985
15. Kitz DS, Lecky JH, Slusarz-Ladden C, Conahan TJ: Inpatient *vs.* day surgery—differences in resource use, patient volume and anesthesia reimbursement. Anesth Analg 66:S97, 1987
16. Ancona-Berk A, Chalmers TC: Cost and efficacy of the substitution of ambulatory for inpatient care. N Engl J Med 304:393, 1981
17. Othersen HB, Jr., Clatworthy HW, Jr.: Outpatient herniorrhaphy for infants. Am J Dis Child 116:78, 1968
18. Federated Ambulatory Surgery Association: Special Study I. Number 520. Alexandria, VA, 1986
19. Hatch LR: Day care surgery—do we and our patients need it? Can Anaesth Soc J 30:542, 1983
20. Kurer FL, Walsh DB: Gynecological laparoscopy: clinical experiences of two anaesthetic techniques. Br J Anaesth 56:1207, 1984
21. Haworth EA, Balarajan R: Day surgery—does it add to or replace inpatient surgery? Br Med J 294:133, 1987
22. Natof HE: Pre-existing medical problems—ambulatory surgery. IMJ 166:101, 1984
23. Meridy HW: Criteria for selection of ambulatory surgical patients and guidelines for anesthetic management—a retrospective study of 1553 cases. Anesth Analg 61:921, 1982
24. Kortilla K, Saarnivaara L, Tarkkanen J, et al: Effect of age on amnesia and sedation induced by flunitrazapam during local anesthesia for bronchoscopy. Br J Anaesth 50:1211, 1978
25. Sear JW, Cooper GM, Kumar V: The effect of age on recovery. A comparison of the kinetics of thiopentone and althesin. Anaesthesia 38:1158, 1983
26. Chung F, Lavelle PA, McDonald S, et al: MMS—a screening test for elderly outpatients. Anesthesiology 69:A900, 1988
27. Steward DJ: Preterm infants are more prone to complication following minor surgery than term infants. Anesthesiology 56:304, 1982
28. Liu LM, Cote CJ, Goudsouzian NG, et al: Life-threatening apnea in infants recover-

ing from anesthesia. Anesthesiology 59:506, 1983
29. Kurth CD, Spitzer AR, Broennle MD, et al: Postoperative apnea in former premature infants. Anesthesiology 63:A475, 1985
30. Welborn LG, Ramirez N, Oh TM, et al: Postanesthetic apnea and periodic breathing in infants. Anesthesiology 65:658, 1986
31. Welborn LG, Hannallah RS, Fink R, et al: High-dose caffeine suppresses postoperative apnea in former preterm infants. Anesthesiology 71:347, 1989
32. Welborn LG, McGill WA, Hannallah RS, et al: Perioperative blood glucose concentrations in pediatric outpatients. Anesthesiology 66:543, 1986
33. Tetzlaff JE, Annand DW, Pudimat MA, et al: Postoperative apnea in a full-term infant. Anesthesiology 69:426, 1988
34. Tait AR, Knight PR: The effects of general anesthesia on upper respiratory tract infections in children. Anesthesiology 67:930, 1987
35. Chripko D, Bevan JC, et al: Decreases in arterial oxygen saturation in paediatric outpatients during transfer to the postanaesthetic recovery room. Can J Anaesth 36:128, 1989
36. Egbert LD, Battit GE, Turndorf H, et al: The value of the preoperative visit by the anesthetist. JAMA 185:553, 1963
37. Leigh JM, Walker J, Janaganathan P: Effect of preoperative anaesthetic visit on anxiety. Br Med J 2:987, 1977
38. Arellano R, Cruise C, Chung F: Timing of the anesthetist's preoperative outpatient interview. Anesth Analg 68:645, 1989
39. Wilson ME, Williams NB, Baskett PJF, et al: Assessment of fitness for surgical procedures and the variability of anaesthetists' judgments. Br Med J 1:509, 1980
40. Tompkins BM, Tompkins WJ, Loder E, Noonan AC: A computer-assisted preanesthesia interview: value of a computer-generated summary of patient's historical information in the preanesthesia visit. Anesth Analg 59, 1980
41. Apfelbaum J, Roizen MF, Stocking C, et al: Initial clinical trials of computerized "Healthquiz" to suggest preoperative laboratory tests. Anesthesiology 69:A717, 1988
42. Roizen MF, Kaplan EB, Sheiner LB, et al: Elimination of unnecessary laboratory tests by preoperative questionnaire. Anesthesiology 61:A455, 1984
43. Kaplan EB, Sheiner LB, Boeckmann AJ, et al: The usefulness of preoperative laboratory screening. JAMA 253:3576, 1985
44. Ogg TW: An assessment of postoperative outpatient cases. Br Med J 4:573, 1972
45. Malins AF: Do they do as they are instructed? A review of outpatient anaesthesia. Anaesthesia 33:832, 1978
46. Lemarbre L, Hudon G, Coche G, Bourassa MG: Outpatient peripheral angioplasty: survey of complications and patients' perceptions. AJR 148:1239, 1987
47. Redman HC: Has the time come for outpatient peripheral angioplasty? AJR 148:1241, 1987
48. Kitz DS, Conahan TJ, Young ML, Lecky JH: Differences among short procedures—selecting patient populations for clinical research in ambulatory surgery. Anesthesiology 69:A901, 1988
49. Fahy A, Marshall M: Postanaesthetic morbidity in outpatients. Br J Anaesth 41:433, 1969
50. Natof HE: Complications associated with ambulatory surgery. JAMA 244:1116, 1980
51. Patel RI, Hannallah RS: Anesthetic complications following pediatric ambulatory surgery: 3 year study. Anesthesiology 69:1009, 1988
52. Brindle GF, Soliman MG: Anaesthetic complications in surgical outpatients. Can Anaesth Soc J 22:613, 1975
53. Collins KM, Docherty PW, Plantevin OM, et al: Postoperative morbidity following gynaecological outpatient laparoscopy. A reappraisal of the service. Anaesthesia 39:819, 1984
54. Dawson B, Reed WA: Anaesthesia for adult surgical outpatients. Can Anaesth Soc J 27:409, 1980
55. White PF, Coe V, Dworsky WA, et al: Disseminated intravascular coagulation following mid-trimester abortions. Anesthesiology 58:99, 1983
56. Ogg TW: Use of anesthesia—implications of day-case surgery and anaesthesia. Br Med J 281:212, 1980
57. Clark AJM, Hurtig JB: Premedication with

meperidine and atropine does not prolong recovery to street fitness after outpatient surgery. Can Anaesth Soc J 28:390, 1981
58. Jakobsen H, Hertz JB, Johansen JR, et al: Premedication before day surgery—a double-blind comparison of diazepam and placebo. Br J Anaesth 57:300, 1985
59. Rita L, Seleny FL, Goodarzi M: Intramuscular midazolam for pediatric preanesthetic sedation—a double-blind controlled study with morphine. Anesthesiology 63:528, 1985
60. Taylor MB, Vine PR, Hatch DJ: Intramuscular midazolam premedication in small children. Anaesthesia 41:21, 1986
61. Raeder JC, Breivik H: Premedication with midazolam in outpatient general anaesthesia—a comparison with morphine, scopolamine and placebo. Acta Anaesthesiol Scand 31:509, 1987
62. Shafer A, White PF, Urquhart ML, Doze VA: Outpatient premedication: use of midazolam and opioid analgesics. Anesthesiology 71:495, 1989
63. White PF: The role of midazolam in outpatient anesthesia. Anesth Rev 12:55, 1985
64. Lichtor JL, Korttila K, Lane BS, et al: The effect of preoperative anxiety and premedication with midazolam on recovery from ambulatory surgery. Anesth Analg 68:S163, 1989
65. Nightingale JJ, Norman J: A comparison of midazolam and temazepam for premedication of day case patients. Anaesthesia 43:111, 1988
66. Feld LH, Negus JB, White PF: Oral midazolam: optimal dose for pediatric premedication. Anesthesiology 71:A1053, 1989
67. Beechey APG, Eltringham RJ, Studd C: Temazepam as premedication in day surgery. Anaesthesia 36:10, 1981
68. Hargreaves J: Benzodiazepine premedication in minor day-case surgery—comparison of oral midazolam and temazepam with placebo. Br J Anaesth 61:611, 1988
69. Pinnock CA, Fell D, Hunt PCW, et al: A comparison of triazolam and diazepam as premedication agents for minor gynecological surgery. Anaesthesia 40:324, 1985
70. Forrest P, Galletly DC, Yee P: Placebo controlled comparison of midazolam, triazolam and diazepam as oral premedicants for outpatient anaesthesia. Anaesth Intensive Care 15:296, 1987
71. Wilton NCT, Leigh J, Rosen D, et al: Intranasal midazolam premedication in preschool children. Anesth Analg 67:S260, 1988
72. Saint-Maurice C, Meistelman C, Rey E, et al: The pharmacokinetics of rectal midazolam for premedication in children. Anesthesiology 65:536, 1986
73. Korttila K, Linnoila M: Psychomotor skills related to driving after intramuscular administration of diazepam and meperidine. Anesthesiology 42:685, 1975
74. White PF, Chang T: Effect of narcotic premedication on the intravenous anesthetic requirement. Anesthesiology 61:A389, 1984
75. Doze VA, Shafer A, White PF: Nausea and vomiting after outpatient anesthesia—effectiveness of droperidol alone and in combination with metoclopramide. Anesth Analg 66:S41, 1987
76. Manchikanti L, Canella MG, Hohlbein LF, et al: Assessment of effect of various modes of premedication on acid aspiration risk factors in outpatient surgery. Anesth Analg 66:81, 1987
77. Wilton NCT, Burn JMB: Delayed vomiting after paravaretum in paediatric outpatient surgery. Can Anaesth Soc J 33:741, 1986
78. Chestnutt WN, Clarke RSJ, Dundee JW: Comparison of nalbuphine, pethidine and placebo as premedication for minor gynaecological surgery. Br J Anaesth 59:576, 1987
79. Epstein BS, Levy M-L, Thein MH, et al: Evaluation of fentanyl as an adjunct to thiopental-nitrous oxide-oxygen anesthesia for short surgical procedures. Anesth Rev 2:24, 1975
80. Horrigan RW, Moyers JR, Johnson BH, et al: Etomidate vs. thiopental with and without fentanyl—a comparative study of awakening in man. Anesthesiology 52:362, 1980
81. Craig J, Cooper GM, Sear JR: Recovery from day-care anaesthesia. Br J Anaesth 54:447, 1982
82. White PF, Sung ML, Doze VA: Use of sufentanil in outpatient anesthesia—determining an optimal preinduction dose. Anesthesiology 63:A202, 1985

83. Pandit SK, Kothary SP: Should we premedicate ambulatory surgical patients? Anesthesiology 65:A352, 1986
84. Nelson PS, Streisand JB, Mulder S, et al: Premedication in children: a comparison of oral transmucosal fentanyl citrate (fentanyl lollipop) and an oral solution of meperidine, diazepam and atropine. Anesthesiology A490, 1989
85. Feld LB, Champeau MW, van Steennis CA, et al: Preanesthetic medication in children: a comparison of oral transmucosal fentanyl citrate *versus* placebo. Anesthesiology 71:374, 1989
86. Brzustowicz RM, Nelson DA, Betts EK, et al: Efficacy of oral premedication for pediatric outpatient surgery. Anesthesiology 60:475, 1984
87. Abramowitz MD, Oh TH, Epstein BS, et al: The antiemetic effect of droperidol following outpatient strabismus surgery in children. Anesthesiology 59:579, 1983
88. Metter SE, Kitz DS: Nausea and vomiting after outpatient laparoscopy: incidence, impact on recovery room stay and cost. Anesth Analg 66:S116, 1987
89. White PF, Shafer A: Nausea and vomiting—causes and prophylaxis. Semin Anesth 6:300, 1987
90. Dundee JW, Chestnutt WN, Ghaly RG, et al: Traditional Chinese acupuncture—a potentially useful antiemetic? Br Med J 293:583, 1986
91. Ghaly RG, Fitzpatrick KT, Dundee JW: Antiemetic studies with traditional Chinese acupuncture—a comparison of manual needling with electrical stimulation and commonly used antiemetics. Anaesthesia 42:1108, 1987
92. Fry ENS: Acupressure and postoperative vomiting. Anaesthesia 41:661, 1986
93. Rita, I, Goodarzi M, Selany F: Effect of low-dose droperidol on postoperative vomiting in children. Can Anaesth Soc J 28:259, 1981
94. O'Donovan N, Shaw J: Nausea and vomiting in day-case dental anesthesia—the use of low-dose droperidol. Anaesthesia 39:1172, 1984
95. Lerman J, Eustis S, Smith DR: Effect of droperidol pretreatment on postanesthetic vomiting in children undergoing strabismus surgery. Anesthesiology 65:322, 1986
96. Eustis S, Lerman J, Smith D: Droperidol pretreatment in children undergoing strabismus repair—the minimal effective dose. Can Anaesth Soc J 33:116, 1986
97. Nicolson SC, Kay KM, Betts EK: The effect of preoperative oral droperidol on the incidence of postoperative emesis after paediatric strabismus surgery. Can J Anaesth 35:364, 1988
98. Valanne J, Korttila K: Effect of a small dose of droperidol on nausea, vomiting and recovery after outpatient enflurane anesthesia. Acta Anaesthesiol Scand 29:359, 1985
99. Millar JM, Hall PJ: Nausea and vomiting after prostaglandins in day case termination of pregnancy—the efficacy of low-dose droperidol. Anaesthesia 42:613, 1987
100. Korttila K, Kauste A, Auvinen J: Comparison of domperidone, droperidol, and metoclopramide in the prevention and treatment of nausea and vomiting after balanced general anesthesia. Anesth Analg 58:396, 1979
101. Madej TH, Simpson KH: Comparison of the use of domperidone, droperidol and metoclopramide in the prevention of nausea and vomiting following gynaecological surgery in day cases. Br J Anaesth 58:879, 1986
102. Cohen SE, Woods WA, Wyner J: Antiemetic efficacy of droperidol and metoclopramide. Anesthesiology 60:67, 1984
103. Hardley AJ: Metoclopramide in the prevention of postoperative nausea and vomiting. Br J Clin Pract 21:460, 1967
104. Clark MM, Storrs JA: The prevention of post-operative vomiting after abortion—metoclopramide. Br J Anaesth 41:890, 1969
105. Lind B, Breivik H: Metoclopramide and perphenazine in the prevention of postoperative nausea and vomiting: a double blind comparison. Br J Anesth 42:614, 1970
106. Diamond MJ, Keeri-Szanto M: Reduction of postoperative vomiting by preoperative administration of oral metoclopramide. Can Anaesth Soc J 27:36, 1980
107. Spelina KR, Gerger HR, Pagels IL: Nausea and vomiting during spinal anaesthesia. Effect of metoclopramide and domperidone: a double-blind trial. Anaesthesia 39:132, 1984

108. Pandit SK, Kothary SP, Pandit VA, et al: Premedication with cimetidine and metoclopramide. Anaesthesia 41:486, 1986
109. Broadman LM, Cerruzi W, Patane PS, et al: Metoclopramide reduces the incidences of vomiting following strabismus surgery in children. Anesthesiology 69:A747, 1988
110. Wyner J, Cohen SE: Gastric volume in early pregnancy—effect of metoclopramide. Anesthesiology 57:209, 1983
111. Palazzo MGA, Strunin L: Anaesthesia and emesis II—prevention and management. Can Anaesth Soc J 31:407, 1984
112. Bailey PL, Bubbers SJM, East KA, et al: Transdermal scopolamine reduces postoperative nausea and vomiting. Anesthesiology 69:A641, 1988
113. Gibbons PA, Nicolson SC, Betts EK, et al: Scopolamine does not prevent postoperative emesis after pediatric eye surgery. Anesthesiology 61:A435, 1984
114. Uppington J, Dunnet J, Biogg CE: Transdermal hyoscine and postoperative nausea and vomiting. Anaesthesia 42:16, 1986
115. Tigerstedt I, Salmela L, Aromaa U: Double-blind comparison of transdermal scopolamine, droperidol and placebo against postoperative nausea and vomiting. Acta Anaesthesiol Scand 32:454, 1988
116. MacKenzie R, Wadhwa RK, Uly NTL, et al: Antiemetic effectiveness of intramuscular hydroxyzine compared with intramuscular droperidol. Anesth Analg 60:783, 1981
117. Warner LO, Rogers GL, Martino JD, et al: Intravenous lidocaine reduces the incidence of vomiting in children after surgery to correct strabismus. Anesthesiology 68:618, 1988
118. Ong BY, Palahniuk RJ, Cumming M: Gastric volume and pH in outpatients. Can Anaesth Soc J 25:36, 1978
119. Manchikanti L, Roush JR: Effect of preanesthetic glycopyrrolate and cimetidine on gastric fluid pH and volume in outpatients. Anesth Analg 63:40, 1984
120. Manchikanti L, Roush JR: Effect of preanesthetic ranitidine and metoclopramide on gastric contents in morbidly obese patients. Anesth Analg 65:195, 1986
121. Sutherland AD, Stock JG, Davies JM: Effects of preoperative fasting on morbidity and gastric contents in patients undergoing day-stay surgery. Br J Anaesth 58:876, 1986
122. Maltby JR, Sutherland AD, Sale JP, et al: Preoperative oral fluids—is a five-hour fast justified prior to elective surgery? Anesth Analg 65:1112, 1986
123. Manchikanti L, Colliver JA, Roush JR, et al: Evaluation of ranitidine as an oral antacid in outpatient anesthesia. South Med J 78:818, 1985
124. Maltby JR, Reid CRG, Hutchinson A: Gastric fluid volume and pH in elective patients. Part II: coffee or orange juice with ranitidine. Can J Anaesth 35:16, 1988
125. Manchikanti L, Grow JB, Colliver JA, et al: Bicitra[R] (sodium citrate) and metoclopramide in outpatient anesthesia for prophylaxis against aspiration pneumonitis. Anesthesiology 63:378, 1985
126. Stock JG, Sutherland AD: The role of H_2 receptor antagonist premedication in pregnant day care patients. Can Anaesth Soc J 32:463, 1985
127. Olsson GL, Hallen B, Hambraeus-Jonzon K: Aspiration during anaesthesia: a computer-aided study of 185,358 anaesthetics. Acta Anaesthesiol Scand 30:84, 1986
128. Morison DH, Dunn GL, Fargas-Babjak AM, et al: A double-blind comparison of cimetidine and ranitidine as prophylaxis against gastric aspiration syndrome. Anesth Analg 61:988, 1982
129. Zeldis JE, Friedman LS, Isselbacher KJ: Ranitidine—a new H_2 receptor antagonist. N Engl J Med 309:1368, 1983
130. Coombs DW: Aspiration pneumonis prophylaxis. Anesth Analg 62:1055, 1983
131. Miller M, Wishart HY, Nimmo WS: Gastric contents at induction of anesthesia—is a 4-hour fast necessary? Br J Anaesth 55:1185, 1983
132. Sutherland AD, Stock JG, Davies JM: Effects of preoperative fasting on morbidity and gastric contents in patients undergoing day-stay surgery. Br J Anaesth 58:876, 1986
133. Doze VA, White PF: Effects of fluid therapy on serum glucose levels in fasted outpatients. Anesthesiology 66:223, 1987
134. Hutchinson A, Maltby JR, Reid CRG: Gastric fluid volume and pH in elective inpa-

tients. Part I: coffee or orange juice *versus* overnight fast. Can J Anaesth 35:12, 1988
135. Splinter WM, Stewart JA, Muir JG: The effect of preoperative apple juice on gastric contents, thirst, and hunger in children. Can J Anaesth 36:55, 1989
136. Sandhar BK, Goresky GV, Maltby JR, et al: Effect of oral liquids and ranitidine on gastric fluid volume and pH in children undergoing outpatient surgery. Anesthesiology 71:327, 1989
137. Meakin G, Dingwall AE, Addison GM: Effect of fasting and oral premedication on the pH and volume of gastric aspirate in children. Br J Anaesth 59:678, 1987
138. Rao TIK, Madhavareddy S, Chinthagada M, et al: Metoclopramide and cimetidine to reduce gastric pH and volume. Anesth Analg 63:1014, 1984
139. Foulkes E, Jenkins LC: A comparitive evaluation of cimetidine and sodium citrate to decrease gastric acidity: effectiveness at the time of induction of anaesthesia. Can Anaesth Soc J 28:29, 1981
140. Hey VMF, Ostick DG, Mazumder JK, et al: Pethidine, metoclopramide and the gastro-oesophageal sphincter. Anaesthesia 36:173, 1981
141. White PF: Anaesthesia for day-case surgery—overview. Curr Opin Anaesth 1:45, 1988
142. Kenefick JP, Leader JR, et al: Laparoscopy: blood-gas values and minor sequelae associated with three techniques based on isoflurane. Br J Anaesth 59:189, 1987
143. Erikksson E, Haggmark T, Saartok T, et al: Knee arthroscopy with local anesthesia in ambulatory patients: methods, results and patient compliance. Orthopedics 9:186, 1986
144. Blitt CD: Monitoring during outpatient anesthesia. Int Anesthesiol Clin 20:17, 1982
145. Raemer DB, Warren BS, Morris R, et al: Hypoxemia during ambulatory gynecologic surgery as evaluated by the pulse oximeter. J Clin Monit 3:244, 1987
146. Stafford M, Jeon A, Pascucci R: Pre- and post-induction blood glucose concentrations in healthy fasting children. Anesthesiology 63:A350, 1985
147. Thomas DKM: Hypoglycaemia in children before operation: its incidence and prevention. Br J Anaesth 46:66, 1974
148. Jensen BH, Wernberg M, Adersen M: Preoperative starvation and blood glucose concentrations in children undergoing inpatient and outpatient anesthesia. Br J Anaesth 54:1071, 1982
149. Conahan TJ III, Williams GD, Apfelbaum J, et al: Airway heating reduces recovery time (cost) in outpatients. Anesthesiology 67:128, 1987
150. Cooper GM: Recovery from anaesthesia. Clin Anaesth 2:145, 1984
151. White PF: Continuous infusions of thiopental, methohexital or etomidate as adjuvants to nitrous oxide for outpatient anesthesia. Anesth Analg 63:282, 1984
152. Hannington-Kiff JG: Measurement of recovery from outpatient general anaesthesia with simple ocular test. Br Med J 3:132, 1970
153. Whitwam JG, Manners JM: Clinical comparison of thiopentone and methohexitone. Br Med J I:1663, 1962
154. Korttila K, Linnoila M: Recovery and simulated driving after intravenous anesthesia with thiopental, methohexital, propranidid, or alphadione. Anesthesiology 43:291, 1975
155. Miller BM, Hendry JGB, Less NW: Etomidate and methohexitone—a comparative clinical study in outpatient anaesthesia. Anaesthesia 33:450, 1978
156. Boralessa H, Holdcroft H: Methohexitone or etomidate for induction of dental anesthesia. Can Anaesth Soc J 27:578, 1980
157. Wagner RL, White PF: Etomidate inhibits adrenocortical function in surgical patients. Anesthesiology 61:647, 1984
158. Figallo EM, McKenzie R, Tantistra B: Anaesthesia for dilation, evacuation, and curettage in outpatients. Can Anaesth Soc J 24:110, 1977
159. White PF, Dworsky WA, Horai Y, et al: Comparison of continuous infusion fentanyl or ketamine *versus* thiopental—determining the mean effective serum concentration for outpatient surgery. Anesthesiology 59:564, 1983
160. White PF: Ketamine update—its clinical uses in anesthesia. Sem Anesth 7:113, 1988
161. Crawford ME, Carl RS, Andersen RS, et al: Comparison between midazolam and thiopentone-based balanced anaesthesia

for day-case surgery. Br J Anaesth 56:165, 1984
162. Berggren L, Eriksson I: Midazolam for induction of anaesthesia in outpatients a comparison with thiopentone. Acta Anaesthesiol Scand 25:492, 1981
163. Verma R, Ramasubramanian R, Sachar RM: Anesthesia for termination of pregnancy: midazolam compared with methohexital. Anesth Angl 63:792, 1985
164. Zuurmond WWA, van Leeuwen L, Helmers JHJH: Recovery from fixed-dose midazolam-induced anaesthesia and antagonism with flumazenil for outpatient arthroscopy. Acta Anaesthesiol Scand 33:160, 1989
165. Forrest P, Galletly DC: Comparison of propofol and antagonized midazolam anaesthesia for day-case surgery. Anaesth Intensive Care 15:394, 1987
166. MacKenzie N, Grant IS: Comparison of the new emulsion formulation of propofol with methohexitone and thiopentone for induction of anaesthesia in day cases. Br J Anaesth 57:725, 1985
167. O'Toole DP, Milligan KR, Howe JP, et al: A comparison of propofol and methohexitone as induction agents for day case isoflurane anaesthesia. Anesthesia 42:373, 1987
168. Johnston R, Noseworthy T, Anderson B, et al: Propofol versus thiopental for outpatient anesthesia. Anesthesiology 67:431, 1987
169. Henricksson BA, Carlsson P, Hallen B, et al: Propofol *versus* thiopentone as anaesthetic agents for short operative procedures. Acta Anaesth Scand 3:62, 1987
170. Raeder JC, Misvaer G: Comparison of propofol induction with thiopentone or methohexitone in short outpatient general anesthesia. Acta Anaesthesiol Scand 32:607, 1988
171. Heath PJ, Kennedy DJ, Ogg TW, et al: Which intravenous induction agent for day surgery? Anaesthesia 43:365, 1988
172. Valanne J, Korttila K: Comparison of methohexitone and propofol for induction of enflurane anaesthesia in outpatients. Postgrad Med 61:138, 1985
173. Sanders LD, Isaac PA, Yeomans WA, et al: Propofol-induced anaesthesia. Anaesthesia 44:200, 1989
174. Doze VA, Westphal LM, White PF: Comparison of propofol with methohexital for outpatient anesthesia. Anesth Analg 65:1189, 1986
175. Millar JM, Jewkes CF: Recovery and morbidity after daycase and morbidity after daycase anaesthesia. A comparison of propofol with thiopentone—enflurane with and without alfentanil. Anaesthesia 43:738, 1988
176. Doze VA, Shafer A, White PF: Propofol *versus* thiopental-isoflurane for general anesthesia. Anesthesiology 69:63, 1988
177. Kay B, Hargreaves J, Sivalingam T, Healy TEJ: Intravenous anaesthesia for cystoscopy—a comparison of propofol or methohexitone with alfentanil. Eur J Anaesthesiol 3:111, 1986
178. DeGrood PMRM, Harbers BM, van Egmond J, et al: Anaesthesia for laparoscopy. Anaesthesia 42:815, 1987
179. Milligan KR, O'Toole DP, Howe JP, et al: Recovery from outpatient anaesthesia: a comparison of incremental propofol and propofol-isoflurane. Br J Anaesth 59:1111, 1987
180. Marais ML, Maher MW, Wetchler BV, et al: Reduced demands on recovery room resources with propofol (Diprivan™) compared to thiopental-isoflurane. Anesth Rev 16:29, 1989
181. Weightman WM, Zacharias M: Comparison of propofol and thiopentone anaesthesia (with special reference to recovery characteristics). Anaesth Intensive Care 15:389, 1987
182. Sigurdsson GH, Lindahl S: Cardiac arrhythmias in intubated children during adenoidectomy. A comparison between enflurane and halothane anaesthesia. Acta Anaesthesiol Scand 27:484, 1983
183. Willatts DG, Harrison AR, Groom JF, et al: Cardiac arrhythmias during outpatient dental anaesthesia: comparison of halothane with enflurane. Br J Anaesth 55:399, 1983
184. Fisher DM, Robinson S, Brett CM, et al: Comparison of enflurane, halothane, and isoflurane for diagnostic and therapeutic procedures in children with malignancies. Anesthesiology 63:647, 1985
185. Pandit UA, Steude GM, Leach AB: Induction and recovery characteristics of iso-

flurane and halothane anaesthesia for short outpatient operations in children. Anaesthesia 40:1226, 1985
186. Cattermole RW, Verghese C, Blair IJ, et al: Isoflurane and halothane for outpatient dental anaesthesia in children. Br J Anaesth 58:385, 1986
187. Kingston HGG: Halothane and isoflurane anesthesia in pediatric outpatients. Anesth Analg 65:181, 1986
188. Wilton NCT, Thomas VL: Single breath induction of anesthesia, using a vital capacity breath of halothane, nitrous oxide and oxygen. Anaesthesia 41:472, 1986
189. Goresky GV, Steward DJ: Rectal methohexitone for induction of anaesthesia in children. Can Anaesth Soc J 26:213, 1979
190. Linton DM, Thornington RE: Etomidate as a rectal induction agent. S Af Med J 64:309, 1983
191. Saint-Maurice C, Laquenie G, Couturier C, et al: Rectal ketamine in paediatric anaesthesia. Br J Anaesth 51:573, 1979
192. Carrel R: Ketamine—a general anesthetic for unmanageable ambulatory patients. J Dent Child 40:288, 1973
193. Hannallah RS, Patel RI: Low-dose intramuscular ketamine for anesthesia pre-induction in young children undergoing brief outpatient procedures. Anesthesiology 70:598, 1989
194. Meyers EF, Charles P: Prolonged adverse reactions to ketamine in children. Anesthesiology 49:39, 1978
195. Hannallah RS, Rosales JK: Experience with parents' presence during anaesthesia induction in children. Can Anaesth Soc J 30:286, 1983
196. Manner T, Kanto J, Iisalo E, et al: Reduction of pain at venous cannulation in children with a eutectic mixture of lidocaine and prilocaine (EMLA® cream)—comparison with placebo cream and no local premedication. Acta Anaesthesiol Scand 31:735, 1987
197. Alexander GD, Skupski JN, Brown EM: The role of nitrous oxide in postoperative nausea and vomiting. Anesth Analg 63:175, 1984
198. Lonie DS, Harper NJN: Nitrous oxide anaesthesia and vomiting—the effect of nitrous oxide anaesthesia on the incidence of vomiting following gynaecological laparoscopy. Anaesthesia 41:703, 1986
199. Melnick BM, Johnson LS: Effects of eliminating nitrous oxide in outpatient anesthesia. Anesthesiology 67:982, 1987
200. Muir JJ, Warner MA, Buck CF, et al: The role of nitrous oxide in producing postoperative nausea and vomiting. Anesthesiology 65:A461, 1986
201. Korttila K, Hovorka J, Erkola O: Omission of nitrous oxide does not decrease the incidence or severity of emetic symptoms after isoflurane anesthesia. Anesth Analg 66:S98, 1987
202. Gibbons P, Davidson, P, Adler E: Nitrous oxide does not affect post-op vomiting in pediatric eye surgery. Anesthesiology 67:A530, 1987
203. Sengupta P, Plantevin OM: Nitrous oxide and day-case laparoscopy: effects on nausea, vomiting and return to normal activity. Br J Anaesth 60:570, 1988
204. Davidson SH: A comparitive study of halothane and enflurane in pediatric anesthesia. Acta Anaesthesiol Scand 22:58, 1978
205. Tracey JA, Holland AJC, Unger L: Morbidity in minor gynaecological surgery—a comparison of halothane, enflurane, and isoflurane. Br J Anaesth 54:121, 1982
206. Carter JA, Dye AM, Cooper GM: Recovery from day-case anaesthesia—the effect of different inhalational anaesthetic agents. Anaesthesia 40:545, 1985
207. Stanford BJ, Plantevin OM, Gilbert JR: Morbidity after day care gynaecological surgery: comparison of enflurane with halothane. Br J Anaesth 51:1143, 1979
208. Azar J, Karambelkar DJ, Lear E: Neurologic state and psychomotor function following anesthesia for ambulatory surgery. Anesthesiology 60:349, 1984
209. Valanne JV, Korttila K: Recovery following general anesthesia with isoflurane or enflurane for outpatient dentistry and oral surgery. Anesth Prog 35:48, 1988
210. Fahy LT: Delayed convulsions after day case anaesthesia with enflurane. Anaesthesia 42:1327, 1987
211. Yasuda N, Targ AG, Eger EI II: Solubility of I-653, sevoflurane, isoflurane, and halothane in human tissues. Anesthesiology 69:A615, 1988

212. Koblin DD, Weiskopf RB, Holmes MA, et al: Metabolism of I-653 and isoflurane in swine. Anesth Analg 68:147, 1989
213. Eger EI II, Johnson BH: Rates of awakening from anesthesia with I-653, halothane, isoflurane, and sevoflurane: a test of the effect of anesthetic concentration and duration in rats. Anesth Analg 66:977, 1987
214. Kestin IG, Dorje P: Anaesthesia for evacuation of retained products of conception. Br J Anaesth 59:364, 1987
215. White PF: Use of continuous infusion *versus* intermittent bolus administration of fentanyl or ketamine during outpatient anesthesia. Anesthesiology 59:294, 1983
216. Ogg TW, Fischer HBJ, Bethune DW, et al: Day care anaesthesia and memory. Anaesthesia 34:784, 1979
217. Cooper GM, O'Connor M, Mark J, Harvey J: Effect of alfentanil and fentanyl on recovery from brief anaesthesia. Br J Anaesth 55:179S, 1983
218. Goroszeniuk T, Whitwam JG, Morgan M: Use of methohexitone, fentanyl and nitrous oxide for short surgical procedures. Anaesthesia 32:209, 1977
219. Collin RIW, Drummond GB, Spence AA: Alfentanil supplemented anaesthesia for short procedures. Anaesthesia 41:477, 1986
220. Phitayakorn P, Melnick BM, Vicinie AF: Comparison of continuous sufentanil and fentanyl infusions for outpatient anaesthesia. Can J Anaesth 34:242, 1987
221. Martin DE, Rosenberg H, Aukburg SJ, et al: Low-dose fentanyl blunts circulatory responses to tracheal intubation. Anesth Analg 61:680, 1982
222. Cork RC, Weiss J, Hameroff SR, Bentley J: Pre-treatment with low-dose fentanyl for rapid sequence intubation. Anesthesiology 59:A344, 1983
223. Sanders RS, Sinclair ME, Sear JW: Alfentanil in short procedures. Anaesthesia 39:1202, 1984
224. Kennedy DJ, Ogg TW: Alfentanil and memory function—a comparison with fentanyl for day case termination of pregnancy. Anaesthesia 40:537, 1985
225. Kay B, Venkataraman P: Recovery after fentanyl and alfentanil in anaesthesia for minor surgery. Br J Anaesth 55:169S, 1983
226. Kallar SK, Keenan RL: Evaluation and comparison of recovery time from alfentanil and fentanyl for short surgical procedures. Anesthesiology 61:A379, 1984
227. Raeder JC, Hole A: Out-patient laparoscopy in general anaesthesia with alfentanil and atracurium—a comparison with fentanyl and pancuronium. Acta Anaesthesiol Scand 30:30, 1986
228. White PF, Coe V, Shafer A, et al: Comparison of alfentanil with fentanyl for outpatient anesthesia. Anesthesiology 64:99, 1986
229. Dachowski MT, Kalayjian R, Angelilo JC, Dolan EA: Continuous infusion of methohexital and alfentanil hydrochloride for general anesthesia in outpatient third molar surgery. J Oral Maxillofac Surg 47:233, 1989
230. Pollard J: Clinical evaluation of intravenous *vs* inhalational anesthesia in the ambulatory surgical unit: a multicenter study. Curr Ther Res 36:617, 1984
231. Melnick BM, Chalasani J, Uy NTL: Comparison of enflurane, isoflurane, and continuous fentanyl infusion for outpatient anesthesia. Anesth Rev 11:36, 1984
232. Jellicoe JA: A comparison of alfentanil, halothane and enflurane for day-case gynaecological surgery. Anaesthesia 40:810, 1985
233. Collins KM, Plantevin OM, Whitburn RH, Doyle JP: Outpatient termination of pregnancy—halothane or alfentanil-supplemented anaesthesia. Br J Anaesth 57:1226, 1985
234. Zuurmond WWA, van Leeuwen L: Alfentanil *vs* isoflurane for outpatient arthroscopy. Acta Anaesthesiol Scand 30:329, 1986
235. Zuurmond WWA, van Leeuwen L: Recovery from sufentanil anaesthesia for outpatient arthroscopy—a comparison with isoflurane. Acta Anaesthesiol Scand 31:154, 1987
236. Wasudev G, Kambam JR, Hazlehurst WM, et al: Comparative study of sufentanil and isoflurane in outpatient surgery. Anesth Analg 66:S186, 1987
237. Simpson JEP, Glynn CJ, Cox AG, et al: Comparative study of short-term recovery of mental efficiency after anaesthesia. Br Med J I:1560, 1976
238. Rising S, Dodgson MS, Steen PA: Isoflu-

rane *v* fentanyl for outpatient laparoscopy. Acta Anaesthesiol Scand 29:251, 1985
239. Moss E, Hindmarch I, Pain AJ, Edmondson RS: A comparison of recovery after halothane or alfentanil in anaesthesia for minor surgery. Br J Anaesth 59:970, 1987
240. Gaskey NJ, Ferriero L, Pournaras L, Seecof J: Use of fentanyl markedly increases nausea and vomiting in gynecological short stay patients. AANA 54:309, 1986
241. Garfield JM, Garfield FB, Philip B, et al: A comparison of clinical and psychologic effects of fentanyl and nalbuphine in ambulatory surgical patients. Anesth Analg 66:1303, 1987
242. Bone ME, Dowson S, Smith G: A comparison of nalbuphine with fentanyl for postoperative pain relief following termination of pregnancy under day care anaesthesia. Anaesthesia 43:194, 1988
243. Pandit SK, Kothary SP, Pandit UA, et al: Comparison of fentanyl and butaphanol for outpatient anaesthesia. Can J Anaesth 34:130, 1987
244. Heneghan C, McAuliffe R, Thomas D, et al: Morbidity after outpatient anaesthesia. Anaesthesia 36:4, 1981
245. Dhamee MS, Gandhi SK, Callen KM, et al: Morbidity after outpatient anesthesia—a comparison of different endotracheal anesthetic techniques for laparoscopy. Anesthesiology 57:A375, 1982
246. Herbert M, Healy TEJ, Bourke JB, et al: Profile of recovery after general anaesthesia. Br Med J 286:1539, 1983
247. Brindle GF, Soliman MG: Anaesthetic complications in surgical outpatients. Can Anaesth Soc J 22:613, 1975
248. Urbach GM, Edelist G: An evaluation of the anaesthetic techniques used in an outpatient unit. Can Anaesth Soc J 24:401, 1977
249. Fragen RJ, Shanks CA: Neuromuscular recovery after laparoscopy. Anesth Analg 63:51, 1984
250. Pearce AC, Williams JP, Jones RM: Atracurium for short surgical procedures in day patients. Br J Anaesth 56:973, 1984
251. Sengupta P, Skacel M, Plantevin OM: Post-operative morbidity associated with the use of atracurium and vecuronium in day-case laparoscopy. Eur J Anaesthesiol 4:93, 1987
252. Bailey DM, Nicholas DG: Comparison of atracurium and vecuronium during anaesthesia for laparoscopy. Br J Anaesth 61:557, 1988
253. Zuurmond WWA, van Leeuwen L: Atracurium versus vecuronium: a comparison of recovery in outpatient arthroscopy. Can J Anaesth 35:139, 1988
254. Skacel M, Sengupta P, Plantevin OM: Morbidity after day case laparoscopy. A comparison of two techniques of tracheal anaesthesia. Anaesthesia 41:537, 1986
255. Trepanier CA: Myalgia in outpatient surgery: comparison of atracurium and succinylcholine. Can J Anaesth 35:255, 1988
256. Zahl K, Apfelbaum JL: Muscle pain occurs after outpatient laparoscopy despite the substitution of vecuronium for succinylcholine. Anesthesiology 70:408, 1989
257. Poler SM, Luchtefeld G, White PF: Comparison of mivacurium (B10900) and succinylcholine during outpatient laparoscopy. Anesthesiology 69:A523, 1988
258. Goldberg ME, Larijani GE, Azad SS, et al: Comparison of tracheal intubating conditions and neuromuscular blocking profiles after intubating doses of mivacurium chloride or succinylcholine in surgical outpatients. Anesth Analg 69:93, 1989
259. Savarese JJ, Ali HH, Basta SJ, et al: The clinical neuromuscular pharmacology of mivacurium chloride (BW B1090U)—a short-acting nondepolarizing ester neuromuscular blocking drug. Anesthesiology 68:723, 1988
260. Cronnelly R, Morris RB: Antagonism of neuromuscular blockade. Br J Anaesth 54:183, 1982
261. King MJ, Milazkiewicz R, Carli F, Deacock AR: Influence of neostigmine on postoperative vomiting. Br J Anaesth 62:403, 1988
262. Edelist G: Prophylaxis and management of post-operative problems. Can Anaesth Soc J 30:558, 1983
263. Fishburne JI, Fulghum MS, Hulka J, et al: General anesthesia for outpatient laparoscopy with an objective measure of recovery. Anesth Analg 53:1, 1974
264. Doenicke A, Kugler J, Laub M: Evaluation of recovery and "street fitness" by EEG and psychodiagnostic tests after anesthesia. Can Anaesth Soc J 14:657, 1967

265. Steward DJ, Volgyesi G: Stabilometry—a new tool for the measurement of recovery following general anaesthesia for outpatients. Can Anaesth Soc J 25:4, 1978
266. Alexander CD, Wetchler BV, Thompson RE: Bipivacaine infiltration of the mesosalpinx in ambulatory surgical laparoscopic tubal sterilization. Can J Anaesth 34:362, 1987
267. Goldberg ME, Rehana J, Gregg C, et al: The heat and moisture exchanger does not preserve body temperature or reduce recovery time in outpatients undergoing surgery and anesthesia. Anesthesiology 68:122, 1988
268. Freeman J: The effectiveness of doxapram administration in hastening arousal following general anesthesia in outpatients. AANA J 54:16, 1986
269. Bridenbaugh LD: Regional anaesthesia for outpatient surgery. Can Anaesth Soc J 30:548, 1983
270. Mulroy MF: Regional anesthesia—when, why, why not? Outpatient Anesthesia. Probl Anesth 2:82, 1988
271. Bridenbaugh LD, Soderstrom RM: Lumbar epidural block anesthesia for outpatient laparoscopy. J Reprod Med 23:85, 1979
272. Pflug AE, Aasheim GM, Foster C: Sequence of return of neurological function and criteria for safe ambulation following subarachnoid block. Can Anaesth Soc J 25:133, 1978
273. Carbaat PAT, van Crevel H: Lumbar puncture headache: controlled study on the preventive effect of 24 hours bed rest. Lancet 22:1133, 1981
274. Flaatten H, Raeder J: Spinal anaesthesia for outpatient surgery. Anaesthesia 40:1108, 1985
275. Mulroy M, Bridenbaugh LD: Regional anesthetic techniques for outpatient surgery. p. 71. In Woo SW (ed): Ambulatory Anesthesia Care. Little, Brown, Boston, 1982
276. Flaatten H, Rodt S, Rosland J, et al: Postoperative headache in young patients after spinal anesthesia. Anaesthesia 42:202, 1987
277. Paluhniak RJ, Cumming M: Prophylactic blood patch does not prevent post-lumbar puncture headache. Can Anaesth Soc J 26:132, 1979
278. Ravindran RS: Epidural autologous blood patch on an outpatient basis. Anesth Analg 63:962, 1984
279. Cohen SE: Epidural blood patch in outpatients—a simpler approach. Anesth Analg 64:458, 1985
280. Aromaa U: Anaesthesia for short-stay varicose vein surgery. Acta Anaesthesiol Scand 21:368, 1977
281. Abdu RA: Ambulatory herniorrhaphy under local anesthesia in a community hospital. Am J Surg 145:353, 1983
282. Ryan JA, Jr., Ayde BA, Jolly PC, et al: Outpatient inguinal herniorrhaphy with both regional and local anesthesia. Am J Surg 148:313, 1984
283. Duvall JO, Griffith DP: Epidural anesthesia for extra-corporeal shock wave lithotripsy. Anesth Analg 64:544, 1985
284. Baker AB, Baker JE: Outpatient anesthesia for dilatation and curettage. Anaesth Intensive Care 7:362, 1979
285. Landeen FH, Epstein L, Haas L: Special regional anesthetic techniques in ambulatory anesthesia. p. 71 In Brown BR (ed): Outpatient Anesthesia. FA Davis, Philadelphia, 1978
286. Olney RW, Lugg PC, Turner PL, et al: Outpatient treatment of upper extremity injuries in childhood using intravenous regional anaesthesia. J Pediatr Orthop 8:576, 1988
287. Patel NJ, Flashburg MH, Paskin S, et al: A regional anesthetic technique compared to general anesthesia for outpatient knee arthroscopy. Anesth Analg 65:185, 1986
288. Sarrafian SK, Ibrahim IN, Breihan JH: Ankle-foot peripheral nerve block for mid and forefoot surgery. Foot Ankle 4:86, 1983
289. Shandling B, Steward DJ: Regional analgesia for postoperative pain. J Pediatr Surg 15:477, 1980
290. Langer JC, Shandling B, Rosenberg M: Intraoperative bupivacaine during outpatient hernia repair in children: a randomized double blind trial. J Pediatr Surg 22:267, 1987
291. Lunn JW: Postoperative analgesia after circumcision. Anaesthesia 34:552, 1979
292. May AE, Wandless J, James RH: Analgesia for circumcision in children. Acta Anaesthesiol Scand 26:331, 1982
293. Yeoman PM, Cooke R, Hain WR: Penile

block for circumcision. Anaesthesia 38:862, 1983

294. Elder PT, Belman AB, Hannallah RS, et al: Postcircumcision—a prospective evaluation of subcutaneous ring block of the penis. Reg Anaesth 9:48, 1984
295. Vater M, Wandless J: Caudal or dorsal nerve block? A comparison of two local anaesthetic techniques for postoperative analgesia following day case circumcision. Acta Anaesthesiol Scand 29:175, 1985
296. Tree-Trakarn T, Pirayavaraporn S: Postoperative pain relief for circumcision in children—comparison among morphine nerve block, and topical analgesia. Anesthesiology 62:519, 1985
297. Fell D, Derrington MC, Taylor E, Wandless JG: Paediatric postoperative analgesia. Anaesthesia 43:107, 1988
298. Reid MG, Harris R, Phillips PD, et al: Day-case herniotomy in children. A comparison of ilio-inguinal nerve block and wound infiltration for postoperative analgesia. Anaesthesia 42:658, 1987
299. Tree-Trakarn T, Pirayavaraporn S, Lertakyamanee J: Topical analgesia for relief of post-circumcision pain. Anesthesiology 67:395, 1987
300. Orandi A: Urological endoscopic surgery under local anesthesia—a cost-reducing idea. J Urol 132:1146, 1984
301. Chang FC, Farha GJ: Inguinal herniorrhaphy under local anesthesia. Arch Surg 112:1069, 1977
302. Lawler RA, Larson C, Rudy T, Biglan A: The comparative incidence of postoperative vomiting in adult and teen unilateral strabismus surgeries performed under general anesthesia or retrobulbar blockade. Anesthesiology 69:A370, 1988
303. Malhotra V, Long CW, Meister MJ: Intercostal blocks with local infiltration anesthesia for extracorporeal shock wave lithotripsy. Anesth Analg 66:85, 1987
304. Sinclair R, Cassuto J, Hogstrom S, et al: Topical anesthesia with lidocaine aerosol in the control of post-operative pain. Anesthesiology 68:895, 1988
305. Muir VMJ, Leonard M, Haddaway E: Morbidity following dental extraction. Anaesthesia 31:171, 1976
306. Vinnik CA: An intravenous dissociation technique for outpatient plastic surgery. Plast Reconstr Surg 67:799, 1981
307. McCarthy FM, Solomon AL, Jastak JT, et al: Conscious sedation: benefits and risks. J Am Dental Assoc 109:546, 1984
308. Campbell RL, Satterfield SD, Dionne RA, et al: Postanesthetic morbidity following fentanyl, diazepam, and methohexital sedation. Anesth Prog 2:45, 1980
309. Lundgren S, Rosenquist JB: Amnesia, pain experience, and patient satisfaction with intravenous diazepam. J Oral Maxillofac Surg 41:99, 1983
310. Lundgren S, Rosenquist JB: Comparison of sedation, amnesia, and patient comfort produced by intravenous and rectal diazepam. J Oral Maxillofac Surg 42:646, 1984
311. Lundgren S: Sedation as an alternative to general anesthesia. Acta Anaesthiol Scand 32:21, 1987
312. White CS, Dolwick MF, Gravenstein N, Paulus DA: Incidence of oxygen desaturation during oral surgery outpatient procedures. J Oral Maxillofac Surg 47:147, 1989
313. Shane SM: Intravenous amnesia for total dentistry in one sitting. J Oral Surg 24:27, 1966
314. McCarthy FM, Solomon AL, Jastak JT, et al: Conscious sedation: benefits and risks. J Am Dent Assoc 109:546, 1984
315. Scamman FL, Klein SL, Choi WW: Conscious sedation for procedures under local or topical anesthesia. Ann Otol Rhinol Laryngol 94:21, 1985
316. Gale GD: Recovery from methohexitone, halothane and diazepam. Br J Anaesth 48:691, 1976
317. White PF, Vasconez LO, Mathes S, et al: Comparison of midazolam and diazepam for sedation during plastic surgery. J Plast Reconstr Surg 81:703, 1988
318. Kawar P, McGimpsey JG, Gamble JAS, et al: Midazolam as a sedative in dentistry. Br J Anaesth 54:1137, 1982
319. Dixon J, Power SJ, Grundy EM: Sedation for local anaesthesia. Comparison of intravenous midazolam and diazepam. Anaesthesia 39:372, 1984
320. McClure JH, Brown DT, Wildsmith JAW: Comparison of the i.v. administration of midazolam and diazepam as sedation dur-

ing spinal anesthesia. Br J Anaesth 55:1089, 1983

321. O'Boyle CA, Harris D, Barry H, et al: Comparison of midazolam by mouth and diazepam i.v. in outpatient oral surgery.' Br J Anaesth 59:746, 1987
322. O'Boyle CA, Barry H, Fox E, et al: Controlled comparison of a new sublingual lormetazepam formulation and i.v. diazepam in outpatient minor oral surgery. Br J Anaesth 60:419, 1988
323. White PF, Shafer A, Boyle WA, et al: Benzodiazepine antagonism does not provoke a stress response. Anesthesiology 70:636, 1989
324. Ghoneim MM, Dembo JB, Block RI: Time course of antagonism of sedative and amnesic effects of diazepam by flumazenil. Anesthesiology 70:899, 1989
325. Jensen S, Knudsen I, Kirkegaard I, et al: Flumazenil used for antagonizing the central effects of midazolam and diazepam in outpatients. Acta Anaesthesiol Scand 33:26, 1989
326. Boldy DAR, English JSC, Hoare AM: Sedation for endoscopy: a comparison between diazepam, and diazepam plus pethidine with naxoxone reversal. Br J Anaesch 56:1109, 1984
327. Tucker MR, Ochs MW, White RP, Jr.: Arterial blood gas levels after midazolam or diazepam administered with or without fentanyl as an intravenous sedative for outpatient surgical procedures. J Oral Maxillofac Surg 44:688, 1986
328. Bailey PL, Moll JWB, Pace NL, et al: Respiratory effects of midazolam and fentanyl: potent interaction producing hypoxemia and apnea. Anesthesiology 69: A813, 1988
329. Dolan EA, Murray WJ, Immediata AR, Gleason N: Comparison of nalbuphine and fentanyl in combination with diazepam for outpatient oral surgery. J Oral Maxillofac Surg 46:471, 1988
330. Gilbert J, Holt JE, Johnston J, et al: Intravenous sedation for cataract surgery. Anaesthesia 42:1063, 1987
331. Schelling G, Weber W, Sackmann M, et al: Pain control during extracorporeal shock wave lithotripsy of gallstones by titrated alfentanil infusion. Anesthesiology 70:1022, 1989
332. White PF: Use of ketamine for sedation and analgesia during injection of local anesthetics. Ann Plast Surg 15:53, 1985
333. Thompson GE, Moore DC: Ketamine, diazepam, and Innovar[R]. Anesth Analg 50:458, 1971
334. Scarborough DA, Bisaccia E, Swensen RD: Anesthesia for outpatient dermatologic cosmetic surgery: midazolam—low-dosage ketamine anesthesia. J Dermatol Surg Oncol 15:658, 1989
335. Philip BK: Hazards of amnesia after midazolam in ambulatory surgical patients. Anesth Analg 66:97, 1987
336. Urquhart ML, White PF: Comparison of sedative infusions during regional anesthesia: methohexital, etomidate and midazolam. Anesth Analg 68:249, 1989
337. MacKenzie N, Grant IS: Comparison of propofol with methohexitone in the provision of anaesthesia for surgery under regional blockade. Br J Anaesth 57:1167, 1985
338. Jessop E, Grounds RM, Morgan M, et al: Comparisons of infusion of propofol and methohexitone to provide light general anesthesia during surgery with regional blockade. Br J Anaesth 57:1173, 1985
339. Negus JB, White PF: Use of sedative infusions during local and regional anesthesia—a comparison of midazolam and propofol. Anesthesiology 69:A711, 1988
340. Philip BK: Supplemental medication for ambulatory procedures under regional anesthesia. Anesth Analg 64:1117, 1985
341. Hallonsten A-L: Sedation by the use of inhalation agents in dental care. Acta Anaesthesiol Scand 32:31, 1987
342. Korttila K: Psychomotor recovery after anesthesia and sedation in the dental office. p. 135. In Dionne RA, Laskin DM (eds): Anesthesia and Sedation in the Dental Office. Elsevier, New York, 1986
343. Korttila K: Postanesthetic cognitive and psychomotor impairment. Int Anesthesiol Clin 24:59, 1986
344. Cashman JN, Power SJ, Jones RM, Adams AP: Assessment of recovery from anaesthesia: what test should we use? Anesthesiology 67:A434, 1987
345. Korttila K: Recovery and driving after brief anaesthesia. Anaesthesist 30:377, 1981

346. Denis R, Letourneau JE, Londorf D: Reliability and validity of psychomotor tests as measures of recovery from isoflurane or enflurane anesthesia in a day-care surgery unit. Anesth Analg 63:653, 1984
347. Daos FG, Virtue RW: Sympathetic block persistence after spinal or epidural analgesia. JAMA 183:285, 1963
348. Roe CF, Cohn FL: Sympathetic blockade during spinal anesthesia. Surg Gynecol Obstet 136:265, 1973
349. Alexander CM, Teller LE, Gross JB, et al: New discharge criteria decrease recovery room time after subarachnoid block. Anesthesiology 70:640, 1989
350. White PF: Pain management after day-case surgery. Curr Opin Anaesth 1:70, 1988
351. Anderson R, Krohg K: Pain as a major cause of postoperative nausea. Can Anaesth Soc J 23:366, 1976
352. Milligan KA, Mowbray MJ, Mulrooney L, et al: Intra-articular bipivacaine for pain relief after arthroscopic surgery of the knee joint in daycase patients. Anaesthesia 43:563, 1988
353. Vallane J, Korttila K, Ylikorkata O: Intravenous diclofenac sodium decreases prostaglandin synthesis and postoperative symptoms after general anaesthesia in outpatients undergoing dental surgery. Acta Anaesthesiol Scand 31:722, 1987
354. Thompson GE, Remington JM, Millman BS, Bridenbaugh LD: Experiences with outpatient anesthesia. Anesth Analg 52:881, 1973
355. Paasuke RT, Davies JM: Anaesthesia for daycare patients—controversies and concerns. Can Anaesth Soc J 33:644, 1986
356. Detmer DE: Ambulatory surgery. N Engl J Med 305:1486, 1981
357. Davis JE: The need to redefine levels of surgical care. JAMA 251:2527, 1984
358. Lahti PT: Early postoperative discharge of patients from the hospital. Surgery 63:410, 1968

Appendix 1-1

Guidelines for Ambulatory Surgical Facilities (Amended by House of Delegates on October 12, 1983)*

PREAMBLE

The American Society of Anesthesiologists endorses and supports the concept of ambulatory surgery and anesthesia and encourages the anesthesiologist to play a role of leadership in the development of this concept in both the hospital and freestanding setting.

1. An Ambulatory Surgical Facility is a hospital-administered or freestanding facility (administratively independent of a hospital), which is established, equipped, and operated primarily for the purpose of performing outpatient surgical procedures.
2. The ASA Guidelines to the Ethical Practice of Anesthesiology and Guidelines for Patient Care in Anesthesiology should be adhered to in all cases except where they are not applicable to outpatient care.
3. A licensed physician, preferably an anesthesiologist, must be in attendance in the facility at all times during patient treatment, recovery, and until discharge.
4. The facility must be established, equipped, constructed, and operated in accordance with the applicable laws in the jurisdiction in which it is located.
5. The staff shall consist of:
   A. An adequate administrative staff.
   B. A professional staff.
      1. physicians, dentists, and podiatrists must be duly licensed, qualified, and should have admitting privileges to a nearby hospital unless prior arrangements exist for transfer of patient to an acute care hospital.
      2. registered nurses, duly licensed and qualified, must be present in proper numbers to adequately care for patients within the surgical facility.
   C. A housekeeping and maintenance

* Courtesy of the American Society of Anesthesiologists, Park Ridge, IL.

staff adequate to insure proper care and cleanliness of the facility.

6. Physicians providing medical care in the facility should be organized into a medical staff which assumes responsibility for credentials review and delineation of clinical privileges. A medical audit committee shall carry on continuing review and evaluation of medical care.
7. Personnel and equipment shall be on hand to handle all emergencies, including cardiopulmonary resuscitation. The facility should also have immediate access to a blood bank where blood or blood products are readily obtainable.
8. Minimal physical requirements of the facility should include:
   A. Properly equipped and constructed operating rooms, sterilizing, instrument storage, pack, and clean-up areas.
   B. An admitting area appropriately designed and equipped for preoperative preparation, examination, holding, and observation of patients.
   C. Adequate space for reception and registration. Ample space for administrative requirements, including proper care of records. Comfortable waiting areas for relatives and/or escorts.
   D. Proper postoperative recovery room facilities.
   E. Accurate, confidential, and current medical records for each patient.
9. Minimal patient care shall include:
   A. Adequate preoperative instructions and preparation.
   B. An appropriate history and physical examination by a physician prior to anesthesia and surgery.
   C. Appropriate preoperative studies as medically indicated.
   D. Anesthesia shall be administered by anesthesiologists, other qualified medical physicians or nonphysician anesthetists under the direct supervision of a medical physician.
   E. Patients who receive general anesthesia shall be evaluated by a physician after recovery from anesthesia, prior to discharge.
   F. Patients who receive general anesthesia must be discharged to the company of a responsible adult.
   G. Adequate postoperative instructions and follow up care.

Appendix 1-2

Perioperative Anesthesia Records

The pages that follow are an example of a perioperative anesthesia record used at a freestanding outpatient surgical facility (Courtesy of Dr. L. H. Chandler, Alaska Surgicenter, Anchorage, AL).

Alaska Surgery Center

DATE	ASSISTANT	SURGEON NAME	ANESTHESIOLOGIST

LAST NAME	FIRST NAME	M.I.	SEX	DOB	AGE	SOCIAL SECURITY NO.

MARITAL STATUS	NO. & STREET	CITY	STATE	ZIP	PHONE

RESPONSIBLE PARTY NAME	NO. & STREET	CITY	STATE	ZIP	PHONE

RESPONSIBLE PARTY EMPLOYER	CODE	EMPLOYER ADDRESS	EMPLOYER PHONE	OCCUPATION

FAC. FEE	INSURANCE CO. NAME	GROUP NO.	POLICY NO.	ADDRESS
ANES. FEE	INSURANCE CO. NAME	GROUP NO.	POLICY NO.	ADDRESS

ALLERGIES	Hb	HCT	WBC	pH	PROTEIN	KETONE	BILIRUBIN	BLOOD	GLUCOSE	HEIGHT	WEIGHT	TEMP	B.P.	PULSE	RESP.

H&P HEART DISEASE	ASTHMA	T.B.	NEUROGENIC DIS.	HI B.P.	HEPATITIS	DIABETES	BLEEDING	STEROID	PREGNANT	DAILY MEDICATIONS

DENTURES	CONTACT LENSES	N.P.O. SINCE	SMOKE	PREVIOUS OPERATIONS

I.V. FLUIDS	AMT.	LOCAL	SITE	NEEDLE	☐ PAINT ☐ SHAVE	MISCELLANEOUS

PROPOSED OPERATION	R.N. INITIALS

PREOPERATIVE MEDICAL EVALUATIONS

PHYS STATUS

DRUGS

O_2

N_2O

$ET.CO_2$

SAO_2

START ANES X

START OP •

END ANES X

200

180

160

140

120

100

80

60

40

FLUIDS GEN ☐ MAC ☐ AX BLOCK ☐ IV REG. ☐ SLA. ☐ LOCAL ☐ INTUBATED ☐ ORAL ☐ NASAL ☐ SIZE ORAL AIRWAY ☐ NASAL AIRWAY ☐

BLOOD LOSS PRECORDIAL STETH. ☐ ESOPHAGEAL STETH. ☐ ECG ☐ B.P. CUFF ☐ PULSE OXIMETER ☐ E.T.CO_2 ☐ TEMP ☐

ROOM / ANESTHESIA TIME	OPERATION TIME	UNIT TOURNIQUET TIME / PRESSURE	PREP SOLUTION	GROUND SITE UNIT COAG
TO	TO	MM/HG		CUT

LASER C-ARM ☐ X-RAY ☐ CATHETERIZATION ☐ DRAIN POSITIONS ☐ SUPINE ☐ PRONE ☐ LAT ☐ LITH HARDWARE IMPLANTS

☐ CAST ☐ SPLINT ☐ BRACE PATIENT RESTRAINT ☐

IRRIGATIONS DRUGS

RAYTEC LAPS TONSIL OTHER NEEDLE INCORRECT SIGNATURES SCRUB NURSE CIRCULATING NURSE

BLADE CORRECT

OPERATION PERFORMED SPECIMEN # ☐ PATH ☐ MICRO ☐ CYTOLOGY

☐ PROV ☐ HUMANA ☐ P.M.L. ☐ F.S.

TIME RETURNED TO R.R. CART AMB W/C AIRWAY ORAL NASAL ET OUT 0_2on L/M OFF

TIME	B.P.	P	R	SAO_2	RES.	CIR.	COL.	L.O.C.	ACT.	DRESS	PAIN	NAUSEA	I.V.	MEDS.	TREATMENT	OBSERVATIONS

DISCH. WITH WHOM POST OP INSTR. SURGEON IV CATH INTACT DISC SCORE Rx

RTO SUPPLIES IV TOTAL DISC TIME

DISCHARGE SUMMARY & REMARKS

PHYSICIAN SIGNATURE DATE

Alaska Surgery Center

DATE	ASSISTANT	SURGEON NAME	ANESTHESIOLOGIST

LAST NAME	FIRST NAME	M.I.	SEX	DOB	AGE	SOCIAL SECURITY NO.

MARITAL STATUS	NO. & STREET	CITY	STATE	ZIP	PHONE

RESPONSIBLE PARTY NAME	NO. & STREET	CITY	STATE	ZIP	PHONE

RESPONSIBLE PARTY EMPLOYER	CODE	EMPLOYER ADDRESS	EMPLOYER PHONE	OCCUPATION

FAC. FEE	INSURANCE CO. NAME	GROUP NO.	POLICY NO.	ADDRESS
ANES. FEE	INSURANCE CO. NAME	GROUP NO.	POLICY NO.	ADDRESS

PROPOSED OPERATION

PHONE PHONE PATIENT TO CALL ASC

NO PHONE NO CALL REQUIRED

POST DISCHARGE FOLLOW-UP

DATE TIME NURSE

DATE TIME NURSE

ANSWERING MACHINE-PATIENT INSTRUCTED TO CALL ASC IF QUESTIONS OF PROBLEMS

PATIENT

PARENT

SPOUSE

OTHER

HOSPITAL HUMANA PROVIDENCE

NO PROBLEMS

PAIN

NAUSEA

VOMITING

BLEEDING

NOTES

Appendix 1-3

Nursing Discharge Record

The following page is an example of a pediatric nursing discharge record after myringotomy with tube insertion/adenoidectomy (Courtesy of Dr. R. S. Hannallah, Children's National Medical Center, Washington, D.C.)

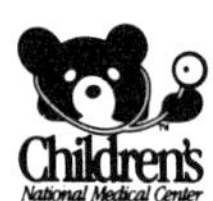

NURSING DEPARTMENT
NURSING DISCHARGE SUMMARY

ADDRESSOGRAPH

Patient's Primary Diagnosis: ______________________

____

Primary Nurse: ______________________

PART I - HOME CARE INSTRUCTIONS: MYRINGOTOMY WITH TUBE INSERTION/ADENOIDECTOMY

NOTE: If you have printed instructions from your private physician, please follow those and use this as a supplement.

ACTIVITY: Limited activity for the first 2-3 days.

DIET:
Continue with clear liquids at home with the addition of milk products, soups, eggs, and soft cereal. Avoid hot, spicy, acidic (orange juice), and rough (example: chips, toast) foods for the first 3-4 days. As recovery progresses, you may include solid foods. If vomiting occurs, do not give liquid or food for one hour; start over with ice chips and build slowly to regular diet

MEDICATIONS:
Acetaminophen (Tylenol, Tempra) ________ mg every ________ hours, if needed for discomfort.
Do not give aspirin or products containing aspirin since these may interfere with blood clotting.
Your doctor may give you ear drops for your child. This medication is ________________. Place ______ drops in each ear ______ times per day for ______ days. This will prevent blood clotting in the ear tubes and decrease irritation of the ear canal. Keep the drops at room temperature.

SPECIAL INSTRUCTIONS:
- Keep ears dry. Use vaseline on cotton balls in ears for baths, showers or shampoo to prevent getting ears wet. Ear plugs may be used when prescribed by the doctor.
- Do not put medication in your child's ear unless prescribed by the doctor.
- Expect minimal drainage from ears for first 72 hours.
- Coughing, gargling, straining, shouting, clearing the throat, or blowing the nose should be kept at a minimum.
- Expect some bleeding or brown mucous from the nose for the first 24 hours.
- You may notice that your child's voice is changed. If it persists by your office visit - bring this to the attention of your doctor.

WHEN TO CALL THE DOCTOR:
- Fever over 102°F/38.4°C, not relieved by Tylenol
- Excessive bleeding or drainage from ears or nose
- Persistent cough
- Persistent pain not relieved by Tylenol

WHERE TO CALL WITH QUESTIONS:
- SHORT STAY UNIT — open 8:00 a.m. to 11:00 p.m., Monday through Friday.
- Clinic/Private Doctor ______________________
- ***IN AN EMERGENCY,*** call ______________________

FOLLOW-UP APPOINTMENT: Make an appointment with ______________________

I have received and understand the above instructions:

____
(Parent Signature)

PART II

DISCHARGED: ☐ Home ☐ Extended Care Facility Other: ______________
VIA: ☐ Ambulatory ☐ Wheelchair ☐ Stretcher ☐ Carried
ACCOMPANIED BY: ☐ Parent: ______________ ☐ Other: ______________
Patient's physical/emotional condition at discharge: ______________________

____

____

Summary of patient/family understanding of discharge instruction *(i.e., by verbalization or demonstration);* ______________

____

____

Date of Discharge: ______________________

Time of Discharge: ______________________

____
(Discharging Nurse's Signature)

*(TO DOCUMENT ANY ADDITIONAL INFORMATION ON ANY ITEM ABOVE, PLEASE INDICATE DATE OF CORRESPONDING **PROGRESS NOTE.**)*
COPY DISTRIBUTION: WHITE - CHART PINK - Parent

CHNMC 113.3

2

Outpatient Facility and Personnel

Jeffrey L. Apfelbaum
Bruce D. Schreider

Modern ambulatory surgical services in the United States are presently undergoing a phenomenal period of growth, expansion, and reorganization. In its Annual Survey of Hospitals, the American Hospital Association estimated that 40.3 percent of all surgical procedures performed in hospitals in 1986 were completed on an outpatient basis. Additionally, several million ambulatory surgical procedures are estimated to have been performed in freestanding, independent facilities and physicians' offices. Experts predict that by the end of the 20th century, the annual number of outpatient surgical procedures in the United States will far exceed the number of inpatient surgical procedures. Clinical experience seems to support these predictions.

The American Hospital Association recently reported that from 1981 through 1986, the number of outpatient surgical procedures performed in hospitals increased by nearly 120 percent while inpatient surgical volume suffered a substantial decrease. This trend is particularly evident in pediatric surgery, with a 30 percent decrease among inpatient procedures in the past decade as a result of substitution of outpatient for inpatient surgical treatment.[1] Like the increase in hospital-based outpatient surgery, the demand for such surgery in freestanding outpatient clinics has also skyrocketed. Nearly 700 freestanding outpatient surgery centers participated in the federal Medicare program in 1987. Given the fact that the first "modern generation" outpatient surgical facility is less than two decades old, and the fact that it was not until 1983 that the American College of Surgeons approved "the concept that certain surgical procedures may be performed in an ambulatory surgical facility,"[2] this unprecedented rate of growth is truly remarkable.

This chapter focuses on the organization and management of the modern ambulatory surgical program in the United States, with particular attention to the historic development of the ambulatory surgical facility, the characteristics of a successful ambulatory surgical program, the classification of modern ambulatory surgical programs, the current role of the anesthesiologist in an ambulatory surgical program, important techniques in the development of an ambulatory surgical program, and the role of office-based surgery.

HISTORIC DEVELOPMENT

It seems as though we have come full circle in ambulatory surgery. Initially, of course, there were no hospitals. Mac-

Alister[3] suggests that physicians constitute one of the oldest professional classes in the history of mankind and that they appear to have practiced surgery generations before the advent of hospitals. Before the development of general anesthesia, most patients who underwent surgery recovered at home.[4] The sedative and analgesic properties of alcohol and opiate derivatives were well-known to the ancient Greeks and Egyptians; these agents were used routinely in the home to provide perioperative relief for wound closures. In time, physicians came to believe that postoperative results were better when patients were treated in a more formal environment, and hospitalization for surgery eventually became the standard of care. One of the most important advances in the field of surgery was the discovery and use of ether anesthesia by Crawford Long in 1842; the first reported clinical use of general anesthesia in a patient was also the first reported general anesthetic administered to an outpatient.

The safety and economic advantages of "same-day home discharge" were first formally advocated at a meeting of the British Medical Association in 1909 when Nicoll and Glasg reported that ambulatory surgical care for some procedures in pediatric patients at the Glasgow Royal Hospital was *at least* as satisfactory as inpatient surgical care.[5] They made the following observations: "we keep similar cases in adults too long in bed," "the treatment of a large number of the cases at present treated indoors constitutes a waste of the resources," and the results obtained on ambulatory patients at a fraction of the cost "are equally good." Nicoll and Glasg concluded that in their experience of nearly 9,000 cases, ambulatory surgical procedures in infants were "amongst the safest and most efficient of all our operations."

In 1919, Waters described what is believed to be the first freestanding ambulatory surgical facility and suggested that this "clinic" was created in response to his observation that surgeons and dentists "objected to going to the hospital because of the time and expense involved."[6] He noted that the clinic's fees were "considerably less than for similar work in hospitals" and predicted that "the future for such a venture . . . is bright." Unfortunately, when Waters left Iowa to establish the Department of Anesthesia at the University of Wisconsin, the enthusiasm for ambulatory surgery diminished.

The modern era of ambulatory surgery began in the United States with the opening of the outpatient surgery program at the Butterworth Hospital in Grand Rapids, Michigan, in 1961.[7] The resurgence of ambulatory surgery continued in the United States through the 1960s with the creation of hospital-based outpatient surgery facilities at the University of California at Los Angeles by Cohen and Dillon and at the George Washington University Medical Center in Washington by Levy and Coakley. Cohen and Dillon established the guidelines for today's standard of safety and ambulatory surgery when they observed that "safety of the patient is not a matter of inpatient versus outpatient. Safety is an attitude and when good practice is followed . . . there is no reason to expect more complications than under the circumstances of hospitalization."[8] Levy and Coakley first described the importance of consumer satisfaction with the process of ambulatory surgery when they observed that over 90 percent of their patients would choose to be an outpatient for future surgical procedures and would highly recommend the process to others.[9]

The fundamental principles of ambulatory surgery as we know it today were first reported by Lahti[10] in 1968. In many respects, this landmark publication provides us with the foundation on which the ambulatory surgical subspeciality is built. To summarize Lahti:

1. Unlike adults, children do not intuitively "know" that they are supposed to be sick following minor surgery and, consequently, they do not act sick.

2. When healthy adults are bedridden for approximately 1 week and intermittently given intramuscular narcotics, they generally require several weeks to recuperate from the experience.

3. Postoperative medications may actually prolong recovery from minor surgery. Patients who know they will be going home shortly after surgery are more relaxed and less afraid compared with inpatients undergoing similar procedures. Outpatients seem to prefer less postoperative medication.

Using many of the concepts developed by these investigators,[5,6,8–10] the freestanding ambulatory surgery facility program in the United States was successfully launched in 1970 with the development of the Phoenix Surgicenter.[11] Described as an innovation in the delivery of surgical care, the Phoenix Surgicenter was a totally self-sufficient freestanding facility designed for the sole purpose of providing quality surgical care. Much of the success of the Phoenix Surgicenter can be attributed to the fact that unlike many of its predecessors, this center was developed with the involvement of anesthesiologists, surgeons, local facilities (hospitals, laboratories, etc.), planning agencies, and major third-party payers. In two short decades, the freestanding outpatient surgery program in the United States has grown from a single center to over 1,000 such facilities performing millions of surgical procedures annually.

Today, with rapid pharmacologic and technologic advances in anesthesia and surgery, the ambulatory setting has become a realistic option for many patients. Outpatient surgery has progressed from a few simple procedures without anesthesia to thousands of different surgical procedures under all types of anesthetics. Simply put, surgical health care is moving away from hospitalization. Indeed, with the recent emphasis on health care cost containment, medical practitioners sometimes find they no longer have a choice regarding site of service: ambulatory surgery is now often mandated by third-party payers, including the federal government.

CHARACTERISTICS OF THE SUCCESSFUL FACILITY

The successful ambulatory surgical facility of the 1990s is quite different from its hospital operating room predecessor; it is often a self-sufficient, independent, and extraordinarily dynamic center that requires direct interaction and close cooperation between anesthesiologist, nurse, surgeon, facility manager, and patient. According to Ring and Wong,[11] to survive, the modern freestanding ambulatory surgical facility

Services Offered by Some Ambulatory Surgical Facilities

"Free" above insurance surgery fees
"Free" above insurance doctor fees
"Free" above insurance laboratory fees
"Free" convenient parking
"Free" transportation to and from surgery center
"Free" postoperative home health care
Overnight accommodation
Conveniently scheduled preoperative assessment appointments
Conveniently scheduled preoperative laboratory appointments
Conveniently scheduled patient education program
Conveniently scheduled child orientation programs
Convenient arrangements for child care

must be a well-organized and autonomous unit that thrives on management innovations. Successful ambulatory surgical programs process patients through their surgical procedures while providing an environment superior to the "customary" hospital milieu; consumers (patients, surgeons, and third-party payers) find advantages sufficient to induce them to use the facility again or, at the very least, to recommend its use to others. Although it is impossible to define the perfect outpatient center, successful ambulatory surgical facilities often possess many similar characteristics.

Consumer-Oriented Care

The 1980s have produced a new age of "consumer awareness," and health care is no exception. While still insisting on the highest quality at the lowest possible price, consumers now additionally demand increased convenience and upgraded service features from their health care providers. As competition in the ambulatory surgical service arena has intensified, successful providers often market and heavily promote their advantages in an attempt to court consumers.

Patients often prefer ambulatory surgical care because it is more convenient, faster, and less of an imposition on them and their families. Upgraded amenities, such as readily accessible parking, conveniently scheduled preoperative laboratory appointments, accommodations for perioperative child care, and postoperative home care visits, give patients the impression that they are the center of attention and not just victims of a bureaucratic hospital environment. Because the ambulatory surgical facility is designed specifically for outpatient surgery, a functional and competent environment that is cheery and nonthreatening can generally be created and presented to the patient.

Surgeons often prefer to perform ambulatory surgery because it allows them to have more control over their patients in an environment that is more personable, pleasant, and convenient than the traditional hospital environment. Many surgeons have become disillusioned with the bureaucracy typically encountered in large hospitals. Delays resulting from the completion of redundant paperwork, or a lack of accountability in determining the cause of erroneous scheduling, incomplete charts, or inadequate preoperative testing have caused many surgeons to leave the hospital environment. Once they have experienced a smaller, more manageable facility dedicated exclusively to the surgical outpatient, many surgeons strongly prefer to stay. Additionally, the absence of hospital "rounds" or "errands" allows the surgeon in the ambulatory surgical facility to establish a more personable, and theoretically less litigious, relationship with the patient and family at the time of surgery. Lastly, an efficiently run ambulatory surgical facility, particularly one located adjacent to a complex of medical offices, can save the surgeon a great deal of time. Many successful ambulatory surgical facilities vigorously promote these advantages to their surgeon consumers.

Third-party payers benefit from the ambulatory surgical setting because it eliminates overnight hospital charges and, in general, provides less expensive surgical care than that of hospitals, presumably because of greater subspecialization and efficiency. Multiple studies have documented savings of 20 to 75 percent with equivalent surgical outcomes for certain operative procedures in selected patients when the site of surgery was moved away from the hospital.[12–14] Insurers were initially skeptical of moving cases to the ambulatory surgical setting, but later encouraged the practice. Now, they often mandate specified surgical procedures be performed on an outpatient basis. Successful ambulatory surgical facil-

Techniques for Direct Marketing to Patients, Physicians, and Third-Party Payers

Television advertising
Radio advertising
Local and regional newspaper and magazine advertising
Direct mailings
Informational brochures
Open house visitations
Journal advertising
"Giveaways" (balloons, refrigerator magnets, calendars)

ities often set the most rigorous standards for their facilities (accreditation from the Joint Commission on Accreditation of Health Care Organizations [JCAHO] and the Accreditation Association for Ambulatory Health Care [AAAHC]) and their physicians (board certification), then market quality of care and cost-effectiveness directly to third-party payers.

Convenient Location

Successful ambulatory surgical facilities are readily accessible to patients, physicians, facility staff (nurses, office personnel, and laboratory technicians) and external facility support services (laundry, trash, central supply, and material management services). Physical constraints resulting from poor facility design or location invariably lead to inefficiencies and loss of revenue.

Creativity and Innovation

Successful ambulatory surgical facilities thrive on innovations generally shunned by traditional hospital environments. For example, the University of Chicago recently opened a freestanding ambulatory surgical facility in one of Chicago's most famous shopping malls, the Water Tower Place. Patient's escorts often receive beepers and are "notified" when the patient is ready to be discharged. For those individuals who prefer not to travel after surgery, convenient overnight accommodations may be arranged at the Ritz-Carlton Hotel. Other successful facilities offer "free" (above insurance) surgery, transportation via limousine to and from the facility, perioperative child care, gourmet meals, postoperative home health care visits, and even breathtaking mountain views from the operating rooms as "incentives" to attract patients. Some facilities offer additional convenience to patients and surgeons with locations in or adjacent to physician's office buildings, clinical laboratories, recovery care centers, or even shopping malls.

Adaptability

Successful programs generally demonstrate the flexibility to adjust as necessary to changing conditions. What works today may not work tomorrow. Changes in medical technology, pharmacology, socioeconomic conditions, and even local competition must be addressed as rapidly as they affect the day-to-day operations of any facility. Successful programs should be adaptable to the needs of their consumers (patients, physicians, and third-party payers) as well as to the procedures performed. In situations in which the facility's viability is dependent on a particular group of surgeons or specialized type of surgery, decreased surgical volume may require radical practice changes. Sometimes the answer is the recruitment of new surgeons, different surgical procedures, or even alternate facility uses.

Staff Satisfaction

In addition to satisfying their consumers, successful facilities are often "staff-oriented." Economies of scale and specialization of workload generally enable successful facilities to recruit and retain a small group of employees (5 to 25). Staff turnover is often extremely low. A typical ambulatory surgical facility has particular appeal to health care professionals because of its daytime operations. Off-hour, holiday, and weekend coverage are virtually eliminated in the efficiently run ambulatory surgical facility. Fluctuations in surgical schedules encourage the use of flexible and part-time staff. In addition to meeting the needs of the facility staff, this scheduling often allows the facility to be more competitive and cost-effective. To offer a quantifiable, economic incentive, some facilities allow all vested employees to share in the year-end profits. This responsiveness to the needs of staff produces a satisfaction level that is usually reflected in a positive work ethic.

Successful ambulatory surgical facilities are in the business of providing operating room services. They do so by striving to achieve the highest quality patient care in an aesthetically pleasing environment that promotes maximum utilization of operating rooms, equipment, and staff.

CLASSIFICATION OF AMBULATORY SURGICAL PROGRAMS

Outpatient surgery in the United States is performed in a variety of settings and is best classified in accordance with the governance of the facility and its specific affiliation with a major health care organization (hospital, third-party payer, or independent). These programs may be described as (1) hospital-integrated, (2) hospital-segregated, (3) freestanding hospital satellite, and (4) freestanding hospital-independent.

The hospital-integrated program is the way modern ambulatory surgery began, and is the method by which most ambulatory surgery in the United States is practiced. In this model, the hospital processes its ambulatory surgery patients separately from other hospital patients but uses the regular hospital operating rooms. Theoretically, the patient never occupies a hospital bed in a defined location and is generally discharged home from the recovery room or a "stepdown" area adjacent to it. The most significant advantage of this type of program is that it allows the hospital to offer ambulatory surgery at minimal financial risk without a significant expenditure of funds. Additionally, surgeons have "the best of both worlds" in terms of flexibility; they are often willing to undertake a greater variety of procedures on sicker patients, particularly procedures that are more complex because they know that, regardless of their findings, they will have the full support of the hospital facilities. The principal disadvantages of this type of program are numerous, and all directly affect the patients, who are often treated as second-class citizens. This type of program often lacks appropriate areas of privacy for patients, including dressing rooms, a preoperative examination area, and a dedicated postoperative recovery area. Ambulatory patients in this system are often unnecessarily exposed to septic or critically ill patients, which may add considerable infection potential as well as psychological stress. The needs of ambulatory patients and their families are frequently sacrificed to care for hospitalized inpatients whose medical problems are often considered to be more serious. For example, the need to perform emergency surgery on an inpatient may "bump" the totally elective patient to a later surgical time slot or even to a different day. The ambulatory surgery patients may be charged excessive rates because they share in-hospital costs, although they receive no substantial benefits. The multitude of disadvantages inherent in this system has led to the reorganization and explosive growth of the ambulatory surgery subspecialty.

In the hospital-segregated facility, surgical procedures are generally performed in a special area of the hospital exclusively assigned to ambulatory surgery. Although this arrangement may totally prohibit the use of these dedicated operating rooms for any purpose other than ambulatory surgery, the hospital may or may not prohibit outpatients from being treated in the regular hospital operating rooms. The hospital-segregated program gives the facility the freedom to have its own nursing, anesthesia, secretarial, and housekeeping staff; innovative management techniques may counteract the inherent disadvantages to which the patients are exposed merely by being in a hospital. In general, this type of facility is able to perform more complicated procedures than a freestanding facility because it has the full "backup" services offered by the hospital (e.g., radiology, pathology, laboratory services, intensive care). The biggest disadvantage is the potentially high cost to the hospital secondary to duplication of staffing and/or equipment needs.

The freestanding hospital satellite is an entirely autonomous, separate, and distinct facility that may or may not be physically attached to a hospital. Because it is controlled by a hospital, charges are generally higher than those at an independent freestanding facility. Depending on the specifics of the physical connection to the hospital (or lack thereof), it may be virtually impossible to share staffing (except surgeons) or equipment. Cooperation between anesthesiologists, management, nurses, surgeons, and patients is critical to the successful operation of this type of facility. Any substantial breakdown encourages a "worst of both worlds" scenario in which the facility acquires the inefficiencies of a large inpatient hospital suite and the duplication of costs for equipment, staffing, and space.

The independent freestanding ambulatory facility is a specialty unit that is physically separate from other health care facilities. Accordingly, registration, laboratory facilities, preoperative assessment, education, and waiting rooms, operating rooms, and postanesthesia recovery rooms appear to make patient care much more convenient. The facilities themselves may be more liberally decorated than traditional hospital environments, often displaying bright colors and murals, and therefore appear less frightening and more attractive to the patient. Because these facilities are much smaller than their hospital counterparts, their governance and management can be accomplished with relative ease. The smaller facility invariably enables the employees to function as a closely knit team. Patients and their families often perceive this "closeness" of the staff and can become a part of it. Only rarely can this degree of personal attention occur in a hospital-based unit. Two major disadvantages of the independent freestanding facility are (1) the high financial costs (with little, if any, guarantees) to the investors, and (2) the lack of rapid direct access to a hospital for the *rare* patient who needs to be admitted.

THE ROLE OF THE ANESTHESIOLOGIST/MEDICAL DIRECTOR

The role of the anesthesiologist in the modern ambulatory surgical facility is extremely controversial. Experts in the administration of this subspecialty (Epstein, Wetchler, and Wong) have been forecasting a need for radical practice changes since the early 1970s. In the fall of 1988, James Arens, M.D., newly elected president of the American Society of Anesthesiologists, addressed the membership on this subject, stating that "it is important for our members to practice medicine and provide care beyond the O.R. if we are to continue to push our specialty ahead."

For most physicians, innovative alterations in their patterns of medical practice are difficult to assimilate. The explosive growth of ambulatory surgery has created new potential roles for the anesthesiologist which demand skills that entail more than simply "giving a good anesthetic."[15] When most anesthesiologists think of innovations in the anesthesia care of their patients, they tend to think of new equipment (e.g., lasers, mass spectrometers, pulse oximeters), new pharmacologic agents (e.g., propofol [Diprivan], mivacurium, sevoflurane), or new monitors (e.g., transesophageal echocardiography, intraoperative electroencephalography, evoked potential monitors). Unfortunately, the importance of other innovations, particularly changes involving administrative direction and leadership, is not fully appreciated.

Ginzberg[16] suggested that traditional hospital management policies have developed under a system of cost-based reimbursement. Under this reimbursement system, hospital administration or other providers of health care (i.e., physicians) were exposed to minimal risk. Different long-term goals in the absence of substantial risk led to the development of a schism between medical staff and hospital management which still exists today in many hospital environments. Himmelstein and Woodhandler[17] suggest that the resulting inefficiencies have led to a substantial increase in cost without benefit to patient care.

The new prospective payment reimbursement system (diagnosis-related groups [DRGs]) has spawned innovations that may minimize this dichotomy between medical staff and facility management. One such innovation may lead facility administrators to ally themselves with anesthesiologists in the management of ambulatory surgical facilities. Ring and Wong[11] point out that both groups have a similar goal: the safe, efficient use of operating room space. Historically, at the first truly successful modern ambulatory surgical facilities, dedicated anesthesiologists were forced to assume administrative and medical responsibilities. When the medical director and facility administrator are the same person, the traditional dichotomy (medical staff versus facility management) is eliminated, thereby allowing for better lines of authority and a more efficient organization.

Practically speaking, the role of an anesthesiologist/administrator/medical director makes a great deal of sense. Anesthesiologists spend more time in operating rooms than any other physician and work closely with all operating room personnel on a daily basis. In the traditional hospital environment, few administrators actually spend time in the operating room, and they rarely understand how operating rooms actually function. In situations in which an omnipresent physician/administrator is given authority to hire and fire, the entire staff generally becomes more responsive to the needs of the facility. Simply put, the operating rooms function more smoothly.

The executive director (anesthesiologist/administrator/medical director) must be impartial, immediately available for decisions, and completely familiar with the day-to-day operations as well as the long-term goals and objectives of the ambulatory surgical facility. This individual essentially acts as a liaison and coordinator between the medical staff, facility staff, and Board of Directors. The executive director is directly responsible to the Board of Directors, although he or she is not a voting member (Fig. 2-1). Whenever possible, the executive director should be a shareholder in the ownership of the ambulatory surgical facility, thereby having a substantial "vested" interest in its successful development, marketing, and operations.

The medical director should be responsible for ensuring the quality of patient care administered in the facility. Through the various committees (quality assurance, utilization review, medical records, pharmacy and therapeutics, credentialing, etc.), the medical director is accountable to the Board of Directors for the quality of clinical ser-

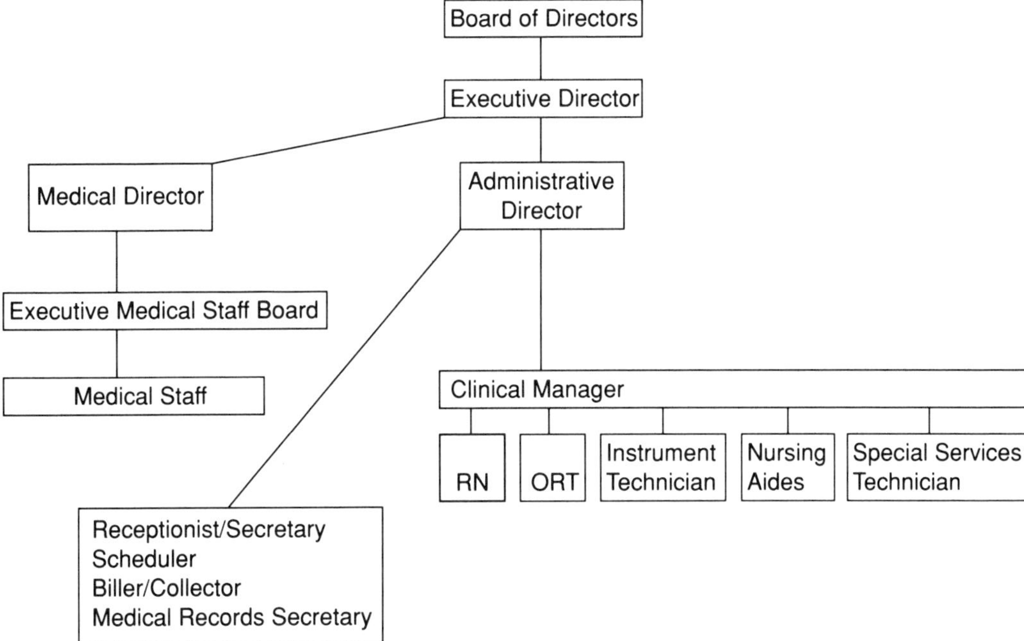

Fig. 2-1. Organization chart depicting staffing needs and lines of authority for an ambulatory surgical center.

vices delivered by the medical staff. Similarly, to the Board of Directors, the medical director represents the opinions, concerns, and grievances of the medical staff. He or she is responsible for enforcing the medical staff bylaws as well as the policies and procedures of the ambulatory surgical facility. Additionally, the medical director implements those policies and procedures applicable to the medical staff that are required to meet accreditation and licensure.

DESIGN AND MANAGEMENT CONSIDERATIONS IN ESTABLISHING AN AMBULATORY SURGICAL PROGRAM

Patient Flow

Generally, patient flow in an ambulatory surgery facility should be arranged to accomplish several goals. First, the flow pattern should maximize the ease of moving patients in and out of the facility, particularly the operating rooms. This should be accomplished without compromising the ability of staff to access operating rooms for stocking and turnover. Second, separation should be maintained between preoperative and postoperative patients, patients visiting to discuss potential surgery, and patients scheduled for preoperative evaluation. Finally, a central registration area should be provided so that all patients and family can be tracked within the facility. In larger facilities, separate waiting areas for preoperative patients, those awaiting pre-evaluation, and for family members may be a good solution. Figures 2-2 and 2-3 are block diagrams of patient flow that represent an almost infinite variety of possibilities.

Preoperative Evaluation and Laboratory Testing Facilities

An efficiently run ambulatory surgery facility should minimize delays in getting cases started. One extremely important

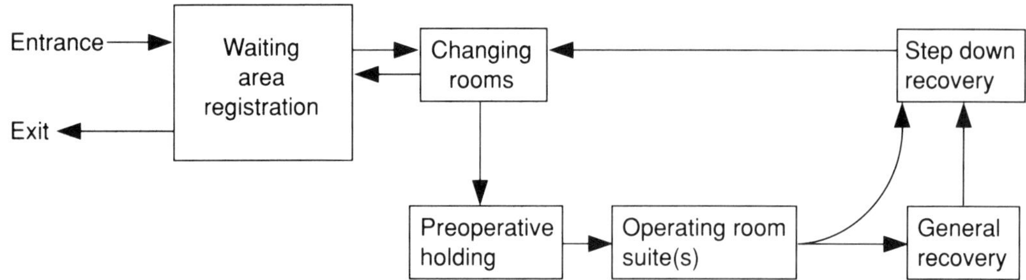

Fig. 2-2. Minimal components of patient flow in an ambulatory surgical facility.

area of consideration is that of preoperative patient assessment and laboratory testing. Lack of necessary medical history, laboratory tests, financial information, and/or pre-approval (when required) constitutes a major source of delay. Generally, these problems can be completely eliminated by patient visits to the facility prior to the scheduled surgery date. The purpose of such patient visits is to gather this information and to arrange for laboratory testing or consultation from other physicians (if indicated) well in advance of the day of surgery. In order to deliver the best possible medical care, the initial preoperative visit must be made far enough in advance of the scheduled surgery date to permit the completion of medical consultation and laboratory testing, as well as the assembly of a medical chart. In the unlikely event that a case is postponed, the facility staff should make every effort to fill the vacant time. Many busy facilities create short waiting lists to accommodate this occasional problem.

There are two major considerations in designing a preoperative evaluation clinic: physical plant and ancillary support (i.e.,

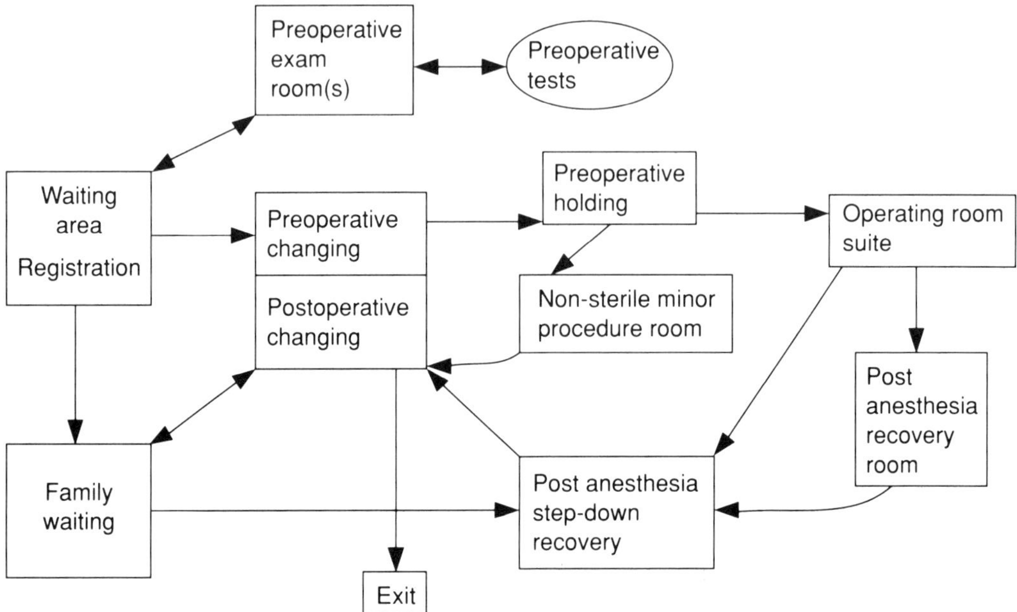

Fig. 2-3. Optimal patient flow in an ambulatory surgical facility.

medical records, laboratory testing, medical consultations). In an office practice, the physical plant is a minor issue because the regular office examination rooms are sufficient for preoperative examinations. Furthermore, in this setting, the office medical chart is usually readily available when needed. A more significant problem is obtaining necessary laboratory data in a timely fashion. Since almost all the surgical procedures scheduled in the office setting will be minor and will be performed on relatively healthy patients, laboratory requirements will be minimal. Still, it will be advantageous to have identified a laboratory that can provide the necessary services promptly.

In the case of freestanding ambulatory surgical facilities, whether hospital satellite or hospital-independent, a specifically designed preoperative evaluation area is absolutely essential. The ideal preoperative evaluation area should be large enough to accommodate as many patients as might have surgery in the facility on a fully scheduled day, allowing for a 20 percent surplus of space to accommodate revisits and mismatches in patient scheduling. The exact amount of time for a patient's preoperative visit must be modified by considerations of patient, nursing, and physician convenience. A good rule of thumb for determining the size of the physical plant allows for 20 to 30 minutes of examination room time per patient on an initial preoperative assessment and for about half that for the rare follow-up visit. Once again, adequate medical records, laboratory testing, and availability of a consulting physician are essential, and mechanisms for the rapid access and use of these services must be in place before the preoperative evaluation clinic initiates services. In hospital-based facilities, the problem of space is often critical. While the sharing of space with other hospital-based functions is often taken as a solution, the access to such shared space for preoperative evaluation and laboratory testing services must be ensured. Inability to process patients efficiently inevitably leads to dissatisfaction by both the patients and the physicians using the ambulatory surgery facility. Dissatisfaction will result in decreased use and often leads to a facility's failure.

In the hospital-based facility, the availability of comprehensive medical records, a full spectrum of readily accessible laboratory tests, and consultation services permit more complicated procedures to be performed on patients with more formidable baseline medical disease. Although medical records are often more comprehensive in hospital-based practice, obtaining them on short notice is sometimes extremely difficult; therefore, the preoperative evaluation visit in a hospital-based practice should be scheduled to allow for adequate time to obtain the necessary medical records. Unfortunately, it is often in the hospital-based setting that it is most convenient for surgeons and patients to schedule preoperative evaluation visits on the same day as the surgery office visit. When the medical records of patients with complex medical problems are not readily available, a comprehensive history and physical examination performed by the patient's surgeon or primary care physician is extremely important. All too often, surgeons believe that merely scheduling their patients for preoperative evaluation relieves them of the responsibility of obtaining adequate medical histories. In complex cases, the ability of the anesthesiologist to adequately assess a patient is severely hampered without a medical history, and attempts to gather this data at the time of the patient's visit can be both frustrating and overly time-consuming. For these reasons, it is sometimes best to forego the apparent convenience of same-day surgery office visits, preoperative evaluations, and laboratory testing in order to maximize facility efficiency.

A further question that comes up in hospital-based facilities is whether patients scheduled for surgery outside the confines of the ambulatory surgical facility should be

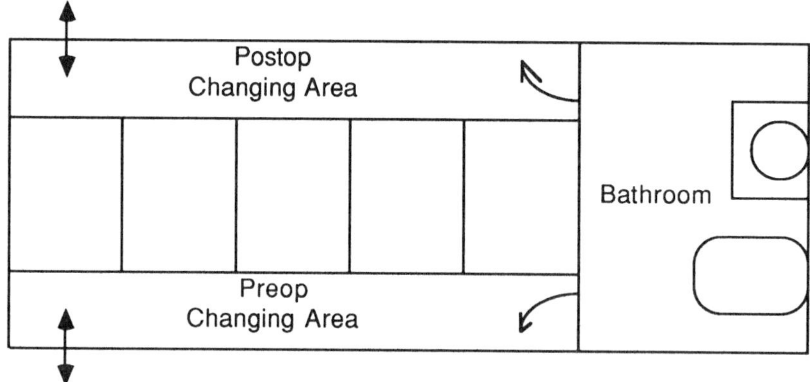

Fig. 2-4. Floor plan for lockers that open onto both the preoperative and postoperative sides of the locker room.

evaluated preoperatively in its clinic. These are either inpatients or patients admitted the same day as their scheduled surgeries ("A.M. admits") who will undergo more extensive surgical procedures that are often more medically complex than those for outpatients. Ambulatory surgery programs have evolved as a mechanism for providing surgical care in a manner that is more efficient, more personalized, and less costly than the traditional hospital surgical environment. For these reasons, most successful hospital-based programs choose to segregate their inpatients and outpatients, not only by their site of surgery, but also by the site of preoperative evaluation.

Changing Rooms

The changing area or patient's locker room is the one place in the ambulatory surgery center where preoperative and postoperative patients may be in close proximity. Whenever possible, contact between these individuals should be avoided. This can be accomplished by any number of designs, but in an ideal setting, lockers have two doors that can be opened by the same key and that connect with either the preoperative or the postoperative side of the locker room (Fig. 2-4). Lockers for all patients should be provided; five to six times as many lockers as there are operating rooms are usually needed. Lavatory facilities should be provided in the changing area as well. Again, it is best to have two separate lavatories to ensure the separation of preoperative and postoperative patients. Duplicate keys for lavatory doors locking from the inside must be available for emergency access.

Lavatories, locker rooms, and any area in which patients may be alone for even the shortest period of time must be equipped with highly visible, easy-to-use nurse call systems, and patients must be instructed in their use whenever they are left alone.

Operating Rooms

The operating rooms in a modern ambulatory surgical facility should be designed to provide an environment that is optimally safe for the patient, efficient for the surgeon, and satisfying to the staff. Highly desirable is a pleasant, nonthreatening environment for the patient in a milieu that allows for the most expeditious use of the facility's resources. Exact code requirements for construction of new ambulatory surgical facilities and renovation of existing hospital facilities vary tremendously among municipalities and states and must therefore be individually obtained before a new construction project is undertaken. Most regulations incorporate standards published in 1974 by the United States Department of Health and Human Services.[18]

In the case of office-based facilities, the design of the operating rooms should reflect as much as possible the particular procedures to be performed in them. Operating rooms capable of supporting virtually all possible operating procedures are not necessary, and such rooms are often more costly than smaller, more specialized designs.

Whatever the anticipated surgical procedure, the operating room should be large enough to allow for gowning of the operating team, easy movement of the circulating nurse and anesthesia team without contamination of sterile areas, space for technologically advanced operating equipment (i.e., lasers, microscopes, laparoscopic insufflators, video equipment), rapid access to the patient with resuscitative equipment, and easy access of a gurney for postoperative patient transportation. Before proceeding with the architectural design of an ambulatory surgical facility, many managers create fully equipped "mock-ups" of the operating rooms for their surgeons to examine.

Technologic advances in the last several years have led to a gradual increase in operating room dimensions: the minimum size recommended for an operating room for general use in a newly constructed ambulatory surgical facility is 400 square feet. Smaller-sized rooms (260 square feet) may be adequate for some specialized procedures, such as cystoscopy or cataract extration, whereas larger rooms (550 square feet) may be advisable for specialized orthopaedic or gynecologic procedures. Ceiling height should be at least 10 feet to accommodate ceiling mounting of operating room lights, and the floor should be seamless and easily cleaned. If possible, the operating room walls should be designed with the patient in mind, that is, it should be cheery, with brightly-colored paint or wallpaper. Some individuals have suggested that operating rooms should be designed with picture windows.[19] Hospital-based facilities may require larger, more complex operating rooms to provide future flexibility of use. In all cases, a clear idea of the potential uses of the operating rooms is essential to ensure that the facility is neither "locked out" of providing services in the future nor "overbuilt" for its present use.

Well-managed, efficient, ambulatory surgical programs are labor-intensive. Depending on the number of operating days per week, the average length of a procedure, the available hours of operating room time per day, and the efficiency of operating room turnover, a well-managed facility should accommodate between 800 and 2,000 patients per operating room per year. At its peak load, a suite of four operating rooms may be required to handle as many as 10 to 20 patients per hour.[11]

Scheduling

There are basically two types of scheduling paradigms: open room (first-come, first-served) and block (preference time). With the open room format, maximum flexibility of staffing and equipment utilization is possible. In larger facilities in which several operating rooms are involved, this type of scheduling also allows for the manipulation of the schedule by managers to maximize the use of equipment and staff. The principal disadvantage of open room scheduling is that it favors those cases that can be scheduled well in advance, such as plastic or ophthalmologic surgery. When operating room space is in short supply, which of course is the goal of every facility, this format puts cases such as last-minute vascular access cases, breast biopsies, and hernia repairs at a distinct disadvantage.

Block scheduling avoids this problem, as it saves operating rooms for those surgeons who consistently use them. Block scheduling more accurately predicts staffing supply, equipment, and instrument needs. The principal disadvantage of block scheduling occurs when surgeons fail to use their "reserved" time. When practicable, a combination of the two methods may create the best system, allowing for both protection of consistent users and flexibility of staffing and equipment use. This hybrid system works best in larger facilities, but can be effective in facilities with as few as two rooms.

Finally, it should be noted that in facilities specializing in a particular type or limited number of types of procedures, many of the advantages of flexibility found with open scheduling are achieved automatically.

Data Acquisition

In order to comply with various codes for quality assurance and to properly bill patients for services rendered, data concerning each patient visit must be collected and saved. Today, such data acquisition almost inevitably presupposes computerization. Before establishing a computerized data acquisition system, just what is expected from the system and how best to accomplish these expectations should be determined. Minimally, such a system should meet governmental and JCAHO requirements for quality assurance and should supply documentation for billing. By collecting and storing additional data on cases performed, various types of other potentially helpful reports (e.g., operating room utilization and surgical service activity reports) can be generated. The larger the facility, the more useful such reports are for analyzing the efficiency of operations and delineating problem areas. Conversely, in small facilities, such as an office-based practice, complicated systems are often unnecessary and costly, not only in capital outlay, but in upkeep as well. Any data that are to be used in the generation of reports and/or bills must be collected and entered by some human agent. Having a physician do this work puts a high price on the collection of such data, and the output must provide information worth this cost. In facilities with large case loads, it becomes economically feasible to hire clerical staff, thereby reducing the cost per item entered.

There are three potentially important areas of data storage and use: case data, including demographics for billing and quality assurance; inventory data, for control of available supplies and reordering; and scheduling data, for optimization of personnel and material usage. To store and retrieve such information, numerous commercially available software packages are available that range from simple billing programs to intricate program sets covering portions of all three areas mentioned. As these programs become more complex and adaptable to practice setups, the need for skilled support staff increases. Simple programs, which require fewer support staff, offer far fewer options and are relatively inflexible. Software can often be customized to fit the needs and operations of a practice more closely. Such software is usually more expensive and requires support staff for data entry but offers significant advantages, particularly to more complex practices.

The following is a brief description of one such customized system for both inpatient and outpatient procedures. This type of program could be adapted easily to serve the needs of a freestanding ambulatory surgical facility. The system processes data from approximately 14,000 cases per year. The data is input from a custom-designed form that is filled out either by an anesthesia staff member for all procedures involving anesthesia or by an operating room nurse for all local procedures (Fig. 2-5). A data set is

ANESTHESIA COMPUTER INPUT DOCUMENT

DATE of procedure: ____________

AGE: ________ years ________ months

SEX: M F (circle one) RACE: ________

ASA STATUS: ________ (1-5)

PRIMARY INPUT ☐

SECONDARY INPUT ☐

PATIENT STATUS ☐ INPATIENT ☐ OUTPATIENT ☐ DAY SURGERY

INSURANCE
1. ☐ MEDICADE / MEDICARE
2. ☐ BLUE CROSS / BLUE SHIELD
3. ☐ OTHER THIRD PARTY
4. ☐ SELF INSURED
5. ☐ I.D.P.A. / G.A.
6. ☐ NONE / UNKNOWN

TIMES: (use 24 hour clock with NO punctuation — 0000 to 2359)

ROOM TIME	**ANES TIME**	**SURG TIME**
START ______ END ______	START ______ END ______	START ______ END ______
		SCHEDULED TIME IN HRS. ______

SURGERY SERVICE: ____________

	training credit
ATTENDING ____________	
RESIDENT ____________	☐
FIRST ASST. ____________	☐
SECOND ASST. ____________	☐

ANESTHESIA

	case credit
ATTENDING ____________	
FIRST ASST. ____________	☐
SECOND ASST. ____________	☐
THIRD ASST. ____________	☐

ROOM: Area ________ (B, G, J, L, S, or O) Number ________

PROPOSED OPERATION ____________ (40 chrs. maximum)

OPERATION DONE ____________

PRE-OP DIAGNOSIS ____________

POST-OP DIAGNOSIS ____________

CPT # ________ BASIC UNITS ________

CASE STATUS
☐ REGULARLY SCHED.
☐ URGENT CASE
☐ EMERGENCY

(CHECK ONE IN EACH CATAGORY)

REGION/PROCEDURE
☐ INTRA-ABDOMINAL
☐ INTRA-THORACIC
☐ INTRA-CRANIAL
☐ VAGINAL DELIVERY
☐ C-SECTION
☐ EMERG. RESUSC.
☐ E.C.T.
☐ PAIN TREATMENT
☐ ALL OTHERS

POSITION
☐ SUPINE
☐ SITTING
☐ JACKKNIFE/LITHOTOMY
☐ LATERAL
☐ PRONE

ANESTHESIA
☐ GENERAL
☐ SPINAL
☐ EPIDURAL
☐ NERVE BLOCK
☐ MONITOR
☐ LOCAL by SURGEON
☐ OTHER ________

AGENT
☐ NITROUS OXIDE
☐ HALOTHANE
☐ ETHRANE
☐ FORANE
☐ PENTATHOL
☐ KETAMINE
☐ LOCAL -caine-
☐ NARCOTIC
☐ OTHER ________

RELAXANTS: ☐ SUX ☐ DTC ☐ PAV ☐ ATR ☐ VEC ☐ NONE ☐ OTHER ________

REVERSAL: ☐ PROSTIG ☐ PYRIDOSTIG ☐ EDROPHONIUM ☐ NONE

(CHECK OR COMPLETE ALL ITEMS THAT APPLY)

AIRWAYS
☐ MASK
☐ OROTRACHEAL
☐ NASOTRACHEAL
☐ CRASH INDUCTION
☐ AWAKE INTUBATION
☐ FIBER OPTIC SCOPE

HEMODYNAMICS
☐ EKG
☐ CVP
☐ ARTERIAL LINE
☐ P.A. CATHETER
☐ DELIBERATE HYPOTENSION
☐ EXTRA CORPOREAL CIRCULATION

SPECIAL TECHNIQUES
☐ INDUCED HYPOTHERMIA
☐ CLOSED CIRCUIT
☐ DOUBLE LUMEN TUBE
☐ EEG MONITORING
☐ N.G. TUBE
☐ FOLEY CATHETER

MISC.
☐ COMPLICATIONS ________
☐ PATHOLOGY SPECIMEN(S)
☐ CHEST TUBE(S)
☐ ANTIBIOTICS
☐ OTHER ________

____

pts. ________

FLUID REPLACEMENT
BLOOD ________ units
F.F.P. ________ units
PLATELETS ________ units
COLLOID ________ cc's
CRYSTALLOID ________ cc's
BLOOD GAS ANALYSES (No.) ________

SURGEON SEARCH FIELDS
#1. ________
#2. ________
#3. ________
#4. ________
(15 chrs. maximum)

Fig. 2-5. Customized form to be filled out by an anesthesia staff member or by the operating room circulating nurse for a surgical procedure.

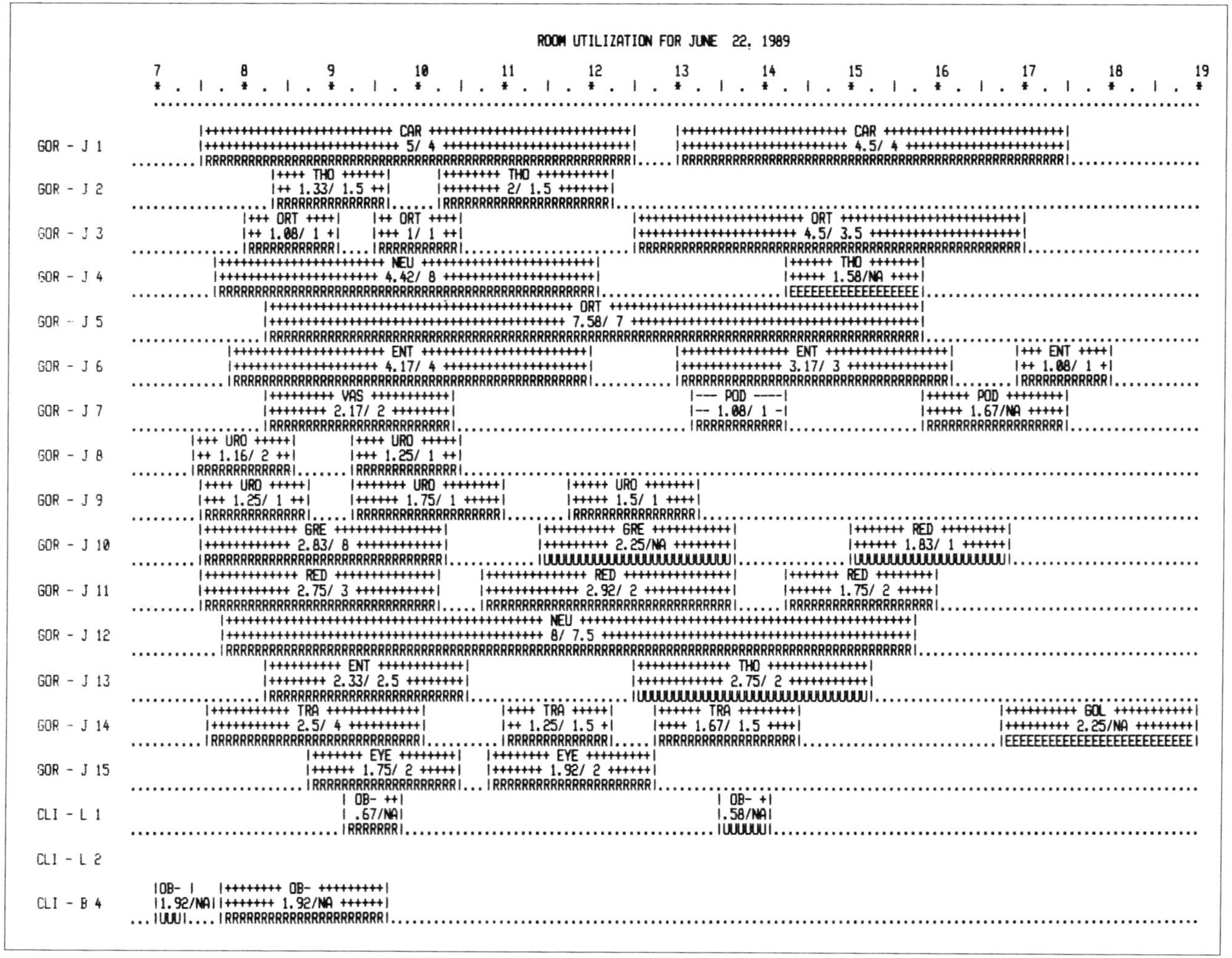

```
                                        ROOM UTILIZATION FOR JUNE  22, 1989

            7       8       9       10      11      12      13      14      15      16      17      18      19
            * . | . * . | . * . | . * . | . * . | . * . | . * . | . * . | . * . | . * . | . * . | . * . | . *

GOR - J 1      |++++++ CAR ++++++|           |++++++ CAR ++++++|
               |++++++ 5/ 4 +++++|           |++++++ 4.5/ 4 +++|
               |RRRRRRRRRRRRRRRRR|           |RRRRRRRRRRRRRRRRR|
GOR - J 2      |++++ THO ++++++|  |++++++++ THO ++++++++++|
               |++ 1.33/ 1.5 ++|  |++++++++ 2/ 1.5 +++++++|
               |RRRRRRRRRRRRRRR|  |RRRRRRRRRRRRRRRRRRRRRRR|
GOR - J 3      |+++ ORT ++++|  |++ ORT ++++|     |+++++++ ORT +++++++|
               |++ 1.08/ 1 +|  |+++ 1/ 1 ++|     |+++++ 4.5/ 3.5 ++++|
               |RRRRRRRRRRRR|  |RRRRRRRRRRR|     |RRRRRRRRRRRRRRRRRRR|
GOR - J 4      |+++++++ NEU +++++++|     |++++++ THO +++++++|
               |++++++ 4.42/ 8 ++++|     |+++++ 1.58/NA ++++|
               |RRRRRRRRRRRRRRRRRRR|     |EEEEEEEEEEEEEEEEEE|
GOR - J 5      |+++++++++++++ ORT +++++++++++++|
               |+++++++++++ 7.58/ 7 +++++++++++|
               |RRRRRRRRRRRRRRRRRRRRRRRRRRRRRRR|
GOR - J 6      |++++++ ENT ++++++|  |++++++ ENT ++++++|  |+++ ENT ++++|
               |+++++ 4.17/ 4 +++|  |+++++ 3.17/ 3 +++|  |++ 1.08/ 1 +|
               |RRRRRRRRRRRRRRRRR|  |RRRRRRRRRRRRRRRRR|  |RRRRRRRRRRRR|
GOR - J 7      |+++++++++ VAS ++++++++++|  |--- POD ----|  |++++++ POD ++++++++|
               |+++++++++ 2.17/ 2 ++++++++|  |-- 1.08/ 1 -|  |+++++ 1.67/NA +++++|
               |RRRRRRRRRRRRRRRRRRRRRRRRR|  |RRRRRRRRRRRR|  |RRRRRRRRRRRRRRRRRRR|
GOR - J 8      |+++ URO +++++|  |++++ URO +++++|
               |++ 1.16/ 2 ++|  |+++ 1.25/ 1 ++|
               |RRRRRRRRRRRRR|  |RRRRRRRRRRRRRRR|
GOR - J 9      |++++ URO +++++|  |+++++++ URO ++++++++|  |+++++ URO +++++++|
               |+++ 1.25/ 1 ++|  |++++++ 1.75/ 1 +++++|  |+++++ 1.5/ 1 ++++|
               |RRRRRRRRRRRRRR|  |RRRRRRRRRRRRRRRRRRRR|  |RRRRRRRRRRRRRRRRR|
GOR - J 10     |+++++++++++++ GRE +++++++++++++++|  |++++++++++ GRE +++++++++++|  |+++++++ RED +++++++++|
               |++++++++++++ 2.83/ 8 +++++++++++++|  |+++++++++ 2.25/NA ++++++++|  |++++++ 1.83/ 1 ++++++|
               |RRRRRRRRRRRRRRRRRRRRRRRRRRRRRRRRRR|  |UUUUUUUUUUUUUUUUUUUUUUUUUU|  |UUUUUUUUUUUUUUUUUUUUU|
GOR - J 11     |+++++++++++++ RED +++++++++++++++|  |+++++++++++++ RED +++++++++++++++|  |+++++++ RED ++++++++|
               |++++++++++++ 2.75/ 3 +++++++++++|  |+++++++++++++ 2.92/ 2 ++++++++++++|  |++++++ 1.75/ 2 +++++|
               |RRRRRRRRRRRRRRRRRRRRRRRRRRRRRRR|  |RRRRRRRRRRRRRRRRRRRRRRRRRRRRRRRRR|  |RRRRRRRRRRRRRRRRRRRR|
GOR - J 12     |+++++++++++++++++++++ NEU +++++++++++++++++++++|
               |+++++++++++++++++++ 8/ 7.5 +++++++++++++++++++|
               |RRRRRRRRRRRRRRRRRRRRRRRRRRRRRRRRRRRRRRRRRRRRRRR|
GOR - J 13     |++++++++++ ENT ++++++++++++|  |+++++++++++++ THO ++++++++++++++|
               |++++++++ 2.33/ 2.5 ++++++++|  |++++++++++++ 2.75/ 2 +++++++++++|
               |RRRRRRRRRRRRRRRRRRRRRRRRRRR|  |UUUUUUUUUUUUUUUUUUUUUUUUUUUUUUUU|
GOR - J 14     |+++++++++++ TRA +++++++++++++|  |++++ TRA +++++|  |++++++ TRA ++++++++|  |++++++++++ GOL ++++++++++++|
               |++++++++++ 2.5/ 4 ++++++++++|  |++ 1.25/ 1.5 +|  |++++ 1.67/ 1.5 ++++|  |+++++++++ 2.25/NA ++++++++|
               |RRRRRRRRRRRRRRRRRRRRRRRRRRRR|  |RRRRRRRRRRRRRRR|  |RRRRRRRRRRRRRRRRRRR|  |EEEEEEEEEEEEEEEEEEEEEEEEEEE|
GOR - J 15     |+++++++ EYE ++++++++|  |++++++++ EYE +++++++++|
               |++++++ 1.75/ 2 +++++|  |+++++++ 1.92/ 2 ++++++|
               |RRRRRRRRRRRRRRRRRRRR|  |RRRRRRRRRRRRRRRRRRRRRR|
CLI - L 1      | OB- ++|       | OB- +|
               | .67/NA|       |.58/NA|
               |RRRRRRR|       |UUUUUU|
CLI - L 2

CLI - B 4      |OB-  |  |++++++++ OB- +++++++++|
               |1.92/NA|  |+++++++ 1.92/NA ++++++|
               |UUU|  |RRRRRRRRRRRRRRRRRRRRRR|
```

Fig. 2-6. Graphic display of operating room activity for 1 day.

TOTAL — ABA REPORT FOR JUNE, 1989 — TOTAL CASES: 1133

REGION/POSITION		TECHNIQUE		AGENT		ASA CAT.		STATUS		TIMES		SCHEDULE	
INTRA-ABDOMINAL:	207	GENERAL:	680	NITROUS OXIDE:	15	I:	288	INPATIENT:	857	ROOM:	2622.062	REG. SCHEDULE:	835
INTRA-THORACIC:	57	SPINAL:	24	HALOTHANE:	75	II:	439	OUTPATIENT:	276	ANES.:	2966.15	URGENT CASE:	143
INTRA-CRANIAL:	26	EPIDURAL:	109	ETHRANE:	124	III:	299	DAY SURGERY:	0	SURG.:	1932.459	EMERGENCY CASE:	155
VAGINAL DELIVERY:	71	NERVE BLOCK:	33	KETAMINE:	10	IV:	99						
C-SECTION:	40	MONITORING:	167	NARCOTIC:	177	V:	8						
RESUSCITATION:	0	OTHER:	120	LOCAL AGENT:	326								
E.C.T. :	5			OTHER ANES.:	406								
PAIN TREATMENT:	0												
ALL OTHERS:	727												
ABA OTHERS:	732												

AGE UNDER 2 years:	39
AGE 2 TO 12 years:	70
AGE 12 TO 70 years:	881
AGE OVER 70 years:	143

MALES:	443
FEMALES:	690

POSITIONS) SUPINE: 851 SITTING: 4 LITHOTOMY: 198 LATERAL: 47 PRONE: 33

****

MONITORING, SPECIAL TECHNIQUES, ETC.

MASK:	146	CLOSED CIRCUIT:	37	ARTERIAL LINE:	169	CRASH INDUCTION:	66
ORAL INTUBATION:	547	HYPOTHERMIA:	0	CVP:	169	DOUBLE LUMEN TUBE:	5
NASAL INTUBATION:	31	HYPOTENSION:	3	P.A. CATHETER:	24	FIBER OPTIC SCOPE:	8
AWAKE INTUBATION:	6	EXTRA CORPOREAL CIRCULATION:	20	COMPLICATIONS:	0		

****

CASES WITH CRNA's: 516 CASES WITHOUT CRNA's: 552

TOTAL UNITS GENERATED:	28616
BASE UNITS GENERATED:	6638
MODIFYING UNITS:	6252
TIME UNITS GENERATED:	15726

Fig. 2-7. American Board of Anesthesiologists report of procedures performed by one department showing the breakdown of information provided by a customized software program.

ROOM UTILIZATION REPORT FOR JUNE, 1989 ROOM: J 1

VARIABLE	MONDAY	TUESDAY	WEDNESDAY	THURSDAY	FRIDAY	SATURDAY	SUNDAY	TOTAL	
TOTAL CASES	10	5	6	7	10	0	0	38	
AVAILABLE PREFERENCE TIME	32.00	32.00	32.00	40.00	40.00	0.00	0.00	176.00	
AVAILABLE UNASSIGNED TIME	25.50	15.76	23.84	28.37	25.42	0.00	0.00	118.89	
AVAILABLE NON-PREF. TIME	58.00	58.00	58.00	72.50	72.50	96.00	96.00	511.00	
TOTAL PREFERENCE TIME	12.50	22.24	14.16	19.13	22.08	0.00	0.00	90.11	
TOTAL UNASSIGNED TIME	13.99	4.67	14.25	6.75	4.58	0.00	0.00	44.24	
TOTAL NON-PREF. TIME	5.74	0.08	2.32	2.50	8.00	0.00	0.00	18.64	
% TOTAL TIME - PREFERENCE	0.388	0.823	0.461	0.674	0.637	0.000	0.000	0.589	
% TOTAL TIME - UNASSIGNED	0.434	0.173	0.464	0.238	0.132	0.000	0.000	0.289	
% TOTAL TIME - NON-PREF.	0.178	0.003	0.075	0.088	0.231	0.000	0.000	0.122	
% AVAILABLE - PREFERENCE	0.391	0.695	0.443	0.478	0.552	0.000	0.000	0.512	
% AVAILABLE - UNASSIGNED	0.549	0.296	0.598	0.238	0.180	0.000	0.000	0.372	
% AVAILABLE - NON-PREF.	0.099	0.001	0.040	0.034	0.110	0.000	0.000	0.036	
TOTAL ROOM TIME	32.24	27.01	30.74	28.38	34.66	0.00	0.00	153.03	
TOTAL ANES. TIME	33.50	29.33	31.66	31.58	37.58	0.00	0.00	163.65	
TOTAL SURG. TIME	23.33	20.83	25.17	19.92	25.00	0.00	0.00	114.25	
AVERAGE ROOM TIME	3.22	5.40	5.12	4.05	3.47	0.00	0.00	4.03	
AVERAGES									
ROOM - SURGERY DIFF.	0.89	1.24	0.93	1.21	0.97	0.00	0.00	1.02	
ANES. - SURGERY DIFF.	1.02	1.70	1.08	1.67	1.26	0.00	0.00	1.30	
ROOM - ANES. DIFF.	-0.13	-0.46	-0.15	-0.46	-0.29	0.00	0.00	-0.28	
USED HOURS									
7:00 to 3:30	0.640	0.695	0.700	0.478	0.552	0.000	0.000	0.576	0.613
7:00 to 5:00	0.697	0.708	0.748	0.545	0.561	0.000	0.000	0.643	0.652
7:00 TO 3:30 ctd:	0.734	0.711	0.732	0.503	0.614	0.000	0.000	0.621	0.659
7:00 to 5:00 ctd:	0.776	0.721	0.774	0.566	0.614	0.000	0.000	0.681	0.690

SCHEDULING ACCURACY SUMMARY FOR JUNE 1989
(alphabetical listing)

SERVICE	TOT # OF CASES	AVG. CASE TIME	RELATIONSHIP BETWEEN ACTUAL AND BOOKED TIMES WITHIN: 10%	25%	ABOVE 150%	AVERAGE DISCREPENCIES: HOURS	PERCENT
CARDIAC	24	4.6	25	66.6	20.8	1	27.2
DENTAL	5	2.7	0	80	0	-1.1	26.1
DERMATOLOGY	7	.9	0	57.1	28.5	.2	20
ENT	66	2.4	27.2	51.5	24.2	.5	26.6
EYE	30	2.1	26.6	70	10	.1	2.6
GOLD	54	3.2	7.4	37	42.5	1	43.5
GREEN	58	3	18.9	41.3	27.5	.4	16.1
HEME	4	1.8	25	75	0	.1	3.5
MISC.	17	.9	11.7	17.6	0	-.8	41.8
NEUROSURGERY	44	4.1	27.2	70.4	4.5	-.3	5.6
OB-GYN	53	1.7	22.6	56.6	13.2	.1	4.6
OPHTH	1	2.5	0	0	100	1	66.6
ORAL SURGERY	11	3.5	18.1	18.1	27.2	.8	31.3
ORTHOPEDICS	99	2.3	20.2	48.4	16.1	.1	3.6
PLASTICS	46	3.8	21.7	56.5	21.7	.5	15.5
PODIATRY	18	1.7	38.8	50	33.3	.4	26.5
RED	55	1.7	30.9	54.5	25.4	.2	14.8
THORACIC	37	1.9	18.9	35.1	13.5	0	.4
TRAUMA	20	1.9	35	75	10	.1	5.7
UROLOGY	64	1.9	23.4	57.8	15.6	.1	3.4
VASCULAR	23	4.7	8.6	26	26	1.2	34.9

Fig. 2-9. A report of the accuracy of scheduling, separated by surgical service.

stored daily so that any one day's cases can be quickly accessed. Quality assurance data regarding each case is gathered and stored in a separate file. From these files, various reports are produced on a daily and monthly basis.

Professional fees for anesthesiologists and surgeons are produced each day. These bills either can be generated as hard copy ready to be sent out, if the facility does its own collections, or can be electronically transferred to an outside agency. This system also produces a graphic representation of the previous day's operating room activity (Fig. 2-6). Displayed for each case are the surgical service, the scheduled time, the actual time used, and whether the case was regularly scheduled, urgent, or emergent. Since the display also shows "down times" between cases, this report enables the facility manager to easily track the efficiency of the facility on a day-to-day basis and to deal with any systematic problems as they arise.

Reports that show utilization efficiency, patient mix, inpatient versus outpatient dis-

←

Fig. 2-8. Typical operating room utilization report for 1 week. Preference time is a block of time reserved for certain surgeons on a regular basis; nonpreference time is allocated for surgery but not reserved for particular surgeons; and unassigned time is the time available at night or on weekends that is not routinely scheduled for surgery.

tribution, and other information required by the system's users are generated each month. In our academic setting, monthly reports indicate (1) cases worked and techniques utilized by each anesthesia staff member, (2) cases worked by groups of attending staff, (3) and types of cases handled (Figs. 2-7). Cases performed are listed by surgical service, attending surgeon, and resident physician. In order to allow the nursing staff to readily modify staffing patterns, a room utilization report shows the use of each operating room (Fig. 2-8). A surgical service activity report indicates the assigned block time and time available to each surgical service. Since inappropriate scheduling can be extremely destructive to facility efficiency, a report of the accuracy of scheduling by various surgeons or surgical services is often helpful in reminding surgeons to reserve space accurately (Fig. 2-9). An important concern to facility managers is budgeting for future operating room utilization, both in funds and staff; one report helpful in this regard compares the number of cases worked in 1 month to the number worked that month of the previous year (Fig. 2-10). This data is presented on a service-by-service basis, with displays of data for both the base year and the comparison year. Other reports, such as those showing patient mix by insurers or a categorization of cases by their start and end times, can be useful in planning and operations management. Running such a system in-house makes accountability possible, as the efficiency of the facility's operating practices are readily available. The disadvantages include the necessity of purchasing costly software and hardware, as well as the problems associated with support of the system.

Recovery Room

Regardless of the simplicity of planned procedures or the health of prospective patients, any facility that provides anesthesia involving loss of consciousness or protective reflexes must provide for full recovery of the anesthetized patient. This includes equipment for resuscitation, pharmacologic support, ventilatory support, and all monitoring equipment. In facilities in which recovery from general anesthesia is not expected, the preoperative holding area or the operating room itself can serve this purpose. For the most part, when planning an ambulatory surgical facility, a general recovery room should be included, since lack of such provision will severely limit the flexibility of the facility and preclude the potential use of general anesthesia. The general recovery room must be completely equipped, regardless of the prospective patient population. In hospital-based facilities it is always tempting to use an existing recovery area as the phase I or general recovery facility for the ambulatory surgery unit. When the hospital's postanesthesia care unit (PACU) has available beds, their use can provide a substantial cost savings. There are, however, serious drawbacks to such an arrangement, mostly related to the difference in care given outpatients and inpatients. Generally, the ambience of a regular hospital PACU is not in keeping with that sought for ambulatory surgical patients. This may seem a trivial point; however, its importance in a world of competitive facilities cannot be overemphasized.

A recovery area more specifically serving ambulatory surgery is usually called the "step-down" recovery unit. Ideally, patients brought to this unit will be alert and easily able to sit, having recovered to this point from general anesthesia, regional anesthesia, or monitored anesthesia care. It is from this unit that patients are discharged. In the step-down unit, patients are given oral fluids, are allowed to become ambulatory, and, in many institutions, are kept until they are able to void. The exact criteria for discharge may vary, but some systematic method of patient assessment is absolutely essential and should be documented in each case. In fact, the application of such a set of criteria is mandated by the JCAHO.

SERVICE	JUL.	AUG.	SEP.	OCT.	NOV.	DEC.	JAN.	FEB.	MAR.	APR.	MAY.	JUN.	TOT.	AVG.
BLUE	-17	-10	4	-40	-40	-20	-30	-32	-36	-47	-43	-35	-346	-28.9
CARDIAC	21	15	13	-3	16	-5	5	4	11	15	19	15	126	10.5
DENTAL	4	6	6	3	5	3	1	4	4	-1	-2	2	35	2.9
DERMATOLOGY	------	1	7	6	2	-3	7	-11	5	3	------	-9	8	.6
ENT	-4	15	-6	14	25	-18	-9	5	23	-11	6	-9	31	2.5
EYE	-8	-3	-2	-21	-4	-9	------	9	9	9	6	-7	-21	-1.8
GOLD	12	-17	-35	-3	7	-4	-6	3	41	-23	25	14	14	1.1
GREEN	-8	-7	-7	-4	-31	-16	13	6	-8	-29	26	8	-57	-4.8
HEME	2	-1	4	-2	5	-3	2	------	1	5	-2	1	12	1
MISC.	2	4	2	-4	-4	-6	4	4	2	------	-4	13	13	1
NEUROSURGERY	-12	5	-9	-14	-1	-16	-1	3	26	-8	-13	-24	-64	-5.4
ORAL SURGERY	-6	-2	-11	-4	-3	-1	-2	-1	-3	6	6	-3	-24	-2
ORTHOPEDICS	-8	48	-7	-6	-9	27	19	2	-19	-24	13	3	39	3.2
PEDIATRICS	-46	-62	-51	-37	-46	-55	-44	-56	-29	-7	------	-1	-434	-36.2
PLASTICS	-12	-11	-14	-2	7	-1	4	-20	-6	-34	1	-25	-113	-9.5
PODIATRY	-2	4	-24	8	-8	-4	3	2	-6	-3	8	-4	-26	-2.2
PSYCHIATRY	1	-9	-21	-3	-5	-5	2	1	-9	------	-3	4	-47	-4
RED	-6	23	4	-6	3	12	15	19	12	4	2	3	85	7
THORACIC	-26	8	-26	-21	-16	-22	-12	4	11	4	14	17	-65	-5.5
TRAUMA	24	32	46	24	27	35	58	23	15	20	13	22	339	28.2
UROLOGY	15	-14	-2	8	-9	-9	7	4	10	14	-16	7	15	1.2
VASCULAR	-10	2	-3	------	1	-17	7	-12	-7	-9	20	7	-21	-1.8
TOTAL	-84	27	-132	-107	-78	-137	43	-39	47	-116	76	-1	-501	xxxxxx
AVERAGE	-3.8	1.2	-6	-4.9	-3.5	-6.2	2	-1.8	2.1	-5.3	3.5	0	xxxxxx	-1.9
OB-GYN	-23	54	18	38	40	-31	59	2	11	27	40	-21	214	17.8
TOTAL	-107	81	-114	-69	-38	-168	102	-37	58	-89	116	-22	-287	xxxxxx
AVERAGE	-4.7	3.5	-5	-3	-1.7	-7.3	4.4	-1.6	2.5	-3.9	5	-1	xxxxxx	-1.1

Fig. 2-10. Operating room case report, separated by service, comparing data for 1 month with data for that same month the previous year.

Perhaps the most important equipment in this area should be a comfortable lounge chair capable of reclining fully so that the patient can assume a Trendelenburg position. The chair should be easily washable and have an integrated IV pole, although this feature may have to be added after purchase. An important feature of the chair is its mobility, since overall facility efficiency and convenience is much enhanced if the recovery chair can be moved easily into the operating room for patient transport postoperatively to the step-down unit. This feature avoids the necessity of an intermediate transport device, such as a wheelchair. For nonambulatory patients, such as those receiving podiatric surgery, the chair can be used to transport patients to the postoperative changing area at the time of discharge. At some institutions, space limitations have led to the use of a single area for preoperative holding and postoperative step-down recovery. This has obvious drawbacks and should be avoided whenever possible.

Floor Plans of Hospital-Independent Facilities

The floor plan of an ambulatory surgical facility that demonstrates many of the design features presented in the previous pages is presented in Figure 2-11.

GUIDELINES FOR A SAME-DAY SURGERY CENTER

At the University of Chicago, our hospital-based, Same-Day Surgical Center functions under the guidelines that follow. These guidelines are presented to demonstrate that even a large, complex, tertiary-care hospital can establish an ambulatory surgical program that can compete effectively with smaller freestanding facilities. Of course, these guidelines can be adapted easily to accommodate various facilities, including those that are hospital-independent.

University of Chicago Same-Day Surgery Center Guidelines

The Same-Day Surgery Center operating rooms represent a new approach to surgical care for our institution. They are much more than replacement rooms for some of our hospital surgical suites. As outpatient surgery continues to grow in relation to inpatient procedures, the Same-Day Surgery Center can serve as a paradigm for future expansion of University of Chicago outpatient surgical centers. In this light, certain goals must be met. The center's surgery suites must provide state-of-the-art care to patients while operating at a high level of efficiency. Turn-around times must be held to an absolute minimum. Delays in patient arrival and workup must be avoided, and medical coverage, both by surgery and anesthesia, must be prompt and efficient.

Given the harsh economic environment in which the institution is forced to compete, and the absolute necessity of expanding our presence in the community, the Same-Day Surgery Center must serve as a pilot program for future outpatient services. To do this effectively, it must be treated from the onset as a ''stand alone'' center and show its profitability as such. To achieve these goals, certain rules and regulations pertaining to the center's use must be observed. Guidelines that we feel will lead in this direction are presented in Appendix 2-1.

If these guidelines are followed, it is possible to achieve an environment that is pleasant and efficient for both patients and staff.

OFFICE-BASED SURGERY

To some extent the growth of office-based surgery has paralleled the growth of the ambulatory surgery movement in general. Ophthalmologic and plastic surgery have been at the forefront of the office-based surgery movement and have pro-

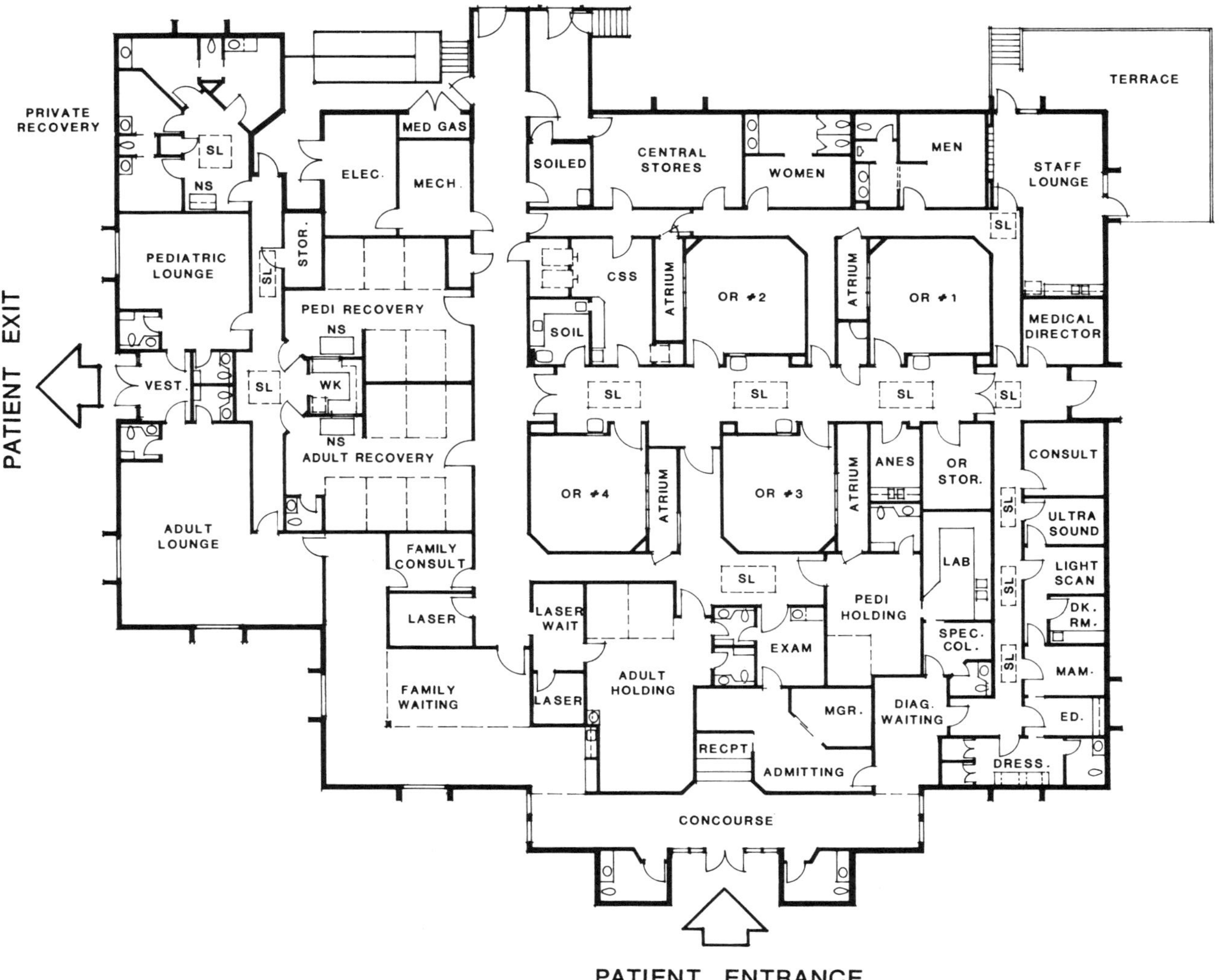

Fig. 2-11. Floor plan for ambulatory surgical center. (Courtesy of The Burford Group, Inc., Architects, Houston, TX, 1989.)

gressed so far as to create their own accrediting association (American Association for the Accreditation of Ambulatory Plastic Surgery Facilities [AAAAPSF]) and subspecialty society (Outpatient Ophthalmic Surgery Society [OOSS]). The principal advantages of office-based surgery are in large part the same as those for other types of ambulatory surgical facilities, that is, patient convenience, surgeon convenience, staff satisfaction, greater economic benefit, and more flexibility. However, the office-based facility clearly skews the distribution of benefits toward the surgeon.

The increased convenience for the surgeon comes primarily from consolidating his or her entire practice in one location, resulting in a substantial savings of time and energy. Because the surgeon has control of the facility schedule, competition with other physicians for optimal surgical operating time is eliminated. Staff may be hired and equipment purchased to suit his or her particular needs. Lastly, paperwork is generally reduced because the rules and regulations for office-based facilities are more streamlined than those for their hospital counterparts.

Patients sometimes prefer office-based surgery because the environment is less threatening than that of a hospital or even a facility designed exclusively for surgery. Since they are already familiar with the office facility, patients are not likely to be alarmed on the day of surgery by new surroundings or personnel. Patients often view office care as more personalized than comparable care provided in a larger facility.

Several studies have suggested that office-based surgery, particularly plastic and ophthalmologic procedures, significantly reduces the overall cost of surgical care. Porterfield and Franklin[12] reviewed over 13,000 plastic surgery procedures performed in their office surgical facility over a 16-year period and concluded a cost savings to the facility, patients, and third-party payers of 30 to 50 percent when compared with identical procedures performed on hospital inpatients. In this review, the authors' comparison of surgical costs did not include the expense of an overnight hospital stay. The OOSS has conservatively estimated that if all ophthalmologic surgical procedures, with the exception of transcranial orbitotomy and exenteration of the orbit, were performed on an ambulatory basis, approximately 1 billion dollars would be save annually.[20]

The principal disadvantage of office-based surgery is the high cost associated with its construction and maintenance. The changing medicolegal environment and mandates from third-party payers (including the federal and some state governments) have led to the requirement for more sophisticated facilities. Previously, office-based surgical facilities stocked barely enough equipment to perform surgery safely and economically. These same facilities are now expending a more intensive effort to meet all the safety standards of competing fully equipped ambulatory surgical facilities. Backup electrical generators, fire-safety equipment, state-of-the-art monitors, defibrillators, and fully equipped "crash" carts are now found in many office-based facilities.

Although many localities and states permit the operation of office-based surgical facilities without accreditation, or in some instances even without licensure, many office-based surgical facilities actively seek accreditation from one of the nationally recognized agencies (the AAAHC, Skokie, Illinois; or the JCAHO, Chicago, Illinois) in order to ensure that they qualify for reimbursement from third-party payers.

Rapid technologic advances that have produced expensive new operating room equipment (e.g., lasers and microscopes), as well as the changing medicolegal environment, have made the expense of designing, building, equipping, and managing the office-based surgical facility much higher in the last decade. Nevertheless, the practice continues to grow, not only because surgeons generally recognize a profit from these facilities, but also, and primarily, because of the tremendous savings in time and the convenience that these specialized facilities offer both to surgeons and to their patients.

SUMMARY

With the rapid pharmacologic and technical advances in anesthesia and surgery, the ambulatory setting has become a realistic option for an increasing number of surgical procedures. Whether an outpatient center is hospital-based or hospital-independent, it provides services—beyond the actual surgical procedure—that are very attractive to patients. Surgeons, too, prefer the smaller, more manageable setting of an ambulatory surgical facility because it is more flexible and less bureaucratic than the traditional hospital. Finally, efficiency and cost-effectiveness are provided without the sacrifice of quality care, making these facilities appealing to third-party payers.

REFERENCES

1. Perrin JM, Valvona J, Sloan FA: Changing patterns of hospitalization for children requiring surgery. Pediatrics 77:587, 1986
2. Ambulatory Surgery Report of the American College of Surgeons, Chicago, IL, 1983
3. MacAlister RA: p. 133. Textbook of European Archaeology. 1921
4. Detmer DE, Buchanan-Davidson DJ: Ambulatory surgery. Surg Clin North Am 62:685, 1982
5. Nicoll JH, Glasg CM: The surgery of infancy. Br Med J 2:753, 1909
6. Waters RM: The down-town anesthesia clinic. Am J Surg (anesthesia suppl) 33:71, 1919
7. Davis JE: The major ambulatory surgical center and how it is developed. Surg Clin North Am 67:671, 1987
8. Cohen DD, Dillon JB: Anesthesia for outpatient surgery. JAMA 196:98, 1966
9. Levy ML, Coakley CS: Survey of "in and out surgery"—first year. South Med J 61:995, 1968
10. Lahti PT: Early postoperative discharge of patients from the hospital. Surgery 63:410, 1968
11. Ring WH, Wong HC: Designing and administering an OP facility. Probl Anesth 2:1, 1988
12. Porterfield HW, Franklin LT: The use of general anesthesia in the office surgery facility. Clin Plast Surg 10:289, 1983
13. Caldamone AA, Rabinowitz R: Outpatient orchiopexy. J Urol 127:286, 1982
14. Siegel AL, Snyder HM, Duckett JW: Outpatient pediatric urological surgery: techniques for a successful and cost-effective practice. J Urol 136:879, 1986
15. Apfelbaum JC: The adult problem patient. Probl Anesth 2:101, 1988
16. Ginzberg E: The destabilization of health care. N Engl J Med 315:757, 1986
17. Himmelstein DU, Woolhandler S: Cost without benefit. N Engl J Med 314:441, 1986
18. Requirements of construction and equipment for hospitals and medical facilities. Health and Human Services Publication HRS-M-HF-84-1, Rockville, MD, 1974
19. Ulrich R: View through a window may influence recovery from surgery. Science 224:420, 1984
20. Williamson DE: Ambulatory cataract surgery. Int Ophthalmol Clin 27:163, 1987

Appendix 2-1

Guidelines for Establishment of an Ambulatory Surgical Program

I. Hours

A. The Same-Day Surgery Center will be open weekdays from 6:30 A.M. until all cases are finished, operating rooms are cleaned, and the next day's cases have been selected.
B. The postanesthetic recovery room will open daily by 8:00 A.M. and remain open until all patients are discharged.
C. Cases will be scheduled to start from 7:30 A.M.to 2:00 P.M. No case should be scheduled to end after 3:00 P.M.
D. When block time is designated as a half day,
   1. morning block time will be from 7:30 A.M. to 11:00 A.M. and
   2. afternoon block time will be from 11:15 A.M. to 3:00 P.M.

II. Patient flow

A. After a patient's surgery is scheduled, an appointment will be made for the patient to come to the Same-Day Surgery Center for a financial interview, preoperative anesthesia and nursing assessments, and laboratory studies, as indicated.
B. In accordance with our current policies, patients will arrive at the Same-Day Surgery Center at least 1 hour before the scheduled surgical start time. At that time, all required paperwork (laboratory reports, consent forms, medical evaluations, history, and physical forms) should be available. Patients arriving after the expected time may have to be deferred to a later surgical time slot or date.
C. Approximately 30 minutes before surgery or anesthesia is begun, the patient will change clothes and be seated in the preoperative holding area or block room.
D. Upon arrival in the preoperative holding area, all patients who will be receiving anesthesia will be required to sign an affadavit stating that they have not had food for a minimum of 8 hours and that they have made arrangements for a re-

sponsible adult to escort them from the Same-Day Surgery Center.

E. Immediately after surgery, all ambulatory patients will be transferred via wheelchair to the step-down postanesthesia recovery area. There, suitability of recovery will be determined by the anesthesiologist involved. Nonambulatory patients will be transferred via gurney to the regular postanesthesia recovery room, where they will stay until they reach ambulatory status. At that time, they will be transferred via wheelchair to the step-down anesthesia recovery area.

F. For discharge, a patient must meet the following criteria:
 1. return to baseline vital signs;
 2. return to baseline orientation;
 3. the patient is able to ambulate (if ambulatory before surgery and the surgical procedure has not altered that status);
 4. the patient has a responsible escort present in the Center;
 5. the patient has no excessive pain, nausea, or bleeding;
 6. the patient is able to tolerate clear fluid intake without significant nausea;
 7. if the site of surgery involved the genitourinary tract, the patient is able to void;
 8. the patient and escort have been provided with oral *and* written postoperative instructions;
 9. the patient and escort are provided with a mechanism that allows them to contact a physician rapidly should medical assistance be necessary; and
 10. the patient is considered suitable for discharge by the anesthesiologist.

III. Quality assurance

A short report documenting extenuating circumstances will be completed by both the attending surgeon and anesthesiologist in the following situations:

1. surgery extending past 3:00 P.M.;
2. surgery taking more than 20 percent of the scheduled time;
3. any hospital admission other than a scheduled 23-hour admission; or
4. any significant perioperative complication.

IV. Patient restrictions

A. Only outpatients or "23-hour admission" patients may be scheduled for procedures in the Same-Day Surgery Center.

B. Patients with concurrent medical problems who require *extensive* monitoring or care are not eligible for surgery in the Same-Day Surgery Center.

C. All patients must have preoperative financial approval from involved third-party payers.

D. In cases in which patients arrive without preoperative evaluations, appropriate laboratory results, or necessary financial clearance, surgery may be postponed at the discretion of the Same-Day Surgery Center coordinator.

V. Scheduling

A. Cases may be scheduled by calling the schedule desk at the same time preoperative and laboratory testing is scheduled. The schedule desk is open from 6:30 A.M. through 6:00 P.M.

B. For purposes of efficiency, patients should have completed their financial review, preanesthesia evaluation, and laboratory testing *at least 3 working days prior to scheduled surgery*.

C. Block time will be held until 10:00 A.M. *3 working days prior to surgery*, i.e.,

Monday schedule closes at 10 A.M. Wednesday,

Tuesday schedule closes at 10 A.M. Thursday,

Wednesday schedule closes at 10 A.M. Friday,

Thursday schedule closes at 10 A.M. Monday, and

Friday schedule closes at 10 A.M. Tuesday.

D. Unassigned time may be scheduled on a first-come, first-served basis until 10 A.M. the working day prior to surgery.

E. Cases to be scheduled after the appropriate closing time must be approved by the Same-Day Surgery Center coordinator.

F. The Same-Day Surgery Center coordinator will have the option of postponing ambulatory surgery if a conflicting case has been scheduled in the main operating room. Repeated occurrences of this nature will result in loss of operating room time for the surgical service involved.

G. No case may be scheduled to start after 2:00 P.M. or to end after 3:00 P.M.

H. Repeated underbooking or overbooking of cases will result in loss of first-come, first-served or block-time priority for the surgical service involved.

I. All scheduling should include 30 minutes for anesthesia induction and emergence, as well as patient and room preparation.

J. No cases of more than 7 hours' duration should be scheduled unless specifically approved by the Same-Day Surgery Center coordinator.

K. Prior to accepting "special equipment" cases, the Same-Day Surgery Center scheduling secretary will check with the Clinical Manager to avoid any potential equipment conflicts. With clearance from the Clinical Manager, the scheduling secretary will then confirm the surgery with the office making the request.

L. All cases will have a scheduled time (i.e., there will be no "to follow" booking permitted).

VI. Scheduling requirements

A. Patient's full name, age, sex, and phone number;
B. Date and time requested;
C. Outpatient or 23-hour admission;
D. Estimated start and finish times;
E. Name of surgeon and first assistant;
F. Anesthetic requested (choice, general, monitored anesthesia care, local);
G. Patient diagnosis;
H. Operation to be performed;
I. Positioning information; and
J. Special requirements (i.e., microscope or x-ray).

VII. Perioperative physician presence

A. Surgical presence
   1. Whenever possible, surgeons should be able to start cases

earlier than booked to help compensate for occasional "no-shows."

2. When a surgeon is unable to be present in the Same-Day Surgery Center within 15 minutes of the scheduled surgery time, the case may be postponed to a later surgical time slot or date at the discretion of the Same-Day Surgery Center coordinator.
3. No surgeon may book a case in the Same-Day Surgery Center during a time when he or she has a major case scheduled in the main operating rooms.
4. During the entire duration of a case in the Same-Day Surgery Center, the attending surgeon must be available to the center within a maximum of 5 minutes.

B. Anesthesia presence
   1. Whenever there is a case in the Same-Day Surgery Center, an attending anesthesiologist must be available in the immediate area of the center.
   2. A medical member of the Department of Anesthesia and Critical Care (certified registered nurse anesthetist, resident, or attending physician) must be present during the entire anesthetic period for each case scheduled to receive anesthesia care (general, regional, or monitored anesthesia).

C. Attending cross-coverage
   1. Attending surgeons or anesthesiologists who are unable to be present for cases in the Same-Day Surgery Center may arrange cross-coverage by another attending physician. In all cases of cross-coverage, the Same-Day Surgery center coordinator must be informed prior to the implementation of that coverage.
   2. Any failure in attending physician coverage will be documented and reviewed by the Same-Day Surgery Center Operating Room Committee, which will have the power to suspend or revoke that physician's privileges in the center.

VIII. Clinical studies

While clinical studies are encouraged, certain rules and restrictions must be observed in the Same-Day Surgery Center:

1. prior approval by the Institutional Review Board is required;
2. informed consent (when appropriate) must be obtained from the patient prior to surgery;
3. all attending physicians involved in the care of the patient must agree to the clinical study; and
4. no studies may be undertaken that will delay or add to case time by more than 15 minutes.

IX. VIP cases

Since there are restrictions on the patients who receive care in the Same-Day Surgery Center, *all patients should be considered "VIPs" and accorded the most courteous and gracious service possible.*

3

Economic and Regulatory Issues

Fredrick K. Orkin

Widely acknowledged among the most dramatic changes in health care delivery in the United States during the 1980s is the movement of almost half of surgery from the hospital to the outpatient setting. When asked to account for this remarkable phenomenon, most physicians and other health care providers cite economic factors, such as the apparent cost savings and cost-effectiveness of this mode of surgical care. Often cited, too, are the greater convenience and satisfaction for both the patient and the surgeon, and the reduced incidence of nosocomial infection, both of which might be characterized as enhanced quality of care. This chapter surveys relevant economic factors and quality of care concerns, considers how they have shaped the growth of outpatient surgery, and looks ahead to how they are likely to influence its future. It is fitting that these topics be included in a comprehensive text on outpatient anesthesia care, because anesthesiologists have been among the prime motivators in the development of outpatient surgical care and will continue to have an important role, especially in relation to economic issues, quality of care, and related regulatory activities.

THE GROWTH OF OUTPATIENT SURGERY

Until the late 19th century, only the poor were treated and housed in structures resembling hospitals; other patients were attended in their homes or physicians' offices. With the introduction of aseptic surgical technique in the 1880s, surgery moved into the hospital and developed as a mode of care for which patients were hospitalized for recuperation as well as for the surgery itself. In the early 20th century, two pioneers, James Nicholl at the Royal Glasgow Hospital for Children and Ralph Waters at the Down-Town Anesthesia Clinic in Sioux City, Iowa, laid the foundations for the rebirth of outpatient surgery and showed the direction for a significant development in surgical care. In the 1960s, outpatient surgery began to take hold with the development of two delivery models: one within the hospital or on the hospital campus, and the other hospital-independent and freestanding. The growth in these two systems has been astronomic. During the past decade, almost all hospitals developed formal outpatient surgery programs, relying on existing surgical and recovery facilities to a

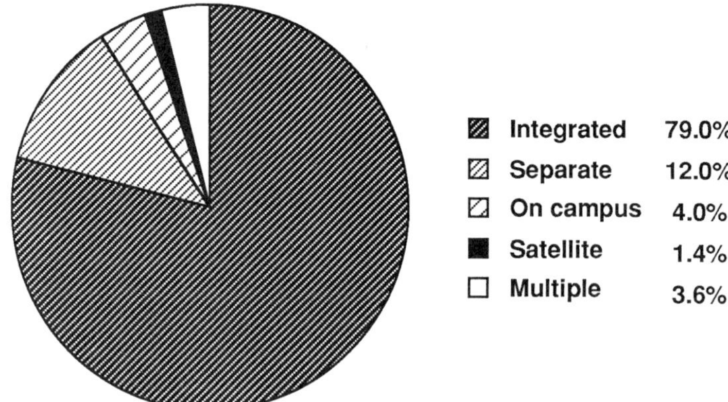

Fig. 3-1. The site of outpatient surgery programs reported by hospitals in 1987. Integrated programs used the same operating suite and postanesthesia care unit as inpatient surgery; separate programs were located apart from inpatient surgical facilities within the hospital; on campus programs were located out of the hospital building, but on the hospital grounds; satellite programs were located two or more blocks from the hospital; and some hospitals used two or more locations (multiple). (From the American Hospital Association,[1] with permission.)

highly variable degree. For example, in 1987, 86 percent of hospitals responding to a national survey reported providing outpatient surgery, with more than one-fifth using other facilities in place of, or in addition to, those used for inpatients (Fig. 3-1).[1]

Even more remarkable has been the rapid growth in outpatient surgery in hospital-affiliated facilities during the past decade. The fraction of total hospital-based surgery performed on an outpatient basis doubled between 1979 and 1983, then increased by almost half again by 1988; moreover, during the period from 1983 to 1988, the number of inpatient procedures decreased despite growth in the general population (Fig. 3-2).[2] In 1987, outpatient surgery comprised 44 percent of all surgery performed in hospital-affiliated facilities.[3] Differing only quantitatively, this trend has affected university hospitals,[4] community hospitals,[5] and urban hospitals,[6] as well as all surgical subspecialties[6] and patients of all ages.[7] It is likely that half of all hospital-affiliated surgery will be undertaken on an ambulatory basis in the early 1990s. Whereas some hospitals already report a 60 percent level of outpatient surgery, this level is predicted to be the national average by 1995.[3]

Ralph Waters' concept of the totally self-sufficient, freestanding surgical center found its prototype in 1970 when anesthesiologists Wallace Reed and John Ford opened the Surgicenter in Phoenix, Ari-

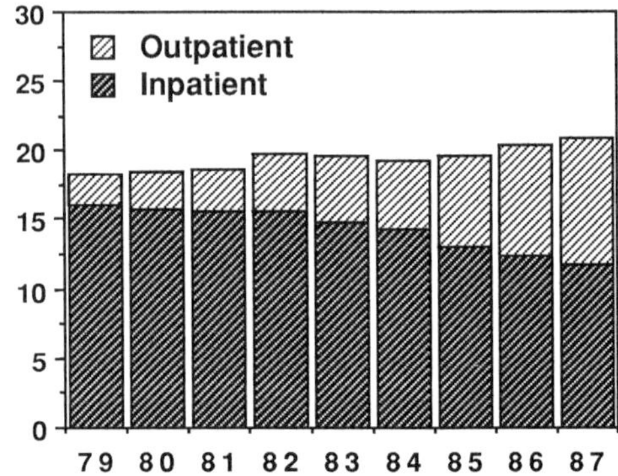

Fig. 3-2. The changing site of non-obstetric surgery in hospital-affiliated facilities during the period from 1979 to 1987, based on annual surveys conducted by the American Hospital Association.[1]

zona.[8] An increasing number of similar freestanding facilities opened in the following years, with 42 in operation by 1975 and 130 by 1980. As with hospital-affiliated units, however, most of the growth occurred during the period between 1983 and 1988 (Fig. 3-3).[9] Approximately 1,247 freestanding facilities are expected to be open in 1990,[9] where about 10 percent of all surgery within the United States will be performed (exclusive of that undertaken in physicians' offices).

Although these two models developed independently, their recent growth has been dynamic and interdependent, with freestanding facilities increasingly claiming outpatient surgical cases that might have been performed in hospital-affiliated facilities. Whereas the freestanding facilities' share of outpatient surgical care (exclusive of that performed in physicians' offices) amounted to only approximately 2 percent of outpatient surgery in 1980, their share is likely to be about 20 percent in 1990. Alternatively, hospitals were the loci for 98 percent of outpatient surgical care in 1980 and probably will have lost one-fifth of their share by 1990.

Augmenting this redistribution of surgical care will soon be another new structure on the medical landscape: located adjacent to a freestanding surgery facility, a recovery center will provide postoperative nursing care for up to 72 hours to patients who require more care than they could receive at home, yet who do not need the sophisticated hospital environment. The prototype recently opened in Fresno, California, and undoubtedly will be quickly emulated, further fueling the growth of hospital-independent, freestanding surgery facilities. Finally, in this dynamic process of redistribution of surgery, a small but increasing amount of outpatient care requiring anesthesia personnel is being performed in surgeons' offices (e.g., ophthalmic, plastic, and hand surgeries). The future role of anesthesiologists in office-based surgical practice is yet to be defined. However, it is obvious that this represents a fertile area

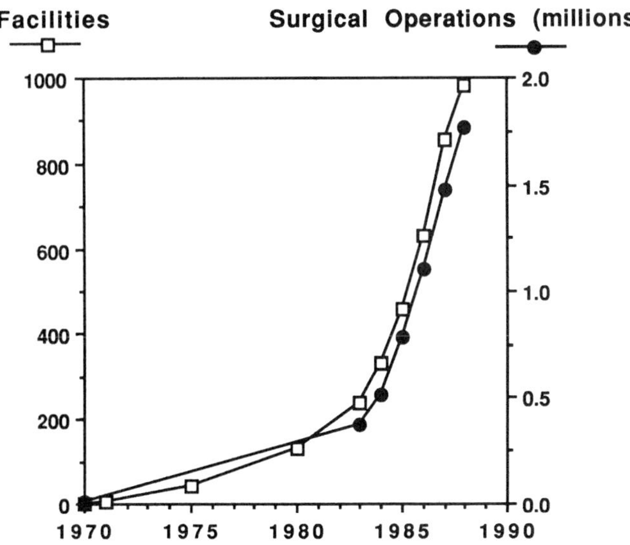

Fig. 3-3. The growth in the numbers of hospital-independent, freestanding surgical centers and the surgical operations performed in them during the period from 1970 to 1988. (Data from SMG Marketing Group, Inc.[9])

for future advancement in outpatient surgical care.

ACCOUNTING FOR THE RAPID GROWTH OF OUTPATIENT SURGERY

The recent growth of outpatient surgery is truly unprecedented, surpassing the growth in the use of other common medical technology and far exceeding the growth in population. What accounts for this phenomenon? A variety of factors have been suggested.[10–13]

Advances in Medical Technology

Outpatient surgical care has clearly benefited from advances in medical technology, including drugs, equipment, surgical procedures, and treatment protocols. Familiar examples in anesthetic practice consist of shorter-acting narcotics (e.g., fentanyl, alfentanil), induction agents (e.g., methohexital, propofol), inhalation anesthetics (e.g., isoflurane), and neuromuscular blocking drugs (e.g., atracurium, vecuronium). Discussed in detail throughout this book, these drugs facilitate the outpatient anesthetic management of patients of all ages and widely varying physical condition. Similarly, recently introduced laser, endoscopic, and arthroscopic equipment enable the surgeon to perform an ever-increasing array of surgical procedures on an outpatient basis. Yet, enhanced medical technology has undoubtedly been a diffuse influence over many years and, on its own, cannot account for the very rapid growth in outpatient surgery during the period from 1983 to 1988 (Figs. 3-2 and 3-3).

Increasing Consumerism and Public Acceptance

Consumerism has been an increasingly potent trend since Ralph Nader forced a car "unsafe at any speed" out of the marketplace 25 years ago. Not unexpectedly, the general public finds outpatient surgery, a mode of care offering enhanced safety, especially appealing. Several anecdotal surveys suggest that the incidence of major complications, infections, and medication errors is lower in the outpatient surgical setting.[12] In a study of outpatient dental surgery, in which it is likely that all deaths were counted, the death rate was 1 in approximately 280,000 patients receiving anesthetics.[14] Another aspect of consumerism favoring the outpatient surgical setting is the enhanced convenience enjoyed by both the patient and surgeon: the outpatient setting values the time of both individuals as much as they do. Patients suffer less disruption in their increasingly mobile, fast-paced lives and retain greater autonomy. The surgeon can efficiently complete less complex cases in the outpatient facility and is spared making postoperative hospital rounds because the patients return to the surgeon's office. Given that the care is provided with fewer complications and greater convenience, the patient and surgeon also enjoy greater satisfaction with outpatient care. Finally, favorable clinical experience accrued over time leads to greater acceptance of this mode of care by the patient, surgeon, and health care insuror. As important as these influences have been, however, they are also diffuse, and alone cannot account for the recent rapid growth in outpatient surgery.

Changing Health Care Economics

The advent of Medicare and expanded availability of private health insurance in the 1960s fueled demand for medical services, with resultant progressively increasing health care expenditures. Although cost-containment has become a very visible national issue in recent years, the delivery of high-quality surgical care at lower cost was the principal goal in the establishment of outpatient surgery facilities in the 1960s and early 1970s, especially for the freestanding units.[8,15] Hospitals also increasingly saw outpatient care as a way to use their beds more appropriately and to treat overcrowding in the operating suite. Undoubtedly, these influences were important in the development of this mode of care over the past 20 years, but alone cannot account for its recent rapid growth.

However, one economic factor deserves special attention because it cannot only explain the recent rapid growth in outpatient surgery but it can also help us understand future changes. That factor is the reimbursement for the outpatient care—principally, the payment made by the health care insuror to the facility in which the care is given—and the size of that payment in relation to payments for equivalent care in alternative settings.[16] Often overlooked is the truism that what is paid for determines what services are available for delivery.

The early outpatient surgery facilities encountered difficulty in securing reimbursement for what was an untested mode of care of unknown quality. In fact, possibly because insurors were leery about outpatient surgical care, the early hospital-based facility was often called a "short procedure unit," rather than an "ambulatory" or "outpatient surgery unit." Initially, private insurors deemed only the healthiest patients having the simplest procedures candidates for this novel setting. With experience, insurors became not only more lenient but also much more supportive of the concept. Later, in the 1970s and early 1980s, insurors promulgated progressively longer lists of surgical procedures deemed appropriate for outpatient care.

Given the pre-eminent position of Medicare in the health care marketplace, outpatient surgery received a decided boost when the Social Security Act was amended in 1980 to authorize Medicare payment for specified surgical procedures performed in outpatients units. Almost 2 years later, the federal Health Care Financing Administration (HCFA) listed 100 surgical procedures for which Medicare would pay; the list has grown substantially since. Significantly, with time, insurors also began to deny payment to the hospital—and, in turn, the surgeon and anesthesiologist—for inpatient care if the procedure could reasonably be performed in the outpatient setting. A waiver was (and continues to be) available for specific situations in which a patient having an ostensibly outpatient procedure requires inpatient care, usually for other medical problems or coexisting disease; however, obtaining the waiver is typically time-consuming and intimidating. Thus, insurors created potent incentives for outpatient surgery through the availability of payment. Payment for services was obviously a necessary circumstance for the development of outpatient surgery, but, by itself, this influence also does not account for the recent utilization phenomenon.

The critical element in promoting the recent growth of outpatient surgery is the relative size of the payments.[16] Once reimbursement was available in a given setting, the actual payment was based on the facilities' charges, which reflected the underlying costs plus a small profit. The hospital, with its higher operating costs (reflecting diverse sophisticated services), necessarily set its operating room and ancillary charges for inpatient surgery higher than those for the same procedures in freestanding centers; charges for hospital-affiliated outpatient surgery were intermediate. Depending on the health insurance plan, patients were responsible for a deductible or copayment bearing a fixed relationship to the payment; thus, patients had an incentive to have their care at the lowest cost facility. The hospital-independent, freestanding facility received another boost in 1982, when Medicare began paying 100 percent of the facility fee, instead of 80 percent with the facility billing the patient for the remainder of the fee. Although the federal government was actually paying according to a discounted, four-level facility fee schedule that recognized different groups of procedures (and which would not be revised for several years), relieving the patient of a payment of perhaps 20 percent represented a substantial incentive to use freestanding surgical facilities.

The greatest incentive to the use of outpatient surgery, however, was created with the inception of the Medicare prospective payment system in 1983, which other insurors have also emulated: hospitals would be paid fixed, prospectively set amounts based on the principal diagnosis (or procedure, in the case of surgery). Uninfluenced by the actual costs incurred in the care of given patients, the payments were modified only to reflect regional wage rate differences and intensity of graduate medical education in the facility. The number of hospital services provided would no longer favorably influence revenue; instead, increased net revenue from inpatient care would depend on increasing patient volume and reducing costs. Faced with fixed payments for inpatient surgery, hospitals escaped such limitations by moving cases to the outpatient setting where payments were still charge-based. Thus, the hospital-affiliated outpatient surgery case load soon grew rapidly, even at the expense of inpatient surgery (Fig. 3-2). Not unexpectedly, outpatient surgery has represented one of the most successful and profitable ways in which hospitals "diversified" around limited fixed payment mechanisms to maximize their revenues.[17]

THE COST-EFFECTIVENESS OF OUTPATIENT SURGICAL CARE

Underlying the incentives for moving surgery to the outpatient setting created by changing reimbursement, as well as the general support for this mode of care, is the perception that outpatient surgery is more "cost-effective" than its inpatient counterpart. This perception is merely part of the larger, intuitively obvious belief that outpatient care is less costly than similar medical services delivered in a hospital. Interestingly, there is little objective support for this belief. This issue was explicitly examined in a survey of the English literature published between 1965 and 1979[18]: of 240 articles purporting to compare outpatient and inpatient care with regard to clinical outcome or costs, 106 were anecdotal or descriptive reports. Of the remaining 134 reports with objective comparative data, only four contained sufficient data concerning both cost and efficacy to permit statistically valid conclusions: two studies suggested potential savings in the outpatient setting with slightly poorer clinical outcome, and two studies showed that outpatient care was as effective as inpatient care and less costly. A recent review of the literature relevant to outpatient surgery revealed that this is actually a complex issue about which little is known.[19]

What is "Cost-Effectiveness"?

Part of the problem in establishing whether outpatient surgery is cost-effective relates to misunderstandings regarding terminology and economic concepts. Medical care, like all goods and services, consumes resources. These resources include not only the time of physicians and nurses but also equipment and facilities. As elsewhere in the economy, resources are limited, and resources used for one activity cannot be used for another. Thus, trade-offs between alternative uses of limited resources are inevitable as we try to obtain the greatest benefit.

The term *cost-effective* connotes a comparison between two (or more) alternative uses of resources with respect to a specific outcome or objective. For example, the objective might be herniorrhaphy and the alternative uses of resources would be the inpatient and outpatient settings. In cost-effectiveness analysis, quantitation is obtained by computing the costs of the resources that are consumed by the alternative uses.[20] Thus, the results of this analysis would be presented succinctly as dollars per herniorrhaphy, but no attempt would be made to quantitate other outcomes (e.g., complications, death, quality of life).

Such analyses are often problematic in health care, partly because "cost-effective" is usually assumed to be synonymous with "cost-saving." Thus, programs that do not save money but that do provide benefit at a reasonable cost would not be considered cost-effective. Another common usage, which is also too rigid for application in health care, is that a cost-effective program saves money and provides an outcome equal to a more expensive program. A more satisfactory definition of a cost-effective strategy is one that has an additional benefit worth the cost.[21] Thus, such a program might cost less and be equally effective, cost more and be more effective (when the added benefit is worth the added cost), or cost less and be less effective (when the added benefit is not worth the added cost). Obviously, the analysis is far simpler if the outcome is fairly specific and there are no other benefits to consider.

Costs Versus Charges

Another source of misunderstanding concerns the distinction between true economic costs incurred in providing a service and the charges (bills) that are levied on the patient or the patient's insuror.[22] Although commonly used interchangeably in the medical literature, there is no set relationship between costs and charges. Whereas economic costs represent the sum of the actual resources consumed in providing the service, charges are list prices generated through empiric accounting procedures that have a goal of maximizing overall institutional reimbursement. Charges usually do not represent what the institution paid, even in nonprofit facilities. For example, charges for laboratory tests may be 20 times their true costs, whereas charges for the use of the operating room are closer to the costs. The difference between costs and charges allows for cross-subsidization among institutional services, uncompensated care (e.g., bad debts, charity care), amortization of equipment, and expansion of facilities.

Charges are often used as surrogates for costs in cost-effectiveness studies because determining resource costs for a given patient or set of patients is generally very difficult, if not herculean. Thus, when reading a study of cost-effectiveness, one must note whether costs or charges are reported and whether the choice is appropriate for the analysis. If a study examines the financial impact of, for example, outpatient versus inpatient surgery on the patient, analysis of charges may be acceptable. However, in most other situations, since the patient's insuror is paying for the care and society ultimately pays the bill, resource costs are more appropriate.

COST-EFFECTIVENESS STUDIES IN OUTPATIENT SURGERY

Evaluating the cost-effectiveness of outpatient surgery requires identification of all costs associated with the care. There are the direct costs of the goods and services needed for the procedure (e.g., supplies, equipment). More difficult to ascertain are the many indirect costs, which include maintenance and depreciation of the facility, rent and leases, and utilities. Especially important among the indirect costs are the various, often forgotten, costs that the patient and the patient's family incur. These include lost income (for both the patient and the person caring for him or her), provisions for child care, arrangements for postoperative home care, transportation (e.g., postoperative visits to the surgeon), meals, and, if necessary, hotel accommodations. Since the burden of care following outpatient surgery has shifted to the patient and the patient's family, accounting for these indirect costs has become especially important. Thus, when reading individual reports in the literature, it is important to identify the perspective taken (insuror, facility, patient and family, or society) and whether costs or charges are being analyzed.

Charge-Based Studies of Clinical Experience

The movement of surgery out of the hospital occurred too rapidly to permit randomized clinical trials comparing similar care delivered simultaneously in the inpatient and outpatient settings. Hence, the majority of papers report clinical experience, with cost savings based on excluding the daily hospital room charge. As noted above, the charges that are "saved" are unlikely to reflect true costs saved. More important, however, is the fact that there have been increased health care expenditures, rather than cost savings, because the bed that the outpatient would have occupied has been used for another patient at the same time. Thus, the growth of outpatient surgery has been accompanied by an increase in the total number of surgical operations performed across all settings and in the surgical operation rate on a per capita basis (Fig. 3-4), thereby expanding the health care system (and related expenditures) and vitiating potential cost savings. That is, unless the hospital shrinks (i.e., decreases its census and related staffing), outpatient surgery per se cannot be cost-saving from a societal perspective.[23]

Typical of these studies are a series of reports that appeared in the urologic literature during the 1980s.[24–30] These reports detail favorable clinical experience with a wide variety of procedures performed on adults and children in the outpatient setting, with savings of 25 to 75 percent based largely on avoiding the overnight hospital charge. Similar reports based on clinical ex-

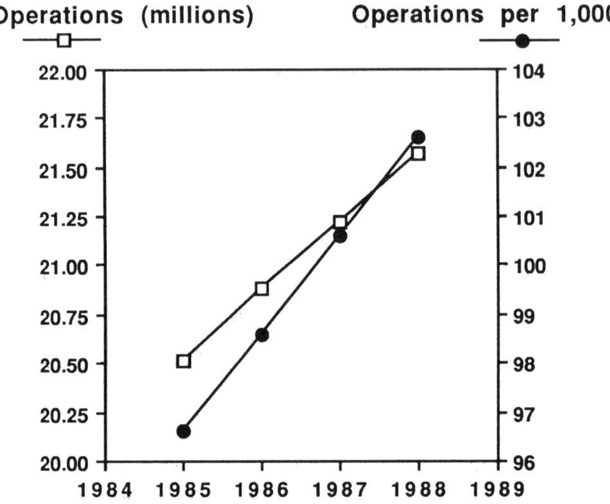

Fig. 3-4. The growth in total non-obstetric surgical operations and in those procedures per 1,000 population. (Procedure data from Figs. 3-2 and 3-3. Population data from US Bureau of the Census: Statistical Abstract of the United States: 1989. 109th Ed. US Government Printing Office, Washington, DC, 1989.)

perience and charges related to breast biopsy,[31,32] anorectal surgery,[33] and thyroidectomy have appeared in the medical literature.[34]

A more satisfying study examined clinical outcomes and Medicare payments for patients having cataract extraction before and after the locus of care shifted from the inpatient to the outpatient setting.[35] Not unexpectedly, the outpatient setting was associated with lower costs in terms of Medicare payments; however, the investigators did not include the patient's out-of-pocket expenses, supplemental insurance payments, or lost wages, if any. Yet, because there were fewer infections and less pain requiring medication, quality of care appeared to be improved.

Charge-Based Clinical Trials

Although clinical trials across surgical facilities have not been undertaken, this methodology has been used to examine potential savings, based on charges, in aspects of outpatient anesthesia care. Because patients who were somewhat hypothermic in the postanesthetic care unit seemed to have longer immediate recovery stays, a randomized clinical trial was conducted examining the influence of active heating and humidification of airway gases.[36] A small but significant difference in postoperative body temperature was associated with a longer recovery stay; the differential cost of this recovery stay was estimated using recovery room charges. Although the findings were not corroborated,[37] the application of this methodology, albeit with charges rather than costs, is important.

Cost-Based Studies of Clinical Experience

Although there are few studies of this type, three are especially interesting. One examined patient satisfaction, clinical outcome, and economic cost associated with herniorrhaphy, tubal ligation, and knee menisectomy in both outpatient and hospital settings.[38] Although the surgical procedures were not further described, one assumes that the patients had inguinal herniorrhaphy, laparoscopic tubal ligation, and open menisectomy; all patients received a standard general anesthetic. The study was undertaken in Canada, which has universal health insurance and a uniform physician fee schedule (with no other billing permitted); institution-related economic costs were obtained through a standard step-down costing procedure which allocates total institutional support costs (e.g., housekeeping, laundry, pharmacy) to patient treatments. Although clinical outcomes were similar across both settings, patient satisfaction and costs differed: a higher proportion of outpatients found their stay too short and would have preferred hospitalization. Outpatient herniorrhaphy and tubal ligation were cost-saving, but menisectomy was not, largely because of higher costs associated with outpatient physiotherapy. Thus, even if a procedure can be accomplished in the outpatient setting, the resultant care is not necessarily more cost-effective or better.

The second example of this type of study is important because it illustrates the often substantial, uncompensated indirect costs borne by the family of a patient having outpatient surgery.[39] As Canadians function under universal health insurance, the investigators examined family expenditures associated with two common pediatric surgical procedures: adenoidectomy performed in the hospital, and strabismus repair in the outpatient setting. Using telephone interviews 24 to 36 hours postoperatively, they inquired about the financial costs associated with the time lost from work, child care, and transportation, among other information. The total work time lost was less and the costs were considerably lower for outpatient surgery. Lost wages constituted a large part of the total indirect costs, largely determined by the time spent with the child, away from work. Interestingly, the parents of inpatients did not return to work after the surgery, whereas one parent typically returned to work following their child's procedure in the outpatient setting. They also found that fathers tended to receive "compassionate time" leave more often than mothers. Besides concluding that outpatient care is cost-effective for the family, the investigators suggested that outpatient facilities should function on weekends to reduce the financial burden placed on working parents.

The third example of this type of study documents economic cost savings resulting from a strategic change in physician practice patterns.[40] Among the changes accompanying the opening of a separate outpatient surgery unit in a university hospital was the use of an algorithm for preoperative laboratory testing that is dependent on the individual patient's characteristics; in contrast, inpatients having the same surgical procedures as outpatients continued to have laboratory testing ordered routinely on admission. The investigators conducted a retrospective review of the costs associated with pelvic laparoscopy and knee arthroscopy in both the outpatient and inpatient settings. Not unexpectedly, fewer laboratory tests were obtained in outpatients with the use of the algorithm, resulting in a savings of approximately 83 percent per patient. Operating room time and recovery time in the postanesthetic care unit were also shorter in the ambulatory setting; since the patients were similar in both settings, these differences may reflect more difficult (and thus prolonged) surgery, with longer immediate recovery, among the inpatients, or perhaps a variety of managerial changes relating to how procedures are scheduled in the outpatient setting. However, a variety of algorithms are available to assist in ordering preoperative testing more appropriately, regardless of the setting in which surgery is performed.[41,42]

Cost-Based Simulation

Given the changes in reimbursement previously discussed, randomized clinical trials comparing aspects of care in similar patient populations across inpatient and outpatient settings may not be possible; such studies may also impose artificial and sometimes inappropriate strictures on clinical care. An alternative approach for some inquiries is a simulation, often using data obtained from other studies.

In one recent application of simulation, the investigators explored the cost implications of the new anesthetic propofol on recovery stay in the postanesthetic care unit.[43] They hypothesized that the more rapid awakening and lower incidence of nausea and vomiting associated with this drug should lead to lower staffing costs due to shorter recovery times. They used data concerning anesthesia and recovery times associated with a variety of procedures undertaken in an outpatient unit in a community hospital and an inpatient operating suite in a university hospital; in each setting, patients received nitrous oxide with either thiopental-isoflurane or propofol anesthesia. The shorter recovery times associated with the use of propofol resulted in simulations suggesting substantial potential for more efficient recovery nurse staffing, the actual savings depending on current staffing patterns, case mix, and volume, as well as underlying staffing criteria.

The other recent cost-based simulation compared outpatient and inpatient cataract extraction.[44] Drawing on their literature survey,[18] the investigators hypothesized that the cost savings alleged to result from substituting outpatient for inpatient surgery results from a reduction and/or complete accounting of services delivered to the outpatient. From a review of inpatient medical records, they developed a list of services provided to patients after cataract extraction (e.g., administering medication, changing dressing, assisting in feeding and ambulation); in turn, they estimated the economic cost of providing each service. They then simulated several outpatient scenarios that differed in degree of family participation; thus, less family support would necessitate more time from a visiting nurse. Outpatient care was less costly only if fewer services were provided or if the accounting failed to note the contributions of the family to care. Thus, at least in part, the savings attributed to outpatient surgery result from shifting the cost of care from the health care industry to the family. This provocative study also questioned whether all inpatient services are necessary and whether similar patient outcomes would result in the hospital if fewer services were provided (as seems to be the case in the outpatient setting).

MAINTAINING QUALITY AS OUTPATIENT SURGERY GROWS

Quality control is important in any productive enterprise. Maintaining quality is especially important in outpatient surgical care because of the active efforts described above to reduce expenditures and, in turn, potentially necessary services. However, despite several decades of research relating to quality of medical care, the term *quality* remains an almost metaphysical entity that expresses the capacity of the health care delivered to meet medical and nonmedical goals that are shaped by patient values.[45] The level of quality achieved is determined by variables associated with the patient, physician(s) and other practitioners, clinical setting, institution, and health care policy. Although the quantification of quality is currently an active research area, quality control activities in the clinical setting principally relate to detecting and treating lapses in quality (e.g., maloccurrences) under the terms *risk management* and *quality assurance*.[46,47]

Rationale for Effective Quality Control Programs

As caring and responsible physicians, we have a professional responsibility to provide high-quality care. The rationale for developing programs to maintain quality is strengthened further by recognizing that the bulk of anesthetic-related maloccurrences are preventable and costly.[46,48] Moreover, since early treatment (if not prevention) is generally less costly than treating a bad outcome, we should work toward identifying problems in the delivery of care at the earliest time. Quality control activities are also mandated by the accreditation and reimbursement agencies on behalf of the public that we serve. In turn, perhaps as part of the consumerism discussed above, the public now expects greater accountability from health care providers in general and near-zero rates of maloccurrence in generally healthy patients undergoing anesthesia care.[49]

Quality Control Terminology

Although we do not have an operational definition of quality that is suitable for the clinical setting, the dimensions of quality have been characterized by the following attributes[50] that may be monitored as we work to maintain quality in the outpatient setting:

Effectiveness: the power of a procedure or treatment to improve health status.

Efficiency: the delivery of a maximal number of comparable units of care for a given health care expenditure.

Accessibility: the ease with which care is obtainable in the face of various potential barriers of a financial, organizational, cultural, or emotional type.

Acceptability: the degree to which the health care delivered satisfies the patient.

Provider competence: an individual's technical and interpersonal skills, or the way the health care delivery system as a whole functions.

Risk management, a term more commonly used in the business world, refers to programs designed to reduce or eliminate injuries (and their related costs) to persons, and to prevent or minimize losses of property, usually related to specified risks. The principal focus of risk management in health care has been reducing malpractice liability payouts.

Quality assurance is a system or program that provides an organized procedure for the evaluation of the level of care provided (quality of care assessment) and the establishment of mechanisms for improvement. A quality assurance program is the mechanism by which we track trends that may suggest deficiencies in quality of care delivered, institute corrective measures, and document their successful correction. Thus, quality assurance and risk management are two overlapping and interrelated activities.

An Integrated Approach to Quality Assurance and Risk Management

In the past, quality assurance involved periodic audits of medical records for specific problems or topics; these were time-consuming and, because they were "hit or miss," often did not have great impact on improving health care. Presently, the principal focus is on continual monitoring and evaluation of the broad array of medical and administrative activities of the health care setting. An effective monitoring and evaluation program is interdisciplinary and fully integrated with other parts of the institution; thus, if the outpatient surgery unit is a hospital-affiliated facility, its quality assurance activities are integrated, through an institution-wide committee, with those of other parts of the institution in which anesthesia and surgical services are provided. In fact, the current edition of the manual of the principal accreditation agency presents surgery and anesthesia standards in one chapter.[51] As a corollary and long-standing principle, policies and procedures should be uniform throughout the institution and not different for the outpatient. Although the orientation of quality assurance programs has been to identify and treat problems, an evolving viewpoint emphasizes the need to look more broadly at the process of delivering care and to exploit opportunities for continuous improvement rather than maintaining minimalist "standards" of care.[52]

The Monitoring and Evaluation Process

Aid in establishing a program of monitoring and evaluation of anesthesia services is found in a recent publication of the principal accreditation agency.[53] The monitoring and evaluation model consists of the following nine steps:

Assign Responsibility. The director, chief, or chairman of the department is responsible for the monitoring and evaluation activities, and should identify and assign relevant components to others in the department.

Delineate the Scope of Care. Identifying the range of surgical and diagnostic procedures performed and patients served is not difficult. The monitoring and evaluation activities should encompass, or at least sample, this spectrum of clinical activity.

Identify the Important Aspects of Care. Priority should be given to those aspects of care that occur frequently or that affect large numbers of patients; that pose serious risk or are less beneficial if not provided correctly or in a timely, appropriate fashion; and that are historically problem-prone. Thus, the monitoring and evaluation activities should encompass high-volume, high-risk, or problem-prone aspects of care.

Identify Indicators Related to These Aspects of Care. An indicator is a defined, measurable event, complication, or outcome that enables estimation of an incidence that, in turn, permits comparison with results in other settings. Characteristics of a good indicator include clear, precise description; measurability, reproducibility, and reliability; and relevance to clinical practice. Among the many indicators suitable for the outpatient setting are unplanned admission to the hospital, unplanned admission to an intensive care unit, failure to emerge from general anesthesia in a specified time, peripheral nerve injury, brain or spinal cord injury, acute myocardial infarction, respiratory arrest, fulminant pulmonary edema, pulmonary aspiration of gastric contents, postdural puncture headache, ocular injury, dental trauma, death, and cardiac arrest. These 14 clinical indicators were chosen for possible use in outcome-based accreditation in the 1990s and are undergoing field testing; in each case, the event must be temporarily related to anesthesia care.

Other outcome-related indicators of special interest in the outpatient setting are wound infection, persisting nausea and vomiting, excessive pain, excessive bleeding (e.g., need for unplanned transfusion), and patient satisfaction. Indicators can also relate to the structure (e.g., qualifications of staff, adequacy of physical facilities) and process (e.g., adherence to established procedures or standards) of care. Examples of indicators relating to the structure and process of care are having a fire extinguisher in need of refilling, proceeding with surgery without a signed patient consent, not having current certification in cardiopulmonary resuscitation, failing to perform an appropriate preanesthetic evaluation, and not having sufficient dantrolene for initial treatment of an episode of malignant hyperthermia in an adult.

Establish Thresholds Related to the Indicators. The threshold is an incidence below which the level of performance monitored by the given indicator is considered "acceptable" and above which further evaluation and remedial action will be taken. For example, the threshold for unplanned hospital admission might be 1.5 percent, reflecting the belief that some hospital admissions from ambulatory surgery are unavoidable, perhaps due to more extensive surgery unforeseen preoperatively, whereas the threshold for peripheral nerve injury and dental trauma should be zero. The thresholds should be chosen or adapted by a consensus process involving the practitioners in the given clinical setting, based on authoritative sources.

Collect and Analyze Data. For each indicator, appropriate data are collected in an ongoing fashion, from predetermined sources and at specified intervals. Because de novo data collection is expensive, emphasis should be placed on existing data sources within the facility or institution, which may be especially appropriate for each indicator. These may include patient records, incident reports, infection control reports, and patient questionnaires, among other less formal sources. Data collection related to structure and process indicators is obviously easier, often merely involving physical inspection of the facility. If the incidence is found to be below the threshold value, attention should be directed to other identified problems; however, that indicator should not necessarily be removed from the monitoring and evaluation activity.

Take Actions to Improve Care. When the incidence of events (indicators) exceeds threshold values, a plan of corrective action is implemented which specifies what is being done, by whom, and when change is expected. Obviously, the corrective action will specify the perceived problem, typically addressing insufficient knowledge, defects in systems, or deficient behavior. Successful resolution involves apprising the staff of the facility and enlisting their interest and support in achieving a solution.

Assess the Effectiveness of the Actions and Document Improvement. After sufficient time has elapsed for change to have occurred, ongoing data collection should indicate whether the corrective action has solved the problem. If the situation is unchanged, the problem and the action taken should be reassessed; new action should be taken and ongoing data collection should continue in a cyclical fashion until the problem is successfully resolved (Fig. 3-5). Satisfactory resolution of the problem, however, should not necessarily result in removal of that indicator from the monitoring and evaluation process.

Communicate Relevant Information. Communicating the results of this process to the staff of the outpatient surgery facility reinforces the changes imposed. If the facility is part of a hospital, the results should also be communicated to the anesthesia departmental and institutional quality assurance programs.

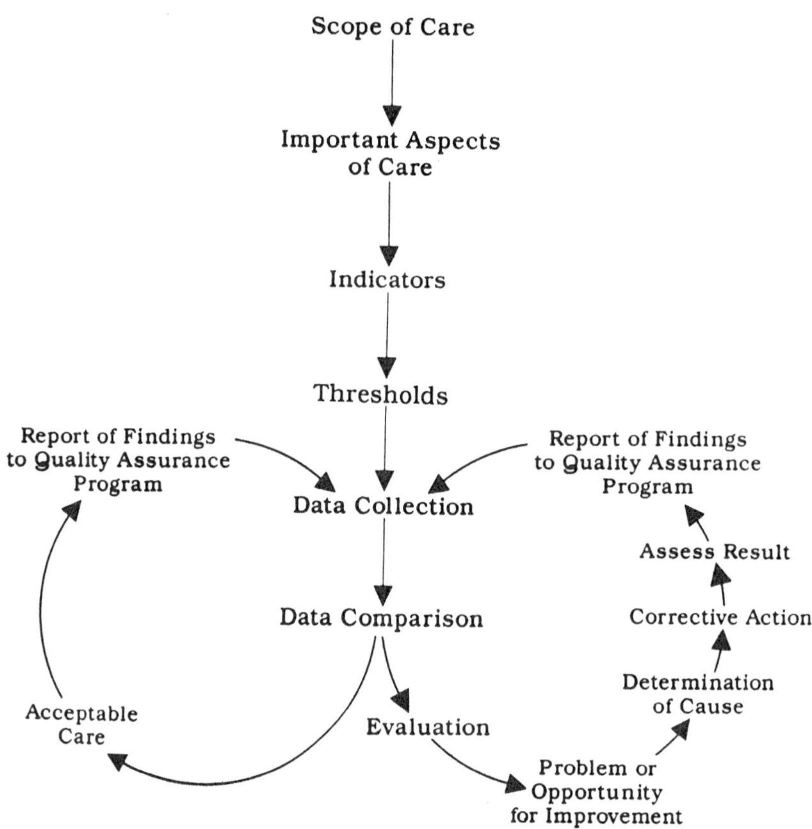

Fig. 3-5. The monitoring and evaluation process (see text). (Modified from Fromberg,[53] with permission.)

Ancillary Activities

Surrounding the monitoring and evaluation process are other activities that are also important in maintaining quality control, including delineating credentials and safety activities.

Credentials for specific clinical privileges are delineated for each practitioner in a clinical setting. It is administratively and ethically incumbent on the director of a given clinical setting to assure that those who provide services in that setting are competent to do so.[54] Delineation of privileges is based on education, training, and current competence. Whereas education and training are easy to document, current competence may be more difficult. One source of documentation is the ongoing monitoring and evaluation process that may yield provider-specific data relevant to the volume and outcome of specific procedures, as well as the process of delivering care (e.g., lack of conformance with departmental policies, persistent failure to perform an appropriate preanesthetic evaluation) and behavioral problems. Among the latter are failure to meet professional responsibilities and drug abuse.[55,56]

Safety activities comprise an ever-increasing number of diverse initiatives, many launched by the specialty of anesthesiology in response to an increased interest in risk management. Arguably, this specialty has done more than any other in this important area, and recent moderation in premium increases for malpractice liability insurance is taken as evidence that these efforts are effective. Examples of these activities include prepurchase expert evaluation of equipment and its inspection before first use; a preanesthetic equipment checkout procedure recommended by an expert panel convened by the U.S. Food and Drug Administration; an ongoing program of equipment maintenance; a periodic inservice equipment education program within the facility; a specific procedure for identifying patients before anesthesia care; and standards for minimal intraoperative patient monitoring.

THE FUTURE CONVERGENCE OF ECONOMICS AND QUALITY CONCERNS

William Roper, the former HCFA Administrator, has noted that Medicare's first decade was characterized by enhanced access to care, the second was characterized by cost containment, and the one we have just entered is characterized by enhanced quality. Indeed, even though economics and quality concerns have been especially important in the development of outpatient surgical care, these two areas have progressed quite independently. Their convergence is approaching, however, especially in ways that will affect the future development of outpatient surgical care.

The New Economics

The progression in changes in facility reimbursement for outpatient surgical care described above created an incentive to move patients out of the hospital and into the outpatient setting, especially to hospital-independent, freestanding facilities. Recall that the most potent incentive was different levels of reimbursement for the same procedure, with the difference related solely to whether the surgery was performed in a hospital as an inpatient, in a hospital-affiliated outpatient facility, or in a hospital-independent freestanding facility.

Health policymakers became aware of this irrational reimbursement situation in mid-1985, at the same time they became aware of the rapid growth in Medicare Part B spending, which includes outpatient surgery, among other outpatient care and all physician payments. They recognized an inherent potential for substantial cost savings in outpatient surgical care if the payments were made from a prospectively defined facility fee schedule and were uniform across surgical sites. Such was the import of changes in the Medicare regulations that became effective in October 1988. To cushion the financial blow for hospital-affiliated outpatient facilities, in the first year the facility fee would represent a blend, with 75 percent of the payment based on actual hospital costs and 25 percent based on the substantially lower fee paid to hospital-independent, freestanding facilities; in the second year, the blend would be 50-50. Thereafter, the facility fee paid to any outpatient surgery facility would be based on a yet-to-be formulated ambulatory prospective payment system based on ambulatory visit groups, which would resemble the diagnosis-related groups used in hospitals. The ambulatory prospective payment system would replace the six payment groups (relating to types of procedures) with several hundred procedure-specific payment groups. In the end, the all-inclusive facility payment for a given surgical procedure would not be influenced by the type of facility in which it was performed, although there would be adjustments for regional wage differences. It is uncertain as we approach 1990 whether physician payments for outpatient care will be part of the payment groups.

Outcome-Based Quality Assessment

Since patient outcome is considerably more difficult and expensive to assess, quality of care was assessed largely with audits that focused on structure and process variables. However, as described above, the emphasis is now on outcome variables, using discrete, objective, and quantifiable events (''indicators'') from which incidences can be calculated. Using batteries of indicators currently being field-tested, the principal accreditation body proposes to begin outcome-based accreditation in the early 1990s.[57] Under this scheme, hospitals would collect similar sets of data that would be evaluated within the institution and submitted to the accreditation agency; the latter would undertake statistical analyses that compare one facility's performance to that of similar institutions. A major barrier yet to be overcome is the development of a technically satisfactory, yet administratively feasible method of case-mix adjustment of the data so that the outcome comparisons are valid.

The Convergence of Economics and Quality Concerns

Formerly independent concerns about rapidly increasing health care expenditures and quality of care are now converging rapidly for a variety of reasons. First, the health care system is expanding rapidly—witness the rapid growth in the per capita rate of surgery that has been fueled, in part, by the growth in outpatient surgery (Fig. 3-4)—and there is intense competition for market share, leading to diffused accountability for the quality of what is delivered. Second, there is excellent documentation on the highly variable rate of performance of a variety of procedures across geographic areas and different institutional settings[58,59]; such information raises the concern that there may be a considerable amount of inappropriate care. Finally, as health insurance premiums have increased rapidly, the cost of health care has become a major issue for both consumers and employers, who have been forced to make comparisons of alternative health insurance plans based on price. However, as price differences have narrowed, the focus is now shifting to quality of care.

Advances in computer technology now enable managed care entities (e.g., health maintenance organizations [HMOs], preferred provider organizations [PPO]) and major corporations (self-insured or major purchasers of private insurance) to track the health care experiences and related costs of their insured members, permitting the identification of high-cost practitioners and institutions. Since additional health care bills following surgery may represent treatment of a complication, it is now feasible to use medical claims data to study patient outcome after surgery.[60,61] Recently, the federal government has initiated a major data collection effort designed to improve health care by distributing outcome information relating to specific medical practices.[62]

Implications for Outpatient Surgical Care

No health care sector will remain unaffected as intense scrutiny of health care costs and patient outcomes converge to make good-quality care cost-effective. Facilities whose costs are higher for similar outcomes (whether because of complications or excessive services) will lose market share to competitors who function more efficiently and produce better results. The marketplace will also determine the level of quality, not necessarily the highest, that will prevail.

Under this scenario, outpatient surgery facilities will survive only by trimming costs and maintaining quality of care. Although platitudinous, these activities will be a challenge because cost accounting, strategic planning, and quality control are not well-developed in most units.

Hospital-affiliated outpatient surgery units will have a more difficult time, at least initially, because they previously received cost-based reimbursement, which effectively shielded them from lean payments in an increasingly competitive environment. With the advent of a separate prospective payment system for outpatient surgery, hospital administrators must identify overhead and other costs associated with this care that were formerly interwoven with inpatient costs; as a result, they will search for ways to physically separate outpatient and inpatient care when they are provided in the same facility. Over the longer term, administrators will want to establish outpatient surgery facilities as distinct financial as well as physical entities. Finally, as was the case with prospective payment for inpatient care, there will be great interest in evaluating the mix of outpatient cases for relative profitability (once the details of the payment mechanism become known), and specializing in given segments of outpatient surgical care. With time, the relative advantage held by hospital-independent, freestanding facilities will fade.

Maintaining quality of care under this scenario will be as important as trimming costs. Undoubtedly, there will be greater emphasis placed on quality assurance and risk management activities. There will also be increased emphasis on practice standards. However, given their contribution to the cost of care, the value of individual standards in improving care must be established lest their incorporation into practice lead to higher costs without enhancement of quality.[52,63]

REFERENCES

1. Survey of Hospital Ambulatory Surgery Programs, 1987. American Hospital Association, Chicago, 1988
2. Hospital Statistics, 1988. p. xxxiv. American Hospital Association, Chicago, 1988
3. Ambulatory care growth continues. Outreach 10:1, 1989
4. Bartlett MK, Battit GE, Rockett AM, et al: The role of surgery on ambulatory patients in one teaching hospital. Arch Surg 114:319, 1979
5. Laffaye HA: The impact of an ambulatory surgical service in a community hospital. Arch Surg 124:601, 1989

6. Lagoe RJ, Milliren JW: A community-based analysis of ambulatory surgery utilization. Am J Public Health 76:150, 1986
7. Lagoe RJ, Bice SE, Abulencia PB: Ambulatory surgery utilization by age level. Am J Public Health 77:33, 1987
8. Ford J, Reed W: The Surgicenter®—an innovation in the delivery and cost of medical care. Ariz Med 26:801, 1969
9. SMG Freestanding Surgery Center Directory: 1988 Edition. SMG Marketing Group, Chicago, 1988
10. Detmer DE: Ambulatory surgery. N Engl J Med 305:1406, 1981
11. Davis JE: Major ambulatory surgery today. p. 33. In Davis JE (ed): Major Ambulatory Surgery. Williams & Wilkins, Baltimore, 1986
12. Detmer DE, Buchanan-Davidson DJ: Ambulatory surgery. p. 31. In Rutkow IM (ed): Socioeconomics of Surgery. CV Mosby, St. Louis, 1989
13. Durant GD: Ambulatory surgery centers: surviving, thriving into the 1990s. MGM J 36:14, 1989
14. Coplans MP, Curson I: Deaths associated with dentistry. Br Dent J 153:357, 1982
15. Davis JE, Detmer DE: The ambulatory surgical unit. Ann Surg 175:856, 1972
16. Davis K, Russell LB: The substitution of hospital outpatient care for inpatient care. Rev Econ Stat 54:109, 1972
17. Sabatino FG: The diversification success story continues: survey. Hospitals 63:26, 1989
18. Ancona Berk A, Chalmers TC: Cost and efficacy of the substitution of ambulatory for inpatient care. N Engl J Med 304:393, 1981
19. Gold B, Orkin FK: Cost-effectiveness of outpatient surgery. Curr Opin Anaesthesiol 1:76, 1988
20. Warner KE, Luce BR: Introduction to cost-benefit and cost-effectiveness analysis. p. 43. In Warner KE, Luce BR (eds): Cost-Benefit and Cost-Effectiveness Analysis in Health Care. Health Administration Press, Ann Arbor, 1982
21. Doubilet MD, Weinstein MC, McNeil BJ: Use and misuse of the term "cost effective" in medicine. N Engl J Med 314:253, 1986
22. Finkler SA: The distinction between cost and charges. Ann Intern Med 96:102, 1982
23. Egdahl RH: Should we shrink the health care system? Harvard Bus Rev 61:125, 1984
24. Caldamone AA, Rabinowitz R: Outpatient orchiopexy. J Urol 127:286, 1982
25. Kaye KW, Clayman RV, Lange PH: Outpatient hydrocele and spermatocele repair under local anesthesia. J Urol 130:269, 1983
26. Nadelson EJ, Cohen M, Warner R, et al: Update: Varicocelectomy—a safe outpatient procedure. Urology 24:259, 1984
27. Shepard B, Hensle TW, Burbige KA, et al: Outpatient surgery in pediatric urology patients. Urology 24:581, 1984
28. Siegel AL, Snyder HMcC, Duckett JW: Outpatient pediatric urological surgery: techniques for a successful and cost-effective practice. J Urol 136:879, 1986
29. Gluck RW, Hanna MK: Magpi hypospadias repair: ambulatory versus inpatient surgery. Urology 30:461, 1987
30. Kaye KW: Modified high varicocelectomy: outpatient microsurgical procedure. Urology 32:13, 1988
31. Saltzstein EC, Mann RW, Chua TY, et al: Outpatient breast biopsy. Arch Surg 109: 287, 1974
32. Doberneck RC: Breast biopsy: a study of cost-effectiveness. Ann Surg 192:152, 1980
33. Smith LE: Ambulatory surgery for anorectal diseases: an update. South Med J 79:163, 1986
34. Steckler RM: Outpatient thyroidectomy: a feasibility study. Am J Surg 152:417, 1986
35. Bloom BS, Krueger N: Cost and quality effects of outpatient cataract removal. Inquiry 25:383, 1988
36. Conahan TJ III, Williams GD, Apfelbaum JL, et al: Airway heating reduces recovery time (costs) in outpatients. Anesthesiology 67:128, 1987
37. Goldberg ME, Jan R, Gregg CE, et al: The heat and moisture exchanger does not preserve body temperature or reduce recovery time in outpatients undergoing surgery and anesthesia. Anesthesiology 68:122, 1988
38. Pineault R, Contandriopoulos A-P, Valois M, et al: Randomized clinical trial of one-day surgery: patient satisfaction, clinical outcome, and costs. Med Care 23:171, 1985
39. Stanwick RS, Horne JM, Peabody DM, et al: Day-care versus inpatient pediatric sur-

gery: a comparison of costs incurred by parents. Can Med Assoc J 137:21, 1987

40. Kitz DS, Slusarz-Ladden C, Lecky JH: Hospital resources used for inpatient and ambulatory surgery. Anesthesiology 69:383, 1988
41. Kitz DS, Gold B, Schwartz JS, et al: Decreasing unnecessary testing in PS I and II patients. Anesth Analg 67:S116, 1988
42. Orkin FK, Gold B: Selection. In Wetchler BV (ed): Anesthesia for Ambulatory Surgery. 2nd Ed. JB Lippincott, Philadelphia (in press)
43. Marais ML, Maher MW, Wetchler BV, et al: Reduced demands on recovery room resources with propofol (Diprivan) compared to thiopental-isoflurane. Anesthesiol Rev 16: 29, 1989
44. Ancona-Berk VA, Chalmers TC: An analysis of the costs of ambulatory and inpatient care. Am J Public Health 76:1101, 1986
45. Steffen GF: Quality medical care: a definition. JAMA 260:56, 1988
46. Orkin FK: Risk management and quality assurance in outpatient anesthesia care. Probl Anesth 2:152, 1988
47. Brown EM: Quality assurance in anesthesiology. Adv Anesth 6:1, 1989
48. Duberman SM, Bendixen HH: Mortality, morbidity and risk studies in anaesthesia. p. 37. In Lunn JN (ed): Epidemiology in Anaesthesia: The Techniques of Epidemiology Applied to Anaesthetic Practice. Edward Arnold, Baltimore, 1986
49. Duberman SM, Bendixen HH: Concepts of fail-safe anesthetic practice. Int Anesthesiol Clin 22:149, 1984
50. Institute of Medicine: Advancing the Quality of Health Care: Key Issues and Fundamental Principles. National Academy of Sciences, Washington, DC, 1974
51. Joint Commission on Accreditation of Healthcare Organizations: Surgical and anesthesia services. p. 269. In Accreditation Manual for Hospitals. 1989. Joint Commission on Accreditation of Healthcare Organizations, Chicago, 1989
52. Berwick DM: Continuous improvement as an ideal in health care. N Engl J Med 320:53, 1989
53. Fromberg R: Monitoring and Evaluation: Anesthesia Services. Joint Commission on Healthcare Organizations, Chicago, 1987
54. Roberts JS, Radany MH, Nash DB: Privilege delineation in a demanding new environment. Ann Intern Med 108:880, 1988
55. Cloutier CB: Confronting the problem of physician impairment. QRB 9:96, 1983
56. Gallegos KV, Browne CH, Veit FW, et al: Addiction in anesthesiologists: drug access and patterns of substance abuse. QRB 14: 116, 1988
57. O'Leary DS: The Joint Commission looks to the future. JAMA 258:951, 1987
58. Wennberg JE, Gittelsohn A: Small area variation in health care delivery. Science 182:1102, 1973
59. Wennberg JE, Freeman JL, Culp WJ: Are hospital services rationed in New Haven or over-utilised in Boston? Lancet 1:1185, 1987
60. Bunker JP, Fowles J: Medical audit by claims data. Am J Public Health 75:1261, 1985
61. Roos LL, Cageorge SM, Austen E, et al: Using computers to identify complications after surgery. Am J Public Health 75:1288, 1985
62. Roper WL, Winkenwerder W, Hackbarth GM, et al: Effectiveness in health care: an initiative to evaluate and improve medical practice. N Engl J Med 319:1197, 1988
63. Orkin FK: Practice standards: the Midas touch or the emperor's new clothes? Anesthesiology 70:567, 1989

4

Anesthetic Considerations

Robert K. Stoelting

An understanding of basic pharmacologic and physiologic principles is useful in achieving desirable goals in the management of anesthesia for outpatients. For example, adjustment of delivered concentrations of a drug based on that drug's pharmacokinetics and pharmacodynamics facilitates the establishment of a rapid induction of anesthesia followed by prompt recovery when administration of the drug is discontinued.[1] Likewise, recognizing the impact of each drug on the function of multiple organ systems permits the anesthesiologist to minimize the alterations in physiologic function that accompany anesthesia.[1]

PHARMACOLOGY

The term *pharmacokinetics* refers to the absorption, distribution, metabolism, and excretion of inhaled or injected drugs (i.e., what the body does to a drug).[2–4] The concentration of a drug at its sites of action (receptors) and variations in plasma concentration of drug among patients is determined by pharmacokinetics. Selection and adjustment of drug dosage schedules and interpretation of measured plasma concentrations of drugs are facilitated by an understanding of pharmacokinetic principles.

Pharmacodynamics is the term used to describe the intrinsic sensitivity of receptors to drugs and the mechanisms by which these effects occur (i.e., what the drug does in the body).[4,5] Intrinsic sensitivity of receptors is established by measuring plasma concentrations of drug present when a specific pharmacologic response (e.g., flat electroencephalogram or 90 percent depression of neuromuscular twitch response) occurs. Variability in intrinsic sensitivity of receptors is evidenced when similar plasma concentrations of drugs produce a therapeutic response in some patients, no response in others, and toxicity in a few.

Chronic exposure to a drug that results in a decreased pharmacologic effect is termed *tolerance*. *Cross-tolerance* commonly develops between drugs of different classes that produce similar effects, such as depression of the central nervous system (CNS). Tolerance that develops abruptly with only a few doses of a drug, such as thiopental, is termed *tachyphylaxis*. The most important factor in tachyphylaxis is the development of neuronal adaptation.

An *additive effect* is present when a second drug acting with the first drug produces an effect equal to algebraic summation. *Synergism* is present when two drugs interact to produce an effect that is greater than the algebraic summation. A drug that activates a receptor is an *agonist*, while a drug that binds to but does not activate the receptor is an *antagonist*. Increasing concentrations of an agonist can overcome competitive antagonism but not noncompetitive antagonism. Termination of drug effect is by metabolism, excretion, or redistribution to inactive tissue sites.

Pharmacokinetics of Injected Drugs

Compartmental Models

Compartmental models depict the distribution of a drug in the body (peripheral compartments) following its intravenous injection (central compartment) (Fig. 4-1). Volume of distribution (Vd), calculated as the dose of drug injected intravenously divided by the resulting plasma concentration before elimination starts, depicts distribution characteristics of a drug in the body. Binding to plasma proteins and poor lipid solubility (e.g., nondepolarizing muscle relaxants) limit passage of drug to tissues, thus maintaining a high plasma concentration and a small calculated Vd. Lipid soluble drugs (e.g., thiopental and fentanyl) are concentrated in peripheral tissues with a resulting low plasma concentration and a calculated Vd that exceeds total body water.

Plasma Concentration Curves

A graphic plot of the logarithm of the plasma concentration of drug versus time following a rapid intravenous injection characterizes the distribution (α) and elimination (β) halftimes of that drug (Fig. 4-2). The distribution phase begins immediately after intravenous injection of the drug and reflects its distribution from the circulation to peripheral tissues. The subsequent elimination phase is characterized by a gradual decline in the plasma concentration of the drug and reflects its elimination from the central vascular compartment, principally by renal and hepatic clearance mechanisms.

Elimination halftime is the time necessary for the plasma concentration of drug to decline 50 percent during the elimination phase. Clearly, renal or hepatic disease that alters Vd and/or clearance will alter the elimination halftime. Drug accumulates in the plasma when drug dose (infusion rate or dosing intervals) exceeds the rate of elimination.

First Pass Effect

Drugs absorbed from the gastrointestinal (GI) tract enter the portal venous blood and thus pass through the liver before entering the systemic circulation for delivery to receptors. This is known as the first pass effect and, for drugs that undergo extensive hepatic extraction and metabolism (e.g., propranolol and lidocaine), this is the rea-

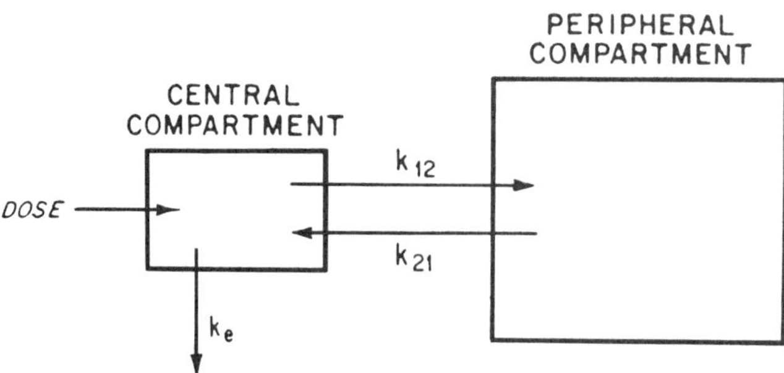

Fig. 4-1. A two-compartment pharmacokinetic model as derived from a biexponential plasma decay curve (see Fig. 4-2). k_{12} and k_{21} are the rate constants that characterize intercompartmental transfer of drugs, and k_e is the rate constant for overall drug elimination from the body. (From Stanski and Watkins,[4] with permission.)

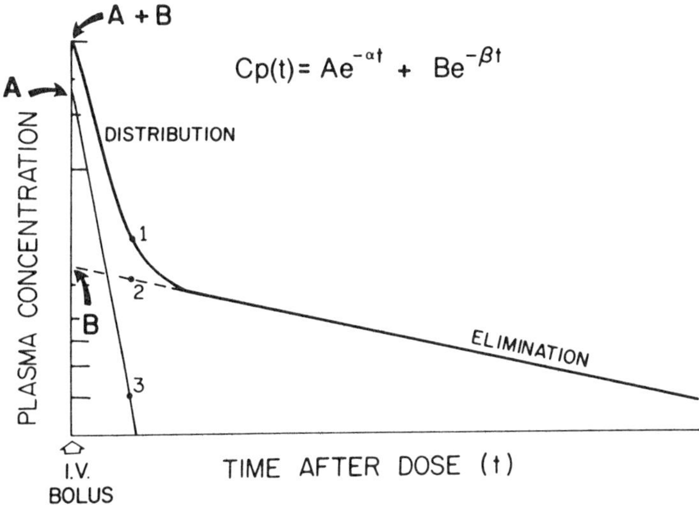

Fig. 4-2. Schematic depiction of the decline in the plasma concentration of drug with time following rapid intravenous injection into the central compartment (see Fig. 4-1). Two distinct phases (e.g., biexponential) characterize this curve, designated as the distribution and elimination phases. (From Stanski and Watkins,[4] with permission.)

son for large differences between effective oral and intravenous doses.[6]

Ionization

The degree of ionization of a drug is a function of its dissociation constant (pKa) and the pH of the surrounding fluid. When pK and pH are identical, 50 percent of the drug exists in the ionized form. Barbiturates tend to be highly ionized at an alkaline pH, whereas opioids and local anesthetics are highly ionized at an acid pH. The nonionized drug molecule is usually lipid soluble and can diffuse across lipid membranes that constitute the blood-brain barrier, renal tubular epithelium, and hepatocytes (Table 4-1).[1] As a result, this drug fraction is pharmacologically active, undergoes reabsorption from renal tubules, is absorbed from the GI tract, and is susceptible to hepatic metabolism. Conversely, the ionized drug fraction cannot easily cross lipid membranes and possesses limited pharmacologic activity.

Protein Binding

A variable amount of most drugs is bound to plasma proteins. Only unbound drug is available to cross cell membranes and act on receptors. As a result, it is the unbound fraction that is principally responsible for pharmacologic effects of the drug. High protein binding results in a small calculated Vd and limited hepatic metabolism.

Clearance

Clearance (Cl) is the volume of plasma cleared of drug, most often by renal and/or hepatic mechanisms. Constant drug infu-

Table 4-1. Characteristics of Drug Fractions

	Nonionized	Ionized
Pharmacologic effect	Active	Inactive
Solubility	Lipid	Water
Cross-lipid barriers	Yes	No
Renal excretion	No	Yes
Hepatic metabolism	Yes	No

(Adapted from Stoelting,[1] with permission.)

sion techniques depend on adjustment of drug delivery to parallel clearance to maintain a desired therapeutic concentration in the plasma. It is important to recognize that individual variations in Vd and clearance may alter the elimination halftime ($t_{1/2}\alpha$ Vd/Cl) of a drug in an individual patient compared with values calculated from normal patients.

Renal Clearance

Renal clearance of drugs involves (1) glomerular filtration, (2) active tubular secretion, and (3) passive tubular reabsorption. The amount of drug that enters the renal tubular lumen depends on the fraction of drug bound to protein and the glomerular filtration rate. Reabsorption from renal tubules removes drug that has entered tubules by glomerular filtration and tubular secretion. This reabsorption is most prominent for lipid-soluble drugs that can easily cross cell membranes of renal tubular epithelial cells to enter pericapillary fluid. A highly lipid-soluble drug such as thiopental is almost completely reabsorbed, so little or no unchanged drug is excreted in the urine. Conversely, production of water-soluble metabolites by virtue of hepatic enzyme activity limits renal tubular reabsorption and facilitates excretion in the urine. Likewise, water-soluble drugs such as long-acting nondepolarizing muscle relaxants undergo extensive renal excretion in the absence of hepatic metabolism.

Renal clearance of drugs is correlated with endogenous creatinine clearance or serum creatinine concentration. The magnitude of elevation of these indices provides an estimate of the downward adjustment in drug dosage to prevent a cumulative drug effect.

Hepatic Clearance

Hepatic clearance of a drug is dependent on hepatic blood flow (perfusion-dependent elimination) and hepatic microsomal enzyme activity (capacity-dependent elimination). The role of metabolism is to convert pharmacologically active lipid-soluble drugs into water-soluble and often pharmacologically inactive metabolites. Increased water solubility reduces the Vd of that drug and its metabolites, thus enhancing renal excretion.

The four pathways of metabolism are oxidation, reduction, hydrolysis, and conjugation. Hepatic microsomal enzymes which also include cytochrome P-450 catalyze most of the oxidation, reduction, and conjugation reactions that lead to metabolism of drugs. Lipid solubility of a drug favors passage across cell membranes, and thus facilitates access of drugs to microsomal enzymes in hepatocytes. Individual variations in hepatic microsomal enzyme activity are genetically determined, accounting for differences (up to sixfold) in rates of drug metabolism among patients. Furthermore, a unique feature of hepatic microsomal enzymes is the ability of drugs to stimulate activity of these enzymes. The resulting enzyme induction speeds the rate of metabolism of certain drugs. Finally, most drugs are metabolized as a constant fraction in a given period of time (first-order kinetics). Rarely, plasma concentration of drug exceeds the capacity of metabolizing enzymes, and metabolism of a constant amount of drug in a period of time occurs (zero-order kinetics).

Nonmicrosomal enzymes principally catalyze reactions responsible for metabolism of drugs by conjugation and hydrolysis. These nonmicrosomal enzymes are present principally in the liver, but are also found in the plasma and GI tract. Nonspecific esterases in the plasma are responsible for hydrolysis of drugs that contain ester bonds (e.g., succinylcholine, atracurium, ester local anesthetics). Individual variation in activity of nonmicrosomal enzymes is similar to that present for microsomal enzymes, except that enzyme induction does not seem to occur.[7] The activity of these enzymes is genetically determined, as emphasized by patients with atypical cholinesterase enzyme and by those who are classified as being rapid or slow acetylators.[8]

Dose-Response Curves

Dose-response curves depict the relationship between dose of drug administered and the resulting pharmacologic effect. These curves are characterized by differences in (1) potency, (2) slope, (3) efficacy, and (4) individual responses (Fig. 4-3).[1] For clinical purposes, the potency of a drug makes little difference as long as the effective dose of the drug can be administered conveniently. The slope of dose-response curves is influenced by the number of receptors that must be blocked before a drug effect occurs. For example, if a drug must occupy a majority of receptors before an effect occurs (e.g., nondepolarizing muscle relaxants), the slope of the dose response curve will be steep.

The maximal effect of a drug reflects its efficacy (i.e., intrinsic activity). Efficacy is reflected by the plateau in dose response curves (i.e., ceiling effect), emphasizing that further increases in dose are not associated with additional therapeutic effect. Differences in efficacy among drugs are depicted by the ability of opioids to relieve intense pain while even large doses of aspirin are effective against only moderate pain. Clearly, efficacy and potency of a drug are not necessarily related.

Individual responses to a drug may vary as a reflection of differences in pharmacokinetics (e.g., bioavailability, renal function, hepatic enzyme function, cardiac output, and patient age) and pharmacodynamics (e.g., receptor responsiveness, drug concentration, and genetics) among patients.[1] Changing pharmacokinetics and/or pharmacodynamics may account for differences in pharmacologic effects of drugs in the same patient at different times. Furthermore, by virtue of altering circulatory, hepatic, and renal function, inhaled anesthetics may influence the pharmacokinetics of injected drugs.[2] Drug interactions may also influence the intensity of drug effect as reflected by therapeutic responses or undesirable side effects.

Pharmacodynamics of Injected Drugs

Receptors

The most common mechanism by which drugs exert pharmacologic effects is by the interaction of the drug with a specific pro-

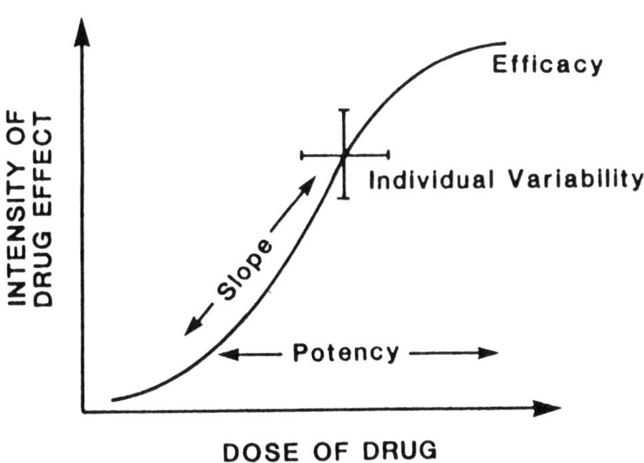

Fig. 4-3. Dose-response curves are characterized by differences in potency, slope, efficacy, and individual responses. (From Stoelting,[1] with permission.)

tein macromolecule (e.g., receptor) in the cell membrane.[9] Conceptually, a receptor consists of three components designated as (1) a recognition site facing the exterior of the cell membrane, (2) a catalytic site oriented toward the interior of the cell, and (3) transducing or coupling proteins (G proteins) necessary for interaction between the recognition and catalytic sites.

Receptors often function as a mechanism for the regulation of the intracellular concentration of adenosine 3′,5′-monophosphate (cyclic AMP). Cyclic AMP is the second messenger. Conceptually, the recognition site interacts with endogenous ligands or drugs. It is likely that this recognition site is the enzyme adenylate cyclase (i.e., the first messenger). This ligand-receptor interaction activates G proteins responsible for activation of the catalytic site leading to conversion of adenosine triphosphate to cyclic AMP. Alternatively, activation of the receptor complex may open channels in cell membranes, allowing ionic fluxes to move along concentration and electrical gradients.

Concentration of Receptors

The concentration of receptors in cell membranes is dynamic either increasing (up-regulation) or decreasing (down-regulation) in response to endogenous concentrations of ligands, plasma concentrations of drugs, or disease states. For example, an excess of catecholamines, as present in the patient with pheochromocytoma, results in a decrease in the concentration of β-receptors (e.g., down-regulation) in an attempt to reduce the magnitude of stimulation. Conversely, interference with activity of receptors as produced by chronic treatment with β-antagonists may result in increased numbers of receptors (i.e., up-regulation) so that an exaggerated response (i.e., hypersensitivity) occurs when the blockade is abruptly reversed by sudden discontinuation of therapy.[10] Increasing age may be associated with decreased responsiveness of receptors despite an unchanged concentration. For example, more isoproterenol is necessary to increase heart rate in elderly patients compared with younger patients.[11]

Characteristics of the Drug-Receptor Interaction

A drug is an agonist if the drug-receptor interaction elicits a pharmacologic effect by virtue of an alteration in the functional properties of receptors. A drug is an antagonist when it interacts with receptors but does not alter the functional properties of receptors, and at the same time prevents the response of receptors to an agonist. If inhibition can be overcome by increasing the concentration of agonist, the antagonist drug is said to produce competitive blockade. Examples of drugs that produce competitive antagonism are nondepolarizing muscle relaxants and β-antagonists. Partial agonists are drugs that bind weakly to receptors so that a maximum concentration produces only modest pharmacologic effects. Examples of partial agonists are the opioid agonist-antagonist drugs.

The affinity of drugs for a specific receptor and its intrinsic activity (e.g., agonist, partial agonist, and antagonist) are closely related to chemical structure. Indeed, minor modifications in drug structure (especially changes in stereoisomerism) can result in dramatic alterations in the drug's pharmacologic effects.

It is traditionally assumed that the intensity of drug effect is proportional to the fraction of receptors occupied by the drug (i.e., receptor-occupancy theory). To explain differences in intrinsic activity between drugs that occupy the same number of receptors but produce responses ranging from stimulation to antagonism, the concept of receptor activation has been proposed.[12] According to this theory, full agonists are able to convert most of the receptors they occupy to the activated state, partial agonists convert only a fraction of the receptors they occupy to the activated state, and antagonists do not activate any of the receptors they occupy to the activated state.

Plasma Drug Concentrations

There is a direct relationship between the intensity of drug effect (i.e., receptor concentration) and plasma concentration of that drug. The plasma concentration of drug is the most practical measurement for monitoring the receptor concentration. Nevertheless, plasma drug concentrations are a reliable monitor only when interpreted in parallel with the patient's clinical response. Furthermore, serial measurements of plasma drug concentrations at selected intervals are more informative than isolated determinations. Clearly, it is misleading to measure plasma concentrations of drugs during rapidly changing periods, such as those that typically follow intravenous injections.

Measurement of plasma concentrations of drugs along with clinical observations serves to verify the appropriateness of the initial loading and maintenance doses. Measurement of plasma concentrations of drugs is particularly useful in avoiding cumulative drug effects in elderly patients and/or in the presence of decreased hepatic or renal clearance. For example, the maintenance dose of a drug must be decreased in the presence of reduced clearance mechanisms to prevent drug accumulation due to a prolonged elimination halftime. This adjustment can be achieved by reducing the size of the maintenance dose or increasing the time interval between doses.

Pharmacokinetics of Inhaled Anesthetics

Pharmacokinetics of inhaled anesthetics describes (1) their uptake (absorption) from alveoli into pulmonary capillary blood, (2) their distribution in the body, and (3) their eventual elimination, principally by the lungs.[1,2] A series of partial pressure gradients beginning at the anesthetic machine serves to drive the inhaled anesthetic across tissue barriers (such as alveoli, capillaries, and cell membranes) to sites of action in the brain. The principal objective of an inhalation anesthetic is to achieve a constant and optimal brain partial pressure (Pbr) of the inhaled anesthetic.

All tissues, including the brain, equilibrate with the anesthetic partial pressure that is present in the perfusing arterial blood (Pa).[13]

$$P\text{A} \leftrightarrows Pa \leftrightarrows Pbr$$

Likewise, arterial blood equilibrates with the alveolar partial pressure (PA) of inhaled anesthetics. This emphasizes the importance of PA as an indirect measurement of Pa and Pbr.[13] This is the reason that PA is used as an index of (1) the rate of induction and recovery from anesthesia, (2) the depth of anesthesia, and (3) the measure of anesthetic equal potency (i.e., minimum alveolar concentration [MAC]). An appreciation of those factors that determine PA and thus Pbr permits control of the doses of inhaled anesthetics delivered to the brain.

Determinants of Alveolar Partial Pressure

The PA, and ultimately the Pbr, of inhaled anesthetics is determined by input (delivery) of the anesthetic to alveoli minus uptake (loss) into the pulmonary capillary blood (Table 4-2).[13] Input of inhaled anesthetics depends on (1) the inhaled partial pressure (PI), (2) the alveolar ventilation (VA), and (3) the characteristics of the anesthetic breathing system. Uptake of inhaled anesthetics from alveoli depends on (1) lipid solubility, (2) cardiac output (CO), and (3) alveolar-to-venous partial pressure difference (A-vD).

Table 4-2. Factors Determining Partial Pressure Gradients for Inhaled Anesthetics

Transfer from anesthetic machine to alveoli
Inspired partial pressure
Alveolar ventilation
Characteristics of anesthetic breathing system
Transfer from alveoli to arterial blood
Blood:gas partition coefficient
Cardiac output
Alveolar-to-venous difference
Transfer from arterial blood to brain
Brain:blood partition coefficient
Cerebral blood flow
Arterial-to-venous difference

(Adapted from Stoelting and Miller,[13] with permission.)

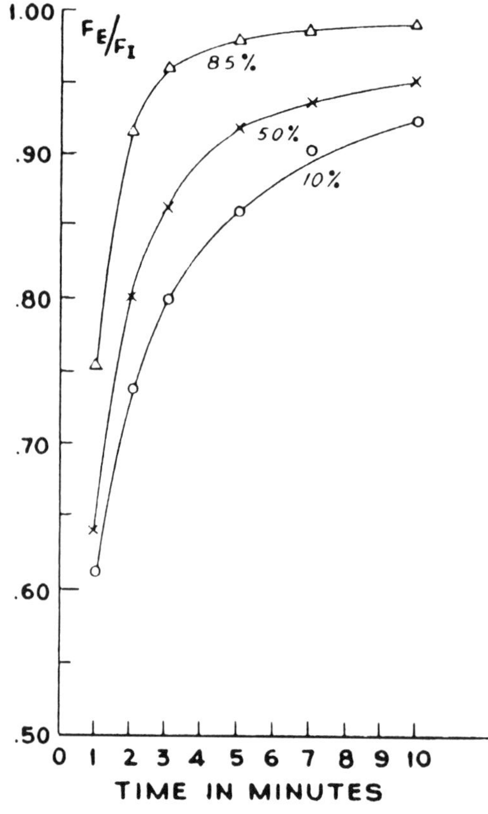

Fig. 4-4. The impact of the inhaled concentration of an anesthetic on the rate at which the alveolar concentration approaches the inspired concentration (FE/FI) is known as the concentration effect. (From Eger,[14] with permission.)

Inhaled Partial Pressure

A high PI delivered from the anesthetic machine is required during initial drug administration. This high initial PI offsets the impact of uptake, accelerating induction of anesthesia as reflected by the rate of increase of the PA and thus the Pbr. With time, as uptake decreases due to saturation of tissues with the anesthetic, the PI is decreased to match reduced anesthetic uptake, maintaining a constant and optimal Pbr. If the PI is maintained constant with time, the PA and Pbr will increase progressively as uptake diminishes.

Concentration Effect. The concentration effect is the impact of PI on the rate of increase of the PA of an inhaled anesthetic (Fig. 4-4).[14] The greater the PI the more rapidly the PA approaches the PI, reflecting greater input to offset uptake. A sufficient range of clinically acceptable inspired concentrations is possible only with nitrous oxide, thus limiting the usefulness of the concentration effect to this drug.

Second Gas Effect. The second gas effect reflects the ability of high volume uptake of one gas (first gas) to accelerate the rate of increase of the PA of any concurrently administered companion (second) gas (Fig. 4-5).[15] For example, the initial large volume uptake of nitrous oxide accelerates the uptake of companion gases, such as volatile anesthetics and oxygen.

Alveolar Ventilation

Increased VA, like PI, facilitates input of inhaled anesthetics to oppose their uptake into arterial blood. The result is a more rapid rate of increase in the PA and induction of anesthesia. Decreased VA has the opposite effect, acting to reduce input and

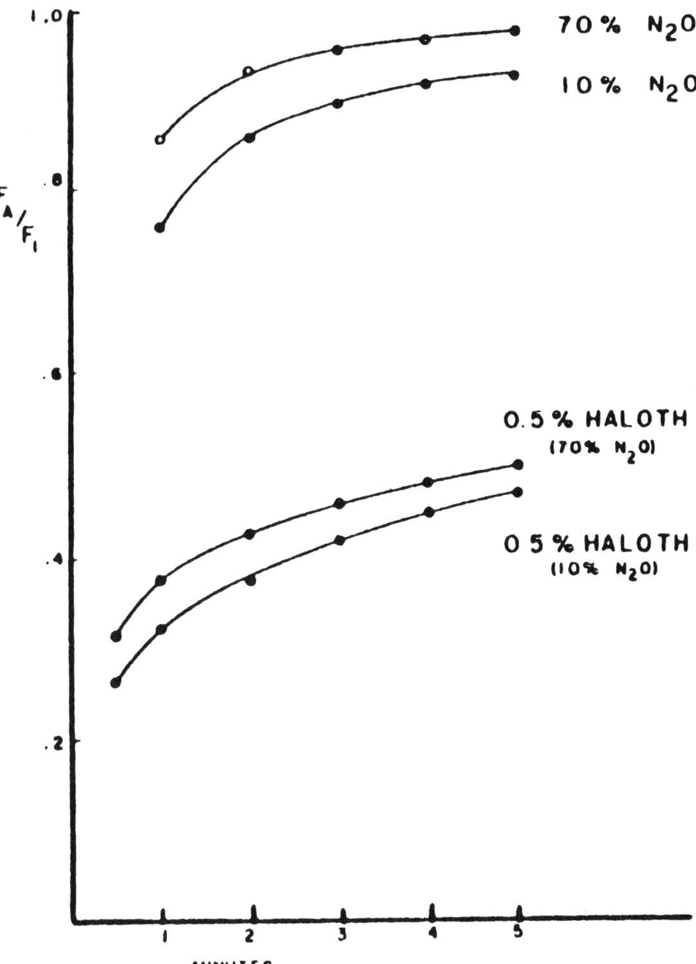

Fig. 4-5. The second gas effect is the accelerated increase in the alveolar concentration of a second gas, halothane (HALOTH), toward the inspired concentration (FA/FI) in the presence of a high inhaled concentration of the first gas (nitrous oxide). (From Epstein et al.,[15] with permission.)

thus slowing achievement of a PA and Pbr necessary for the induction of anesthesia. In addition to increased input produced by hyperventilation of the lungs, the concomitant reduction in $PaCO_2$ acts to decrease cerebral blood flow which could offset the effect of increased input on PA by decreasing delivery of anesthetic to the brain.

Inhaled anesthetics influence their own uptake by causing hypoventilation, thus reducing input.[2] This acts as a negative feedback mechanism that prevents establishment of an excessive depth of anesthesia when a high PI is administered. This protective mechanism is lost when mechanical ventilation of the lungs replaces spontaneous ventilation.

Anesthetic Breathing System

Characteristics of the anesthetic breathing system that influence the rate of increase of the PA are (1) volume of the breathing circuit, (2) solubility of inhaled anesthetics in the components of the breathing system, and (3) gas inflow from the anesthetic machine. The volume of the anesthetic breathing circuit acts as a buffer to slow achievement of the PA and thus the Pbr. This buffer effect is negated by delivering high gas flows (5 to 10 L/min) from the anesthetic machine into the breathing circuit at the start of the anesthetic. Solubility of inhaled anesthetics in the components of the anesthetic breathing system initially slows the rate at which the PA increases and, like the volume of the breathing system, is negated by high initial gas flows from the anesthetic machine.

Solubility

Solubility of inhaled anesthetics in blood and tissues is denoted by the partition coefficient (Table 4-3).[1,2,16] A partition coefficient is a distribution ratio that describes how an inhaled anesthetic distributes itself between two phases (e.g., blood and gas) at equilibrium (i.e., when the partial pressures are identical). The partition coefficient may also be thought of as reflecting the relative capacity of each phase to accept anesthetic. Solubility of anesthetics in fluids and tissues is temperature dependent. Unless otherwise stated, partition coefficients are at 37°C (100.4°F).

Blood : Gas Partition Coefficient. The rate at which the PA approaches the PI is principally determined by solubility of the anesthetic in blood. When the blood : gas partition coefficient is high, a large amount of anesthetic must be dissolved in blood (i.e., an inactive reservoir) before the Pa equilibrates with the PA. For example, the high solubility of methoxyflurane slows the rate at which the PA and Pbr increase; thus, induction of anesthesia is slow (Fig. 4-6).[17] The impact of high blood solubility on the rate of induction of anesthesia can be offset, to some extent, by increasing the PI. When blood solubility is low, as with nitrous oxide, minimal amounts of inhaled anesthetic must be dissolved before equilibrium is reached; thus, the rate of increase of PA and Pa is prompt, and achievement of a Pbr is rapid (Fig. 4-6).[17]

Table 4-3. Comparative Solubilities of Inhaled Anesthetics

	Blood : gas partition coefficient
Methoxyflurane	12
Halothane	2.4
Enflurane	1.9
Isoflurane	1.4
Nitrous oxide	0.47
Sevoflurane	0.6
Desflurane (I-653)	0.42

Nitrous Oxide Transfer to Closed Gas Spaces. The blood : gas partition coefficient of nitrous oxide (0.47) is 34 times greater than that for nitrogen (0.014). This differential solubility means that nitrous oxide can leave the blood to enter an air-filled cavity 34 times more rapidly than nitrogen can leave the cavity to enter blood.[18] As a result of this preferential transfer of nitrous oxide, the volume or pressure of the air-filled cavity increases. Passage of nitrous oxide into an air-filled cavity that is surrounded by a compliant wall (e.g., intestine, pneumothorax, pulmonary blebs, or air emboli) causes the volume of the gas space to expand. Conversely, passage of nitrous oxide into an air-filled cavity surrounded by a noncompliant wall (middle ear, nasal sinuses) causes an increase in intracavitary pressure.

The magnitude of volume or pressure increase in an air-filled cavity produced by nitrous oxide is determined by (1) the partial pressure of nitrous oxide in the blood perfusing the cavity, (2) the blood flow to the cavity, and (3) the duration of nitrous oxide administration. A pneumothorax or air emboli expands rapidly in the presence of nitrous oxide and administration of this anesthetic is contraindicated when these conditions are present (Fig. 4-7).[18] Con-

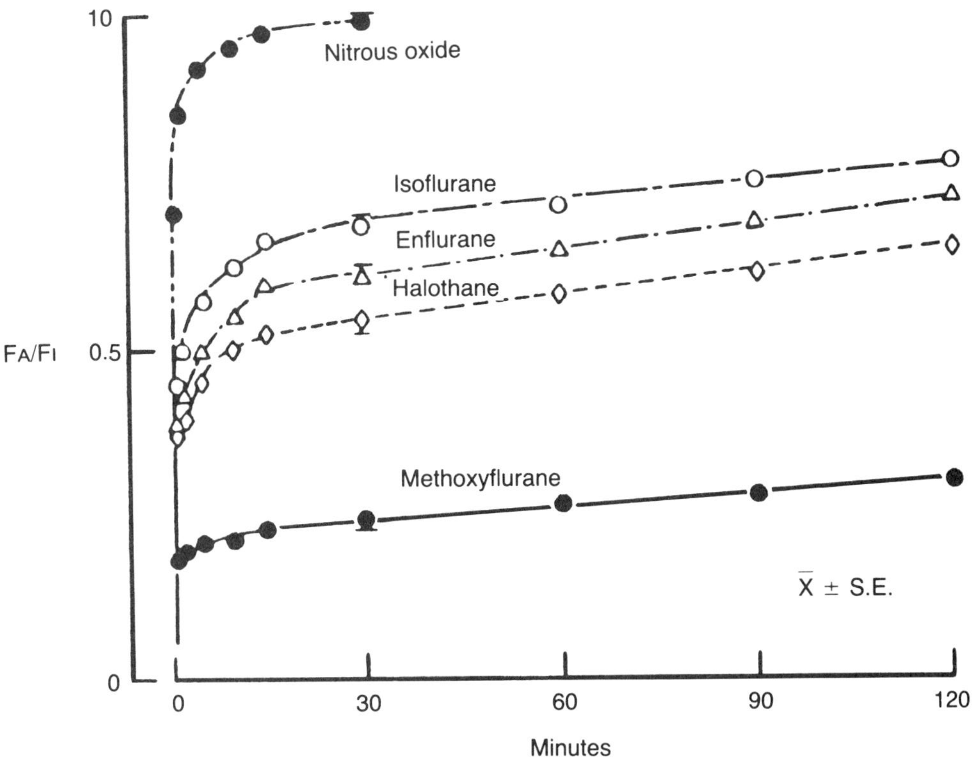

Fig. 4-6. The increase in the ratio of the alveolar to the inspired concentrations of anesthetic (FA/FI) was plotted against time (means for all data ± SE for 30-minute values). (From Carpenter et al.,[17] with permission.)

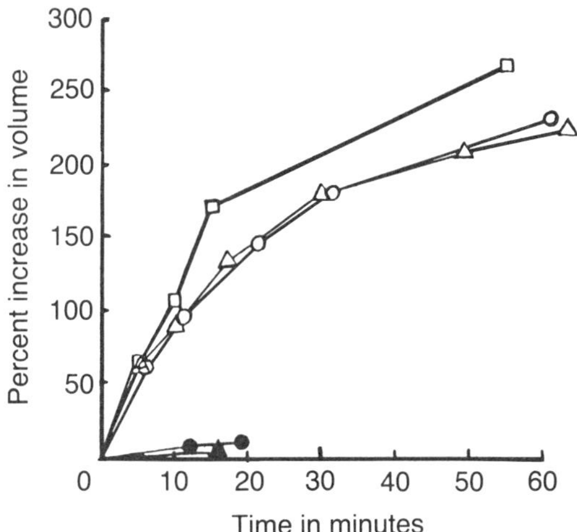

Fig. 4-7. Inhalation of 75 percent nitrous oxide rapidly increases the volume of a pneumothorax (open symbols). Inhalation of oxygen (solid symbols) does not alter the volume of a pneumothorax. (From Eger and Saidman,[18] with permission.)

versely, increase in bowel gas volume produced by nitrous oxide is slow and does not ordinarily influence use of this anesthetic.

Nitrous oxide diffuses into the middle ear more rapidly than it leaves, and middle ear pressures may become excessive if eustachian tube function is compromised by inflammation. Furthermore, middle ear pressure may become negative after discontinuation of nitrous oxide, leading to serous otitis. Nausea and vomiting following anesthesia may be due to multiple mechanisms, but the possible role of altered middle ear pressures due to nitrous oxide should be considered.

Tissue: Blood Partition Coefficients. Tissue: blood partition coefficients determine the time necessary for equilibration of tissues with Pa. This time can be predicted by calculating a time constant (amount of inhaled anesthetic that can be dissolved in tissue divided by tissue blood flow) for each tissue. One time constant on an exponential curve represents 63 percent equilibration, and three time constants are considered to represent nearly complete equilibration.[2] Brain: blood partition coefficients for volatile anesthetics are approximately 2 minutes, and the calculated time constant is approximately 5 minutes. Therefore, equilibration between the brain and blood for volatile anesthetics requires approximately 15 minutes (i.e., three time constants). Three time constants for less soluble nitrous oxide equal approximately 6 minutes. Equilibration of the Pbr and P_A can be accelerated by initially administering a high PI.

Cardiac Output

The CO influences uptake and, therefore, P_A by carrying away more or less anesthetic from the alveoli. A high CO in a frightened or febrile patient results in more rapid uptake, so the rate of increase in the P_A and, thus, the induction of anesthesia is slowed. A low CO speeds the rate of increase of the P_A because there is less uptake to oppose input. Conceptually, a change in CO is analagous to the effect of a change in solubility. For example, doubling CO increases the capacity of blood to hold anesthetic just as solubility increases the capacity of the same volume of blood.

Volatile anesthetics that depress CO can exert a positive feedback response that contrasts with the negative feedback response on spontaneous ventilation exerted by these drugs. For example, depression of CO due to an excessive dose of volatile anesthetic results in an increase in the P_A which further increases anesthetic depth and, thus, cardiac depression. The administration of a volatile anesthetic that depresses CO plus controlled ventilation of the lungs results in a situation characterized by unopposed input of anesthetic (e.g., VA) combined with decreased uptake (e.g., CO). The net effect of this combination of events can be an unexpected rapid increase in P_A and an excessive depth of anesthesia.

Distribution of CO will influence the rate of increase of the P_A. For example, fractional rather than proportional increases in CO with highly perfused tissues receiving a large portion of the CO results in a more rapid induction of anesthesia than if flow was increased proportionally to all tissues. Infants have a relatively greater perfusion of vessel-rich group tissues than do adults, and consequently show a faster rate of increase of the P_A toward the PI.[19]

An intrapulmonary shunt or a right-to-left intracardiac shunt slows the rate at which the Pa approaches the P_A of an inhaled anesthetic.[20] Although the effect of this change will be to slow induction of anesthesia, it seems unlikely that the magnitude of the effect would be clinically significant. Furthermore, a left-to-right tissue shunt, as produced by vasodilation during inhalation of volatile anesthetics, results in arterialization of peripheral venous blood, which will offset the impact of a right-to-left shunt.[21]

Alveolar to Venous Partial Pressure Difference

The A-vD reflects tissue uptake of inhaled anesthetics. Highly perfused tissues (e.g., brain, heart, and kidneys) receive about 75 percent of the CO (Table 4-4).[1] As a result of the small mass and high blood flow, these vessel-rich group tissues equilibrate rapidly and uptake of a volatile anesthetic is greatly decreased after approximately 15 minutes. For this reason, the PI delivered from the anesthesia machine can be reduced while maintaining an optimal PA, and thus Pbr, of the volatile anesthetic. The PI to PA after equilibration of the vessel-rich group tissues reflects principally continued uptake of anesthetic into skeletal muscles and fat.

Recovery From Anesthesia

Recovery from anesthesia is depicted by the rate of decline in the PA (e.g., Pbr) of the inhaled anesthetic. Although similarities exist between the rate of induction and recovery as reflected by changes in the PA of the inhaled anesthetic, there are important differences between the two events. For example, failure of certain tissues to equilibrate with the PA of the inhaled anesthetic means that the rate of decline of the PA during recovery from anesthesia will be more rapid than the rate of increase of the PA during induction of anesthesia. Specifically, continued uptake of anesthetic into tissues such as skeletal muscles and fat contributes to the decline in the Pa of the inhaled anesthetic when the PI is abruptly reduced to zero at the conclusion of anesthesia. Another difference between induction and recovery from anesthesia is the role of metabolism in speeding the rate of decline in the Pa of inhaled anesthetics, such as methoxyflurane and halothane (Fig. 4-8).[17,22]

Table 4-4. Body Tissue Compartments

	Body mass (percent of 70-kg adult)	Blood flow (percent of cardiac output)
Vessel-rich group	10	75
Muscle group	50	19
Fat group	20	6
Vessel-poor group	20	<1

(Modified from Stoelting and Miller,[13] with permission.)

Diffusion Hypoxia

Diffusion hypoxia describes the high volume outpouring of nitrous oxide into the alveoli at the conclusion of anesthesia when the PI of this anesthetic is abruptly reduced to zero.[23] This outpouring of nitrous oxide can dilute the alveolar oxygen concentration and can result in up to a 10 percent decrease in PaO_2. Prevention of diffusion hypoxia is achieved by filling the lungs with oxygen at the conclusion of anesthesia.

Pharmacodynamics of Inhaled Anesthetics

The mechanism by which inhaled anesthetics produce progressive and occasionally selective depression of the CNS is not known.[1,2] Most evidence is consistent with inhibition of synaptic transmission in the CNS produced by an action of inhaled anesthetics at lipophilic sites in cell membranes. However, a single theory to explain the mechanism of anesthesia seems unlikely.

Meyer-Overton Theory

Correlation between lipid solubility of inhaled anesthetics and anesthetic potency (i.e., MAC) suggests that anesthesia occurs

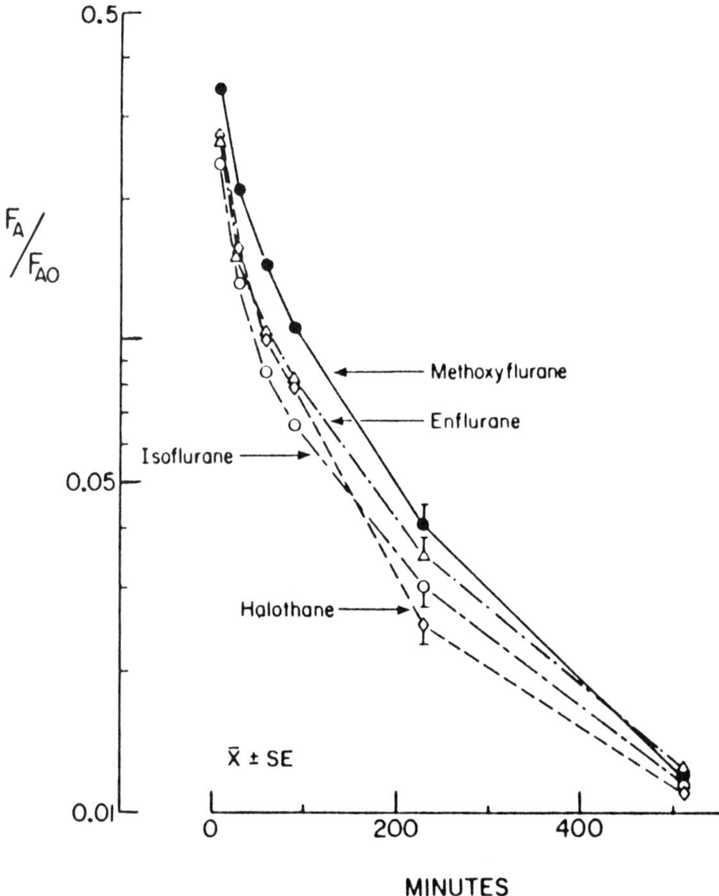

Fig. 4-8. The decline in the alveolar concentration is expressed as the ratio of the PA at a given time (FA) to the alveolar concentration immediately before discontinuation of anesthetic administration (FAO) and is plotted against time (means for all data ± SE for 2- and 4-days values). Note that FA/FAO is plotted on a logarithmic scale. (From Carpenter et al.,[17] with permission.)

when a sufficient number of anesthetic molecules dissolve in lipid cell membranes (Table 4-5).[1,24,25] Conceptually, expansion of cell membranes by dissolved anesthetic molecules could exert pressure on ionic channels necessary for sodium flux and the subsequent development of action potentials necessary for synaptic transmission. Evidence supporting this theory is partial antagonism of anesthesia produced by high atmospheric pressure (40 to 100 atm) that

Table 4-5. Comparative Potencies of Inhaled Anesthetics in Adults

	Minimum alveolar concentration
Nitrous oxide	104%[a]
Halothane	0.74%
Enflurane	1.68%
Isoflurane	1.15%
Methoxyflurane	0.16%
Sevoflurane	2.6% (estimated)
Desflurane (I-653)	7.2%[b]

[a] Determined in a hyperbaric chamber.
[b] Determined in dogs.

presumably compresses lipid membranes back to their preanesthetic contour.[26] Nevertheless, not all lipid-soluble drugs are anesthetics.

Receptor Theory

Existence of receptors in the CNS as sites and mechanisms of action of inhaled anesthetics is suggested by the steep dose-response curve for inhaled anesthetics (e.g., 1 MAC prevents movement in 50 percent of subjects, while 1.3 MAC prevents movement in at least 95 percent of subjects).[27] A crucial degree of receptor occupancy is characteristic of a steep dose-response curve. Marked reductions in MAC (up to 90 percent) produced by α-2 agonists further suggest a receptor site of action for inhaled anesthetics.[28]

Neurotransmitter Availability

γ-Aminobutyric acid (GABA) is the most common inhibitory neurotransmitter in the CNS. In vitro studies have demonstrated the ability of inhaled anesthetics to impair the breakdown of GABA (halothane at a greater extent than enflurane).[29] Conceivably, the accumulation of GABA in the CNS could reduce synaptic transmissions characteristic of anesthesia.

PHYSIOLOGY

Anesthesia produces alterations in the physiologic function of all organ systems. Traditionally, the greatest emphasis has been on circulatory and pulmonary physiology and the impact of anesthetic drugs.[1] There is increased awareness that endocrine function and the hormonal response to stress are influenced by anesthesia. Even in induction doses, etomidate produces transient suppression of adrenocortical function.[30] Changes in renal and hepatic physiology accompany anesthesia, but are transient and only rarely clinically significant in otherwise healthy patients.

Circulation

The cardiac cycle consists of a period of relaxation (diastole) followed by a period of contraction (systole) (Fig. 4-9).[31] Each cardiac cycle is initiated by spontaneous generation of an action potential in the sinus node. Heart valves open passively along a pressure gradient and close when a backward pressure gradient develops due to a high pressure in the pulmonary artery and aorta (Table 4-6).[1]

As blood flows through the systemic circulation, its pressure decreases progressively as it travels to the right atrium (Fig. 4-10).[31] Venous return is more important than myocardial contractility in controlling CO. The intrinsic ability of the heart to adjust its stroke volume in response to changes in venous return is known as the Frank-Starling law of the heart. Venous return is directly related to blood pressure and inversely proportional to systemic vascular resistance. Tissue blood flow is dependent on metabolic oxygen needs which influence perfusion by appropriate changes in resistance to flow. The autonomic nervous system plays a prominent role in the regulation of blood pressure and cardiac output. Baroreceptor reflex responses, principally via the carotid sinus, sense changes in blood pressure and evoke changes in autonomic nervous system activity designed to maintain blood pressure in a normal range.

Cardiac dysrhythmias most often reflect altered automaticity of pacemaker cardiac cells or altered conductivity of cardiac impulses through the specialized conduction system of the heart. Enhanced automaticity most likely reflects activation of the

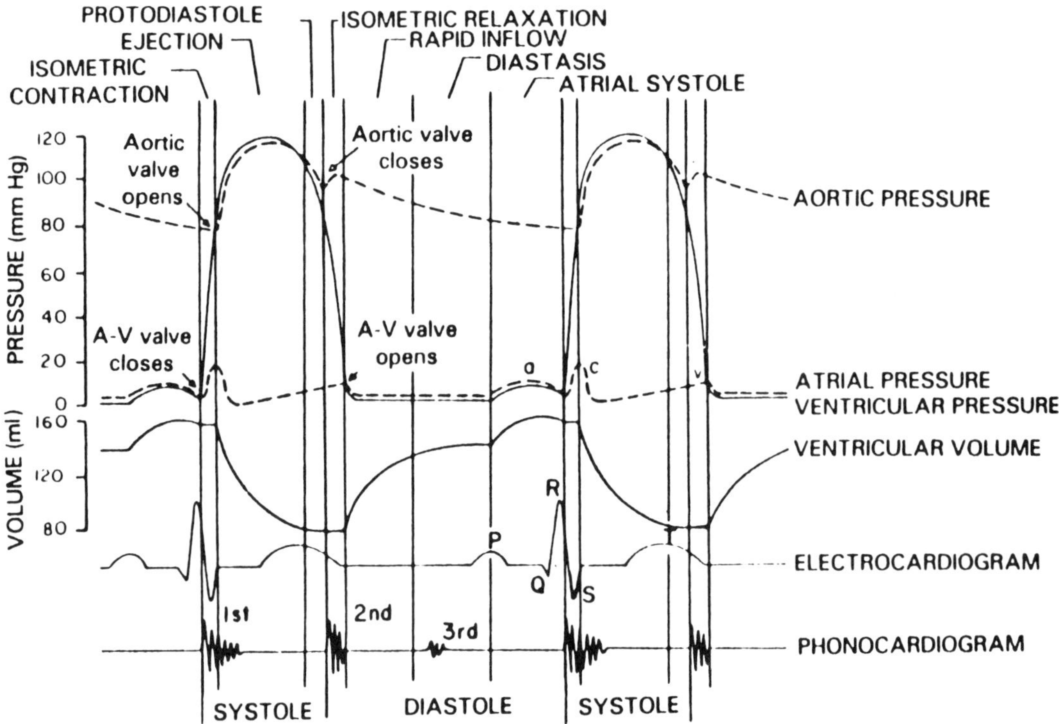

Fig. 4-9. Events of the cardiac cycle, including changes in intravascular pressures, ventricular volume, ECG, and phonocardiogram. (From Guyton,[31] with permission.)

autonomic nervous system by events such as arterial hypoxemia, acidosis, or increased circulating concentrations of catecholamines. Electrolyte abnormalities, particularly potassium, should always be considered when unexpected cardiac dysrhythmias occur.

Lungs

The lungs are responsible for accepting gases from the atmosphere and for the subsequent distribution of these gases to the alveoli. The amount of gas in the lungs has been divided into four different lung capacities which represent the sum of various lung volumes (Fig. 4-11 and Table 4-7).[1] Minute ventilation is the tidal volume times the rate of breathing, while VA is the portion of the minute ventilation capable of participating in gas exchange with pulmonary capillary blood. Control of ventilation is designed to make the necessary adjustments in VA to maintain an optimal and unchanging concentration of hydrogen ions, oxygen, and carbon dioxide. Fine control of ventilation is provided by the respiratory center under the influence of chemical stimuli (especially carbon dioxide) and a peripheral

Table 4-6. Normal Pressures in the Systemic Circulation

	Mean value (mmHg)	Range (mmHg)
Systolic blood pressure	120	90–140
Diastolic blood pressure	80	70–90
Mean arterial pressure	92	77–97
Left ventricular end-diastolic pressure	6	0–12
Left atrial pressure	8	2–12
Right atrial pressure	5	3–8

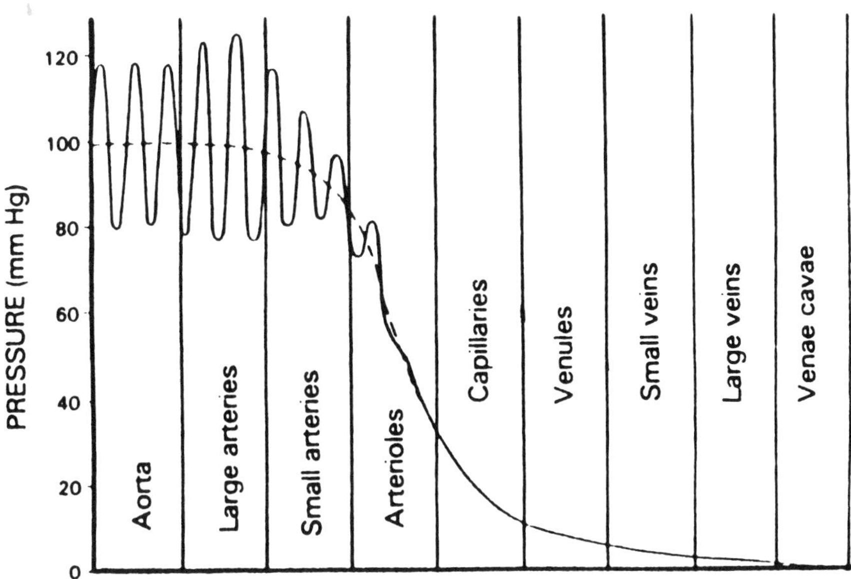

Fig. 4-10. Blood pressure declines as the blood travels from the aorta to large veins. (From Guyton,[31] with permission.)

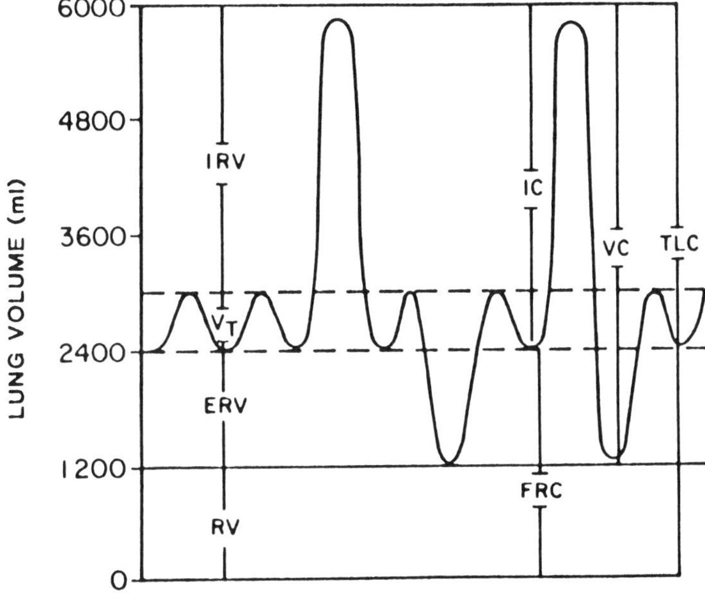

Fig. 4-11. Schematic diagram of breathing excursions at rest and during maximum inhalation or exhalation. The amount of gas in the lungs is categorized as inspiratory reserve volume (IRV), tidal volume (V_T), expiratory reserve volume (ERV), residual volume (RV), inspiratory capacity (IC), functional residual capacity (FRC), vital capacity (VC), and total lung capacity (TLC). (From Stoelting,[1] with permission.)

Table 4-7. Lung Volumes and Capacities

	Normal adult value (ml)
Tidal volume	500
Inspiratory pressure volume	3,000
Expiratory reserve volume	1,200
Residual volume	1,200
Inspiratory capacity	3,500
Functional residual capacity	2,400
Vital capacity	4,500
Total lung capacity	5,900

chemoreceptor system (carotid body responsive to changes in PaO_2).

Oxygen leaves alveoli to enter pulmonary capillary blood, and carbon dioxide enters alveoli from pulmonary capillary blood by diffusion. The ratio of VA to pulmonary capillary blood flow ($\dot{V}/\dot{Q}$) determines the effectiveness of gas exchange, especially for oxygen. The fraction of pulmonary blood flow that is not exposed to ventilated alveoli is designated as an intrapulmonary shunt.

Nearly all of the oxygen transported from alveoli to tissues is carried in chemical combination with hemoglobin. The shape of the oxyhemoglobin dissociation curve assures transfer of large amounts of oxygen to tissues with small changes in PaO_2 (Fig. 4-12).[1] A shift of the curve to the left due to alkalosis or hypothermia reduces release of oxygen from hemoglobin to tissues. Under resting conditions, approximately 5 ml of oxygen is released to the tissues from every 100 ml of blood, resulting in a total delivery of 250 ml of oxygen to tissues each minute when the CO is 5 L/min. At the same time, approximately 200 ml of carbon dioxide is delivered by CO to the alveoli for elimination by VA.

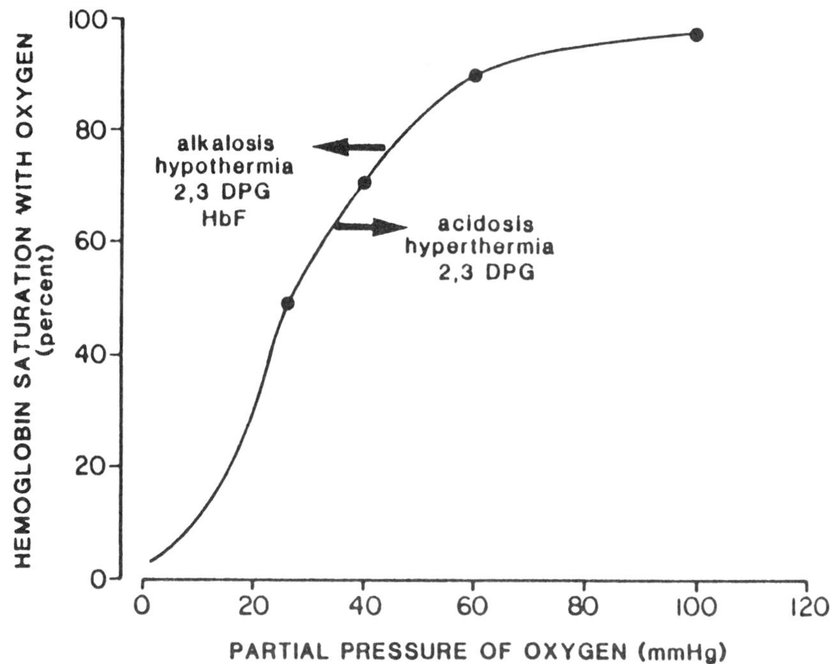

Fig. 4-12. Oxyhemoglobin dissociation curve for adult hemoglobin (HbA) at pH 7.4 and 37°C (100.4°F). Changes in arterial pH, body temperature, concentration of 2,3-disphosphyglycerate (2,3-DPG), and presence of different types of hemoglobin (fetal hemoglobin [HbF]) shift the oxyhemoglobin dissociation curve to the left or right of its normal position. (From Stoelting,[1] with permission.)

REFERENCES

1. Stoelting RK: Pharmacology and Physiology in Anesthetic Practice. JB Lippincott, Philadelphia, 1987
2. Eger EI II: p. 146. Anesthetic Uptake and Action. Williams & Wilkins, Baltimore, 1974
3. Hug CC: Pharmacokinetics of drugs administered intravenously. Anesth Analg 57:704, 1978
4. Stanski DR, Watkins WD: Drug Disposition in Anesthesia. Grune & Stratton, Orlando, FL, 1982
5. Hull CJ: Pharmacokinetics and pharmacodynamics. Br J Anaesth 51:579, 1979
6. Routledge PA, Shand DG: Presystemic drug elimination. Annu Rev Pharmacol Toxicol 19:447, 1979
7. Stoelting RK, Peterson C: Phenobarbital or diazepam therapy and plasma cholinesterase activity. Anesthesiology 42:356, 1975
8. Uetrecht JP, Woosley RL: Acetylator phenotype and lupus erythematosus. Clin Pharmacokinet 6:118, 1981
9. Maze M: Clinical implications of membrane receptor function in anesthesia. Anesthesiology 55:160, 1981
10. Fraser J, Nadeau J, Robert D, Wood AJJ: Regulation of human beta receptors by endogenous catecholamines. Relationship of leukocyte beta-receptor density to the cardiac sensitivity to isoproterenol. J Clin Invest 67:1777, 1981
11. Feldman RD, Limbird LE, Nadeau J, Robertson D, Wood AJJ: Alterations in leukocyte beta-receptor affinity with aging. A potential explanation for altered beta-adrenergic sensitivity in the elderly. N Engl J Med 310:815, 1984
12. Papadimitriou A, Worcel M: Dose-response curves for angiotensin II and synthetic analogues in three types of smooth muscle. Existence of different forms of receptor sites for angiotensin II. Br J Pharmacol 50:291, 1974
13. Stoelting RK, Miller RD: Basic principles. p. 9. In: Basics of Anesthesia. 2nd Ed. Churchill Livingstone, New York, 1989
14. Eger EI II: Effect of inspired anesthetic concentration on the rate of rise of alveolar concentration. Anesthesiology 24:153, 1963
15. Epstein RM, Rackow H, Salanitre E, Wolf G: Influence of the concentration effect on the uptake of anesthetic mixtures: the second gas effect. Anesthesiology 25:364, 1964
16. Eger EI II: Partition coefficients of I-653 in human blood, saline and olive oil. Anesth Analg 66:971, 1987
17. Carpenter RL, Eger EI II, Johnson BH, et al: Pharmacokinetics of inhaled anesthetics in humans: measurements during and after the simultaneous administration of enflurane, halothane, isoflurane, methoxyflurane and nitrous oxide. Anesth Analg 65:575, 1986
18. Eger EI II, Saidman LJ: Hazards of nitrous oxide anesthesia in bowel obstruction and pneumothorax. Anesthesiology 26:61, 1965
19. Salanitre E, Rackow H: The pulmonary exchange of nitrous oxide and halothane in infants and children. Anesthesiology 30:388, 1969
20. Stoelting RK, Longnecker DE: Effect of right-to-left shunt on rate of increase in arterial anesthetic concentration. Anesthesiology 36:352, 1972
21. Williamson DC, Munson ES: Correlation of peripheral venous and arterial blood gas values during general anesthesia. Anesth Analg 61:950, 1982
22. Carpenter RL, Eger EI II, Johnson BH, et al: The extent of metabolism of inhaled anesthetics in humans. Anesthesiology 65:201, 1986
23. Fink BR: Diffusion anoxia. Anesthesiology 16:511, 1955
24. Merkel G, Eger EI II: A comparative study of halothane and halopropane anesthesia. Including method for determining equipotency. Anesthesiology 24:346, 1963
25. Doorley BM, Waters SJ, Terrell RC, Robinson JL: MAC of I-653 in beagle dogs and New Zealand white rabbits. Anesthesiology 69:89, 1988
26. Halsey MJ, Smith B: Pressure reversal of narcosis produced by anesthetics, narcotics and tranquilizers. Nature 257:811, 1975
27. Quasha AL, Eger EI II, Tinker JH: Determination and application of MAC. Anesthesiology 53:315, 1980
28. Vickery RG, Sheridan BC, Segal IS, Maze M: Anesthetic and hemodynamic effects of the stereoisomers of medelomidine, an

alpha$_2$-adrenergic agonist, in halothane-anesthetized dogs. Anesth Analg 67:611, 1988

29. Cheng S-C, Brunner EA: Effects of anesthetic agents on synaptosomal GABA disposal. Anesthesiology 55:34, 1981
30. Wagner RL, White PF, Kan PB, et al: Inhibition of adrenal steroidogenesis by the anesthetic etomidate. N Engl J Med 310:1415, 1984
31. Guyton AC: Textbook of Medical Physiology. 7th Ed. WB Saunders, Philadelphia, 1986

5

Surgical Considerations for Outpatient Procedures

Richard C. Schultz
Michael A. Marschall

Outpatient operative procedures have become progressively more commonplace and more comprehensive in the past 20 years. This is largely the result of improved anesthetic and surgical techniques, increasing numbers of both hospital-based and freestanding outpatient centers, and economic influences encouraging limited hospitalization perioperatively.

FINANCIAL CONSIDERATIONS

Important in this age of diagnosis-related groups is the economic advantage of avoiding prolonged hospitalization before or after operative procedures. Companies are increasingly advocating outpatient management in their health plans, largely as a cost-cutting measure.[1] Many health insurers eliminate the need (and cost) of a second surgical opinion when the procedure is performed on an outpatient basis. Hospital corporations are now also promoting this concept within their own centers and are thus competing with independent freestanding units.

A recent study addresses the potential economic advantage of reduced hospitalization in mastectomy patients.[2] Although not strictly outpatients, an early discharge was usually obtained within 72 hours after surgery, with wound and drain care administered at home. The hospital charges were reduced 39 percent without a change in complication rate. The trend toward elective outpatient surgery is accelerating as increasing numbers of procedures and services are offered in the competitive marketplace.

CONDITIONS AFFECTING OUTPATIENT STATUS

With the exception of patients undergoing suction-assisted lipectomy, those requiring multiple blood transfusions, close observation, or intensive postoperative pain control are not scheduled on an outpatient basis. Classes have been devised for levels of surgical care,[3] but these have minimal clinical validity as enough overlap exists to make the judgment and experience of the surgeon as meaningful as any other criterion.

Although chronologic age is a consideration in the selection of candidates for outpatient surgery, the psychological make-up of the individual is of equal importance.[4] Highly excitable or extremely insecure personalities who are otherwise healthy may make unsuitable candidates for outpatient surgery. Elderly patients sometimes feel more comfortable returning quickly to family and support groups, thus avoiding the isolation and loss of autonomy associated with hospitalization. Each candidate, however, should have an adequate support system in case of possible complications and the subsequent need to be able to contact the surgeon rapidly.[5]

TYPES OF OUTPATIENT SURGICAL FACILITIES

The surgeon may now select from among three types of outpatient surgical facilities. The least sophisticated of these is an office-based operatory in which simple procedures under local anesthesia are performed. This setting requires a minimum of technology to function satisfactorily, although workable and accurate monitoring and resuscitative equipment are always recommended. A second type of facility is the hospital-based operating room that is joined to some form of same-day surgery unit with specialized personnel. The full range of anesthetic techniques are available to the surgeon in this setting, as are the other equipment benefits of a hospital operating suite. An advantage of this type of unit is its proximity to hospital services, such as laboratory, blood bank, and radiography department, as well as its proximity to the hospital itself should admission become necessary. Finally, the freestanding center embodies the newest concepts in ambulatory health care in an era of medical economic reform. The Phoenix Surgicenter has served as a prototype since its inception in the early 1970s. This facility began with a full anesthesiology staff and representative surgeons from many disciplines. In the few years they have been operating, freestanding outpatient centers have proved to be safe, economic, and versatile, providing valuable services to both physicians and patients.[6,7] As of 1989, the Joint Commission for the Accreditation of Hospitals (JCAH) has recognized 54 freestanding facilities, the Accreditation Association for Ambulatory Health Care (AAAHC) recognizes 114, and the American Association for the Accreditation of Ambulatory Plastic Surgery Facilities recognizes another 320.

LABORATORY REQUIREMENTS

Preoperative laboratory studies usually include a hematocrit, as any abnormality here could alter both the surgical outcome and anesthetic management. Urinalysis remains inexpensive, and few surgeons would offer an elective operative procedure in the face of a serious abnormality or urinary tract infection. The coagulation profile is undoubtedly overused in the absence of any symptoms or signs of blood dyscrasia by either history or physical examination and should probably be obtained on a selected basis. As in most areas of medicine, an adequate history and physical examination usually provides a greater indication of hidden underlying abnormalities than an unselected battery of laboratory tests. Chest radiography and ECG screening also fall under this category, and usually need to be performed only when underlying pathology is known or suspected.

The surgeon must carefully weigh the appropriateness of outpatient treatment, considering the standards and capabilities of the facilities in the community in which he or she practices, as well as the capacities of the patient.

COMMON OUTPATIENT SURGICAL PROCEDURES

An array of procedures from all surgical disciplines are currently adaptable to ambulatory surgery.

Up to 75 percent of otolaryngologic procedures may be undertaken safely in the outpatient setting. These include middle ear surgery, nasal procedures, laryngeal procedures (often using endoscopy and lasers), tonsillectomy, adenoidectomy, and some specific neck surgery.[8] A large percentage of urologic procedures, including urethotomy, may be safely performed in ambulatory surgical centers, as can numerous pediatric procedures, including distal hypospadias repair. The economic savings in these circumstances are significant; complication rates are similar to hospitalized patients undergoing the same procedure; and the benefits of reduced hospitalization of the pediatric patient are obvious.[9,10]

Even more technical and demanding urologic surgery, such as microsurgical vasovasostomy, can be safely performed as an outpatient procedure, with estimated savings over inpatient management in excess of 61 percent.[11] The elective esthetic procedures of the plastic surgeon are ideal circumstances for outpatient management.[12,13] In addition, a large number of reconstructive procedures, including tissue expansion, breast reconstruction, otoplasty, and various biopsies, are similarly amenable to outpatient management. Even osseous procedures, such as advancement genioplasty, may be undertaken safely by experienced teams in the ambulatory setting.[14] Almost all reconstructive hand surgery can be performed on an ambulatory basis using general or regional anesthesia and tourniquet control. Numerous other procedures, such as dilatation and curettage, fiberoptic endoscopy, arthroscopy, biopsies, and most ophthalmologic procedures, are also appropriate for the outpatient setting. With the introduction of new surgical techniques that allow for less invasive procedures, the outpatient experience will be more widely applied in all surgical disciplines.

Ophthalmic Surgery

Ophthalmic surgery has benefited greatly from recent technologic advances in microsurgery, suture materials, implant materials, and laser surgery. The ophthalmologist can safely perform glaucoma, strabismus, cataract, and intraocular lens surgery as well as retinal, coroneal, and oculoplastic procedures on an outpatient basis without the additional risk of morbidity that accompanies hospital stays.[15] Outpatient cataract procedures have achieved such a record of safety that European physicians are beginning to use the ambulatory setting for this procedure in a climate where the financial concerns of inpatient management are not a factor.[16]

Endoscopy and Laser Surgery

Arthroscopic orthopaedic procedures have all but revolutionized the management of many joint diseases and are generally performed on an outpatient basis. Laser surgery in some anatomic areas provides a less traumatic operative procedure, enabling outpatient management of formerly difficult problems. For example, inoperable patients with esophageal carcinoma have been successfully palliated by endoscopic Nd:YAG laser; this is done as an ambulatory procedure in the majority of cases.[17] Colonscopy and polypectomy can be performed safely on an outpatient basis, with a complication rate similar to that of hospitalized patients.[18] In addition to laparoscopic procedures, uterine curettage, therapeutic evacuation abortion, and cold knife conization have been performed by the gynecologist on ambulatory patients without additional morbidity.[19]

Various anorectal procedures, including fissures, hemorrhoids, condolomata, endoscopies, and biopsies, may be successfully performed on outpatients with a minimum of morbidity.[20] Again, advances in laser surgery have contributed to new and appropriate outpatient procedures in both anorectal surgery and gynecology.

Pediatric Surgery

Pediatric surgery has benefited tremendously from the increase in outpatient surgery. Procedures for correction of pediatric inguinal hernia, umbilical hernia, and undescended testis probably account for over 90 percent of major outpatient pediatric operations.[6] These procedures can be performed in the outpatient setting, on pediatric patients of almost any age, without additional morbidity. There is an obvious overlap between surgical procedures best suited for inpatient management and those that can safely be performed on an outpatient basis. A recent study of pediatric patients undergoing tonsil and adenoid surgery identified certain criteria, including intraoperative and postoperative factors, that would allow for early discharge and outpatient management. Other patients were managed as inpatients because they were at risk for complications such as hemorrhage, dehydration, and emesis.[21] Some of the factors influencing the choice of inpatient or outpatient surgery are the complexity of the surgery, the duration of the surgery, expected blood loss, anesthetic techniques appropriate for the procedure, and the underlying health and psychologic suitability of the patient.

PROVIDING AN OPTIMAL SURGICAL EXPERIENCE

Although many surgeons perform minor and even relatively major operative procedures without the assistance of an anesthesiologist, the team approach provides the highest level of care possible. Nuances in the smooth management of local anesthetic procedures can be achieved by a team, with each member contributing his or her experience and responsibility. With an anesthesiologist in attendance, the surgeon is free to concentrate on the procedure without the need to closely monitor vital signs or titrate sedative and analgesic medication. Most patients, when properly informed, will accept the added expense of an anesthesiologist.

For an outpatient surgical center to function optimally, the surgeon should have a firm understanding of the planned operative procedure, as well as the anesthetic techniques available to the ambulatory patient. A joint perioperative consultation between the surgeon and anesthesiologist ensures the highest quality of care and patient satisfaction. The most appropriate anesthetic techniques are chosen according to input from the patient, the demands of the operative procedure itself, and the goals of the surgeon and anesthesiologist.

The preoperative consultation with the patient should not only elaborate the surgical outcome, risks, and complications, but should consider the anesthetic side effects, recovery period, and provision for postoperative pain management. An important aspect of local or regional anesthesia success is the quality of preoperative counseling provided by both the anesthesiologist and the surgeon. This can probably be best accomplished at a separate interview with the patient on a day preceding the surgical procedure, with additional time set aside the day of surgery for final clarification. Personal communication between the surgeon and anesthesiologist regarding the procedure and its duration helps the patient both intraoperatively and postoperatively, so that when possible, shorter-acting agents may be used to speed recovery and discharge.

Patients opting for outpatient surgery should be knowledgeable and cooperative, and should have a complete understanding of both the procedure and the choice of anesthesia. Recovery requirements should be discussed, as should appropriate options if complications arise. Patients should be accompanied home by a responsible adult and, when a general anesthetic has been used, should have provisions for at least 24 hours of additional support while at home. The individual responsible for the patient during this period must also be aware of the most likely complications and of how to contact the physician promptly should anything untoward arise.

With this careful preoperative preparation, a certain number of patients may be found not to be suitable candidates for outpatient procedures. These individuals may demonstrate unrealistic expectations of either the operative outcome or the anesthetic management. The patient may also not be a reasonable candidate on the basis of underlying physical limitations or risk factors. Similarly, if a suitable support system for postoperative care is not available, the patient should not undergo the more complex outpatient surgical procedures, particularly when a general anesthetic is to be used.

SELECTING ANESTHETIC TECHNIQUES

Local Anesthetic

Many surgical patients are best served by local anesthesia alone, avoiding all forms of sedation. Obviously, this approach is used primarily for less extensive surgical procedures. The patient must be informed beforehand of precisely what is about to take place in surgery and what sensations he or she is likely to experience. Overly excitable and severely hypertensive patients are unsuitable candidates. More potent local anesthetic agents (i.e., 2 percent lidocaine as opposed to 1 percent lidocaine) can make the experience more pleasant. Safety regarding total dosage of anesthetic agent is usually not a problem since the volume required for injection is typically minimal in such cases. Unless there are special concerns related to selected patients these cases typically do not require pulse oximetry, although some outpatient facilities require this as a matter of routine. The advantages to straight local anesthesia are significant: fewer drugs are used, thus there is less risk to the patient; the surgeon can more easily and legally communicate with the patient during the surgical procedure, thus being able to change or add to the procedure previously discussed. After vital signs have been found to be satisfactory, the patient may leave the facility almost immediately following termination of the procedure; and both time and cost savings are realized.

For more involved procedures, local anesthesia can be combined with intravenous sedation to provide the best operative experience for both the patient and surgeon. Sedation with a degree of amnesia is desirable. When used intravenously and appropriately titrated, diazepam (Valium) and the newer benzodiazepine midazolam (Versed) provide acceptable levels of sedation and amnesia with a high degree of safety. The advantages of midazolam include a short halflife, less venoirritation, marked amnestic effects, a less painful injection, and less postoperative residual drug effect. A recent series verified this and attested to the safety of midazolam, reporting a less than 3 percent incidence of nausea with no respiratory complications from over-sedation.[22]

Recently, lorazepam has been used sublingually as an alternative to diazepam during oral surgical procedures. It provides acceptable sedation, although it is associated with more side effects than either diazepam or a placebo. These side effects include giddiness and prolonged psychomotor impairment.[23] Several recent studies have pointed to the added safety of using a pulse oximeter during and after procedures done with intravenous sedation. It provides a reliable and noninvasive means of defining hypoxemia. Hemoglobin desaturation as detected by the pulse oximeter may be unrelated to changes in blood pressure, pulse rate, and rhythm.[24] The quantity of intravenous medication given can be accurately and safely titrated based on oxygen saturation, improving anesthetic management. In addition, hypoxemia may occur at any time during the procedure, or even in the recovery room; pulse oximetry is a valuable adjunct in the immediate postoperative period as well.[24]

Local anesthetic toxicities should be familiar to the anesthesiologist and surgeon, and may be of particular importance in procedures such as facelifts or truncal suction-assisted lipectomy, in which large quantities of local anesthetic agents are used. Should it occur, treatment of toxicity should be prompt and effective, with a defibrillation unit, an oxygen source, endotracheal tube, and cardiac resuscitative and anticonvulsant drugs readily available.

Ketamine is an intravenous agent producing "dissociative" anesthesia with the potential for producing an essentially cataleptic state. Its usefulness to the surgeon lies in its ease of administration, lack of cardiorespiratory depression, and rapid emergence after discontinuance. Its biggest drawback undoubtedly remains the incidence of unpleasant psychic reactions on emergence. In general, this is felt to be manageable through careful preoperative counseling as well as by preoperative and intraoperative medication with a benzodiazepine. White recommends the selective use of ketamine in outpatient anesthesia for brief surgical procedures in children and adults; as an inducing agent in children, given intramuscularly or rectally; and as a supplement for local or regional procedures in adults. White also suggests that it may be successfully used for endoscopic procedures and in the emergency room setting for closed reduction of fractures and for suture removal.[25] He recommends the use of an antisialagogue prior to ketamine administration to reduce the incidence of airway difficulties. The surgeon is cautioned against the use of ketamine with cocaine or epinephrine because of its tendency to decrease uptake of catecholamines, which could possibly cause untoward cardiac irritability.[26]

General Anesthesia

When a general anesthetic is used, to prevent additive cardiac or systemic toxicity from combined agents, the anesthesiologist should be aware of whether additional local anesthetic with or without epinephrine will be used by the surgeon. In addition, emergence from general anesthesia should be smooth and controlled, with no bucking, thrashing, or transient hypertension. These events can logically contribute to the incidence of postoperative hematoma or, in the extreme, wound separation. An antiemetic can be given prior to emergence to lessen the possibility of postoperative nausea and emesis, thereby facilitating an early and comfortable discharge.

In certain operative circumstances, postoperative pain can be reduced through the administration of 0.5 percent bupivacaine as a nerve block at the time of wound closure. A bupivacaine block of the ilioinguinal and iliohypogastric nerves has been found to decrease the postoperative requirement for analgesics after discharge in the pediatric patient undergoing inguinal herniorrhaphy.[27] Recovery periods should be as short as possible to diminish prolonged nursing care and to lower the incidence of postoperative nausea, emesis, and disorientation.

POSTOPERATIVE OBJECTIVES

Postanesthetic and surgical goals should be the prompt return to normal "ambulatory" or "street-ready" status. The recovery areas should be quiet and equipped, as any recovery room, with resuscitative equipment and trained nursing personnel. Observations of abnormal responses or delays in functional return should be communicated to the surgeon and the anesthesiologist. As soon as patients become fully responsive and oriented, they should be allowed to dress, take liquids, and void. If a formal postrecovery area exists, the patients should be allowed to sit with friends or relatives in a somewhat less controlled setting. This, however, does not preclude the necessity of being discharged in the company of a friend or relative. Ideally, the patient is examined by the surgeon or the anesthesiologist immediately prior to discharge. When the anesthesiologist supervises the recovery area, the discharge can often be appropriately made by the anesthesiologist alone. Wound management guidelines are given both verbally and in writing, as are instructions for dealing with potential emergencies. A follow-up appointment is always given with the discharge information.

POSTOPERATIVE COMPLICATIONS

Postoperative complications requiring hospitalization are rare. In a prospective analysis of over 32,000 patients, Natof found that only 35 patients required immediate hospitalization following ambulatory surgery, but only 3 of the 35 cases were classified as urgent. The most common complication was hemorrhage, followed by infection and persistant nausea and vomiting. In Natof's study, 138 hemorrhagic complications were noted, and 50 infectious complications were diagnosed.[28]

Certain procedures have unique complications that should be considered in perioperative management. As experience has been gained in fiberoptic bronchoscopy, its use for outpatient transbronchial biopsy has become increasingly widespread. However, the danger of delayed pneumothorax following this procedure is real, and careful postoperative screening for this complication is critical. It is felt that 1 hour of observation is sufficient to allow safe discharge for the asymptomatic patient. When this precaution is exercised, the complication rate is no different than when the procedure is performed on an inpatient basis.[29] Suction-assisted lipectomy has been reported to be complicated by hematoma, fat embolism, hemorrhage with shock, necrotizing fascitis, and death. Late complications may include thrombotic episodes and even thromboembolism.[30,31] Patients undergoing urologic procedures should be monitored for hemorrhage and the possibility of acute urinary retention in the immediate postoperative period.

The subcutaneous administration of local anesthetic agents at the chest wall with long needles, such as in augmentation mammaplasty, may lead to pleural injury and pneumothorax which manifest postoperatively. The ophthalmologic patient should be cautioned for the onset of visual disturbances, blindness, or extreme postoperative pain, indicative of retrobulbar hematoma. Postoperative hypertension markedly increases the risk for hematoma formation after rhytidectomy.[32] Proper anesthetic management of these patients should include not only close intraoperative monitoring of blood pressure changes, but also postoperative monitoring to avoid the possibility of hematoma in the immediate postoperative period.

SUMMARY

In conclusion, ambulatory surgery is becoming an increasingly popular means of delivering health care. Its safety record is secure, and it continues to demonstrate multiple benefits for the surgeon, anesthesiologist, and patient. A wide variety of operative procedures are amenable to outpatient management, and the list continues to expand. To optimize this concept and to provide the highest level of health care possible, the surgeon–anesthesiologist relationship should be characterized as cooperative and conferring. The surgeon's greatest concerns with this approach to surgery remain with the welfare of the patient after he or she leaves the facility. Generically, these concerns relate to postoperative pain, bleeding, and infection. As the practice of surgery partly remains an art, such complications are minimized to a large extent through thoughtful planning and experience.

REFERENCES

1. U.S. corporations offer incentives to encourage outpatient surgery. Same Day Surg 5:140, 1981
2. Edwards MJ, Broadwater JR, Bell JL, et al: Economic impact of reducing hospitalization for mastectomy patients. Ann Surg 208:330, 1988
3. Detmer DE, Buchanan-Davidson DJ: Ambulatory surgery. Surg Clin North Am 62:685, 1982
4. Davis JE: Surgical complications. p. 106. In Davis JE (ed): Major Ambulatory Surgery. 2nd Ed. Williams & Wilkins, Baltimore, 1986
5. Orkin FK: Selection. p. 93. In Wetchler B (ed): Anesthesia for Ambulatory Surgery. 1st Ed. JB Lippincott, Philadelphia, 1985
6. Cloud DT: Major ambulatory surgery of the pediatric patient. Surg Clin North Am 67:805, 1987
7. Schultz RC: Outpatient surgery from antiquity to the present. p. 11. In Schultz RC (ed): Outpatient Surgery. 1st Ed. Lea & Febiger, Philadelphia, 1979
8. Gussack GS, Hudson WR: Major ambulatory surgery of the otolaryngologic patient. Surg Clin North Am 67:819, 1987
9. Andronaco RB, Warner RS, Cohen MS: Optical urethrotomy as ambulatory procedure. Urology 24:268, 1984
10. Shepard B, Hensle TW, Burbige KA, Lieberman I: Outpatient surgery in pediatric urology patient. Urology 24:581, 1984
11. Kaye KW, Gonzalez R, Fraley EE: Microsurgical vasovasostomy: an outpatient procedure under local anesthesia. J Urol 129:992, 1983
12. Peacock EE: Major ambulatory surgery of the plastic surgical patient. Surg Clin North Am 67:865, 1987
13. Schultz RC: Plastic and reconstructive surgery. p. 79. In Schultz RC (ed): Outpatient Surgery. Lea & Febiger, Philadelphia, 1979
14. Spear SL, Mausner ME, Kawamoto HR: Sliding genioplasty as an anesthetic outpatient procedure: a prospective two center trial. Plast Reconstr Surg 80:55, 1987
15. McCracken JS: Major ambulatory surgery of the ophthalmic patient. Surg Clin North Am 67:881, 1987
16. Davies PD, Limacher E, Powell K: Outpatient cataract surgery 1982–1986. Eye 1:728, 1987
17. Lightdale CJ, Zimbalist E, Winawer JJ: Outpatient management of esophageal cancer with endoscopic Nd:YAG laser. Am J Gastroenterol 82:46, 1987
18. Norfleet RG: Colonscopy and polypectomy in nonhospitalized patients. Gastrointest Endosc 28:15, 1987
19. Berkus M, Daly JW: Cone biopsy: an outpatient procedure. Am J Obstet Gynecol 137:953, 1980
20. Stern H, McLeod R, Cohen Z, Ross T: Ambulatory procedures in anorectal surgery. Adv Surg 20:217, 1987
21. Raymond CA: Study questions safety, economic benefits of outpatient tonsil/adenoid surgery. JAMA 296:311, 1986
22. Baker TJ, Gordon HL: Midazolam (versed) in ambulatory surgery. Plast Reconstr Surg 82:244, 1988
23. Van Der Bijl P, Roelofse JA, Dev Joubert JJ: Comparison of sublingual lorazepam with intramuscular diazepam as sedative during oral surgery. J Oral Maxillofac Surg 24:559, 1988
24. Singer R, Thomas PE: Pulse oximeter in the ambulatory anesthetic surgical facility. Plast Reconstr Surg 82:111, 1988
25. White PF: Ketamine—its use as an intravenous anesthetic. Clin Anesthesiol 2:43, 1984
26. White PF: Invited comment. Ann Plast Surg 15:53, 1985
27. Langer JC, Shandling B, Rosenberry M: Intraoperative bupivacaine during outpatient

hernia repair in children: a randomized double blind trial. J Pediatr Surg 22:267, 1987
28. Natof HE: Complications. p. 321. Wetchler Bernard (ed): Anesthesia for Ambulatory Surgery. JB Lippincott, Philadelphia, 1985
29. Ahamd M, Livingstone DR, Golish JA, et al: The safety of outpatient transbronchial biopsy. Chest 90:403, 1986
30. Alexander J, Takeda D, Sander G, Goldberg J: Fatal necrotizing fascitis following suction-assisted lipectomy. Ann Plast Surg 21:562, 1988
31. Garga TJ, Courtiss EH: The risks of suction lipectomy. Their prevention and treatment. Clin Plast Surg 11:457, 1984
32. Rees TD, Lee YC, Coburn RJ: Expanding hematoma after rhytidectomy. Plast Reconstr Surg 51:149, 1973

6

Nursing Considerations in Outpatient Surgery

Linda Dickey White
Helen McKebery
John Zelcer

Professional nursing is the promotion, conservation, and restoration of the individual's patterns of physical well-being and psychosocial behavior for the purpose of achieving an optimum level of health. A formal nursing philosophy considers that each patient is a unique individual who should be respected as a person, regardless of nationality, race, creed, color, or status,[1] and who has rights and needs that should be recognized and met in ways that are appropriate to the person and the situation. This chapter focuses on the role of nursing and explores the administrative and practical aspects of nursing care that are pivotal to the competent and successful management of an ambulatory surgical unit.

Ambulatory surgical units are committed to providing perioperative care to all patients. To this end, each facility should develop a "mission" statement that will guide the provision of services and establish a sound philosophic approach to patient care. The statement should reflect the values and attitudes held by management and staff regarding the purpose and goals of the unit.

With an understanding of the changing health care environment and the varying needs of outpatients and their families, the roles of perioperative nursing in the ambulatory surgery unit include

1. providing courteous, safe, and cost-effective perioperative care using the team approach;
2. developing an individualized plan of care that incorporates the principles of nursing process (assessment, planning, implementation, and evaluation);
3. advocating support for and dignity of the individual patient and his or her right to respectful and participatory care;
4. facilitating collaboration with other health care professionals to enhance the level of care received by the patients;
5. individually acknowledging responsibility for one's own actions and judgments as well as one's own professional growth and development; and
6. sharing responsibility for the development of a better working relationship among the members of the health care team.

In addition to creating this philosophical statement, it is imperative that it be operationalized when designing a business plan, establishing the organization of services, hiring and orienting personnel, and developing a marketing strategy.

The mission statement begins by addressing the changing and varied needs of patients. While essential for major surgery, inpatient practices may have a detrimental impact on an outpatient's well-being when applied in the ambulatory setting. Inpatient services may lead to excessive dependence on medical authority, social withdrawal from obligations at home and at work, and passivity or implicit exemption from responsibility for the individual's own medical progress.[2] This pattern of dependence may compromise a patient's ability to assist in the medical progress to the extent that he or she cannot or will not get better without direct medical help and support.

In contrast to this focus on dependence, ambulatory surgery emphasizes "wellness." The patient is regarded as a well person coming to the hospital for a minor procedure in an atmosphere that is positive, cheerful, and nonthreatening. A distinctive feature of the ambulatory setting is the expectation that patients will have a degree of independence and that they will accept some responsibility for their own care. This concept is reinforced in the first mission statement.

ORGANIZATION OF SERVICES

It is the responsibility of nursing management to organize patient services to flow smoothly and efficiently (Fig. 6-1). When designing the facility, factors to consider include how patients will reach the unit, the registration process, and the management of preoperative testing. Well-organized preoperative processing is essential in achieving customer satisfaction with the unit. In addition, all personnel must demonstrate their commitment to customer service and their enthusiasm for meeting the needs of patients and visitors. The patient's initial contact with the unit occurs during the preoperative phase of care, and it must be emphasized that all staff members are responsible for creating a positive first impression.

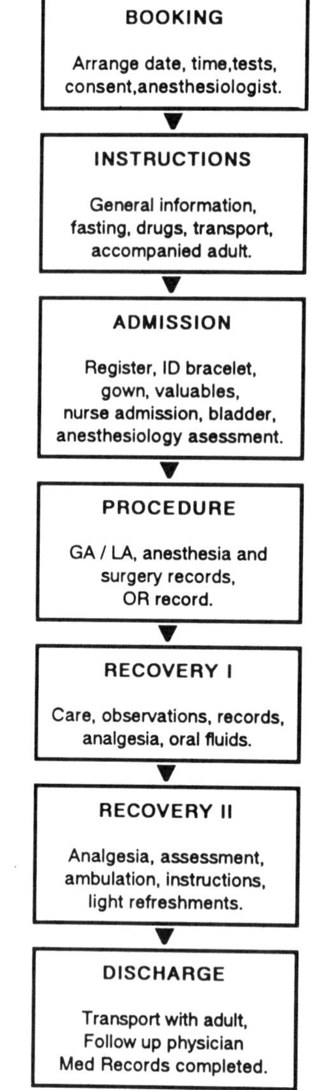

Fig. 6-1. Flowchart of perioperative care. (Courtesy of Dr. John Zelcer, University of Melbourne, Melbourne, Victoria, Australia.)

Of critical importance to the surgeon is the unit's facilitation of surgical procedures. Policies must be developed regarding the types of procedures that will be done, evaluation of patient's physical status, and how procedures will be scheduled.

Scheduling is both a source of frustration as well as a challenge to the smooth running of the ambulatory surgical unit. Typical issues that influence scheduling include the nature of the procedure, expected or actual degree of difficulty, anesthetic requirements, operating room utilization, staff resources (including temporary loss of staff through duties or illness), surgeon availability, equipment availability, and even such simple factors as transportation within the unit. The most common scheduling systems use block, modified block, or open scheduling formats. The decision regarding a scheduling format should be based on the particular needs of those using the facility as well as what similar facilities in the area offer.

A major concern for the anesthesiologist is the process for obtaining laboratory data. Policies are needed to determine which tests will be required, if tests will be performed prior to surgery or on the day of surgery, and how far in advance of the procedure are test results valid.

Once preoperative services are established, intraoperative needs must be addressed. Policies and procedures are created that embrace the Association of Operating Room Nurses (AORN) recommended practices, the Joint Commission on Accreditation of Healthcare Organizations (JCAHO) standards, and regulations outlined by the Occupational Safety and Health Administration (OSHA). Although the nursing service is responsible for identifying policies and procedures, the medical staff must be in agreement and must comply with stated requirements.

Safety is of major importance during the intraoperative period. Nursing responsibilities focus on creating and maintaining an environment that is safe for patients as well as staff. There are also specific safety issues of which nurses should be aware, including fire and evacuation drills, technical safety regulations, such as requirements in selecting, setting up, and operating electrical equipment, and professional issues involving the correct assembly and use of the anesthetic apparatus and minimum standards for patient monitoring.[3]

In addition, OSHA regulations clearly delineate the steps that must be taken by health care providers to assure their own safety as well as the safety of the patient when dealing with body fluid and body substance isolation. Guidelines for universal precautions must be in effect in every ambulatory surgical setting.

Postoperative care is provided by qualified postanesthesia care nurses. Policies and procedures are also needed to assure that patients receive quality care during this phase of their stay. In addition to policies governing nursing services, anesthesiologists must specify policies regarding postanesthesia medical management and discharge criteria.

PERIOPERATIVE NURSING MANAGEMENT

Preoperative Care

The preoperative phase of care begins with the decision to have surgery. The surgeon's office contacts the ambulatory surgery unit to schedule the procedure and register the patient. The admitting process then begins as registration personnel begin to collect data which form the basis of the patient's medical record. Information is obtained to later contact the patient to complete the preregistration process. A patient information brochure should be mailed to the patient at this time to acquaint patients with services available, directions to the unit, and instructions for preoperative preparation, including fasting instructions and what forms and medical information will be required of them the day of surgery.

On the day prior to surgery, a registered nurse contacts the patient to confirm the date of surgery, validate preregistration information, and answer any questions the patient or family members may have. In some instances, the nurse may obtain a history and collect physical assessment data which is reviewed on the day of surgery by the medical staff. When the patient arrives on the day of surgery, he or she verifies and signs registration papers, presents laboratory results or receives tests, and is examined by the anesthesiologist. Nursing personnel review all data to determine a plan of care for the patient. Nursing care plans are mandated by JCAHO and must address any identified problems that are unique to a particular patient as well as standardized care provided to all patients. Care plans reflect the components of the nursing process, assessment, planning, nursing interventions, and evaluation. The assessment and planning aspects of care are completed preoperatively.

The nursing assessment begins with the verification of the preoperative checklist (Fig. 6-2). The nurse obtains and records vital signs, a medication history, and discusses the patient's chief complaint. A more thorough history and physical may also be obtained for later validation by the physician. It is most efficient if the same questions are not asked repeatedly by several different practitioners as it is important to avoid duplication by nurses and physicians. Teamwork should be emphasized as a means of achieving the goal of efficient data collection and retrieval.

Intraoperative Care

The intraoperative phase of care begins when the patient is escorted into the operating room suite and the nurse implements the care plan. Care is delivered in accordance with the surgical procedure preference card, the individual needs of the patient, and the standards of care established by the ambulatory surgery unit. In addition to previously addressed safety issues, appropriate policies for intraoperative care might include positioning, prepping, and draping for procedures; the counting of needles, sponges, and instruments; monitoring requirements; the care and handling of specimens; and cleaning protocols.

Postoperative Care

When the patient is transferred to the postanesthesia care unit (PACU), the postoperative period begins.

The recovery period and progress to full ambulation is one of the key phases of patient management in ambulatory surgical care. Potential acute disorders such as hypoxemia, cardiovascular problems, nausea and vomiting, and other emergence phenomena dictate that services in an ambulatory setting must be equivalent to those applicable to inpatients.[4,5]

Staffing must be adequate to meet both qualitative and quantitative needs. A minimum level requires that nurses be qualified in recovery room care and that nurse-patient ratios be 1:1 for every unconscious patient and 1:3 for all other patients in the postanesthesia care phase.[6]

The postanesthesia recovery phase may be described as two phases. Phase 1 applies to those patients who have had a general anesthetic or regional anesthesia with sedation, and are still not fully responsive to stimuli. Nursing intervention is similar to that in the standard PACU and requires intensive assessment of vital signs, airway management, and attention to specific postanesthesia and postsurgical needs. Evaluation and monitoring will be enhanced by routine use of pulse oximetry.

Phase 2 ("step-down") refers to those patients who have been discharged from phase 1 or who have had local anesthesia with minimal or no sedation, that is, they are conscious. In this case, patients are frequently transferred to a reclining chair, family members are often present, and the patient is encouraged to wake up, move about, and prepare for ambulation. Anticipation and management of nausea, dizziness, pos-

DAY PATIENT
PRE-ANAESTHETIC/PROCEDURE INFORMATION

PATIENT I.D.

D/P

DAY PATIENT PRE-ANAESTHETIC INFORMATION

1. MEDICAL HISTORY

Have you ever had any of the following complaints?

	YES	NO
High Blood Pressure		
Heart Attack		
Angina		
Stroke		
Rheumatic Fever		
Blood Clot in the Legs or Lungs		
Kidney Disease		
Diabetes		
Anaemia		
Shortness of Breath		
Bronchitis		
Asthma		
Pneumonia or Tuberculosis		
Hepatitis or Jaundice		
Eczema		
Hay Fever		
Other Serious Illness		
Nervous Breakdown		
Epilepsy or Other Fits		
Prosthetic Joints		
Heart Valve Replacement or Pacemaker		
Recent Cold		

If yes to any of the above, give further details ....

2. SURGICAL HISTORY

	YES	NO
Have you had previous operations?		

Details ....

	YES	NO
Have you a bleeding tendency or bruise easily?		
Have you had a blood transfusion?		

Dates ....

Have you had any reaction to blood transfusion?

Details ....

Have you taken any Aspirin in the past week?

3. ANAESTHETIC HISTORY

	YES	NO
Have you ever had an anaesthetic?		
Have your or your family had an anaesthetic complication?		

Details ....

4. MEDICATIONS

Have you received any of the following?

	CURRENT	PREVIOUS
Drugs for Diabetes		
Drugs for Hypertension		
Drugs for Heart Disease		
Diuretics		
Anticoagulants		
Drugs for "Nerves"		
Drugs for Psychiatric Illness		
Drugs for Epilepsy		
Drugs for Asthma		
Cortisone		
Other		

If yes to any of above, give details

Current	Previous
....	....

5. ALLERGY

Are you allergic to any of the following:

	YES	NO
Penicillin		
Sulphonamides		
Tetanus Toxoid		
Aspirin		
Narcotics		
Other Drugs		
Iodine or Skin Preps		
Adhesive Plaster(s)		
Food Allergy		
Anything Else		

If yes to any of above give details: ....

6. OTHER

Females are you pregnant?

If yes, give E.D.C. ....

	YES	NO
Caps, crowns or dentures?		
Do you smoke?		

How many per day? ....

Daily average intake of alcohol ....

	YES	NO
Do you have any reason to believe that you may have been exposed to the virus which causes Acquired Immune Deficiency Syndrome (AIDS)?		
Have you used recreational drugs?		

P101

Fig. 6-2. Preanesthesia information record. (Courtesy of St. Vincent's Private Hospital, Melbourne, Australia.)

tural hypotension, and pain as well as attention to general patient safety are important nursing responsibilities during this phase.[7]

Pain management in the ambulatory PACU must balance efficacy against side effects, particularly sedation, nausea, or vomiting. The anesthesiologist and PACU nurse can provide a good level of analgesia with small incremental intravenous doses of opiate, which can later be supplemented by oral analgesics for prolonged pain relief.

Discharge criteria should be formally established and in each case patient documents must confirm that these criteria were met. Postanesthesia care and discharge are the responsibility of the anesthesiologist, who should evaluate and certify that the patient is fit to leave.

Discharge Checklist

Patient breathing normally
Blood pressure and pulse stable
Patient alert and oriented
Wound satisfactory, dressings checked
Analgesia satisfactory
Patient tolerating fluids
Patient has voided
Patient ambulant
Postoperative medications prescribed
Nursing and anesthesiologist assessment complete
Discharge instructions given
Follow-up appointment set
Documentation completed and signed

Postoperative instructions must include specific warnings about driving, alcohol, using machinery, and signing legal documents or making major life decisions. Follow-up calls to the patient during the first 24 hours provide an opportunity to confirm satisfactory recovery, discuss any patient concerns, and re-enforce postoperative instructions. It also provides useful quality assurance information to feedback to recovery room staff.

During the postoperative period, the final phase of the nursing process, evaluation, is completed as the plan of care is evaluated and analyzed to assure that outcome standards have been met. On the day after surgery, a registered nurse contacts the patient for a follow-up conversation. Patients are asked about their physical well-being, if they have experienced any postoperative complications, and if they have any questions. A questionnaire should follow 1 to 2 weeks later to survey patient satisfaction with the surgical experience, including feedback of service received and interactions with staff. The data received can assist in identifying problems or offering suggestions to improve services. In addition, these questionnaires can become an intricate part of the ambulatory surgery unit's quality assurance program.

FINANCIAL MANAGEMENT

Just as the mission statement refers to the importance of cost containment, the continually escalating costs of health care make awareness of budget both a vital and inevitable requirement of the nurse manager. Budget considerations include labor costs, operational costs, and capital expenditures. Ambulatory surgical costs may be less than those in an inpatient setting primarily because the procedures are less complex, patients are healthier and require less intensive monitoring, and fixed costs may be lower. It is, however, necessary to monitor costs and regularly evaluate budget variances in order to maintain a cost-effective operation.

Labor costs are determined by the unit's staffing structure. First, decisions must be made regarding the number of employees needed and the skill requirements for personnel. As in any business, it is imperative that the right person be assigned to the right job to assure efficiency and enhance employee satisfaction. Salaries, benefits, and working conditions must be competitive within the community.

Operational costs are influenced by the daily expenses incurred by the process of providing ambulatory surgical services. Standards of care influence purchases, as do surgeon requests and patient needs. A thorough understanding of costs is essential when establishing charges for services. Charges are also impacted by fixed reimbursement for certain services, payor mix, and community rates. The management team may employ or consult a business manager regarding these issues.

Capital equipment needs arise in relation to the variety of procedures that are performed and the necessity of maintaining emergency equipment. Selection of appropriate equipment must meet minimum requirements for preoperative, intraoperative, and postoperative care; must comply with safety standards; and must be appropriate to the scope of procedures likely to be performed. A formalized system for evaluating capital requests is helpful and may alleviate allegations from surgeons that favoritism influences capital expenditures.

EDUCATION

Education is a critical component in the equation for customer and staff satisfaction with the ambulatory surgery unit. Patient education is vital to the success of an ambulatory facility, particularly when such facilities are new to a community and expectations have been influenced by conventional inpatient experiences. Patient education includes detailed instructions for arrival at the facility; explanations of the need for complete medical records, including current medications and allergies, and the need for an accompanying adult when returning home; management of children (both of patients and as patients); details of the expected length of stay; and explanations of anesthesia and surgery.

The ambulatory surgery unit may also want to extend itself beyond its physical location. Health promotion programs may be offered to increase community awareness of the role and nature of ambulatory surgical care. Nursing and medical staff can support these efforts by being prepared to speak to voluntary organizations in both the hospital and the community at large. A variety of topics can be discussed that involve ambulatory surgical care.

In addition to educating the patient consumers, it is important to provide continuing education to the staff. Managers must remain current with trends in ambulatory care management and changes in reimbursement for services. An informed staff can anticipate future needs and respond proactively to prepare for change.

The professional staff must also maintain their clinical competence through continuing education. It may be appropriate for the ambulatory surgery unit to sponsor speakers and programs to provide educational opportunities for community practitioners. Programs may include such subjects as procedures that are best done in the ambulatory setting, the facilitation of rapid emergence from anesthesia,[8,9] early ambulation, minimizing requirements for postoperative pain relief, and the avoidance of complications such as emesis.

The surgeon's office nurse or receptionist must also be familiar with the ambulatory surgical unit, its staff, and its scope of services. This includes an appreciation of perioperative needs, such as NPO status, taking appropriate medications, and arranging transportation. Since the safety and well-being of the patient are intimately bound to many of these issues, it is important for the surgeon's office staff to have a good working relationship with the staff at the outpatient facility. An effective way for the physician to educate the staffs and to build a rapport between them is to invite the office staff to the facility for periodic updates. In addition, the physician's office staff is a valuable, informal source of feedback from patients, and communication between the two staffs can be helpful in providing efficient, high-quality care.

LEGAL CONSIDERATIONS

A more detailed discussion on the legal aspects of ambulatory surgery is presented in Chapter 20; however, some basic principles that involve nursing service are highlighted here.

All patients must give written, informed consent for their anesthetic and surgical procedures. The importance of an appropriate explanation to the patient, accurate documentation of both consent and all other records, and recognition of the individual rights of the patient, including the right to refuse treatment, must be appreciated by all staff members. Requirements in an ambulatory facility that impact on patient safety include the patient's written confirmation of the need to have a responsible adult accompany them home and verification of fasting status.

The nursing staff should attempt to be informed of specific legal issues relevant to nursing practice, including professional negligence, documentation, scope of practice, liability insurance, and employment contracts.[10,11]

QUALITY ASSURANCE

The regulatory requirements for "ongoing quality assurance programs designed to . . . systematically monitor and evaluate the quality and appropriateness of patient care"[12] provide valuable objective information on which to base improvements in standards and performance.

The reality of these programs is that they must be individually designed according to the particular needs of each facility.[13] This means that a general hospital-based ambulatory facility will most likely be part of the broader quality assurance program, whereas a freestanding unit must develop its own program. While the paperwork for staff sometimes seems onerous, intelligent and enthusiastic implementation, with constructive response to critical feedback, help make the program work more effectively. Involving staff in the preparation and assessment of requirements also helps to develop their own levels of competence.

The standard of care requires that all elements of patient management meet or exceed expected community and peer group standards. In ambulatory surgery, this includes evaluating preoperative assessment, preparation for surgery, the operative procedure, postanesthesia care, discharge protocols, follow-up, and mechanisms for patient feedback.

Quality assurance programs should be capable of yielding highly accurate data on overall facility utilization, case mix, outcome, patient satisfaction, room scheduling, delays, infection rate, equipment utilization, and incident reports. However, the most important feature of any quality assurance program is a means for implementing and monitoring change based on the outcome of the evaluation process. Appropriate peer review, education, and quality assurance programs should be an automatic and integral part of every ambulatory surgical unit.

SUMMARY

The ambulatory surgical unit provides a congenial environment in which patients and staff are permitted a degree of individual expression. Some indications of the success of this style of patient care include the positive response of patients and their families, both before and after their procedures, the quick and enthusiastic adaptation of new staff, and the preferential selection of the ambulatory surgery facility for appropriate procedures by both surgeons and anesthesiologists.

These responses occur because the environment facilitates attention to individual needs, engenders a positive attitude in which it is anticipated that the patient will do well, and allows close contact between physicians, nurses, and patients. The environment adds value to nursing professionalism and ultimately is a more satisfying approach to elective patient surgical care.

REFERENCES

1. Nursing Service Philosophy, Day Surgery Unit. Box Hill Hospital, Melbourne, 1989
2. Turner BS: p. 40. Medical Power and Social Knowledge. Sagoe Publications, London, 1987
3. Centers for Disease Control: Recommendations for prevention of HIV transmission in health-care settings. MMWR 36:suppl #2S, 3S, 1987
4. Cullen DJ: The recovery room. Semin Anesth 1:333, 1982
5. Joint Commission on Accreditation of Hospitals: Accreditation Manual for Hospitals. Joint Commission on Accreditation of Hospitals, Chicago, 1981
6. Faculty of Anaesthetists, Royal Australasian College of Surgeons: Guidelines for the care of patients recovering from anesthesia. Policy Statement (2-83), February 1983
7. Fraulini K: Postanesthesia care. p. 325. In Fraulini K: After Anesthesia. Appleton & Lange, East Norwalk, CT, 1987
8. Marais ML, Maher MW, Wetchler BV, et al: Reduced demands on recovery room resources with propofol (Diprivan) compared to thiopental-isoflurane. Anesthesiol 16:29, 1989
9. Doze VA, Shafer A, White PF: Nausea and vomiting after outpatient anesthesia: effectiveness of droperidol alone and in combination with metoclopramide. Anesth Analg 66:S41, 1987
10. Creighton H: Law Every Nurse Should Know. WB Saunders, Philadelphia, 1981
11. Brent NJ: Legal considerations in postanesthesia nursing. p. 435. In Fraulini KE (ed): After Anesthesia. Appleton & Lange, East Norwalk, CT, 1987
12. Joint Commission on Accreditation of Hospitals (JCAH): Ambulatory Health Care Standards Manual, 1986
13. Burden N: A program of quality assurance in the ambulatory setting. J Post Anesth Nurs 2:106, 1987

7

Preoperative Assessment of Pediatric Outpatients

Frederic A. Berry

In recent years, ambulatory surgery has become a standard practice in the care of infants and children. In the early 1980s, it was well-recognized that a considerable percentage of pediatric surgery could be performed on an outpatient basis, and much of that care has now become mandatory. However, there is nothing new about the concept of outpatient surgery. In 1909, Nicoll reported a series of 8,994 pediatric surgical procedures that had been performed by his group on an ambulatory basis.[1] The group's reasons for doing so were similar to those cited today.

ADVANTAGES OF AMBULATORY SURGERY

The three major advantages to ambulatory surgery are emotional, medical, and financial. Although the infant or child may be the focus of the procedure, the whole family undergoes the surgical experience. There is an increasing appreciation of the risks as well as the benefits of surgery, and the vast majority of families are well-informed about the dangers of anesthesia. Also, many parents understand that their child is about to undergo an unpleasant, if not uncomfortable or frankly painful, procedure in which the discomfort may extend into the postoperative period. All of these factors create either a recognized or unrecognized degree of strain on the parents and often on the entire family. The advantage of an ambulatory surgery facility is that many of the surgical procedures can be performed more expeditiously in an outpatient facility than in a hospital. The result is a reduction in the time that the child and the family are exposed to the potential unpleasantness of the medical setting. In addition, this limited exposure is less threatening to the child than is a hospital stay. Most children do not understand, and if they do, are not particularly pleased about the upcoming total disruption in their normal routine. They do not appreciate the short- or long-term benefits of the surgical procedure about to be performed. Therefore, the parents' ability to explain to the child that they will be going to the hospital on the morning of the procedure and leaving that afternoon reduces the negative impact of the overall experience. The medical advantages for the child include a reduction in exposure to hospital infections. This reduction in nosocomial infections is of particular potential significance to children with chronic illnesses or to those who may be immunosuppressed because of malignancy or transplants.

DISADVANTAGES OF AMBULATORY SURGERY

The disadvantages of ambulatory surgery are (1) its unsuitability for some patients, (2) its potential morbidity for children in the early stages of an illness, and (3) possible complications. Even though many insurance companies mandate that certain procedures be done on an outpatient basis, this mandate does not take into consideration the fact that certain parents and/or children are not suitable candidates for outpatient anesthesia and surgery. Some parents are so upset and overwhelmed by the surgical experience that they may be unwilling or unable to accept important roles, e.g., the preparation of the child for surgery and identification of postsurgical complications. The psychological price they pay might be excessive and could offset the benefits of ambulatory surgery.

Another potential disadvantage is that a child may be in the prodromal stage of an illness (see the later discussion concerning the child with a runny nose). The short time allotted for the evaluation of these patients is sometimes not adequate to identify early symptoms of illness. This may lead to operating on children who may be in the prodromal stage of a serious infection, or it may result in the delay or cancellation of surgery in a patient who subsequently is found to have no illness. Unfortunately, these outcomes cannot be completely eliminated even with the best of intentions and information.

The third potential problem is managing complications following anesthesia and surgery. Complications may not be present or recognized at the time of discharge. On the patient's release, the responsibility for evaluating the child and seeking medical evaluation shifts to the family. While it is very difficult to inform the family of all potential complications that may arise, adequate postoperative instruction should contain enough information to help the family understand the most frequent postanesthetic problems, such as nausea and vomiting, difficulty in breathing, and unexplained fever. In addition to monitoring the patient's progress vigilantly, the family must be encouraged to seek medical help if they have any questions about their child.

AMBULATORY SURGERY IN THE NORMAL NEONATE

The age at which the normal neonate (defined as an infant in the first 30 days after birth) can be treated in an ambulatory setting is open to debate. One of the issues involved is whether the patient is a normal full-term newborn. The conceptual or gestational age of a full-term infant is 38 to 40 weeks. However, the major question in determining when an infant is in an acceptable physiologic state for anesthesia and surgery depends on how the infant fared through the transition from the fetal to the neonatal state.[2] It takes several days after parturition for the cardiopulmonary, hepatic, and renal systems to adjust to the increased blood flow and to the need to perform normal physiologic functions independent of the mother. For the normal full-term neonate, this is effectively accomplished in the first 72 hours after birth.

Certain surgical procedures, such as eye surgery and hernia repair, two of the most frequent reasons for ambulatory surgery in the full-term neonate, fall under the "urgent" category* and cannot be postponed, even as a precautionary measure, for very long. At what point should these infants be considered for outpatient surgery? Unfor-

---

* The occurrence of hernias in premature infants is higher than in the full-term infant population, and their hernias become incarcerated more frequently. Therefore, even though the surgery is scheduled on an "elective" basis, it may well fall into the "urgent" category. That is, it needs to be done within a short time interval, but it can be done on what is defined as an "elective" schedule.

tunately, there is no available scientific data to assist the clinician on this issue. Each case must be decided based on the clinician's evaluation of the infant, the parents, and the medical situation as a whole. We accept full-term infants at 2 weeks. If there is any doubt as to satisfactory outcome, the infant should be admitted for overnight postoperative observation.

SUDDEN INFANT DEATH SYNDROME AND APNEA OF INFANCY

One of the major concerns in infants is sudden infant death syndrome (SIDS), which is the most common cause of death between the ages of 1 month and 1 year.[3] It would appear that SIDS is not a problem during the first month after birth. Despite an enormous amount of study, the etiology of this syndrome remains undiscovered.[4] Another condition of unknown etiology is "apnea of infancy," which is characterized by one or more episodes of cyanosis, limpness, and apnea requiring resuscitation or vigorous stimulation. These episodes may cause death. Unfortunately, there is no diagnostic test that will identify, on a consistent basis, infants who have apnea of infancy. In one study, 62 percent of the infants with this syndrome had an abnormal arousal response to hypoxia.[5] In addition, these infants had a slightly different arousal response to hypercapnia in that it required a higher inspired carbon dioxide concentration for arousal to occur. Infants who have apnea of infancy do have a higher incidence of repeat apneic episodes. There is no concrete evidence in the literature that either apneic episodes or SIDS[6] are associated with anesthesia or surgery, but a recent case report raises the question.[7] It should also be apparent that an apneic episode resulting in death could coincide with the postoperative period without there being a cause and effect relationship between surgery and mortality.

AMBULATORY SURGERY IN THE PREMATURE NURSERY GRADUATE

Premature nursery graduates may have a host of potential problems after discharge; these include apnea, idiopathic respiratory distress syndrome, residual lung disease, and anemia. The issues are many and complex, and it may be very difficult to sort out which infant is suitable for the ambulatory setting.

Apnea and periodic breathing remain the most persistent, difficult problems in the evaluation and management of premature nursery graduates. For purposes of discussion, apnea is defined as a respiratory pause of 20 seconds or longer that may or may not be accompanied by bradycardia; and periodic breathing is defined as a pattern of three or more periods of apnea lasting 3 to 15 seconds each separated by less than 20 seconds of normal respiration. An increase in periodic breathing has been found in infants with "near miss" SIDS. In addition, there is concern that the reduction of ventilation and oxygenation with periodic breathing may result in prolonged apnea. Normal infants have periodic breathing, but it occurs in less than 0.5 percent of total sleep time.

Retrospective and prospective studies have reported varying incidences of apnea.[8,9] Some of these studies, however, have been confounded by the fact that they included infants with pre-existing medical diseases as well as infants undergoing laparotomies and neurosurgical procedures.[10] In general, these infants would be eliminated from consideration for ambulatory surgery in the first several months after birth. Premature infants with a history of apnea who are otherwise normal or who have minimal residual lung disease are at risk for developing apnea postoperatively. However, some premature infants without a previous history of apnea may develop it in the postoperative period.

Apnea is thought to be related to immature brain stem function. The issue is at what age does the central nervous system (CNS) mature so that apnea is no longer a concern. One study of herniorrhaphy in otherwise normal infants reported neither apnea nor periodic breathing in either premature infants greater than 44 weeks' conceptual age or full-term infants greater than 37 weeks' conceptual age.[11] Among the full-term infants, seven were operated on between 38 and 40 weeks' conceptual age and had no apnea or periodic breathing. Among the premature infants less than 44 weeks' conceptual age, 14 of 22 developed periodic breathing, but none had apnea or bradycardia.

There has been recent interest in the administration of caffeine (10 to 20 mg/kg) to control postoperative apnea in the premature nursery graduate.[12] Caffeine increases the ventilatory response to CO_2 and decreases periodic breathing. Theophylline has also been used for this purpose, but apparently has more side effects than caffeine. The elimination halflife of caffeine is prolonged in newborns; therefore, only one dose is needed for the perioperative period. Welborn et al. reported an elimination of apnea following treatment with caffeine in premature nursery graduates having hernia repair.[12] However, they recommend that infants less than 44 weeks' conceptual age be monitored for apnea and bradycardia following general anesthesia. Therefore, most pediatric anesthesiologists feel that apnea and bradycardia are major concerns in patients less than 44 weeks' conceptual age, and therefore, on an arbitrary basis, recommend that premature infants who are 50 weeks' conceptual age or less need to have their anesthesia and surgery in a hospital setting. Some investigators have extended this period to 60 weeks' conceptual age,[10] but they include patients having complicated surgery; in my opinion, these recommendations should not include premature infants having superficial surgery.

Pulmonary Function

A long-term study of premature infants who were given pulmonary function tests between the ages of 6 and 10 years has demonstrated differences in flow rates which are suggestive of an increase in large airway resistance.[13] This finding has been reported in premature infants whether or not they have had respiratory distress syndrome. The issue is not clear whether the flow rates would mature into the normal range in the later catch-up growth period of these children; however, these findings are of relatively minor clinical significance.

Residual Lung Disease

Of much more significance is the history of respiratory distress syndrome even when it is not complicated by bronchopulmonary dysplasia (BPD). There are many studies that demonstrate residual pulmonary function derangements in the first year of life in infants who have apparently successfully recovered from respiratory distress syndrome.[14] They have residual lung disease of both the large and small airways with varying degrees of decrease in compliance and increase in airway resistance. Any infant who has been intubated and ventilated should be considered to have residual lung disease. In addition, these children may continue to have hyperreactive airways.[15] As it is extremely difficult to perform pulmonary function tests on these small infants preoperatively, the clinician would be better served to consider all infants with a history as outlined above to have hyperreactive airways and to treat them accordingly. Consistent with this approach is the use of glycopyrrolate preoperatively to decrease airway secretions, dilate the large airways, and block the vagus. In addition, use of a less irritating inhalation agent, such as halothane, minimizes the incidence of airway reactivity. Such techniques as administering intravenous lidocaine to blunt the airway reflexes during extubation are also useful. Another potential problem in any infant who has been intubated and ventilated is the development of subglottic stenosis. This has been reported to occur in as many as 20 percent of infants who were intubated and ventilated.[16] Although these infants are asymptomatic on leaving the nursery, they subsequently develop problems with respiratory infections because of airway hyperreactivity, decreased lung function, and secretions. Consequently, it is important to carefully question the parents of infants who were ventilated at birth regarding subsequent respiratory complications. Perhaps neonates requiring intubation and ventilation should undergo bronchoscopy before they are discharged from the nursery.

Bronchopulmonary Dysplasia

The infant who has BPD represents a special problem. Such infants have an increased risk of sudden unexplained death after discharge from the neonatal intensive care unit.[17] Whether or not this falls into the category of SIDS is not completely clear. Regardless, the etiology of these deaths is not well-understood, and for that reason mortality is extraordinarily difficult to prevent. It has been shown that some infants with BPD have an inability to reverse a hypoxic episode in the face of CNS arousal and ventilatory responsiveness to hypoxia that is relatively normal. In other words, they have abnormal pulmonary response to hypoxia. This abnormal response may lead to prolonged apnea, hypoxia, bradycardia, and sometimes death. Pneumograms and sleep studies have not been able to identify those infants at risk for developing SIDS or postneonatal death. Thus, the infant with BPD presents two problems: (1) decreased pulmonary function with airway hyperreactivity and, at times, significant residual lung disease causing hypoxia and CO_2 retention and (2) apnea and unexpected sudden death.

It is difficult to develop rigid criteria to determine who may undergo surgery in the ambulatory setting and who requires hospital admission. As a precautionary measure, infants with BPD who have any degree of significant decrease in pulmonary function would be better served by a hospital setting for their postsurgical care. Likewise, infants who require supplemental oxygen need to be admitted to the hospital. It is difficult to perform pulmonary function studies in these infants and, furthermore, to correlate pulmonary function tests with the anesthetic and surgery experience. Consequently, these infants need to be evaluated in advance of surgery to avoid cancellation and disappointment when they arrive on the day of surgery at the ambulatory center.

Acceptable Hematocrit

One of the issues in the assessment of premature nursery graduates is what constitutes an acceptable hematocrit. This issue is complicated by a lack of agreement on what to consider a normal hematocrit. For a long time, the arbitrary number of 30 percent was considered an acceptable hematocrit reading. However, with the increase in incidence of the acquired immunodeficiency syndrome and hepatitis, as well as the experience gained from Jehovah's Witnesses avoiding transfusions, a new appreciation for what can be considered an acceptable hematocrit has emerged. The standards are still arbitrary. No studies have documented the relationship between hematocrit and outcome. The question of acceptable hematocrit level is further complicated by another factor: the premature nursery graduate may have more than one medical problem. That is, the infant may have BPD or some form of residual lung disease in addition to anemia. There are no magic formulas to decide what an acceptable hematocrit is for these infants. As an arbitrary guideline, many pediatric anesthesiologists accept a hematocrit in the mid-20s for elective surgery in the ex-premature infant.

MEDICAL PROBLEMS IN OLDER CHILDREN

Early in the history of ambulatory surgery, many felt that only American Society of Anesthesiologists (ASA) I and II patients should be considered eligible for outpatient procedures. However, it became evident that ASA III patients would also qualify and benefit from the ambulatory setting. It is useful to keep in mind the definition of ASA III physical status: severe systemic disturbance or disease from whatever cause, even though it may not be possible to define the degree of disability with finality.

Cardiac Presentations

From time to time, two separate cardiac issues will confront the anesthesiologist in the ambulatory surgery unit. One of these is the child who recently has been discovered to have a heart murmur, and the other is the child with known heart disease, either congenital or acquired.

Heart Murmurs

The child with a heart murmur may present more of an intellectual than a practical problem, depending on the condition of the child. The intellectual problem is that of trying to decipher whether the murmur is functional or "innocent," or is due to acquired or congenital heart disease. The practical problem may be compounded if the heart murmur is discovered on the day of surgery and if the child is asymptomatic. There are two opinions as to what to do with "innocent" murmurs. The question itself consists of two parts: (1) whether to proceed with surgery or delay it until after evaluation of the murmur, and (2) whether to administer prophylactic antibiotics. One opinion is that if a child is active, shows none of the stigmata of heart disease, such as clubbing and cyanosis, and the murmur is felt not to represent congenital or acquired heart disease, surgery can proceed as in any other normal child and prophylactic antibiotics are not indicated. If the child is asymptomatic but there is suspicion that the murmur may be due to congenital or acquired heart disease, surgery is performed and prophylactic antibiotics are administered, because the danger of developing subacute bacterial endocarditis might represent a greater risk to the child than the potential allergic response to the antibiotic. After surgery, the murmur is evaluated.[18] On the other hand, there are those who think that any child with a newly discovered murmur needs to be fully evaluated before anesthesia and surgery, even if the child has no signs or symptoms of heart disease and is fully active. In the opinion of the author, it is best to proceed with surgery and evaluate the murmur afterward.

Congenital or Acquired Heart Disease

If a child has known heart disease, is being followed by a cardiologist, and has been stable for a period of a month prior to scheduled surgery, it may be acceptable to proceed with surgery in the ambulatory setting. However, the appropriateness of treating such a patient on an outpatient basis depends on the clinical experience and judgment of the anesthesiologist. Pertinent medical history includes a list of medications and medical records, including cardiologic evaluation. A recent history and physical evaluation should be available to ensure the stability of the heart disease and the absence of intercurrent infections. The child should continue all medications up to and including the morning of surgery. Although some anesthesiologists do not feel comfortable administering anesthesia to children with heart disease in the ambulatory setting, most anesthesiologists feel comfortable with this clinical situation.

A short discussion of the pathophysiology of the various congenital heart lesions is appropriate, both to assist in the evaluation of the patient the day of surgery and to help the anesthesiologist understand the blood flow characteristics of the lesion (or lesions) as well as the clinical implications from the anesthetic standpoint. There are several different classification systems for congenital heart disease. Campbell and Schwartz use a classification system that is determined by the answers to four basic questions.[19] These questions are (1) Is there an abnormal pathway for blood flow (shunting) through an intracardiac, extracardiac, or combined defect? (2) Is there a reduction of blood flow due to a supravalvular, subvalvular, or primary valvular abnormality? (3) What are the consequences (e.g., congestive heart failure, myocardial oxygen imbalance) of abnormal cardiovascular pressures or volumes that result from shunting or an obstruction to blood flow? (4) What are the consequences on the pulmonary and systemic vasculature (e.g., pulmonary arterial hypertension) and on pulmonary and systemic blood flow (e.g., hypoxemia)?

Using this system of questions, the pathophysiologic classification of congenital heart lesions can be separated into three groups, two involving shunting and one involving obstruction to blood flow. In the two groups in which there are problems with shunting of blood, the major consequence of the shunt is the alteration of pulmonary blood flow. If it is increased, volume and/or pressure overload to the pulmonary circulation may result. If pulmonary blood flow is decreased, varying degrees of inability to oxygenate the blood occurs. The two major consequences of obstruction to blood flow are increased cardiac workload required to overcome the obstruction and varying degrees of reduced circulation distal to the obstruction.

These pathophysiologic problems of the heart lead to the two major clinical states that need to be evaluated on physical examination: cyanosis and congestive heart failure. Congestive heart failure occurs most commonly in shunt lesions with increased pulmonary blood flow that results in pulmonary vascular congestion and, later, pulmonary hypertension. The most frequent cause of this lesion is a ventricular septal defect. Less frequent causes of pulmonary venous congestion are either myocardial dysfunction or obstructive lesions. The other major sign is cyanosis, which occurs most commonly in lesions in which pulmonary blood flow is decreased (tetralogy of Fallot) or when there is mixing of systemic and pulmonary venous return (transposition of the great vessels).

At times, the anesthesiologist may deal with a child who has a congenital heart defect and, knowing what specific lesion is involved, can enhance the understanding of the pathophysiology. It is important to recognize that heart surgery is sometimes only palliative, and even with corrective surgery the final result may not be a normal heart, but a heart which still has some residual pathophysiologic alteration of function. The basic information the anesthesiologist requires is the status of the pulmonary blood flow and the presence or absence of an obstructive heart lesion. Practically, if pulmonary blood flow is increased, controlled ventilation with positive end-expiratory pressure may be effective in decreasing pulmonary vascular resistance, thus stabilizing pulmonary blood flow. On the other hand, in conditions in which there are a reduction in pulmonary blood flow and an obstructive lesion of the right ventricle plus an interventricular shunt, attempts are made to maintain or increase systemic vascular resistance in order to avoid increasing the right to left shunt, which would magnify the problem. Hyperventilation with a high $F_{I}O_2$ is also important in the cyanotic patient, but maintenance of airway pressures as low as possible are needed to accomplish ventilation. Excessive positive pressure will further reduce pulmonary blood flow. In general, the basic factors to keep in mind are that the preload needs to be augmented in almost every congenital heart disease, and the heart rate needs to be maintained within a normal range.[20] Tachycardia is not a useful hemodynamic state in these patients.

Ambulatory surgery should only be considered on children who have stable heart problems, although their activity may be limited. If there is any question about the stability of the heart disease, hospital admission is suggested, regardless of how simple the surgery.

Prophylactic Antibiotics

Children with acquired or congenital heart disease should have antibiotic coverage to minimize the risk of developing subacute bacterial endocarditis. The American Heart Association has guidelines for the administration of antibiotics, but these are somewhat at variance with some of the other concerns in the pediatric patient, such as the desirability of avoiding intramuscular medications. The basic guideline is that oral antibiotics should be given whenever possible. If the child will allow intravenous administration, the antibiotic can be given intravenously. Intramuscular or intravenous antibiotics before induction in uncooperative children are discouraged, since they can be given rapidly intravenously after induction of anesthesia. Children who have an allergy to penicillin and who may require vancomycin represent a particular problem, because vancomycin needs to be administered over a 20- to 30-minute period to avoid hypotension. The usual recommendations by the American Heart Association then call for another dose of antibiotics 6 hours after the procedure. In the case of intravenous antibiotics, this is difficult to accomplish in the ambulatory setting, since all patients will have been discharged by that time. Therefore, there is a need either to shorten the time interval for the administration of the antibiotics or to administer the antibiotics orally in the postoperative period.

Asthma

Asthma has the highest frequency of any major disease among children. The current prevalence rate among children in the United States is 7.6 percent, with most asthmatics having their first attack before their third birthday.[21] The history of asthma is often vague, and when parents are asked if their child has asthma, they frequently reply in the negative. However, with further questioning, such as "Does your child have bronchitis or asthmatic bronchitis?" the response is often positive. Another valuable question is "Does your child wheeze with a cold or does your child ever wheeze with heavy exercise or when out in the cold?" This questionings can elicit the history of asthma and helps the clinician evaluate and plan the anesthetic management for the child. A recent study indicates that the epidemiology of asthma is clearly changing, with an increase in prevalence, hospitalization rate, and mortality rate.[21] Since hospitalization and mortality appear to be increasing more rapidly than prevalence, the suggestion is that the severity of asthma is increasing. Another interesting factor is that boys have approximately twice the incidence of asthma as girls.

Once it is established that the child has asthma or an asthma-like tendency, certain information must be obtained,[22] namely, the frequency of asthma attacks and the type of medication the child takes. Some children have infrequent asthma attacks and are not on any regular medication. Other children have intermittent attacks and only take their asthma medication as needed. A third group has moderately severe to severe asthma and receives continuous therapy. At the present time, continuous therapy consists of a whole spectrum of drugs, including theophylline, systemic steroids, systemic β-agonist, inhalational β-agonist, inhalational steroids, and cromolyn.[23] When children are on a chronic medication, it is essential that they maintain their normal scheduled medication on the day of surgery. If a child has an intermittent type of asthma and uses an inhaler, he or she is encouraged to bring the inhaler and take a treatment 30 minutes or so before surgery. The patient is re-evaluated at the time of surgery to determine if the asthmatic condition is stable. If the child is having an asthma episode which is unresponsive to his or her usual medication, surgery should be cancelled and rescheduled. Some children are never completely free of wheezing. Therefore, it is important to establish a baseline of the normal physical in the child so this can be used at the time of surgery.

Premedication is not usually given to children before surgery, but this group of patients needs special consideration. Patients with reactive airway disease are usually given an anticholinergic, such as glycopyrrolate, to dilate the large airways and block the vagus nerve. It takes a larger dose of glycopyrrolate to block the vagus than it does to dry secretions. Therefore, oral glycopyrrolate is given in a dose of 0.05 mg/kg PO. Glycopyrrolate is a better drying agent and causes less tachycardia than atropine. The type of induction should be tailored to the child rather than the asthma.

Because asthma may be triggered in the perioperative period, it would be prudent to start an intravenous line in cooperative children before induction, both for hydration and as a route for the administration of various medications to treat bronchospasm. In uncooperative children, this can be delayed until after induction. The general feeling is that halothane is the agent of choice in an asthmatic, but in a child who has malignant hyperthermia susceptibility, nontrigger agents can be used with equal success. In these patients, it would be particularly important to use large doses of anticholinergics as well as intravenous lidocaine prior to intubation to minimize the tracheal irritation by the endotracheal tube. In the asymptomatic asthmatic, there are no special considerations other than being aware that asthma can occur at any time.

Asthma is not the only cause of wheezing. Unexpected wheezing during surgery may be the result of regurgitation and aspiration, and this needs to be differentiated from an asthma attack. Often, asthma will quickly respond to β-agonist and deepening of anesthesia, whereas aspiration with bronchospasm usually does not respond well to either. If an asthma attack begins during surgery, the general course is to deepen the anesthetic by either inhalational techniques or lidocaine, 1.5 mg/kg IV. In addition, the use of an inhaler of a β-2 agonist is also quite effective. These inhalers will deliver a metered dose of an agent that is effective in the treatment of bronchospasm. If the bronchospasm continues to worsen in spite of intubation, ventilation, and bronchodilator therapy, consideration should be given to the intravenous administration of steroids, such as 1 mg/kg dexamethasone. It takes approximately 20 to 30 minutes for both glycopyrrolate and dexamethasone to reach their peak effect. If the asthma attack clears, the patient can then be extubated and followed closely. The child should not be discharged until the asthma is in a stable condition. If there is any question about the child's condition, admission to a hospital is indicated. If the bronchospasm continues (this is extremely rare), consideration should be given to leaving the child intubated and ventilated during transport to a hospital.

The Child With a Cold

The child with a runny nose remains an enigma for the anesthesiologist.[24] The incidence of runny nose and respiratory infection in infants and children is quite high, particularly in the preschool group where it is not unusual for 1- to 5-year-old children to have 2 to 4 viral respiratory infections per year.[25] This age group usually presents with a runny nose. The differential diagnosis of a runny nose is (1) upper respiratory infection (URI), (2) flu syndrome, (3) prodromal stage of a serious bacterial infection, (4) allergic rhinitis, (5) vasomotor rhinitis, and (6) nothing. Automatic cancellation of surgery for children with a cough and runny nose would result in many normal children having their surgery delayed or cancelled. Because many children with allergic rhinitis have a runny nose on almost a continuous basis, scheduling surgery for a time when they do not have a runny nose is almost impossible, which can be frustrating for the parents and the health care team. Therefore, the clinician should consider the likelihood of a differential diagnosis involving a runny nose and proceed accordingly.

The most frequent differential is between allergic rhinitis and an infectious process. Parents are of great help in distinguishing between the child's usual runny nose and the early stages of a respiratory infection. The other problem is to distinguish between a URI of the nasopharynx (the classic URI) and a respiratory infection, such as a flu syndrome, which may involve both the upper and lower respiratory tracts. Flu syndrome may be complicated by bronchospasm and pneumonia, and may result in a respiratory tract that remains hyperreactive for 4 to 6 weeks.[26,27]

It is difficult, if not impossible, to differentiate between many of the conditions early in their clinical course. The clinician is faced with a medicolegal dilemma. The studies by Tait and Knight have shown that even in the presence of an active viral infection of the upper respiratory tract, anesthesia for the placement of tympanostomy tubes, where there was no endotracheal tube and the anesthetic course was approximately 20 minutes, resulted in no increased incidence of complications.[28] Furthermore, the symptoms improved in the children who had anesthesia and surgery compared to a group of children with the same medical background in whom surgery was cancelled. The list below includes the criteria Tait and Knight used for diagnosing a URI: (1) sore or scratchy throat, (2) sneezing, (3) rhinorrhea, (4) congestion, (5) malaise, (6) nonproductive cough, (7) fever of less than 38°C (101°F), and (8) laryngitis. If a child had any two of these symptoms, he or she was diagnosed as having a URI. However, combinations of 1 and 5, 2 and 3, 3 and 6, or 4 and 6 required one additional symptom for the diagnosis of a URI.

Tait and Knight's study has been well thought-out and executed. However, children with allergic rhinitis and vasomotor rhinitis frequently have various combinations of these same signs and symptoms; thus, it is often difficult in the prodromal period to differentiate between allergic rhinitis and an infection. Also, the physical examination may not assist in clarifying the diagnosis. Therefore, it is useful to discuss the problem with the parents and to get them to help in the decision-making process.

Parents should also be informed of the potential for a reactive airway and the complications that may occur with anesthesia so that they may assist in determining whether to delay surgery. The two major points that assist in the differential are the presence of fever and the parents' observation that their child is experiencing the usual runny nose or something different. If the operative procedure is for tympanostomy tubes, Tait and Knight suggest that surgery can be accomplished without any added danger.[28]

Some investigators differ with Tait and Knight on this issue.[24] It has been demonstrated that children with a history of a respiratory infection have a decrease in oxygen saturation in the immediate postanesthesia period.[29] Therefore, these children may need closer supervision on the way to the recovery room as well as in the recovery room. If the respiratory infection is a simple nasopharyngitis without any extension into the lower airway and without bacterial infection, a short 20-minute procedure without endotracheal intubation may be appropriate. No information is available for procedures of longer duration or in situations in which the child might be intubated. In either situation, if the child is suspected of having a respiratory infection, it would be advisable to cancel surgery.

If the child has had a significant respiratory infection within the previous several weeks, there is the potential for an increased incidence of perioperative complications. A significant respiratory infection is arbitrarily defined as one that lasts 3 to 7 days and that is associated with fever, cough, and malaise. These children have hyperreactive airways and are subject to anesthetic problems, such as those reported by McGill et al.[30] In adults, it takes approximately 5 to 6 weeks after a respiratory tract infection involving the lower airways for pulmonary mechanics to return to normal.[26] Similar findings have been noted in children.[27] Therefore, if one is aware that a child has had a lower-tract respiratory infection characterized by a cough and a temperature of at least 38°C (101°F), it would appear prudent to wait until 4 weeks after the last day of acute illness to perform elective surgery.

If an infant or child presents for ambulatory surgery with a runny nose and cough that have developed within the last 12 to 24 hours, and if the parents say this is the usual state for their child, current opinion would be to proceed with elective surgery, even if it involves endotracheal intubation and surgery of approximately 2 hours duration.

In cases of mild URI, almost all patients are at risk of developing a hyperreactive airway. Therefore, it is suggested that such patients be premedicated with oral glycopyrrolate before induction of anesthesia. If this is not possible, the glycopyrrolate should be administered intravenously after anesthesia is induced. The clinician must also be prepared for the full spectrum of problems, including laryngospasm and bronchospasm, in this group of patients.

Anesthetizing children who have a mild URI exposes all of the people in the facility to a viral infection. This may or may not make any difference to the average person, but may cause problems in immunosuppressed patients, in those with chronic illnesses (such as diabetes), and in the elderly.

Down Syndrome

Atlantoaxial instability in children with Down syndrome is a rare but potentially risky problem for the anesthesiologist. Among children with Down syndrome, studies have reported a 10 to 20 percent incidence of atlantoaxial instability and a 5 to 10 percent incidence of subluxation/dislocation, with neurologic injury and/or death occurring in the involved patients.[31–33] Persons with Down syndrome and no instability can undergo anesthesia and surgery without major concern.

There is no consensus about the usefulness of cervical x-rays in predicting which child with Down syndrome may develop problems. Some investigators have recommended cervical x-rays if there is a history suggestive of dislocation.[34]

In a review of cases, however, Davidson found that nearly all dislocations were preceded by physical signs that were present several weeks before the episode of dislocation and that a neurologic examination is more valuable in predicting potential or impending dislocation than the currently recommended radiologic studies.[35] The most frequent findings in these neurologic exams were hyperreflexia and secondary incontinence. Approximately 95 percent of all patients who develop neurologic sequelae will have a positive history of neurologic problems for approximately 1 month before they are diagnosed; consequently, the history should reveal some change in physical status for those patients most at risk for dislocation.

Apparently, the major danger with atlantoaxial instability is that of flexion of the neck. Therefore, it would seem appropriate to maintain the head and neck in the neutral or slightly extended position during intubation and in the perioperative period when the patient is unconscious or semiconscious due to the anesthetic agents. During laryngoscopy, an assistant should help to maintain the head in a slightly extended position, such as is done in trauma patients when there is concern about the cervical spine. The question of whether to use a Thomas collar is difficult to answer since Thomas collars are not usually designed for the smaller child, and the application of one might result in flexion which would defeat the purpose of holding the head in the neutral or extended position. A small pad under the shoulders and base of the neck would help to maintain the head in the neutral or slightly extended position.

The ambulatory care unit nurses and the child's parents need to be advised about the possibility of an injury occurring in the postoperative period, and they should be told to contact the pediatrician or anesthesiologist if there are any signs of brisk deep tendon reflexes, extensor plantar responses, ankle clonus, difficulty in walking, or gait abnormalities.

The anesthesiologist must maintain a high index of suspicion concerning any patient with Down syndrome. Atlantoaxial instability is a rare problem but one that may lead to disaster, and a high level of awareness will help to minimize the chance of a bad outcome.

ADVANTAGES AND DISADVANTAGES OF PREMEDICATION

Premedication is used both as a means of sedation and as an anticholinergic. The major uses of anticholinergics are in the asthmatic child and the child with a sensitive airway. Sensitive airways may be found in infants with BPD or residual lung disease, or in those recovering from respiratory tract infection. The objective of an anticholinergic is to reduce the airway secretions and to block the vagus nerve, thereby reducing the airway hyperreactivity that may be associated with administration of general anesthesia. Glycopyrrolate and atropine are useful for this purpose, but glycopyrrolate may have advantages, as it is a better drying agent and causes less tachycardia. Anticholinergics can be given orally as well as parenterally.

Anticholinergics are also used in infants less than 6 to 8 months of age, because infants of this age group seem to have an active cholinergic nervous system and easily develop bradycardia. In addition, secretions that are present in the relatively small airway of the infant can be bothersome in airway management. Therefore, it is the opinion of many pediatric anesthesiologists that infants in this age group should be given an anticholinergic.

The other purpose for premedication is that of sedation of the child. The practice of pediatric anesthesia has changed, and in many institutions parents are now allowed to accompany the child and be present for the induction of anesthesia. In that situation, the parents relax the child and often obviate the need for sedation. In some institutions and clinics, however, the parents are not allowed to accompany the child to the operating room, and the use of premedication can ease the anxiety of separation from the parents. Sedative premedication is effective in approximately 50 to 80 percent of children, depending on the agents used. The other 20 percent remain either anxious, tearful, or otherwise unappreciative of their proposed surgical experience. The literature is replete with innumerable techniques for premedication of children.[36–40] These include the use of intramuscular, oral, nasal, and rectal sedation. The general consensus is that intramuscular injections are undesirable and that all attempts should be made to use one of the other techniques. There has been interest in transmucosal fentanyl in a lollipop form to sedate children, making them more amenable to the induction of anesthesia. However, some parents and health care workers feel a certain aversion to using either lollipops or intranasal drugs, reasoning that children may relate this to recreational drug use that they have seen in magazines or on television.

The new premedications having high general acceptance by both parents and children are oral and rectal techniques. Rectal premedication, such as midazolam, is primarily reserved for children under the age of 5 years. Oral premedication (e.g., midazolam 0.5 mg/kg) can be given to any child who will swallow the medication. The major point to remember with any kind of premedication is that sufficient time must be allowed to pass between administering the drug and the child's separation from the parents. Approximately 1 hour is required after oral administration to accomplish the desired premedicative effect.

One of the compromises between premedication and induction techniques is the use of drugs such as rectal methohexital, which is an induction agent. Rectal methohexital in a 5 or 10 percent solution at a dose of 30 mg/kg will be effective in 95 percent of children within 5 to 10 minutes,[41] and will last approximately 1 hour.

One of the major problems with the administration of premedication is knowing exactly when to give it. Timing the administration of premedication to account for the hour needed for it to take effect prior to the commencement of surgery and its required duration throughout the procedure can be difficult. The use of methohexital overcomes this difficulty. However, one of the stated disadvantages of methohexital and all the various premedications is that the child will sleep longer in the recovery room. Hospital administrators and some nurses do not like this because they are interested in rapid discharge. Oral midazolam, 0.25 to 0.75 mg/kg PO, may provide for the rapid onset of sedation (less than 30 minutes) without prolonging the recovery room stay.[42] Parents and children are not interested in setting "world speed records" for patients' stays in the recovery room. The bottom line is that the child deserves and needs a gentle surgical experience.

SUMMARY

One of the major challenges for the anesthesiologist is the rapid assessment of outpatients. Insurance companies and the US government are dictating medical care, and this has resulted in many marginal patients being forced to receive their care in an ambulatory setting. Insurance companies and the federal government have set the policy, and the anesthesiologist is responsible for the consequences. This chapter has attempted to point out some of the major issues for the anesthesiologist who has to assess children with pre-existing diseases who are presenting for elective surgery on an ambulatory basis.

The Joint Commission for the Accreditation of Hospitals has appropriately stated that there is no such thing as routine laboratory work for the surgical patient. What is required is *indicated* laboratory work based on a careful history and physical examination. For example, a healthy ASA I or II child who is scheduled for an elective hernia repair but who is developing and growing normally and is eating and playing normally requires no preoperative laboratory tests. On the other hand, an ASA III premature nursery graduate who has some degree of residual lung disease needs a hematocrit and possibly a chest x-ray. Preoperative evaluation of the oxygen saturation with a pulse oximeter will often avoid the need for arterial blood gases and provide a baseline for assessing postanesthetic recovery.

The clinician is left with making judgment calls based on experience and the policies of the ambulatory surgery unit. Clinical judgment would indicate that the patient with a congenital heart defect should be examined by a cardiologist and that the cardiologist should be aware of the child's impending surgery in order to make recommendations regarding the cardiac status of the patient and the need for any additional studies. On the other hand, the decision to proceed with elective hernia repair in an otherwise healthy child in whom a heart murmur was discovered during the preoperative assessment is a judgment that is made based on experience. While a clinical decision to proceed in these circumstances is not uncommon, some clinicians feel that every child with a heart murmur needs to have a complete evaluation by a cardiologist before any type of elective surgery.

The issue of the child with Down syndrome and the need for a neurologic examination and cervical spine films has not yet been resolved. The knowledge that these children may be susceptible to atlantoaxial instability will at least encourage the anesthesiologist to discuss with the parents and surgeon the potential for subluxation and neurologic involvement. Guidelines on the potential problems that may be encountered in these patients can be useful to surgeons in arranging for appropriate evaluation of these children and determining whether they are good candidates for ambulatory surgery. This again touches on the difficult area of judgment and responsibility, and demonstrates the need to have all discussions and considerations well-documented in the chart. Certainly, there are those anesthesiologists who would not anesthetize an otherwise asymptomatic neurologically normal Down syndrome child who has not had a formal neurologic examination and cervical spine films. The paucity of data on this subject makes it extraordinarily difficult, if not impossible, to set what some would consider to be guidelines, much less the standard of care.

The bottom line in preoperative assessment of pediatric outpatients is to stay within one's limitations, to discuss fully any concerns with both the surgeon and the parents, and to involve the parents in the decision-making process. Regardless of how careful the entire medical team may be, there may still be complications from surgery and anesthesia. Parents need to be aware of these. When adequate time has been spent with patients and parents, the anesthesiologist will become comfortable with assessing each case, not by a set of rigid rules but on an individual basis, following the guidelines of good clinical practice.

REFERENCES

1. Nicoll JH: The surgery of infancy. Br Med J II:753, 1909
2. Berry FA: Basic considerations. p. 57. In Berry FA (ed): Anesthetic Management of

the Difficult and Routine Pediatric Patient. Churchill Livingstone, New York, 1986

3. Valdes-Dapena MA: Sudden infant death syndrome: a review of the medical literature 1974–1979. Pediatrics 66:597, 1980
4. Southall DP: Role of apnea in the sudden infant death syndrome. A personal view. Pediatrics 80:73, 1988
5. van der Hal AL, Rodriguez AM, Sargent CW, et al: Hypoxic and hypercapneic arousal responses and prediction of subsequent apnea in apnea of infancy. Pediatrics 75:848, 1985
6. Steward DJ: Is there risk of general anesthesia triggering SIDS? Possibly not! Anesthesiology 63:326, 1985
7. Tetzlaff JE, Annand DW, Pudimat MA, Nicodemus HF: Postoperative apnea in a full-term infant. Anesthesiology 69:426, 1988
8. Liu LMP, Cote CJ, Goudsouzian NG, et al: Life-threatening apnea in infants recovering from anesthesia. Anesthesiology 59:506, 1983
9. Steward DJ: Preterm infants are more prone to complications following minor surgery than are term infants. Anesthesiology 56:304, 1982
10. Kurth CD, Spitzer AR, Broennle AM, Downes JJ: Postoperative apnea in former premature infants. Anesthesiology 66:483, 1987
11. Welborn LG, Ramirez N, Oh TH, et al: Postanesthetic apnea and periodic breathing in infants. Anesthesiology 65:658, 1986
12. Welborn LG, DeSoto H, Hannallah RS, et al: The use of caffeine in the control of post-anesthetic apnea in former premature infants. Anesthesiology 68:796, 1988
13. Coates AL, Bergsteinsson H, Desmond K, et al: Long-term pulmonary sequelae of premature birth with and without idiopathic respiratory distress syndrome. J Pediatr 90:611, 1977
14. Bryan MH, Hardie MJ, Reilly BJ, et al: Pulmonary function studies during the first year of life in infants recovering from the respiratory distress syndrome. Pediatrics 52:169, 1973
15. Bader D, Ramos AD, Lew CD, et al: Childhood sequelae of infant lung disease: exercise and pulmonary function abnormalities after bronchopulmonary dysplasia. J Pediatr 110:693, 1987
16. Jones R, Bodnar A, Roan Y, et al: Subglottic stenosis in newborn intensive care unit graduates. Am J Dis Child 135:367, 1981
17. Garg M, Kurzner SI, Bautista D, Keens TG: Hypoxic arousal responses in infants with bronchopulmonary dysplasia. Pediatrics 82:59, 1988
18. Newburger JW, Rosenthal A, Williams RG, et al: Noninvasive tests in the initial evaluation of heart murmurs in children. N Engl J Med 308:61, 1983
19. Campbell FW, Schwartz AJ: Anesthesia for noncardiac surgery in the pediatric patient with congenital heart disease. American Society of Anesthesiologists Refresher Course Lectures in Anesthesiology. Vol 14. 1986
20. Moore RA: Anesthesia for the pediatric congenital heart patient for noncardiac surgery. Anesthesiol Rev 8:23, 1981
21. Gergen PJ, Mullally DI, Evans R III: National survey of prevalence of asthma among children in the United States, 1976 to 1980. Pediatrics 81:1, 1988
22. Willson DF: The child with asthma. p. 273. In Berry FA (ed): Anesthetic Management of the Difficult and Routine Pediatric Patient. Churchill Livingstone, New York, 1986
23. Ekwo E, Weinberger M: Evaluation of a program for the pharmacologic management of children with asthma. J Allergy Clin Immunol 61:240, 1978
24. Berry FA: The child with the runny nose. p. 349. In Berry FA (ed): Anesthetic Management of the Difficult and Routine Pediatric Patient. Churchill Livingstone, New York, 1986
25. Betts EK: Case no. 10. p. 374. In Wetchler BV (ed): Anesthesia for Ambulatory Surgery. JB Lippincott, Philadelphia, 1985
26. Empey W, Laitinen LA, Jacobs L, et al: Mechanisms of bronchial hyperreactivity in normal subjects after upper respiratory tract infection. Am Rev Respir Dis 113:131, 1976
27. Collier AM, Pimmel RL, Hasselblad V, et al: Spirometric changes in normal children with upper respiratory infections. Am Rev Respir Dis 117:47, 1978

28. Tait AR, Knight PR: The effects of general anesthesia on upper respiratory tract infections in children. Anesthesiology 67:930, 1987
29. DeSoto H, Patel RI, Soliman IE, Hannallah RS: Changes in oxygen saturation following general anesthesia in children with upper respiratory infection signs and symptoms undergoing otolaryngological procedures. Anesthesiology 68:276, 1988
30. McGill WA, Coveler LA, Epstein BS: Subacute upper respiratory infection in small children. Anesth Analg 58:331, 1979
31. Tishler JM, Martel W: Dislocation of the atlas in mongolism: preliminary report. Radiology 84:904, 1965
32. Martel W, Tishler JM: Observations on the spine in mongolism. Am J Roentgenol Radium Ther Nucl Med 94:630, 1966
33. Pueschel SM, Scola FH: Epidemiologic, radiographic and clinical studies of atlantoaxial instability in individuals with Down syndrome. Pediatrics 80:555, 1987
34. Moore RA, McNicholas KW, Warran SP: Atlantoaxial subluxation with symptomatic spinal cord compression in a child with Down's syndrome. Anesth Analg 66:89, 1987
35. Davidson RG: Atlantoaxial instability in individuals with Down syndrome: a fresh look at the evidence. Pediatrics 81:857, 1988
36. Raybould D, Bradshaw EG: Premedication for day case surgery. Anaesthesia 42:591, 1987
37. VanDerWalt JH, Nicholls B, Bentley M, Tomkins DP: Oral premedication in children. Anaesth Intensive Care 15:151, 1987
38. Henderson JM, Brodsky DA, Fisher DM, et al: Pre-induction of anesthesia in pediatric patients with nasally administered sufentanil. Anesthesiology 68:671, 1988
39. Leiman BC, Walford A, Rawal N, et al: The effects of oral transmucosal fentanyl citrate premedication on gastric volume and acidity in children. Anesthesiology 67:A489, 1987
40. Nelson PS, Streisand JB, Mulder S, et al: Premedication in children: A comparison of oral transmucosal fentanyl citrate (fentanyl lollipop) and an oral solution of meperidine, diazepam and atropine. Anesthesiology 67:A490, 1987
41. Kestin IG, McIlvaine WB, Lockhart CH, et al: Rectal methohexital for induction of anesthesia in children with and without rectal aspiration after sleep. Anesth Analg 67:1102, 1988
42. Feld LH, Urquhart ML, Feaster WW, White PF: Premedication in children: oral *versus* intramuscular midazolam. Anesthesiology 69:A745, 1988

8

Anesthesia for Pediatric Outpatients

David J. Steward

Over the past two decades, the concept of outpatient surgery for infants and children has become firmly established. Outpatient pediatric surgery under general anesthesia, originally described in a few pioneering centers, has become the standard mode of treatment for many surgical lesions of childhood. Indeed, it is now more of a problem to convince hospitals and insurance agencies that there are some children who have to be hospitalized for "minor" surgical procedures.

Much has been written concerning the advantages of pediatric outpatient surgery to the patient, the parents, and the health care system.[1,2] This information is available in chapter 7 and will not be repeated here. Rather, this chapter defines the present practices for pediatric outpatient surgery as reported by some of those currently active in this field.

PRESURGERY PROCEDURES

Preparation of the Child

While many units perform all preoperative testing immediately prior to the planned operation, some infants and children may need to see the anesthesiologist in advance of the day of surgery. The outpatient surgical staff should be provided with clear criteria as to which patients will be suitable for general anesthesia. In addition, a consultation service should be provided, not only to determine that patients meet the criteria, but also to answer questions from the children and their parents. Such a service can be provided by a regular weekly anesthesiology clinic. In addition, the use of written instructions (see Appendix 8-1) can be a valuable adjuvant.

Preoperative Fasting

Written instructions for preoperative fasting should be clearly provided to the parents prior to the day of surgery, and compliance with these should be confirmed when the child arrives at the outpatient unit.

A standard practice has been to curtail oral fluid intake for 4 or more hours preoperatively, but evidence is now emerging which suggests that fluids can be safely given to healthy children up to 2 hours before anesthesia. A study of gastric contents after induction demonstrated no difference in volume or pH in children given a standard volume of fluid 2, 4, or 6 hours before anesthesia.[3] Another study suggested that patients given a drink of orange juice 2 hours preoperatively had a lower volume of gastric contents than those who did not drink for 4 hours preoperatively.[4] The pH of gastric contents was the same in both groups; presumably, the ingestion of fluid stimulated gastric emptying into the duodenum.

In light of these studies, and because it is well-known that fluid restriction more rapidly produces significant physiologic disturbance in infants and young children than in adults, some centers are modifying their fasting routines. This minimizes the discomfort for the patient and reduces the need for intraoperative intravenous fluid therapy.

Infants under 2 years of age should be given clear fluids until 3 hours before surgery. Other feedings must be discontinued at least 6 hours before the induction of anesthesia. Infants who are breast-fed should complete the last feeding 4 hours preoperatively and may be offered clear fluid 3 hours preoperatively. Children over 2 years of age should have no solid food on the day of surgery, but may have reasonable amounts of clear fluid up to 3 hours preoperatively. If the patient arrives at the outpatient unit having clearly contravened the fasting instructions, the operation should be rescheduled for another day.

On Arrival for Surgery

The patient should be admitted, and routine nursing observations made (i.e., body weight, temperature, heart rate, and blood pressure). Suitable attractive hospital clothes should be provided; most children will accept these readily. The rare child who does not wish to undress should be allowed to wear his or her own clothes until time to go to the operating room. It is important to respect the modesty of children, uncovering them only as needed to complete an adequate physical examination.

It is accepted practice to require a hemoglobin (or hematocrit) estimation and urinalysis before outpatient surgery. Hemoglobin values in healthy, stable infants and children are considered "valid" for 4 to 6 weeks. The value of routine preoperative hemoglobin estimations in healthy infants and children is unproven, and the added risk of well-conducted general anesthesia in the presence of mild anemia is unknown. While in some jurisdictions it is a legal requirement to perform a preoperative hemoglobin estimation, elsewhere it is considered reasonable to spare children venipuncture (or an equally painful finger prick) unless they have a history of anemia or appear to be anemic. All infants and any children with systemic diseases, a history of bleeding, or other indications of anemia should have a preoperative hemoglobin test to define their hemoglobin level.

Routine chest x-rays are not required by most outpatient units, as the cost-benefit ratio of these is in great doubt for pediatric patients.

Once all preparations are complete, patients should be taken to a play area and allowed to amuse themselves until the time of their surgery. "Special" children, the immune deficient or those who are very upset, for example, may need greater care and should wait with their parents in a separate area.

Premedication

Many centers do not prescribe premedication for the outpatient, and the value of such therapy in preventing lasting psychological trauma to the child is uncertain.[6,7] It is considered preferable to use proven psychological preparation of the child for his or her outpatient experience.[8,9] This may include tours of the ambulatory surgery unit, the viewing of videotapes and puppet shows, and other play therapy. The parents also should be provided with all the information necessary to play their leading role in preparing their child for surgery. Procedures used in the British Columbia's

Children's Hospital are found in Appendix 8-1. Such information contained in brochures should tell children the truth about their visit and reassure them that there will be no "big hurts." To be useful to the parents, leaflets should provide information about the availability of parking, requirements of registration, and so forth, but should avoid being too detailed as to overwhelm. In addition, it is helpful to provide children of appropriate age with specially prepared pictures or storybooks about operations.

Premedication may be useful for some children in facilitating separation from parents and for induction of anesthesia.[5] If it is considered necessary to administer pharmacologic premedication, some general principles are important. First, avoid intramuscular injections, this is often the child's worst memory of the procedure. Second, avoid the use of narcotic analgesics, as these have a tendency to increase the incidence of postoperative nausea and vomiting.[10] Oral premedication has recently been shown to be as effective as intramuscular therapy.[11] Oral diazepam (0.2 to 0.4 mg/kg) can be ordered for the child and can be given at home by a suitably reliable parent 2 hours prior to surgery. Triclofos has also been reported useful to facilitate induction for selected patients.

While the use of sedative premedication is of dubious value, many practitioners feel that anticholinergic drugs are indicated for pediatric patients. Vagal activity may be marked following administration of cholinergic drugs (e.g., succinylcholine, halothane) or instrumentation of the airway. Atropine may be mixed with intravenous or rectal induction agents, or may be given intravenously once inhalation induction is achieved. If there is any doubt about the ease of intravenous access, atropine should be given orally (1 hour before surgery) or intramuscularly (30 minutes before surgery).

When the time for their surgery arrives, older children should be walked to the operating room. Even toddlers may prefer to be helped along on their feet rather than whisked up and carried. If parents are to accompany the child into an induction area, it is important to explain to them beforehand what will happen and when they should leave. The benefits to the child of having parents present during induction have not been convincingly demonstrated; hence, the practice is limited. When practical, the parents' presence may comfort the child.

METHODS FOR GENERAL ANESTHESIA

The method chosen for general anesthesia for the pediatric outpatient should be one that will ensure maximum safety, provide a rapid recovery, and result in minimal postoperative morbidity. The requirements of the planned surgical procedure must, of course, be met.

Induction of anesthesia in pediatric patients has frequently been achieved by inhalational methods, although intravenous or rectal barbiturates have been increasingly used in recent years. Studies have suggested that the method chosen for induction will have little effect on the speed of recovery or the incidence of postoperative minor morbidity.[12,13] This being so, a method of induction appropriate to each child can be selected.

Inhalation induction of anesthesia is usually preferred for small infants and is indicated for any child with an abnormal airway. In addition, some children may request an inhalation induction. Such requests should be met. All published objective comparative studies of inhalation induction of anesthesia in pediatric patients support the widely held contention that halothane is the most suitable drug.[14,15] Isoflurane and enflurane both produce a higher incidence of coughing, breath holding, and laryngospasm and require a longer period to achieve surgical anesthesia. Arterial oxygen saturation levels have been demonstrated to be more consistently maintained during induction with halothane than with isoflurane.[16]

Inhalation Induction

Halothane induction in the unpremedicated outpatient may be achieved in several ways.

In infants, the mask can be held above the face and halothane delivered with 50 percent nitrous oxide allowed to flow down over the mouth and nose until the mask is tolerated. Small infants usually seem to enjoy the smell of halothane and lie quietly during this procedure. Concentrations of up to 3 percent halothane are required to induce anesthesia, but these should be reduced once the induction is completed and before controlled ventilation is applied. The use of more than 1 percent halothane, especially with controlled ventilation, may result in severe hypotension in infants.

Older children who have elected to have an inhalation induction may be allowed to hold the mask to their faces and will often cooperate well. The use of clear masks and artificial scents ("fruit flavors") may make this induction more acceptable.[17] The use of fruit flavors to mask the smell of isoflurane does not affect the incidence of respiratory complications during induction.[18]

A "single breath" induction of anesthesia with halothane may be appropriate for older, cooperative children who have elected an inhalation induction.[19] The essential maneuver should be practiced first using a reservoir bag filled only with oxygen. The patient is instructed to take in a big breath, breathe all the way out (i.e., to residual volume), and stop. The mask is then applied to allow the patient to inhale oxygen via the anesthesia circuit from residual volume. The practice having been perfected, the circuit and an adequate-sized reservoir bag are primed with a mixture containing 5 percent halothane in 50 percent nitrous oxide with oxygen. Induction is achieved by having the patient inspire this mixture from residual volume. After the first "single breath," the inspired concentration of halothane should be reduced to 3 percent and the induction continued. This method can be spectacularly successful for a cooperative child.

Intravenous Induction

Intravenous induction of anesthesia may be preferable to inhaled anesthesia for many children. The few studies that have been performed indicate that intravenous induction may result in less emotional disturbances than those that follow an inhalation induction.[20,21] This may presuppose that each method is equally skillfully applied. (The use of the method with which the anesthesiologist is most familiar and most skilled must always be considered optimal.) Thiopental in doses 5 mg/kg in older children (more than 5 years of age) or 6 to 7 mg/kg in younger patients will produce rapid pleasant hypnosis.[22] A 27-gauge "butterfly" needle is preferable, and needle and syringes should be kept from sight. Preparation of the skin with a eutectic mixture of lidocaine and prilocaine (EMLA cream) beneath an occlusive dressing for 1 hour before venipuncture makes the process painless but may not, of course, alleviate needle phobia.[23] If the anesthesiologist chooses to establish a continuous intravenous infusion with a cannula, this can be done once the child is anesthetized, as venipuncture is much easier once the veins are well-dilated. Many patients who have not had excessive preoperative fasting and are having minor surgical procedures may not require intravenous infusions. The butterfly needle used for induction should, however, be taped into place to provide for venous access, should this be required. The use of an intravenous barbiturate to induce anesthesia does not significantly prolong the recovery of children following anesthesia or increase the incidence of minor morbidity postoperatively.[12]

Propofol (Diprivan) has been used to induce anesthesia in pediatric outpatients. A dose of 2.5 to 3.0 mg/kg is recommended and will induce hypnosis with minimal cardiovascular effects.[24,25] Recovery is rapid and complete following propofol, and it is suggested that the drug may have a useful antiemetic effect during the postoperative period—features that are certainly advantageous for the outpatient. Local pain on injection may be relieved by infusing a dose of 0.2 mg/kg lidocaine into the vein and occluding the vessel for 20 seconds, or by adding a similar amount of lidocaine to the propofol solution.[25]

Rectal barbiturates are useful to anesthetize the child who is too young to cooperate with intravenous or inhalation induction and who may become frightened at separation from the parents.[13] Optimally, rectal induction should be performed in an area adjacent to the operating room where the parents may stay with the child until he or she falls asleep. This area should be discretely equipped with oxygen and suction, and with all facilities necessary to establish an airway and institute controlled ventilation. Methohexital (1 percent) in a dose of 15 mg/kg has been shown to be as effective as larger doses of a 10 percent solution (S. Kaller, personal communication). This is due to the larger volume recruiting a greater area of rectal mucosa for systemic absorption of the drug.[26] Atropine (0.02 mg/kg) may be added and also given rectally at the same time. The drug should be administered from a syringe using the well-lubricated tip of a 10-gauge catheter. A small amount of air should be included in the syringe to flush the total dose into the rectum. Once the drug has been administered, the child may be returned to the parents to hold until the onset of sleep, usually within 4 to 8 minutes. It is wise to place a diaper on the child or to place one discretely on the parent's lap in case of any leakage of the drug and/or rectal contents.

Once asleep, the patient is placed in a lateral position. The anesthesiologist then ensures a good airway and transfers the patient to the operating room. The induction should now be continued with nitrous oxide and halothane, bearing in mind that ventilation may become depressed until the surgery commences.

For short procedures, inhaled anesthesia with nitrous oxide and halothane may suffice. Whenever indicated, however, endotracheal intubation should be performed. Provided that laryngoscopy is gently performed and that an endotracheal tube of the correct diameter is used, postintubation sequelae are rare. The correct size endotracheal tube will pass easily through the glottis and subglottic space and allows a slight leak when the circuit is pressurized to 20 cm/H_2O. Pediatric endotracheal tubes should be meticulously secured and supported to prevent movement or kinking.

A T-piece circuit is preferred for children with a body weight of less than 20 kg. The fresh gas flow should equal 2.5 times the minute ventilation during spontaneous breathing. Minute ventilation of the anesthetized child can be approximately determined by multiplying the observed respiratory frequency × body weight in kilograms × 5. During controlled ventilation, a lower fresh gas flow rate may be used to maintain normocapnia. Flow rates of 1,000 ml + 100 ml/kg for children weighing less than 30 kg and 2,000 ml + 50 ml/kg for children weighing more than 30 kg are required.[27] Minute ventilation should be set at least two times the fresh gas flow rate. For children over 20 kg body weight, an adult circle absorber system may be used.

INDUCTION AND MAINTENANCE FOR GENERAL ANESTHESIA

Inhaled Anesthetic Agents

Many pediatric anesthesiologists prefer to use the volatile inhaled agents for outpatients. Recovery is rapid and predictable, and most children will be suitable for discharge after 1 hour. Halothane has long been a favorite agent, and there is no evidence to suggest that recovery is significantly more rapid or complete if isoflurane or enflurane is used. The incidence of halothane-induced hepatic dysfunction is rare in infants and children,[28] and most pediatric anesthesiologists believe that its efficacy and safety justify its continued routine use. Laryngospasm on extubation following halothane anesthesia is a major concern. This should be prevented by electing to extubate the patient either while still adequately anesthetized or when fully awake. In patients at increased risk of larynospasm (e.g., blood or secretions in the pharynx) or those for whom coughing must be avoided (e.g., following ocular procedures), lidocaine (1 to 1.5 mg/kg IV) should be given 3 minutes prior to extubation.[29]

Isoflurane has been used for pediatric outpatients, but the higher incidence of airway complications and the longer induction time are disadvantages.[15] Isoflurane may be more suitable for patients who require local infiltration of epinephrine-containing solutions or who are taking high doses of theophylline. Serious arrythmias may occur with halothane in such patients. Recovery following isoflurane anesthesia is also rapid and complete.

Many consider that optimal management for infants and children can be achieved by the combined use of an intraoperative volatile anesthetic agent and a regional analgesic technique to control postoperative pain.

Intravenous Anesthetic and Analgesic Agents

Although inhalation methods are more commonly used for pediatric patients, techniques have been described in which intravenous drugs have been used as adjuncts to maintain anesthesia. For example, fentanyl has been used to supplement nitrous oxide anesthesia.[30] More recently, the use of an infusion of alfentanil has been suggested.[31] Propofol has been used by infusion to maintain anesthesia in adults, but there is little experience with such techniques in children.[32] In some studies, recovery after the use of short-acting intravenous narcotics has been demonstrated to be more rapid than after the use of volatile agents, but the use of some narcotics may be followed by a more delayed recovery and discharge as a result of the increased incidence of postoperative nausea and vomiting.

If the operation is likely to be followed by discomfort that cannot be effectively controlled by a regional analgesic technique (e.g., tonsillectomy), the use of an appropriate narcotic analgesic intraoperatively to control pain on awakening is indicated.

Neuromuscular Blocking Agents

Succinylcholine is commonly used to facilitate intubation. The problem of masseter spasm and its possible relationship to malignant hyperpyrexia syndrome has generated much discussion in the literature, but many still consider succinylcholine to be useful in aiding intubation for short procedures. It is notable that masseter spasm is virtually unknown following induction with thiopental; indeed, such a sign under those circumstances is significantly prognostic of malignant hyperpyrexia syndrome, and should prompt both the discontinuation of anesthesia and re-evaluation of the case. However, halothane is known to sensitize skeletal muscle to the effects of succinylcholine, and when these drugs are used together, a much higher incidence of masseter spasm has been described, possibly even as high as 1 in 100 cases. I prefer not to administer succinylcholine after induction of anesthesia with halothane but choose to intubate such patients under deep halothane anesthesia, provided this could be achieved without excessive cardiovascular depression. When I use intravenous thiopental to induce anesthesia, I follow this with succinylcholine if intubation is required for a short procedure (e.g., adenoidectomy).

If succinylcholine is used for pediatric outpatients, the problem of postoperative muscle pains must be addressed.[33] Although the incidence of muscle pains may be lower in younger age groups, some children as young as 4 years of age have pains, and these should be prevented. This can be achieved by the administration of d-tubocurarine 0.05 mg/kg IV prior to succinylcholine. When d-tubocurarine is used, the dose of succinylcholine should be increased by 70 percent to ensure adequate relaxation.

The use of nondepolarizing muscle relaxants to provide continued neuromuscular block is seldom indicated in pediatric outpatient surgery, and most anesthesiologists have avoided their use. If such agents are used, a shorter-acting drug, vecuronium or atracurium, would be preferred, and the child should be carefully assessed for residual muscle weakness prior to discharge.

MONITORING DURING ANESTHESIA

It is most important to monitor all pediatric patients carefully. Disastrous changes in physiologic parameters can occur extremely rapidly and must be immediately detected if serious consequences are to be avoided. Any tendency to downplay the importance of meticulous monitoring in the healthy child undergoing minor surgery must be rejected; many malpractice suits center on patients such as these. Essential monitors for every case are the precordial stethoscope, pulse oximeter, blood pressure cuff, and thermistor temperature probe.

The precordial stethoscope is still a useful tool despite the advent of much more sophisticated devices. Continuous monitoring of heart and breath sounds remains the most rapid and reliable means to diagnose problems of ventilation. Changes in heart sounds provide an early indication of altered cardiac function.

The pulse oximeter is an invaluable additional monitor that should be used for every patient, since it rapidly detects minor changes in systemic oxygenation that might otherwise be missed.[34]

A suitably sized blood pressure cuff should be applied (i.e., one that occupies two-thirds of the upper arm). An automated blood pressure monitor (e.g., Dinamap) may be used, but the anesthesiologist should be aware that the data presented may be outdated by 3 minutes or more. I prefer a Doppler flowmeter positioned over the radial artery and set to run continuously at a barely audible level. Any change in pulse volume can be immediately detected by this means.

Body temperature should be monitored. A thermistor placed in the axilla will accurately demonstrate trends in core temperature, provided the probe is adjacent to the axillary artery and the arm adducted.[35]

The ECG is usually monitored as a matter of routine, but is not very useful in pediatric patients. The ECG must never be relied on to indicate patient well-being. Serious hypotension and significant hypoxemia may occur and cause brain damage before any changes in the ECG are apparent.

Intraoperative Fluid Therapy

Many infants and children who have had fluids up to 3 or 4 hours preoperatively, who are having minor surgery, and who are predicted to resume fluid intake soon after the operation do not require fluids. Those who have inadvertently experienced prolonged preoperative fasting, who are having procedures that may result in blood loss (e.g., tonsillectomy and adenoidectomy), or who may be nauseated postoperatively (e.g., strabismus correction, orchiectomy) should be given an intravenous infusion during surgery. A balanced electrolyte solution, such as Ringer lactate, is preferred, and it should be infused at a rate judged to replace existing deficits and to provide adequate fluid maintenance on the day of surgery. In cases of expected blood loss, appropriately larger volumes of fluid should be given.

PROCEDURES REQUIRING SPECIAL CONSIDERATION

Tonsillectomy and adenoidectomy are now frequently performed on an outpatient basis. The patients should be carefully screened to exclude any evidence of preoperative obstruction causing sleep apnea as well as any factors that might cause increased bleeding (e.g., a coagulopathy or a history of recurrent severe tonsillitis); such patients require overnight admission. Patients for tonsillectomy and adenoidectomy should receive generous intraoperative fluid therapy both to replace deficits and intraoperative blood losses and to provide for a period of limited intake after surgery. Meperidine (1.5 mg/kg IM) should be given before emergence from anesthesia, and acetaminophen (10 mg/kg) can be given as required in the postanesthesia recovery room.

Strabismus surgery is associated with a high incidence of nausea and vomiting. It has been demonstrated that droperidol (75 mg/kg) may reduce the incidence of this, but to be fully effective it must be given before the eye is manipulated.[36] Patients who are required to be alert and cooperative postoperatively (e.g., those with adjustable sutures) should not receive droperidol but may be helped by the administration of metaclopramide (0.15 mg/kg IV) immediately before the end of anesthesia.[37]

POSTOPERATIVE MANAGEMENT

The surgical outpatient recovery phase can be managed optimally in two phases: initial recovery in the postanesthesia recovery room and ongoing recovery in the outpatient unit until the patient is fit for discharge.

The patient should remain in the recovery room until full return of normal consciousness, full resumption of motor functions, return of normal and stable cardiorespiratory function, and until initial pain therapy is judged effective. In many children's hospitals, the parents are allowed and encouraged to be present as their child awakens. Recovery during this early phase should be observed and recorded using a postanesthesia scoring system,[38] and vital signs should be examined periodically (Table 8-1). The duration of stay required in the recovery room will depend on the procedure performed, the immediate postoperative progress, and the presence of any postoperative complications. It is useful to establish guidelines for minimal periods of stay for standard procedures and then to modify these as required in special circumstances.

Table 8-1. Postanesthesia Scoring System

Consciousness	
Awake	2
Responding to stimuli	1
Not responsing	0
Airway	
Coughing on command or crying	2
Maintaining good airway	1
Airway requires maintenance	0
Movement	
Moving limbs purposefully	2
Non-purposeful movements	1
Not moving	0
Total	—

Oral fluids are encouraged as soon as the patient expresses any interest. We find popsicles to be acceptable to most children and consider them a good form of therapy, both during recovery and at home.

Pain Management

Effective relief of postoperative pain is extremely important if the physiologic and psychological effects of the operation are to be minimized. Pain delays physical recovery, increases the incidence of postoperative morbidity (e.g., nausea and vomiting[39]), and results in more severe emotional upset.[40]

Regional analgesia is ideal for the management of postoperative pain in the pediatric outpatient. If the block is administered during general anesthesia, the patient can emerge painfree and comfortable, early ambulation can be achieved, and the side effects of systemic analgesic drugs can be avoided. Hence, a regional block should be performed whenever it is permitted by the surgical site. Alternatively, the incision may be infiltrated with a local anesthetic solution or a topical anesthetic may be applied to a mucous membrane (e.g., after division of tongue tie).

For short surgical procedures, the regional block should be established before the operation commences. This provides adequate time for the block to become established before awakening and may also reduce the need for general anesthetic agents and hence speed recovery. Bupivacaine is the most commonly used agent and may be given in doses of 2 to 3 mg/kg.

Regional Blocks

Ilioinguinal and iliohypogastric nerve blocks may be used for herniotomy and other operations in the inguinal region.[41] A dose of 1 to 3 ml of 0.5 percent bupivacaine can be used to block the nerves in the deep muscle layers just medial to the anterior superior iliac spine. Rarely, a weakness of muscles supplied by the femoral nerve may occur and cause difficulty in walking; presumably, this is due to tracking of the local anesthetic solution into the femoral nerve sheaths. The child and his or her parents should be reassured that this weakness will fully recover in a few hours.

Bilateral block of the tenth intercostal nerves will provide excellent analgesia following umbilical hernia repair. These nerves can be readily blocked using 1 to 2 ml 0.5 percent bupivacaine below the tenth rib in the mid-axillary line.

Caudal blocks using 0.75 ml/kg of 0.125 percent bupivacaine have been demonstrated to provide good analgesia following hypospadius repair, orchiopexy, and other perineal procedures.[42] The use of this technique has been successful in providing good pain relief without muscle weakness, retention of urine, or any significant hypotension due to sympathetic block.

Block of the dorsal nerves of the penis[43] or simple local application of lidocaine jelly[44] provides pain relief following circumcision.

When no specific nerve block is indicated, simple infiltration of the incision with bupivacaine will provide a useful measure of relief[45] but may slightly delay wound healing, especially if tissues are not healthy.[46] This latter effect is probably of no clinical significance for most elective pediatric surgery, and local anesthetic infiltration may in fact improve the final appearance of the scar by preventing keloid formation.[46]

When regional analgesia is impractical or fails to provide complete pain relief, the anesthesiologist must resort to systemic analgesic drugs. It is then important to select the drug that will provide optimal pain relief and minimal side effects (see Ch. 19).

Systemic Analgesic Drugs

Acetaminophen (Tylenol) may be administered orally or rectally in a dose of 10 mg/kg and will provide analgesia following minor superficial surgery. This drug does not cause any increase in nausea or vomiting.

Codeine (1.5 mg/kg), administered either intramuscularly or orally, is suitable for children having more extensive surgery but not so extensive that it merits the use of potent narcotic analgesic drugs. Codeine has a wide margin of safety and causes little respiratory depression, but it may increase the incidence of nausea and vomiting. Codeine cannot be given intravenously.

Meperidine (Demerol), administered intramuscularly in doses of 1 to 1.5 mg/kg, is useful for patients who may have considerable postoperative discomfort (e.g., following tonsillectomy). The drug should be given while the patient is still anesthetized so that he or she is comfortable on emergence from anesthesia.

COMPLICATIONS DURING RECOVERY

Airway problems are of special concern. Laryngeal spasm occurs frequently in pediatric patients,[47] and prevention should be the aim. The incidence of laryngospasm may be reduced by the use of anticholinergic premedication, careful suctioning of the pharynx prior to extubation, avoiding extubation in light planes of anesthesia, and use of intravenous lidocaine before removal of the tube.[48] Once laryngospasm occurs, the jaw should be supported and gentle continuous positive pressure oxygen administered via a tight-fitting facemask. Air entry should be monitored using a stethoscope; the oxygen saturation should also be monitored. If air entry fails to improve and the saturation falls, reintubation should be performed immediately.[47] This may be facilitated by intravenous or intramuscular succinylcholine, but if the child is severely hypoxic and bradycardic, reintubation should be performed without the use of muscle relaxants.

Postintubation stridor should not occur if gentle laryngoscopy and insertion of the correct size tube have been performed.[48] Rarely, however, it may present with no apparent cause or may appear in an infant who has had a recent upper respiratory infection. Mild degrees of stridor should be treated by administration of humidified oxygen. Persistent or more severe stridor requires the use of racemic epinephrine delivered by intermittent positive pressure.[49] Any pediatric outpatient who develops stridor must be closely observed for at least 2 hours after the stridor resolves. Consideration should be given to overnight admission for any child who develops stridor that fails to respond rapidly to simple measures, especially if there is any prior history of croup.

Nausea and vomiting have been reported to occur more frequently in pediatric patients[50] than in adults and are especially troublesome after ear, nose, throat, and eye procedures. The incidence of nausea and vomiting may be reduced by avoiding unnecessary narcotic drugs, aspirating the stomach prior to extubation, and administering specific antinausea drugs. Patients who are having strabismus surgery should be pretreated with droperidol (75 μg/kg) before the eye muscles are manipulated to minimize postoperative vomiting, and they should receive acetaminophen orally or rectally for postoperative pain. I am hesitant to give droperidol to patients having tonsillectomy, as this may cause excessive sedation when combined with potent narcotic analgesics; dimenhydrinate (Gravol) in doses of 1 to 2 mg/kg is safer and may be even more effective.

CRITERIA FOR DISCHARGE

Once initial recovery is complete, the patient should be returned to the surgical outpatient unit to recover fully before discharge. The patient should remain in the unit until judged fit for discharge and until the parents are happy to proceed home. The child should be recovered to normal ambulatory status and should be accepting and retaining clear fluids by mouth. The vital signs should be stable and there should be no significant nausea or vomiting. If the journey home is to be by private automobile, there should be someone in attendance to care for the patient in addition to the driver of the car. The motion of the automobile commonly causes nausea and vomiting. If only one parent is available, the journey home should be by taxicab. Written instructions should be given for postoperative care, together with emergency telephone numbers (see Appendix 8-2). This information should be available in different languages, as necessary, to ensure that the correct information is communicated. A follow-up telephone call should be placed on the first or second postoperative day to document full recovery and record any delayed complications.

SUMMARY

Pediatric outpatient surgery is now established as an ideal method of care for many infants and children who require surgical procedures that demand no special postoperative care. The success of pediatric outpatient programs depends on the development of clear criteria for patient selection, good preoperative assessment, the use of a simple and safe anesthesia regimen, and the provision of optimal postoperative analgesia. It is vital that the parents be well-informed so they may cooperate fully in the process.

Over the past decade, the variety of surgical procedures considered suitable for the pediatric outpatient has steadily increased as improved methods of anesthesia and supportive care have been introduced.

Recent trends in the management of pediatric outpatient anesthesia are toward a further relaxation of the duration of preoperative oral fluid restriction, increased use of intravenous anesthetic agents, and more extensive use of regional analgesic techniques in the prevention of postoperative pain. Regional analgesia permits rapid ambulation and hastens return to full activity, while obviating the need for systemic analgesic therapy that may result in unwanted side effects.

REFERENCES

1. Davenport HT, Shah CP, Robinson GC: Day surgery for children. Can Med Assoc J 105:498, 1971
2. Steward DJ: Outpatient pediatric anesthesia. Anesthesiology 43:268, 1975
3. Farrow-Gillespie A, Christensen S, Lerman J: Effect of the fasting interval on gastric pH and volume in children. Anesth Analg 67:S59, 1988
4. Splinter WM, Stewart JA, Muir JG: The effect of preoperative apple juice on gastric contents, thirst, and hunger in children. Can J Anaesth 36:55, 1989
5. Bruzstowitz RM, Nelson DA, Betts EK, et al: Efficacy of oral premedication for pediatric outpatient surgery. Anesthesiology 60:475, 1984
6. Desjardins R, Ansara S, Charest J: Pre-

anesthetic medication in paediatric day-care surgery. Can Anaesth Soc J 28:141, 1981
7. Hodges RJH: Induction of anesthesia in children. Lancet 1:82, 1960
8. Jackson K: Psychological preparation as a method of reducing the emotional trauma of anesthesia in children. Anesthesiology 12:293, 1951
9. Vernon DTA, Bailey WC: The use of motion pictures in the psychological preparation of children for induction of anesthesia. Anesthesiology 40:68, 1974
10. Booker PD, Chapman DH: Premedication in children undergoing day care surgery. Br J Anaesth 51:1083, 1979
11. Nicholson SC, Betts EK, Jobes DR, et al: Comparison of oral and intramuscular preanesthetic medication for pediatric inpatient surgery. Anesthesiology 71:8, 1989
12. Steward DJ: Experience with an outpatient anesthesia service for children. Anesth Analg 52:877, 1973
13. Goresky GV, Steward DJ: Rectal methohexitone for the induction of anaesthesia in children. Can Anaesth Soc J 26:213, 1979
14. Pandit UA, Steude GM, Leach AB: Induction and recovery characteristics of isoflurane and halothane for short outpatient operations in children. Anaesthesia 40:1226, 1985
15. Fisher DM, Robinson S, Brett CM, et al: Comparison of enflurane, isoflurane, and halothane for diagnostic procedures in children with malignancies. Anesthesiology 63:647, 1985
16. Phillips AJ, Brimacombe Jr, Simpson DL: Anesthetic induction with isoflurane or halothane. Oxygen saturation during induction with isoflurane or halothane in unpremedicated children. Anaesthesia 43:927, 1988
17. Yamashita M, Motokawa K: "Fruit flavoured" mask induction for children. Anesthesiology 64:837, 1986
18. Lewis RP, Eastley RJ, Wanless JG: "Fruit flavoured" mask for isoflurane induction in children. Anaesthesia 43:1052, 1988
19. Ruffle JM, Snider MT: Onset of hypnosis with halothane induction using single breath, triple breath, and conventional techniques. Anesthesiology 61:A498, 1984
20. Kay B: Outpatient anaesthesia, especially for children. Acta Anaesth Scand Suppl 25:421–1966
21. Hodges RJH: Induction of anaesthesia in young children. Lancet 1;82, 1960
22. Jonmarker C, Westrin P, Larsson S, Werner O: Thiopental requirements for induction of anesthesia in children. Anesthesiology 67:104, 1987
23. Broadman LM, Soliman IE, Hannallah RS, McGill WA: Analgesic efficacy of eutectic mixture of local anaesthetics (EMLA) vs intradermal infiltration prior to venous cannulation in children. Can J Anaesth 34:S56, 1987
24. Patel DK, Keeling PA, Newman GB, Radford P: Induction dose of propofol in children. Anaesthesia 43:949, 1988
25. Mirakhur RK: Induction characteristics of propofol in children: comparison with thiopentone. Anaesthesia 43:593, 1988
26. Forbes RB, Vandewalker GE: Comparison of two and ten percent rectal methohexitone for induction of anaesthesia in children. Can J Anaesth 35:345, 1988
27. Rose DK, Byrick RJ, Foese AB: Carbon dioxide elimination during spontaneous ventilation with a modified Mapleson D system: studies in a lung model. Can Anaesth Soc J 25:353, 1978
28. Walton B: Halothane hepatitis in children. Anaesthesia 41:575, 1986
29. Gefke K, Andersen LW, Friesel E: Lidocaine given intravenously as a suppressant of cough and laryngospasm in connection with extubation after tonsillectomy. Acta Anaesth Scand 27:111, 1983
30. Epstein BS, Levy ML, Thein MH, et al: Evaluation of fentanyl as an adjunct to thiopental-nitrous oxide-oxygen anesthesia for short surgical procedures. Anesthesiol Rev 2:24, 1975
31. Youngberg JA, Subaiya C, Graybar GB, et al: Alfentanil for day surgery in children: an evaluation. Anesth Analg 63:284, 1984
32. Roberts FL, Dixon J, Lewis GTR, et al: Induction and maintenance of propofol anaesthesia; a manual infusion scheme. Anaesthesia 43:14, 1988, (suppl.)
33. Bush GH, Roth F: Muscle pains after suxamethonium chloride in children. Br J Anaesth 33:151, 1961
34. Cote CJ, Goldstein EA, Cote MA, Hoaglin DC: A single blind study of pulse oximetry in children. Anesthesiology 68:184, 1988
35. Bissonnette B, Sessler DL, LaFlamme P:

Temperature monitoring sites in infants and children. Anesth Analg 68:S29, 1989

36. Lerman J, Eustis S, Smith DR: Effect of droperidol pretreatment on post anesthetic vomiting in children undergoing strabismus surgery. Anesthesiology 65:322–325, 1986
37. Broadman LM, Cerruzi W, Patane PS, et al: Metoclopramide reduces the incidence of vomiting following strabismus surgery in children. Anesthesiology 69:A747, 1988
38. Steward DJ: A simplified scoring system for the post operative recovery room. Can Anaesth Soc J 22:111, 1975
39. Anderson R, Krohg K: Pain as a major cause of postoperative nausea. Can Anaesth Soc J 23:366, 1976
40. Vernon DTA, Schulman JL, Foley JM: Changes in children's behaviour after hospitalization. Am J Dis Child 111:581, 1966
41. Shandling B, Steward DJ: Regional analgesia for postoperative pain in pediatric outpatient surgery. J Pediatr Surg 15:477, 1980
42. Wolf AR, Valley RD, Fear DW, et al: Bupivacaine for caudal analgesia in infants and children: the optimal effective concentration. Anesthesiology 69:102, 1988
43. Bakon AK: An alternative block for postcircumcision pain. Anaesth Intensive Care 5:63, 1977
44. Tree-Trakarn T, Pirayavaraporn S: Postoperative pain relief for circumcision in children: comparison among morphine, nerve block, and topical analgesia. Anesthesiology 62:519, 1985
45. Dinley J, Dickson RA: The control of pain after Keller's operation by the instillation of local anaesthetic before closure. J Bone Joint Surg 58B:356, 1976
46. Chavph M, Hameroff SR, O'Dea K, Peacock EE: Local anesthetics and wound healing. J Surg Res 27:367, 1979
47. Roy WI, Lerman J: Laryngospasm in paediatric anaesthesia. Can J Anaesth 35:93, 1988
48. Baraka A: Intravenous lidocaine controls extubation laryngospasm in children. Anesth Analg 57:506, 1978
49. Koka BV, Jeon IS, Andre JM, et al: Post intubation croup in children. Anesth Analg 56:501, 1977
50. Jordan WS, Graves CL, Elwyn RA: New therapy for post intubation laryngeal edema and tracheitis in children. JAMA 212:585, 1970
51. Rowley MP, Brown TCK: Postoperative vomiting in children. Anaesth Intensive Care 10:309, 1982

Appendix 8-1*

Getting Ready for Day Care

FASTING INSTRUCTIONS FOR CHILDREN

Infants Up to 6 Months of Age

Breast-fed infants must be finished feeding 4 hours before the scheduled time of the procedure and have nothing more after that, not even water.

Bottle-fed infants on solid foods can have solid food up to 8 hours before the scheduled time of the procedure, formula or milk up to 6 hours before the scheduled time of the procedure; or clear fluids up to 3 hours before the scheduled time of the procedure.

Do not give anything at all to eat or drink (not even a sip of water) after that.

Children 7 to 24 Months of Age

The child should be given a nutritious snack at bedtime the night before, then *no* solid food on the day of the procedure.

The child can have formula, milk, or breast milk up to 6 hours before the scheduled time of the procedure; or a small drink (1 cup) of clear fluid 3 hours before the scheduled time of the procedure.

Do not give anything at all to eat or drink (not even a sip of water) after that.

Children 25 Months of Age and Older

The child should be given a nutritious snack at bedtime the night before, then *no* solid food on the day of the procedure.

The child may have a small drink (1 cup) of clear fluid 3 hours before the scheduled time of the procedure.

Do not allow anything after that (not even a sip of water, candy, or gum).

ITEMS TO TELL PARENTS TO BRING TO THE HOSPITAL

Parents should be instructed to bring the following items to the hospital on the day of their child's surgery:

1. a sample of the child's urine in a clean container;
2. the history form given to the parents by the doctor's, or dentist's office (to be filled in before coming to the hospital);
3. medical card;

---

* Adapted from British Columbia's Children's Hospital: Getting your child ready for day care. Vancouver, British Columbia, Canada, with permission.

4. a favorite toy or blanket marked with the child's name;
5. an empty bottle (if the infant uses a special nipple);
6. a housecoat and slippers (if the child has these);
7. loose-fitting clothing or pajamas for discharge (if the type of surgery makes this necessary); and
8. personal care items—tooth brush, toothpaste, comb, etc. (if the child is staying overnight).

AFTER THE PROCEDURE

Instruct parents that all children who have had a general anesthetic or sedation will go the main recovery room before returning to the day care unit or to their overnight room. The length of stay in the recovery room depends on the type of procedure, anesthetic, or sedation given. If the child becomes upset in the recovery room, a nurse will call the parents to come in to be with the child.

Because of unexpected delays and individual differences in recovery time, it is difficult to give the parents precise discharge time in advance. The staff will give the parents an approximate time only. The day care nurse will tell when their child is ready to go home and will review written discharge instructions with them. It is strongly advised that one adult drives while the other cares for the child. If only one parent is available, taking a taxicab should be considered.

An anesthetic or sedation can disturb balance and judgment for up to 24 hours. During that time, instruct parents not to allow the child to ride a bicycle or to engage in other physical activities of this sort.

IN THE DAY CARE UNIT

Space is limited in the day care unit, which cannot accommodate more than two adults with each patient. Request that parents not bring other children.

Parents should bring their child to the day care unit 1 to 1.5 hours before the scheduled procedure. This allows time for admission routines and for the child to be examined by an anesthesiologist.

A blood sample will be taken by finger prick. This and the urine sample will be tested in the laboratory.

Weight, height, temperature, pulse, and blood pressure measurements will be taken.

The child will change into a hospital gown, but may wear his or her own housecoat and slippers.

Children may play in the play area until they go for their procedure. Parents are requested to be with them during this time. Children are not usually sedated because they are generally happier playing and then walking to the operating room. A child will be put into a bed only if sedation or a particular treatment is needed.

Ask that parents tell their child honestly that they cannot go into the operating area but that they will be waiting in the day care unit. It is strongly recommended that parents be present either in the day care unit or in the overnight room when their child returns from the recovery room.

Appendix 8-2*

Helping the Child After a General Anesthetic

POSTOPERATIVE CARE INSTRUCTIONS TO PROVIDE TO PARENTS

What to Expect

Caution parents that the child may be quite sleepy or dizzy on the day of the anesthetic and that this is to be expected. Some children may appear quite alert and active. The effects of the anesthetic may vary according to the length of the anesthetic and the type of surgical procedure performed. The child may complain of a sore throat or nose and stiff muscles following the anesthetic, and there may be some hoarseness and a croupy cough.

Activity

The child should be expected to be less steady than usual. This lack of coordination can last for about 24 hours; therefore, the child's activities should be supervised closely to prevent falls or injuries during that time. Instruct parents that the child should not ride a bicycle or engage in other potentially dangerous activities for 24 hours.

Give parents specific instructions regarding how soon the child may resume normal activities. There may be limitations related to the surgery.

Fever

A slight fever is not uncommon after an anesthetic, but if it persists or exceeds 38.5°C (101°F) advise parents to contact their surgeon or pediatrician. Fever may be caused by lack of fluids. The parents should be sure the child is drinking plenty of fluids; they are more important than solid food on the day of surgery.

Diet

At the hospital, the parents will begin to give their child clear fluids such as water, diluted apple juice, or popsicles. Inform them that when the child is keeping down clear fluids, the diet may be gradually increased to include small amounts of easily digested foods, such as soups or cereals. Infants may resume breast feeding or for-

* Adapted from British Columbia's Children's Hospital: Helping your child . . . after a general anesthetic. Vancouver, British Columbia, Canada, with permission.

mula once they have kept down water or juice.

Small frequent meals are better than one large meal to make up for the missed breakfast. Hard to digest foods like pizza, hot dogs, and french fries should be avoided. (If the parents promised their child a hamburger as a treat, the promise should be kept another day.)

Warn parents that the child may become nauseous after the anesthetic. If the child vomits on the way home or at home the parents should not be alarmed. The child should be given nothing to drink for 1 hour, then should again receive fluids with small amounts of ice chips or water, a teaspoonful at a time if necessary. If vomiting persists for more than 24 hours or is very severe, the doctor should be contacted.

Usually, children may resume a regular diet by the next day unless the surgeon orders otherwise.

Breathing

No problems should be anticipated. If the child develops wheezing, has difficulty breathing, or has croup, the doctor or emergency department should be contacted. If required, the anesthesiologist should also be contacted. Parents should bring the child to the emergency room if concerned about their child's condition.

If the parents have questions or problems specifically related to the child's surgery, they should contact the surgeon.

9

Preoperative Assessment of Adult Outpatients

Michael F. Roizen
Gita Rupani

The rationale behind the development of outpatient surgical units was patient convenience, with the added benefit of reducing costs for both patient and hospital. Initially, only "healthy" patients were scheduled for outpatient surgery. Now our era of cost containment mandates outpatient surgery for a more diverse group. No longer are patients who fit the American Society of Anesthesiologists' physical status class I or II descriptions the only ones anesthetized in the outpatient setting. Consequently, some anesthesiologists are questioning if the brief 2-minute interview just prior to induction, along with the results of the hematocrit and urinalysis, are adequate measures for preoperative evaluation. As the patient population has changed, questions about which laboratory tests to obtain preoperatively have surfaced. In this chapter, we will evaluate the relative roles of the history, physical examination, and laboratory testing in outpatient surgery. After an examination of the current system of preoperative evaluation, several alternatives are offered.

PREOPERATIVE EVALUATION: THE GOALS

Preoperative evaluation has three goals: (1) to perform medical assessments to optimize perioperative outcome, (2) to obtain informed consent, and (3) to reduce patient anxiety while improving perioperative management by acquainting the patient with facilities, protocol, and personnel involved in the surgical procedure. We will not discuss the latter two goals in any detail except to say that a solid body of data supports the concept of faster recovery when a facility visit and discussion of procedures are provided (refer to Ch. 10 and Egbert et al.,[1,2] Wolfer and Davis,[3] and Anderson[4]).

Preoperative medical assessments provide an important opportunity for physicians to reduce perioperative morbidity by optimizing preoperative status and planning perioperative management. Because perioperative mortality and morbidity increase with the severity of pre-existing disease,[5–12] careful evaluation and treatment should reduce their occurrence.[7,13,14] Consequently, medical care and patient outcome improve given a reliable and effective method for assessing patients preoperatively and a selection of laboratory tests based on that assessment.

RELATIVE VALUE OF HISTORY, PHYSICAL EXAMINATION, AND LABORATORY TESTING

Studies show that the history and physical examination are the best means of screening for disease. (The elements of an appropriate history and physical examination are reviewed below.) Unindicated laboratory testing, on the other hand, provides little additional information to that obtained through the other two methods of assessment. Delahunt and Turnbull[15] retrospectively evaluated patients who were assessed preoperatively for varicose vein stripping or inguinal herniorrhaphy. For 803 patients undergoing 1,972 tests, only 63 abnormalities were uncovered in those patients whose history or physical findings had not indicated the need for tests; in no instance did the discovery of these abnormalities influence patient management. Rossello et al.[16] retrospectively evaluated 690 admissions for elective pediatric surgical procedures. History and physical examination indicated the probability of abnormalities in all 12 patients in whom an abnormality was found through laboratory testing. Clinical diagnosis, not laboratory testing, was the apparent basis for any change in operative plans.

Several studies have compared outcome in hospitalized patients who were given routine laboratory screening tests to supplement the history and physical examination, and those who were not. Wood and Hoekelman[17] found that 28 of 1,924 children examined had changes in preoperative clinical courses (all had surgery postponed) because of abnormal history, physical examination, or laboratory examination results. Three of those 28 patients whose surgery was postponed had abnormal laboratory tests that were not indicated by the history or physical examination. Thus, the history or physical examination dictated appropriate laboratory tests for all but 3 of 1,924 patients. The abnormalities discovered for these three patients pertained to their chest radiographs. (These children were part of a study comparing perioperative outcome at two hospitals, one that required chest radiographs as a screening test for elective surgery in children and one that did not.) There were no differences noted in anesthetic or perioperative complications between the two groups. Therefore, Wood and Hoekelman recommended that chest radiographs not be obtained routinely for apparently healthy children.

Another study also found the value of screening tests to be dubious. Durbridge et al.[18] compared 1,500 patients randomly assigned to groups that either were or were not given screening tests on admission. No benefit resulted from the 8,363 tests that were performed with respect to length of hospital stay or patient outcome.

Even in a referral population, history and physical examination determine more than 90 percent of the clinical course when a patient is referred for consultation concerning cardiovascular, neurologic, or respiratory diseases.[19]

Other studies have also demonstrated that the history and physical examination accurately indicate all areas in which subsequent laboratory testing proves beneficial to patients. For example, Rabkin and Horne[20,21] examined the records of 165 patients having "new" (i.e., a change from a previous tracing) abnormalities on ECG that were potentially "surgically significant" (i.e., that might affect perioperative management or outcome). In only two instances were the anesthetic or surgical plans altered by the discovery of new abnormalities on ECG. Thus, for these 165 patients, for whom the benefits of a laboratory test should have been maximal (i.e., when a new abnormality is detected in the course of preoperative assessments), the history or physical examination determined case management. Even in one of the two instances of altered case management—a patient having atrial fibrillation—physical examination should have indicated that an ECG needed to be performed. A history or physical examination was not available for the other patient. Although a great deal is heard about silent myocardial ischemia,[22] the history and physical examination predicted every patient whose ECG showed abnormalities.

Initially, laboratory screening seems a

logical step in patient care: if abnormalities could be identified before overt disease occurred, disability would be prevented; however, the value of laboratory testing has recently been called into question. The annual cost of preoperative testing and evaluation in the United States is over $40 billion, 60 percent of which could potentially be saved by eliminating extraneous testing. Worse than wasteful, this extra testing is causing iatrogenic disease by pursuit and treatment of borderline and false positive test results. In addition, laboratory testing is increasing medicolegal risk and decreasing the efficiency of practice.

Why are laboratory screening tests less beneficial than other methods of assessing patients? They have at least four disadvantages. First, routine laboratory tests are not the best means of evaluating patients preoperatively. In fact, the literature reports that they are often unnecessary and secondary to history and physical examination in screening for disease. Although laboratory screening tests can aid in optimizing a patient's preoperative condition once a disease is suspected or diagnosed, they have several shortcomings: they frequently fail to uncover pathologic conditions; they detect abnormalities, the discovery of which does not necessarily improve patient care or outcome; and they are inefficient in screening for asymptomatic diseases. Finally, most abnormalities discovered on preoperative screening, or even on admission screening for nonsurgical purposes, are not recorded (other than in the laboratory report) or appropriately pursued.

An increasing body of literature indicates that screening tests may not be the most effective way of evaluating patients preoperatively. Korvin et al.[23] reviewed biochemical tests given routinely to 1,000 patients on hospital admission. None of the tests produced a new diagnosis that was unequivocally beneficial to the patient. In an ambitious, controlled trial of multiphasic screening in 1,500 patients, Olsen and coworkers[24] found no difference in morbidity between control groups and groups having screening tests.

Screening testing in the elderly is no better at identifying clinically silent disease, and may be worse for the patients evaluated. Domoto et al.[25] examined the yield and effectiveness of a battery of 19 screening laboratory tests performed routinely in 70 intellectually and functionally intact elderly patients (average age, 82.6 years) who resided at a chronic care facility. The 70 patients underwent 3,903 screening tests. "New abnormal" results occurred primarily in 5 of the 19 screening tests; most of these "new abnormalities" were only minimally outside the normal range. Only four (0.1 percent of all tests ordered) led to change in patient management, none of which, Domoto et al. concluded, benefited any patient in an important way.

Wolf-Klein and colleagues[26] retrospectively studied the results of annual laboratory screening on a population of 500 institutionalized and ambulatory elderly patients (average age, 80 years). From the 15,000 tests performed, 756 new abnormalities were discovered, 690 of which were ignored. Sixty-six of the new abnormalities were evaluated; 20 new diagnoses resulted, 12 of which were treated. Two patients of the 500 ultimately may have benefited from eradication of asymptomatic bacteriuria (although eradication of asymptomatic bacteriuria has not been shown to improve the quality of, or extend, life[27–30]). Wolf-Klein et al. made no attempt to determine how many patients, if any, were harmed by pursuit or treatment of abnormalities on screening tests.

Levinstein et al.[31] examined the usefulness of 8 years of screening laboratory tests in 121 institutionalized elderly patients (average age, 89 years).They found that all potentially beneficial discoveries from laboratory testing came from measurement of the complete blood cell count electrolytes, blood urea nitrogen (BUN), glucose, thyroxine levels in blood, and urinalysis. By just obtaining these tests, 74 percent of the cost of tests could be saved. (We estimate this 74 percent figure to be high by 7 to 13 percent, as not all of the charges for tests result in cost savings, but data indicate that 87 to 93 percent of the charge reduction results in cost savings.[32])

In summary, the studies cited above point to the inadequacy of routine laboratory tests as an independent means to assess patients preoperatively. It has been shown that many of these laboratory tests are considered superfluous to patient care management. Because history and physical examination are considered the most effective ways to screen for disease, a battery of laboratory tests should be ordered based on indications from both.

Second, testing nonselectively may pose extra risk to the patient. Unnecessary testing may lead physicians to pursue and treat borderline and false positive laboratory abnormalities. This statement does not imply that all screening tests should be discontinued—some are beneficial, such as the mammogram and Papanicolaou smear for every woman over the age of 40, and the stool-for-occult-blood test in all adults over the age of 40. But the majority of screening tests is not justified. And these indiscriminately ordered tests lead to false positive results.

Few studies have examined whether increased tests and the follow-up of false positive tests adversely affect patients. Roizen[33] retrospectively examined adverse effects on patients who had chest x-rays taken. In this study population of 606 patients, 386 extra chest x-rays were ordered without being indicated. In those 386 patients, one elevated hemidiaphragm and probable phrenic nerve palsy were found that may have resulted in improved care for that patient. In addition, three lung shadows were found which resulted in three sets of invasive tests, including one thoracotomy, without discovery of any disease. These procedures caused considerable morbidity, including one pneumothorax and 4 months of disability, for those patients.

In another study, Turnbull and Buck[34] examined the charts of 2,570 patients undergoing cholecystectomy to determine the value of preoperative tests. History and physical examinations successfully indicated all tests that ultimately benefited the patients, with four possible exceptions. Again, in those four patients it is doubtful if any benefit actually occurred. Among them was one patient who had emphysema detected only by chest x-ray; he had preoperative physiotherapy without subsequent postoperative complication. Two patients had unsuspected hypokalemia (3.2 and 3.4 mEq/L, respectively) and received treatment prior to operation. Data now in the literature[35–39] indicate no harm occurs to patients undergoing operation with this degree of hypokalemia, and severe potential harm may be caused by treating such patients with oral and/or intravenous potassium (Table 9-1). The fourth patient in whom possible benefit occurred received a blood transfusion prior to cholycystectomy for an asymptomatic hemoglobin concentration of 9.9 g/dl. Since cholycystectomy is not normally associated with major blood loss, it is concluded that this patient also received no benefit—and

Table 9-1. Risk of Potassium Supplementation

	Oral (%)	IV alone (%)	Oral and IV (%)	All routes (%)
No. of patients	1,910	2,192	819	921
Death	3 (0.2)	3 (0.15)	1 (0.1)	7 (0.14)
Life-threatening and death*	6 (0.3)	7 (0.35)	14 (1.7)	28 (0.57)
Hyperkalemia	74 (3.9)	34 (1.6)	71 (8.7)	179 (3.6)
Other side effects	53 (2.8)	18 (0.8)	33 (4.0)	283 (5.7)

* One patient in 200 dies or has a life-threatening reaction to potassium supplementation.
(Modified from data in Lawson.[38])

only the risk of transfusion—from the preoperative laboratory test and its pursuit. Thus, it is not clear that any patient in this study benefited from preoperative screening tests done without indication.

In a study of the effects of 9,270 screening tests, Levinstein et al.[31] found that at most only two patients (who had eradication of asymptomatic bacteriuria) benefited. At least one patient was seriously harmed from pursuit and treatment of abnormalities on screening tests; this woman developed atrial fibrillation and congestive heart failure after institution of thyroid therapy for borderline low thyroxine and free thyroxine index (FTI) tests. It is unclear if these investigators examined other patients for potential harm arising from pursuit and treatment of abnormalities on screening tests.

Third, when random laboratory tests yield abnormal results that are neither pursued nor noted, the medicolegal risk for physicians increases. Extra testing—that is, testing which is not warranted by indications on a medical history—does not serve as medicolegal protection against liability. A series of studies[33,40] shows that 30 to 95 percent of all unexpected abnormalities found on preoperative laboratory tests are not noted on the chart preoperatively. Many reports for preoperative radiographs, for example, are not in the chart before anesthesia is administered. This lack of notation occurs not only at university medical centers but also at community hospitals. Data show that failing to pursue an abnormality appropriately poses a greater risk to medicolegal liability than does failing to detect that abnormality.[41] In this way, extra testing results in extra medicolegal risk to physicians.

Finally, random preoperative testing is inefficient for operating room schedules. According to hospital administrators in the United States, surgeons say that they order preoperative tests to satisfy the anesthesiologist: they find it easier to order all the tests and let the anesthesiologist sort them out. Surgeons also believe that it is more efficient to order batteries of tests than to have the anesthesiologist, who sees the patient a few hours before surgery, try to get the tests on an emergency basis. These surgeons apparently do not realize that abnormalities arising from tests done in this battery fashion are not discovered until the night before or the morning of surgery, if at all. Abnormal results on these tests then delay or postpone schedules as extra effort and time are wasted in consultant reviews of false positive or slightly abnormal results.

PREDICTIVE VALUE OF AN "ABNORMAL" RESULT ON A LABORATORY TEST

Understanding what constitutes an "abnormal" laboratory test result requires an appreciation of the way "normal" values are determined. A normal range is based on the typical distribution of the Gaussian curve.[42,43] For example, assuming a Gaussian distribution and hemoglobin values of 13.5 to 16.7 g/dl for healthy men, one can expect 5 percent of "normal" healthy men to have a test result outside that range.

Of prime importance in preoperative evaluation is knowing the percentage of abnormal laboratory test values that truly indicates disease. If the anesthetic management of a patient is altered because of test abnormality, that abnormality should indicate a condition that (1) poses a significant risk of perioperative morbidity that can be lessened by preoperative treatment, (2) is undiscoverable through history-taking and physical examination, and (3) is sufficiently prevalent in the population to justify the risk of performing a follow-up test. To make it cost-efficient, the test should be sufficiently sensitive ("positivity in disease") and specific ("negativity in health").[44]

It is important to assess the significance of false positive and false negative results and the prevalence of disease in the test population in relation to abnormal laboratory test results. For example, let us assume that the sensitivity ("positivity in disease") of a test is 75 percent; that is, 75 of 100 people who actually have pneumonia, for instance, will have "pneumonia" written as the diagnosis on their chest roentgenogram reports. Let us also assume that the specificity ("negativity in health") of a test is 98.3 percent; that is, 983 of 1,000 people who actually do not have pneumonia will have "without evidence of pneumonia," "normal," or a similar comment on their chest roentgenogram reports. Third, let us assume that 0.5 percent of the asymptomatic population about to undergo routine elective surgery has pneumonia. Given the above assumptions, what is the likelihood that a person whose chest roentgenogram report reads "pneumonia" will actually have pneumonia?

If we tested 100,000 individuals and 500 (0.5 percent) were diseased, 375 would have abnormal roentgenograms. Of the 99,500 healthy individuals, 1,691 (1.7 percent) would have abnormal roentgenograms. Thus, of 2,066 patients with a diagnosis of pneumonia based on their chest roentgenograms, 1,691 (82 percent) would be false positives. Therefore, it is entirely possible that 82 percent of the chest roentgenograms in otherwise asymptomatic individuals that indicate "infiltrate compatible with pneumonia" will actually predict a totally healthy person.

Only patients who have abnormal test results and who actually have disease benefit from laboratory testing (true positives). Let us assume that 1.5 percent of the chest radiographs in the less than 40 years of age population are positive, and that for each true positive, perioperative mortality is decreased by 50 percent. If we use the 82 percent predictive false positive rate (see above), the number of patients benefiting per 1,000 roentgenograms is 2.7 (true positives = 1.5 percent − [1.5 percent × 0.82] × 1,000 = 2.7 patients). Therefore, a reduction in operative mortality of 50 percent, or 1 per 10,000 (i.e., 2.7 × 0.5 × 0.0002) gives 0.00027 fewer deaths per 1,000 operations when preoperative chest roentgenograms are obtained. Translating this figure into the present value of years of life saved per 1,000 roentgenograms yields the following: 0.00027 fewer deaths per 1,000 operations × 22.62 years saved per life saved = 0.0061 years of life. (The 22.62 is the present value of 60 more years of life for a 20-year-old; refer to Roizen[33] and Newhauser.[44]) At the University of Chicago, this 0.0061 years of life saved would cost $70,000 (an anterior-posterior and lateral chest roentgenogram costs $70, not including fees for consultations, repeated roentgenograms, and other laboratory tests or procedures). Therefore, each year of life saved by obtaining chest roentgenograms costs about $11,400,000 (i.e., $70,000 ÷ 0.0061). We are forced to conclude that screening for an asymptomatic disease with a low prevalence rate is a very expensive, and possibly risky, procedure.

LABORATORY TEST ABNORMALITIES IN HEALTHY POPULATIONS

Chest Roentgenograms

What abnormalities on chest roentgenograms would influence anesthetic approach? Certainly it may be important to know about the existence of tracheal deviation; mediastinal masses; pulmonary nodules; a solitary lung mass; aortic aneurysm; pulmonary edema; pneumonia; atelectasis; new fractures of vertebrae, ribs, or clavicles; dextrocardia; and cardiomegaly before proceeding to anesthesia and surgery. However, a chest radiograph probably would do no better at detecting the degree of chronic lung disease requiring alteration of anesthetic technique than

Table 9-2. Screening Chest Roentgenograms: Incidence of Abnormal Test Results, the Discovery of Which Might Change Anesthetic Management

Age (yr)	Series	No. of patients examined	Abnormalities[a] (%)	New abnormalities[b] (%)
0–14	Farnsworth et al.[45]	350	8.9	0.3
0–18	Brill et al.[46]	1,000	1.9	0.7
0–19	Sagel et al.[47]	521	0	0
0–19	Sane et al.[48]	1,500	5.4	2.2
0–19	Wood & Hoekelman[17]	749	4.7	1.2
1–20	Rees et al.[49]	46	0	0
20–29	Sagel et al.[47]	894	1	
21–30	Rees et al.[49]	62	3	
≤30	Loder[50]	437	10.1	0.2
≥30	Maigaard et al.[51]	1,256	≤4.5	0
30–39	Sagel et al.[47]	942	2.3	
30–69	Loder[50]	515	≤6.0	
31–40	Rees et al.[49]	93	13	
≤40	Catchlove et al.[52]	29	0	0
≤40	Collen et al.[53]	15,978	2.1	
≤40	Sagel et al.[47]	2,357	1.3	1.3
≤40	Combined[c45–48,50–52]	6,422	4.0	0.8
40–49	Sagel et al.[47]	928	7.1	
40–59	Collen et al.[53]	21,489	7.4	
41–50	Rees et al.[49]	119	19	
≥40	Sagel et al.[47]	3,689	23.9	6.0
>40	Catchlove et al.[52]	50	0	0
≥40	Thomsen et al.[54]	1,823	2.3	0.2
50–59	Sagel et al.[47]	833	20.3	
51–60	Rees et al.[49]	121	40.0	
60–69	Sagel et al.[47]	977	29.7	
>60	Collen et al.[53]	7,196	19.2	
61–70	Rees et al.[49]	134	43.3	
≥69	Loder[50]	48	≤72.9	
≥70	Sagel et al.[47]	832	41.7	
≥70	Törnebrandt and Fletcher[55]	100	37	8.1?
71–80	Rees et al.[49]	76	61.8	
≥81	Rees et al.[49]	16	68.8	
0–90	Delahunt and Turnbull[15]	860		0
0–?90	Petterson and Janower[56]	1,530	9.8	1.3
0–?90	Royal College[57]	3,052	3.8	

[a] These data constitute a summary of the data presented in various articles, edited to select abnormalities that might change anesthetic management.

[b] Abnormalities not already known by history or physical examination.

[c] Combined studies in the under 40 years of age population excluding two studies, Rees et al.[49] and Collen et al.[53]

would the history and physical examination. The prevalence of conditions that a chest roentgenogram might detect are listed in Table 9-2. From the data in Table 9-2, it can be concluded that abnormalities are rare in the asymptomatic individual. In fact, risks to the patient when a chest radiograph is performed probably exceed benefits to asymptomatic patients less than 60 years of age. This analysis is, of course, predicated on maximizing benefit to society, as one cannot predict in advance which patients will benefit or which will be harmed.

Electrocardiograms

Data on the incidence of ECG abnormalities were gathered from studies of either working patient populations[53,58] or epidemiologic surveys of healthy people.[46,59,60] Electrocardiographic abnormalities that may alter anesthetic management are as follows: atrial flutter or fibrillation; first-, second-, or third-degree atrioventricular block; ST-T changes suggesting myocardial ischemia or recent pulmonary embolism; premature ventricular and atrial contractions; left or right ventricular hypertrophy; short PR interval; Wolff-Parkinson-White syndrome; myocardial infarction; prolonged QT segment; and tall

Table 9-3. Percentage of Patients Having Abnormalities Determined by Screening Electrocardiograms[a]

Age (yr)/ Sex	Series	No. of patients examined	Total abnormalities[b] (%)	Specific Abnormalities (%)			
				LVH	MI	ST-T changes	AV block
16–19/M	Ostrander et al.[60]	216	20.3	17.8	0	0.9	1.4
16–19/F	Ostrander et al.[60]	242	5.9	1.3	0	4.2	0.4
20–29/M	Ostrander et al.[60]	452	14.0	7.1	0.2	6.0	0.7
20–29/F	Ostrander et al.[60]	577	11.3	0.2	0.2	9.9	1.0
20–29/M	Collen et al.[53]	3,000	9.6				
20–29/F	Collen et al.[53]	4,000[c]	9.3				
>30/Either	Maigaard et al.[51]	1,256	<4.5		0.1		
30–39/M	Ostrander et al.[60]	676		3.0	0	6.9	1.3
30–39/F	Ostrander et al.[60]	699		0.4	0.1	11.6	1.6
30–39/M	Collen et al.[53]	4,000[c]	12.1				
30–39/F	Collen et al.[53]	5,000[c]	11.7				
35–44/M	Kannel et al.[59,61]			2.9			
35–44/F	Kannel et al.[59,61]			0.9			
40–49/M	Ostrander et al.[60]	468	24[c]	4.1	1.7	16.1	1.5
40–49/F	Ostrander et al.[60]	474	21[c]	0.6	0.8	17.2	0.6
40–49/M	Collen et al.[53]	4,000[c]	17.6				
40–49/F	Collen et al.[53]	5,000[c]	15.6				
45–54/M	Kannel et al.[59,61]			4.8			
45–54/F	Kannel et al.[59,61]			3.6			
50–59/M	Ostrander et al.[60]	330	30[c]	3.3	5.1	20.8	1.2
50–59/F	Ostrander et al.[60]	327	40[c]	3.4	0.9	32.4	2.1
50–59/M	Collen et al.[53]	5,000[c]	24.9				
50–59/F	Collen et al.[53]	6,000[c]	20.7				
55–64/M	Kannel et al.[59,61]			10.1			
55–64/F	Kannel et al.[59,61]			4.1			
<60/Either	Rabkin and Horne[20,21]	309	13.5	2.5	1.6	11.0	1.0
>60/Either	Rabkin and Horne[20,21]	503	24.4	2.2	1.9	13.0	0.6
60–69/M	Ostrander et al.[60]	177		8.4	9.0	37.1	4.5
60–69/F	Ostrander et al.[60]	196		10.2	6.1	42.4	4.1
60–69/M	Collen et al.[53]	2,000[c]	35.1				
60–69/F	Collen et al.[53]	3,000[c]	29.7				
64–74/M	Kannel et al.[59,61]			7.1			
65–74/F	Kannel et al.[59,61]			9.6			
>70/M	Collen et al.[53]	1,000[c]	52.2				
>70/F	Collen et al.[53]	1,000[c]	41.2				
70–79/M	Ostrander et al.[60]	100		7.9	9.9	46.5	7.9
70–79/F	Ostrander et al.[60]	119		11.8	2.5	43.8	6.7
>80/M	Ostrander et al.[60]	26		11.5	7.7	46.2	19.2
>80/F	Ostrander et al.[60]	43		16.3	4.7	58.2	9.3

Abbreviations: LVH, left ventricular hypertrophy; MI, myocardial infarctions; ST-T changes, ST-T segment changes on ECG; AV, atrioventricular.

[a] All studies are 12-lead, except for that of Collen et al.[53] which is a 6-lead study.

[b] These data constitute a summary of data given in several series, edited to select abnormalities that might change anesthetic management.

[c] Values are approximations that represent "best guess" numbers from data not explicitly stated in the reports.

Table 9-4. Number and Percentages of Patients Having a New Abnormality with a Previous Electrocardiogram[a]

	New abnormality with a previously normal ECG		New abnormality with a previously abnormal ECG	
Age (yrs)	<60	≥60	<60	≥60
No. of patients/total number	18/180	42/192	24/129	81/310
% New abnormality	10%	21.9%	18.6%	26%
Abnormality (%)				
T wave	11 (6.1)	18 (9.4)	10 (7.8)	19 (6.1)
ST-T segment	7 (3.9)	9 (4.7)	6 (4.7)	20 (6.4)
Dysrhythmias				
SVT or PVCs	3 (1.7)	7 (3.6)		8 (2.6)
Others, including PACs	3 (1.7)	6 (3.1)	1 (0.8)	1 (0.3)
QRS duration		8 (4.2)	2 (1.6)	14 (4.5)
LVH	3 (1.7)	4 (2.1)	5 (3.9)	7 (2.3)
Q wave	4 (2.2)	3 (1.6)	1 (0.8)	7 (2.3)
Ventricular conduction defects	5 (2.6)	1 (0.8)	7 (2.3)	
AV block	2 (1.0)	3 (2.3)	1 (0.3)	

Abbreviations: SVT, supraventricular tachycardia; PVCs, premature ventricular contractions; PACs, premature atrial contractions; LVH, left ventricular hypertrophy; AV, atrioventricular.

[a] Numbers in parentheses are percentages of patients. Two-thirds of patients had a previous ECG within 2 years of their new ECG.

(Data from Rabkin and Horne.[20,21])

peaked T waves. A question might be raised about the incidence in which these abnormalities are identified on a 12-lead preoperative ECG and later overlooked on a standard monitor lead I or modified chest lead V_5 in the operating room immediately prior to induction of anesthesia. As interesting as this issue is, existing studies do not address it. None of the studies on the incidence of ECG abnormalities exclude patients with histories or physical examinations indicating cardiac problems, nor do they distinguish those findings that are evident on monitor leads from those evident only on 6- or 12-lead ECGs (Table 9-3).

How useful is it to repeat ECGs if the patient has had an ECG within the past 2 years? The studies of Rabkin and Horne[20,21] address this question. Data (Table 9-4) indicate that new abnormalities occur with perhaps 25 to 50 percent of the frequency of all abnormalities. Thus, one would be justified in obtaining screening ECGs prior to elective surgery on all patients over 40 years of age, even in those who recently had an ECG.

Hemoglobin, Hematocrit, and White Blood Cell Counts

Wasserman and Gilbert[62] found that of 28 patients having uncontrolled polycythemia (hemoglobin > 16 g/dl) who underwent major surgery, 22 (79 percent) had complications and ten (36 percent) died. That group was compared with a group of 53 patients who had controlled polycythemia (hemoglobin ≤ 16 g/dl) and major surgery; 15 (28 percent) had complications and three (5 percent) died. In both groups, most of the complications were related to polycythemia (e.g., hemorrhage or thrombosis). Although the study has deficiencies (e.g., it was a retrospective study, no time frame was given, " minor" surgery was excluded, and it contained no statement as to why polycythemia was controlled preoperatively in some patients and not in others), its results indicate that knowledge and pretreatment of polycythemia decreases perioperative morbidity and mortality.

No such evidence exists for normovolemic anemia. Rothstein[63] concluded that in patients under 3 months of age, hemoglobin should be over 10 g/dl, whereas in children over 3 months of age, hemoglobin of 9 g/dl is adequate. Slogoff[64] concluded that in adults a hematocrit of 20 percent (hemoglobin of approximately 7 g/dl) is adequate. However, no data confirm the hypothesis that treatment of moderate or mild normovolemic anemia prior to surgery involving no major blood loss in asymptomatic patients decreases perioperative morbidity or mortality. Similarly, no data exist regarding the possible harm from abnormal white blood cell (WBC) counts found preoperatively. Therefore, the following ranges of "surgically acceptable values" have been arbitrarily devised: for hematocrit, 29 to 57 percent for men or 27 to 54 percent for women; and for WBC count, 2,400 to 16,000/m^3 for both men and women. When values fall outside these ranges, we recommend that an alternative diagnosis is sought before anesthesia or surgery is begun.[65] How many healthy patients have this degree of abnormality? None was found in the 223 patients for whom tests were not indicated by history.[66] The other limited available data are provided in Table 9-5. If we assume that 10 percent of all abnormalities are outside the "surgically acceptable" range,[69] and if the benefit-risk analysis described in the chest roentgenogram section is used, either preoperative hematocrit or hemoglobin levels should be determined for all women and for men over 60 years of age. White blood cell counts appear to be rarely, if ever, indicated.

Blood Chemistries, Urinalysis, Clotting Studies

What blood chemistries would have to be abnormal, and how abnormal would they have to be to indicate altering perioperative management? Abnormal liver or renal function might change the choice and dose of anesthetic or adjuvant drugs. Approximately 1 in 700 supposedly healthy patients is actually harboring hepatitis, and 1 in 3 of those will become jaundiced.[72,73] However, we have found no healthy asymptomatic patient who denies exposure to hepatitis who has become jaundiced after an uneventful operation (Roizen, unpublished data from 600 patients in a prospective study of the "HealthQuiz"). These data imply that either the screening history suffices or the incidence of asymptomatic hepatitis is decreasing.

Table 9-5. Abnormalities Discovered by Screening Hemoglobin Tests and White Blood Cell Counts

Age (yr)/Sex	Series	No. of patients examined	Hemoglobin abnormalities (%)	WBC count abnormalities (%)
<19/Either	Wood & Hoekelman[17]	1,924	0.8	
<40/M	Collen et al.[53]	6,941	1.9	2.6
<40/F	Collen et al.[53]	9,037	12.6	2.6
≥18/Either	Parkerson[67]	392	18.8	10.7
40–59/M	Collen et al.[53]	11,832	3.1	2.2
40–59/F	Collen et al.[53]	9,657	10.1	2.2
≥60/M	Collen et al.[53]	4,062	5.6	1.7
≥60/F	Collen et al.[53]	3,134	5.5	1.7
Unspecified/Either	Kaplan et al.[66]	293	0[a]	0[a]
Unspecified/Either	Gold and Wolfersberger[68]	3,375	0.33	
Unspecified/Either	Carmalt et al.[69]	278	30.4[b]	
Unspecified/Either	Huntley et al.[70]	119	23	
Unspecified/Either	Williamson[71]	982	3.2	

[a] Surgically significant abnormalities.

[b] Carmalt et al. found that 24.5 percent were new abnormalities; two patients had hemoglobin values <8 g/dl, 17 had values of 8 to 10 g/dl, and 21 had values of 10 to 12 g/dl.[69]

Available data on screening blood chemistries are presented by Roizen.[33] Unexpected abnormalities are reported in 2 to 10 percent of patients screened, and these abnormalities lead to many additional studies which, in approximately 80 percent of cases, have no significance for the patient. Unexpected abnormalities that are significant arise in 2 to 5 percent of patients studied, and of these abnormalities, approximately 70 percent are related to blood glucose and BUN levels. The 9 to 20 additional tests on the screening simultaneous multichannel analyses (SMAs) 12 to 20 panels lead to very few important discoveries affecting anesthesia. In fact, the false positive rate is so high (i.e., 96.5 percent for calcium) that the cost-benefit value of most of these tests (even when free) is negative, as is the benefit-risk analysis.

If a screening test for hepatitis is desired (because its incidence is 0.14 percent and because the potential legal problems of postanesthetic jaundice are to be avoided), three tests, namely, serum glutamic oxaloacetic transaminase (SGOT), blood glucose, and BUN, are indicated; and then the latter two, only for patients over the age of 60 years. In fact, if our data on asymptomatic liver disease can be generalized, no blood chemistry tests are indicated in patients younger than 60 years.

Abnormalities are commonly found on urinalysis. However, these abnormal results usually do not lead to beneficial changes in management, and of the results that do, most could have been obtained with history or BUN and glucose determinations, which are already recommended for all patients over 60 years of age. Thus, urinalysis, although initially inexpensive, becomes an expensive test to justify on a cost-benefit basis.

Although measurement of the partial thromboplastin time (PTT) and the prothrombin time (PT) are useful tests to screen patients with a history of bleeding, their value as screening tests in asymptomatic patients has never been shown.[33] Thus, the tests listed in Table 9-6 are the most one could recommend for asymptomatic individuals; however, within this patient group, history is a more reliable means of screening for indications for testing.

Any possible benefit of routinely ordering an unselected battery of screening tests is negated by the factors we have discussed. Laboratory screening tests appear to be both an extra cost to society and an extra risk to patients. Several studies in addition to ours show that testing based on indications of disease found in a patient's history is capable of detecting all of the significant abnormalities revealed by routine screening tests. (Significant abnormalities are those whose discovery ultimately benefits the patient.) This practice also avoids some of the risk of nonselective testing. Recently, many professional societies (including the American College of Surgeons, the American

Table 9-6. Screening Studies That Should Be Performed on Asymptomatic Healthy Patients Scheduled to Undergo Non-Blood Loss "Peripheral" Surgical Procedures

	Tests indicated	
Age (yr)	For men	For women
Under 40	None	Hemoglobin or hematocrit
40–59	ECG BUN/glucose	Hemoglobin or hematocrit ECG BUN/glucose
Over 60	Hemoglobin or hematocrit ECG Chest radiograph BUN/glucose	Hemoglobin or hematocrit ECG Chest radiograph BUN/glucose

Society of Anesthesiologists, the American College of Physicians [Clinical Efficacy Project], the American College of Pediatricians, and the American Society of Radiologists) and national organizations such as the Food and Drug Administration panel on preoperative chest x-rays, the National Institutes of Health Consensus Panel on Dental Anesthesia, and the Blue Cross/Blue Shield Medical Necessity Panel have also endorsed the concept of reducing screening tests preoperatively in favor of selectively ordering tests based on a patient's history. Thus, the aim to increase efficiency, the weight of scientific evidence, and organizational endorsements, combined with the changes that have occurred in health care reimbursement (capitational care) and in medicolegal liability (higher risk from not pursuing abnormalities than from failure to diagnose), make this an ideal time to change the current pattern of preoperative medical assessments from one of ordering batteries of tests to one of ordering tests selectively based on medical history. How can we do that efficiently and without major increase in costs? Several strategies are possible.

THE HISTORY AND PHYSICAL EXAMINATION IN THE OUTPATIENT SETTING

A survey of current methods of preoperative evaluation in outpatient surgical units indicates that in some instances, no established practices are used to evaluate a patient prior to induction of anesthesia. Others use a variety of procedures, and the following list indicates some possible evaluation practices.

1. No evaluation—the patient is seen immediately preoperatively on the gurney or in the waiting room, and routine laboratory tests (or tests as indicated in Table 9-7) are obtained by surgeons.
2. No evaluation—the patient is seen the morning of surgery in the presurgery screening area, with routine testing or testing as suggested in Table 9-7.
3. The patient is telephoned by a secretary, nurse, or an anesthesiologist preoperatively with a questionnaire, and laboratory testing may be routine or directed by the patient's answers to the questions.
4. The patient is telephoned by the anesthesiologist who will give anesthesia, and laboratory testing is completed as in procedure 3.
5. The patient is screened by the surgeon and, if indicated, is called by a nurse or anesthesiologist, and laboratory testing is completed as in procedure 3.
6. The patient is screened by the surgeon, seen if indicated, and laboratory testing is completed as in procedure 3.
7. The patient is seen in the preoperative clinic the day(s) prior to surgery by a nurse or an anesthesiologist, and laboratory testing is completed as in procedure 3.
8. The patient is seen in the preoperative clinic the day(s) prior to surgery by the anesthesiologist who will administer anesthesia, and laboratory testing is completed as in procedure 3.

Clearly, some of the above methods do not allow a history and physical examination to be done by the anesthetist prior to laboratory testing. If other tests are required, surgery is often delayed. In fact, in our hospital in 1986, the second most common cause of postponement of surgery was the need to pursue (often with a consultant who was not yet available) abnormal or borderline abnormal laboratory tests. Therefore, the process of preoperative evaluation must be made more effective by timely history-taking so that only necessary and appropriate tests are obtained. This process will, of course, reduce the costs of preoperative evaluation by eliminating unnecessary tests. There are three possible solu-

Table 9-7. Simplified Strategy for Preoperative Testing

	Test to be obtained (preoperative conditions suspected)												
	HGB												
	M	F	WBC	PT/ PTT	PLT, BT	Elect	Creat/ BUN	Blood-Glucose	SGOT/ALK PTASE	X-Ray	ECG	Pregnancy	T/S
Surgical procedure With blood loss	X	X											X
Without blood loss													
Neonates	X	X											
Age <40 yr		X											
40–59 yr		X									±		
≥60 yr	X	X								X	X		
Cardiovascular disease							X			X	X		
Pulmonary disease										X	X		
Malignancy	X	X	*	*						X			
Radiation therapy			X							X	X		
Hepatic disease				X					X				
Exposure to hepatitis									X				
Renal disease	X	X				X	X						
Bleeding disorder				X	X								
Diabetes						X	X	X			X		
Smoking ≥20 pk-yr history	X	X								X			
Possible pregnancy												X	
Diuretic use						X	X						
Digoxin use						X	X				X		
Steroid use						X		X					
Anticoagulant use	X	X		X									

Note: Not all diseases are included in this table. Please use your own judgment on patients with diseases not included.

Symbols: ±, maybe; *, leukemias only; X, obtain.

Abbreviations: HGB, hemoglobin; PLT, platelet count; BT, bleeding time; Elect, Na^+, K^+, Cl^-, CO_2, proteins; Creat/BUN, creatinine or BUN; SGOT/ALK PTASE, serum glutamic oxaloacetic transaminase phosphatase; T/S, blood typing and screen for unexpected antibodies.

(Data from Roizen et al.,[40] Kaplan et al.,[74] and Blery et al.[75])

tions to the problem of timely history-taking in the outpatient setting. All of them have been studied or are in the process of being studied and appear to be acceptable to certain practice situations.

First, the surgeon who sees the patient prior to the scheduled procedure can obtain the history and perform the physical. Second, a clinic can be set up in the outpatient facility to perform these two tasks early enough to ensure that the appropriate laboratory tests or consultations can be obtained without delaying schedules. Third, a questionnaire answered by the patient can be used to indicate appropriate laboratory tests.

A question that might arise regarding the first solution is: can the appropriate testing be generated easily from the surgeon's preoperative visit? One study found that it could. At the University of California, San Francisco (UCSF), Kaplan and coworkers[66] found that even a partial history conveyed enough information to indicate correctly all but 22 abnormalities in over 2,785 preoperative blood tests obtained (counting the CBC and SMA of six variables as one test). Knowing the admission diagnosis, previous discharge diagnoses, and scheduled operation, and using previously determined indications for laboratory testing were enough to enable detection of virtually all abnormalities that would have been revealed by routine screening. Of the approximately 60 percent of 2,785 routine tests not indicated by the admission diagnosis, previous discharge diagnoses, or scheduled operation, only four tests revealed abnormalities of potential perioperative significance. Furthermore, on reviewing the charts of the four patients with abnormalities, we found no discernible alterations in patient care. Indeed, in one instance, abnormal test results were described in the discharge summary as normal. Cost savings from such reduced testing were estimated to exceed 50 percent of current patient charges and hospital costs.[32] (Extrapolating these data to 20 years of testing at UCSF, Kaplan and coworkers[66] estimated that, at most, one perioperative morbidity might have been associated with this reduction in laboratory costs of over $6 million [in 1982 dollars].) Further, it appeared that more individuals would have been hurt than helped by this extra testing.[40]

The third approach to the problem of timely history-taking for the selection of appropriate preoperative tests is the patient questionnaire. Our studies[33,76] determined that the responses of patients to written questions can identify all laboratory tests that will have abnormal results in those patients. After the patient answers the questionnaire, a plastic overlay reveals the tests that are indicated. If the patient cannot answer the questions, a standard group of tests is ordered. However, most physicians will not perform, or do not assign their assistants to perform, this "low tech" task of placing an overlay on a questionnaire. Because the questionnaire method is only effective if a health professional assists and interprets the results, the additional expense for such a professional decreases cost-effectiveness. Also, the cost of a health professional is not borne by the same party benefiting financially from the reduction in testing. Thus, the quality of care and potential cost-saving aspects of the system are negated by the immediate cost and inconvenience of determining from questionnaire responses which laboratory tests to select. To circumvent this problem, we are now using an automated system to integrate a patient's history with suggestions for testing.

This modification to the health questionnaire approach now makes possible the practice of more efficient, higher quality medicine. With this sytem, "HealthQuiz" (obtained from HealthQual, Inc., ℅ ARCH, 1215 E. 58th St., Chicago, Illinois, a University of Chicago related corporation), the patient uses a small computerized box to answer questions (with Yes, No, or Not Sure) concerning his or her health history (Fig. 9-1). Recommendations contained in the algorithm regarding testing are based on indications predetermined and agreed on by the surgeon and anesthesiologist and on results published in the literature. A computer chip contains the algorithm (initially developed by a group of internists, surgeons, anesthesiologists, and laboratory medicine physicians working together at UCSF from 1979 to 1982) that uses these answers to determine which tests would be most productive. The chip is removable and can be updated or changed based on study results. Once the surgeon and anesthesiologist have agreed on indications, the electronic quiz can be taken by the patient to suggest the tests that are needed. HealthQuiz is given on a relatively inexpensive, hand-held computer, whose technology, graphics, and voice properties make it simple for patients to answer questions about their health. After the patient has answered all the questions, HealthQuiz generates a printout of the answers, a symptom summary, and suggested laboratory tests based on the agreed upon indications and the patient's answers. This printout directs the physician to significant facts in a patient's history, and after examining it, the physician, surgeon, or anesthesiologist can override suggested

HEALTHQUAL PATIENT SUMMARY PREOP-1.1 Page 1
COPYRIGHT 1988 JAN 14, 1989
IDENTIFICATION NUMBER: 120362880

PATIENT NAME: ______________________________

PHYSICIAN: ______________________________

PRESENT COMPLAINT: ______________________________

The patient's answers to the HealthQuiz may suggest disease in the following systems as indicated by the following symptoms:

SYSTEM	SYMPTOMS
PULM	RECENT URI ______________________

SOME ITEMS PERTINENT TO ANESTHESIA CARE ARE:

Patient wears dentures.
Patient has capped teeth.
Patient wears contact lenses.
Patient has allergies. **
Patient has previously had Anesthesia.

SUGGESTED LABORATORY TESTS

HCT DIFF
EKG

Consider stool for occult blood

If operation involves insertion of a prosthesis or foreign material, you might obtain a URINALYSIS to rule out a urinary tract infection.

THE PATIENT REPORTS THAT HE/SHE HAS HAD THE FOLLOWING TESTS RECENTLY:

Patient's stool has been checked for blood in the last year.
Patient has had a pap smear in the last year.
Patient has had a mammogram in the last year.

Fig. 9-1. HealthQuiz printout. (© University of Chicago.)

tests or select additional ones before ordering preoperative tests. The time required to complete HealthQuiz and print out its results is less than 10 minutes.

One of the advantages of HealthQuiz is that it never forgets what questions to ask the patient, which affords the opportunity to obtain more details about significant items in a history. What are some of the questions considered important in taking a history? Below is a checklist of items which has been helpful in planning perioperative care, assessing risk, and selecting laboratory tests.[33,45,66,76]

HealthQuiz asks the patient questions relevant to all areas in the checklist below. The greatest significance of HealthQuiz is that it is one of many examples of "smart technology" that are being applied to the practice of medicine. Smart technology refers to the use of new configurations of chips, microprocessors, circuit boards, memory banks, and software that supercede earlier high-tech equipment, and allow clinicians to inexpensively practice more efficient, less costly, and higher quality medicine. It is likely that examples of "smart tech" will not only reduce costs but will also improve the quality of surgical care and serve as a paradigm for future changes in our practice. HealthQuiz is a helpful tool in this regard, in that it quickly and economically records a patient's medical history and coordinates that information with recommended laboratory tests. The advantage in this is clear: by reducing preoperative laboratory testing to that indicated by history and physical examination, an anesthesiologist can reduce risk both to the patients and the medical facility. However, whether the physical examination is supplemented by a pencil-and-paper questionnaire, a history and chart, or a smart-tech computer-generated history with test suggestions, improvements in test ordering can be realized (and in our practice are done many times daily) easily and virtually effortlessly.

Items to Consider When Planning Perioperative Care, Assessing Risk, and Selecting Laboratory Tests

Examination

1. Patient gender
2. Potential of pregnancy
3. Patient age
4. Status of teeth and gums
5. Presence of arthritis that may involve airway structures
6. Presence of contact lenses, false eyes, etc.
7. Past anesthetic history of patient and blood relatives

Patient or family history of any of the following:

8. Cancer
9. Blood dyscrasia or anemia
10. Bleeding diathesis
11. Transfusion requirements
12. Allergies
13. Lung diseases
14. Upper respiratory infections, coughs, productive coughs
15. Cardiac diseases and related risk factors including hypertension and its treatment
16. Abnormal cardiac rhythms
17. Exercise tolerance
18. Gastrointestinal diseases and symptoms of hiatal hernia
19. Diabetes and other metabolic or endocrine diseases
20. Hepatitis exposure
21. Liver problems
22. Alcohol usage
23. Gallbladder disease
24. Renal and electrolyte disorders
25. Urinary symptoms
26. Dialysis
27. Appetite, bowel, or bladder changes
28. Weight changes
29. Neurologic disorders or symptoms
30. Headaches and sweating

31. Pain
32. Medication and drug usage, including steroids
33. Prior surgery
34. Smoking

To the data obtained from this history-taking is added information from the physical examination of the following areas:

35. Airway, including the ability to move neck, and open mouth
36. Cardiac and cardiovascular system
37. Lungs
38. Major organs in the abdomen
39. Neurologic and musculoskeletal systems

W. Edwards Deming, an American management theorist whose ideas are influential in successful Japanese companies today, suggested that if, with constant effort, quality did not improve, it was time to change the way things were done. In preoperative medical assessment, we have reached the point at which the system being used needs re-evaluation. We have already improved care with a system change to oximetry, another example of "smart technology." A patient-directed history-taker is another change in the system which deserves consideration. With smart technology, medical assessments in an outpatient setting can be performed more efficiently, thereby attaining a higher quality of medicine.

SUMMARY

Outpatient surgery has become an economic mandate for many procedures. Consequently, those with concurrent diseases are having surgery as outpatients. For these higher-risk patients, the 2-minute examination performed 5 minutes before induction of anesthesia may not be appropriate. The use of batteries of routine preoperative laboratory tests is widespread, yet much data suggest that such tests do not improve do not provide medicolegal protection, and probably increase risk for the patient. Tests performed without indication often generate abnormal results; such results are falsely positive, leading to extra testing and, ultimately, remedies that are not needed and that may pose extra risk to the patient (a "Starling" function curve[40] of benefits and harm when indications for preoperative testing are increased). Over $60 billion was spent in the United States in 1988 on preoperative evaluation, much of which resulted in false positive screening test results and subsequent follow-up. Sixty percent of preoperative laboratory testing can be eliminated if testing is directed by timely history taking. We have suggested some methods for accomplishing this goal in an outpatient setting. The history and physical examination remain the best measures of screening for disease and of forming medical assessments.

REFERENCES

1. Egbert LD, Battit GE, Turndorf H, Beecher HK: The value of the preoperative visit by an anesthetist. JAMA 185:553, 1963
2. Egbert LD, Battit GE, Welch CE, Bartlett MK: Reduction of postoperative pain by encouragement and instruction of patients. N Engl J Med 270:825, 1964
3. Wolfer JA, Davis CE: Assessment of surgical patients' preoperative emotional condition and postoperative welfare. Nurs Res 19:402, 1970
4. Anderson EA: Preoperative preparation for cardiac surgery facilitates recovery, reduces psychological distress, and reduces the incidence of acute postoperative hypertension. J Consult Clin Psychol 55:513, 1987
5. Vacanti CJ, Van Houten RJ, Hill RC: A statistical analysis of the relationship of physical status to postoperative mortality in 68,388 cases. Anesth Analg 49:564, 1970
6. Lewin I, Lerner AG, Green SH, et al: Physical class and physiologic status in the prediction of operative mortality in the aged sick. Ann Surg 174:217, 1971

7. Goldman L, Caldera DL, Nussbaum SR, et al: Multifactorial index of cardiac risk in noncardiac surgical procedures. N Engl J Med 297:845, 1977
8. Keats AS: The ASA classification of physical status—a recapitulation. Anesthesiology 49:233, 1978
9. Rehder K: Clinical evaluation of isoflurane: complications during and after anaesthesia. Can Anaesth Soc J, suppl. 29, S44, 1982
10. Cohen MM, Duncan PG: Physical status score and trends in anesthetic complications. J Clin Epidemiol 41:83, 1988
11. Ziffren SE, Hartford CE: Comparative mortality for various surgical operations in older versus younger age groups. J Am Geriatr Soc 20:485, 1972
12. Marx GF, Mateo CV, Orkin LR: Computer analysis of postanesthetic deaths. Anesthesiology 39:54, 1973
13. Okelberry CR: Preadmission testing shortens preoperative length of stay. Hospitals 49:71, 1975
14. Duckett JB: Preoperative assessment of the patient for outpatient anesthesia. p. 21. In Brown BB, Jr. (ed): Outpatient Anesthesia. FA Davis, Philadelphia, 1978
15. Delahunt B, Turnbull PRG: How cost effective are routine preoperative investigations? N Z Med J 92:431, 1980
16. Rossello PJ, Cruz AR, Mayol PM: Routine laboratory tests for elective surgery in pediatric patients. Bull Assoc Med Puerto Rico 72:614, 1980
17. Wood RA, Hoekelman RA: Value of the chest x-ray as a screening test for elective surgery in children. Pediatrics 67:447, 1981
18. Durbridge TC, Edwards F, Edwards RG, et al: Evaluation of benefits of screening tests done immediately on admission to hospital. Clin Chem 22:968, 1976
19. Sandler G: Costs of unnecessary tests. Br J Med 2:21, 1979
20. Rabkin SW, Horne JM: Preoperative electrocardiography: its cost-effectiveness in detecting abnormalities when a previous tracing exists. Can Med Assoc J 121:301, 1979
21. Rabkin SW, Horne JM: Preoperative electrocardiography: effect of new abnormalities on clinical decisions. Can Med Assoc J 128:146, 1983
22. London MJ, Hollenberg M, Wong MG, et al: Intraoperative myocardial ischemia: localization by continuous 12-lead electrocardiography. Anesthesiology 69:232, 1988
23. Korvin CC, Pearce RH, Stanley J: Admission screening: clinical benefits. Ann Intern Med 83:197, 1975
24. Olsen DM, Kane RL, Proctor PH: A controlled trial of multiphasic screening. N Engl J Med 294:925, 1976
25. Domoto K, Ben R, Wei JY, et al: Yield of routine annual laboratory screening in the institutionalized elderly. Am J Public Health 75:243, 1985
26. Wolf-Klein GP, Holt T, Silverstone FA, et al: Efficacy of routine annual studies in the care of elderly patients. J Am Geriatr Soc 33:325, 1985
27. Dontas AS, Kasviki-Charvarti P, Chem L, et al: Bacteriuria and survival in old age. N Engl J Med 304:939, 1981
28. Boscia JA, Kobasa WD, Knight RA, et al: Epidemiology of bacteriuria in an elderly ambulatory population. Am J Med 80:208, 1986
29. Boscia JA, Kobasa WD, Knight RA, et al: Therapy vs no therapy for bacteriuria in elderly ambulatory nonhospitalized women. JAMA 257:1067, 1987
30. Nordenstam GR, Brandberg CA, Oden AS: Bacteriuria and mortality in an elderly population. N Engl J Med 314:1152, 1986
31. Levinstein MR, Ouslander JG, Rubenstein LZ, Forsythe SB: Yield of routine annual laboratory tests in a skilled nursing home population. JAMA 258:1909, 1987
32. Finkler SA: The distinction between cost and charges. Ann Intern Med 96:102, 1982
33. Roizen MF: Routine preoperative evaluation. p. 225. In Miller RD (ed): Anesthesia. 2nd Ed. Churchill Livingstone, New York, 1986
34. Turnbull JM, Buck C: The value of preoperative screening investigations in otherwise healthy individuals. Arch Intern Med 147:1101, 1987
35. Hirsch IA, Tomlinson DL, Slogoff S, Keats AS: The overstated risk of preoperative hypokalemia. Anesth Analg 67:131, 1988
36. Vitez TS, Soper LE, Wong KC, Soper P: Chronic hypokalemia and intraoperative dysrhythmias. Anesthesiology 63:130, 1985

37. Harrington JT, Isner JM, Kassirerr JP: Our national obsession with potassium. Am J Med 73:155, 1982
38. Lawson DH: Adverse reactions to potassium chloride. Q J Med 43:433, 1974
39. Lawson DH, Hutcheon AW, Jick H: Life threatening drug reactions amongst medical in-patients. Scott Med J 24:127, 1979
40. Roizen MF, Kaplan EB, Schreider BD, et al: The relative roles of the history and physical examination and laboratory testing in preoperative evaluation for outpatient surgery: the "Starling Curve" of preoperative laboratory testing. Anesthesiol Clin North Am 5:15, 1987
41. Robertson WM: Medical Malpractice: A Preventive Approach. University of Washington Press, Seattle, 1985
42. Kreig AF, Gambino R, Galen RS: Why are clinical tests performed? When are they valid? JAMA 233:76, 1975
43. Robbins JA, Mushlin AI: Preoperative evaluation of the healthy patient. Med Clin North Am 63:1145, 1979
44. Newhauser D: Cost-effective clinical decision making. Pediatrics 60:756, 1977
45. Farnsworth PB, Steiner E, Klein RM, et al: The value of routine preoperative chest roentgenograms in infants and children. JAMA 244:582, 1980
46. Brill PW, Ewing ML, Dunn AA: The value (?) of routine chest radiography in children and adolescents. Pediatrics 52:125, 1973
47. Sagel SS, Evens RG, Forrest JV, et al: Efficacy of routine screening and lateral chest radiographs in a hospital-based population. N Engl J Med 291:1001, 1974
48. Sane SM, Worsing RA, Jr., Wiens CW, et al: Value of preoperative chest x-ray examinations in children. Pediatrics 60:669, 1977
49. Rees AM, Roberts CJ, Bligh AS, et al: Routine preoperative chest radiography in noncardiopulmonary surgery. Br Med J 1:1333, 1976
50. Loder RE: Routine preoperative chest radiography: 1977 compared with 1955 at Peterborough District General Hospital. Anaesthesia 33:972, 1978
51. Maigaard S, Elkjaer P, Stefansson T: Vaerdien af praeoperativ rutinerøntgenundersøgelse af thorax og EKG. (English abstract: Value of routine preoperative radiographic examination of the thorax and ECG.) Ugeskr Laeger 140:769, 1978
52. Catchlove BR, Wilson RM, Spring S, Hall J: Routine investigations in elective surgical patients: their use and cost effectiveness in a teaching hospital. Med J Aust 2:107, 1979
53. Collen MF, Feldman R, Siegelaub AB, Crawford D: Dollar cost per positive test for automated multiphasic screening. N Engl J Med 283:459, 1970
54. Thomsen HS, Gottlieb J, Madsen JK, et al: Rutinemaessig røntgenundersøgelse af thorax iden kirurgiske indgreg i universal anaestesi. (English abstract: Routine radiographic examination of the thorax prior to surgical intervention under general anesthesia.) Ugeskr Laeger 140:765, 1978
55. Törnebrandt K, Fletcher R: Pre-operative chest x-rays in elderly patients. Anaesthesia 37:901, 1982
56. Petterson SR, Janower ML: Is the routine preoperative chest film of value? Appl Radiol Jan-Feb:70, 1977
57. Royal College of Radiologists Working Party on the Effective Use of Diagnostic Radiology: Preoperative chest radiology. National study by the Royal College of Radiologists. Lancet 2:83, 1979
58. Collen MF (ed): Multiphasic Health Testing Services. Wiley, New York, 1978
59. Gordon T, Kannel WB: The Framingham, Massachusetts study twenty years later. p. 123. In Kessler II, Levin ML (eds): The Community as an Epidemiologic Laboratory: A Casebook of Community Studies. John Hopkins Press, Baltimore, 1970
60. Ostrander LD, Jr., Brandt RL, Kjelsberg MO, Epstein FH: Electrocardiographic findings among the adult population of a total natural community, Tecumseh, Michigan. Circulation 31:888, 1965
61. Kannel WB, McGee D, Gordon T: A general cardiovascular risk profile: the Framingham study. Am J Cardiol 38:46, 1976
62. Wasserman LR, Gilbert HS: Surgical bleeding in polycythemia vera. Ann NY Acad Sci 115:122, 1964
63. Rothstein P: What hemoglobin level is adequate in pediatric anesthesia? Anesthesiol Update 1:2, 1978
64. Slogoff S: Anesthesia considerations in the

anemic patient. Anesthesiol Update 2:7, 1979

65. Kowalyshyn TJ, Prager D, Young J: Review of the present status of preoperative hemoglobin requirements. Anesth Analg 51:75, 1972
66. Kaplan EB, Sheiner LB, Boeckmann AJ, et al: The usefulness of preoperative laboratory screening. JAMA 253:3576, 1985
67. Parkerson GR, Jr.: Determinants of physician recognition and follow-up of abnormal laboratory values. J Fam Pract 7:341, 1978
68. Gold BD, Wolfersberger WH: Findings from routine urinalysis and hematocrit on ambulatory oral and maxillofacial surgery patients. J Oral Surg 38:677, 1980
69. Carmalt MHB, Freeman P, Stephens AJH, et al: Value of routine multiple blood tests in patients attending the general practitioner. Br Med J 1:620, 1970
70. Huntley RR, Steinhausser R, White KL, et al: The quality of medical care: techniques and investigation in the outpatient clinic. J Chronic Dis 14:630, 1961
71. Williamson JW, Alexander M, Miller GE: Continuing education and patient care research: physician response to screening test results. JAMA 201:118, 1967
72. Wataneeyawech M, Kelly KA, Jr.: Hepatic diseases unsuspected before surgery. NY State J Med 75:1278, 1975
73. Schemel WH: Unexpected hepatic dysfunction found by multiple laboratory screening. Anesth Analg 55:810, 1976
74. Kaplan EB, Boeckmann AS, Roizen MF, Sheiner LB: Elimination of unnecessary preoperative laboratory tests. Anesthesiology 57:A445, 1982
75. Blery C, Szatan M, Fourgeaux B, et al: Evaluation of a protocol for selective ordering of preoperative tests. Lancet 1:139, 1986
76. Roizen MF, Kaplan EB, Sheiner LB, et al: Elimination of unnecessary laboratory tests by preoperative questionnaire. Anesthesiology 61:A455, 1984 (abstr)

10

Premedication for Adult Outpatients

J. Lance Lichtor

The outpatient, whether young or elderly, who must wait at home for surgery can be just as frightened as the inpatient awaiting surgery in a hospital bed. What seems like a minor procedure to the anesthesiologist and surgeon is a major one to the patient whose anxiety can exceed that of an individual giving a speech before a large audience. To allay this anxiety, a visit with an anesthesiologist prior to surgery can be useful.[1] Or, like the inpatient, the outpatient may receive a premedicant to calm him or her before anesthesia and to ameliorate or prevent certain adverse effects of anesthetics. This premedication differs from that given to inpatients, however, because early patient ambulation and discharge on the same day of surgery is an essential goal for outpatients. This does not mean that premedication should be avoided. Under certain circumstances, premedication in some patients may actually facilitate the essential goal of early ambulation and discharge. In patients who are to undergo a regional or local anesthetic procedure, a premedicant may actually supplement the analgesia provided by the local anesthetic. Like their inpatient counterparts, outpatients may also be at risk for aspiration of stomach contents during their surgery. Certain premedicants or anesthetic techniques that precipitate postoperative nausea and possibly vomiting must be avoided because these conditions can prolong the hospital stay. Conversely, certain premedicants may help to reduce the nausea that results from anesthesia and/or surgery.

What, then, are the goals for premedicating outpatients? Anxiety relief, elevation of gastric pH, a reduction of gastric fluid volume, and the prevention of nausea are the most common. Although some outpatients request amnesia, it may not be a desirable goal because the effects of drugs that reliably produce amnesia can extend beyond an operation and may delay discharge from the hospital. Narcotics are useful for analgesia, but because they can also precipitate nausea, unless the patient is in pain preoperatively, analgesia is better achieved intraoperatively or postoperatively. For bronchoscopy or an examination of the mouth, anticholinergics, which also help to reduce nausea, may be worthwhile; otherwise, the dryness in the mouth that they produce can be quite uncomfortable. A new preparation for administration of these drugs has been developed and will be discussed. The prevention of wound infections is also desirable; although antibiotics are usually ordered by the surgeon, it is the anesthesiologist who usually administers them.

In this chapter, data about anxiety in outpatients awaiting surgery is reviewed and the prophylactic methods of relieving that anxiety are considered. The effect of drug therapy on aspiration of stomach contents by outpatients will also be described. In a discussion of premedication of the elderly ambulatory patient, attention is given to the use of benzodiazepines and H_2 receptor antagonists. The pros and cons of the use of narcotics and anticholinergics and their role in postoperative nausea are reviewed separately. Finally, a discussion of antibiotic prophylaxis concludes the chapter.

ANXIETY AND PREMEDICATION

Incidence of Anxiety

Patients who are scheduled to undergo surgery tend to be anxious. This anxiety is present long before the patient is seen in the preoperative holding area. In one study, 52 consecutive patients completed the Profile of Mood States (POMS)[2]—a questionnaire used to assess anxiety—both the afternoon before surgery and in the preoperative holding area (approximately 1 hour prior to surgery) before any preanesthetic medication was administered.[3] Anxiety levels in the preoperative holding area, although relatively high, were predicted by levels measured the previous afternoon and were not significantly different. In another study, anxiety levels were measured daily before admission to several days following surgery; levels were high before admission, between admission and surgery, and following surgery and were not restricted to the day before surgery[4] (Fig. 10-1).

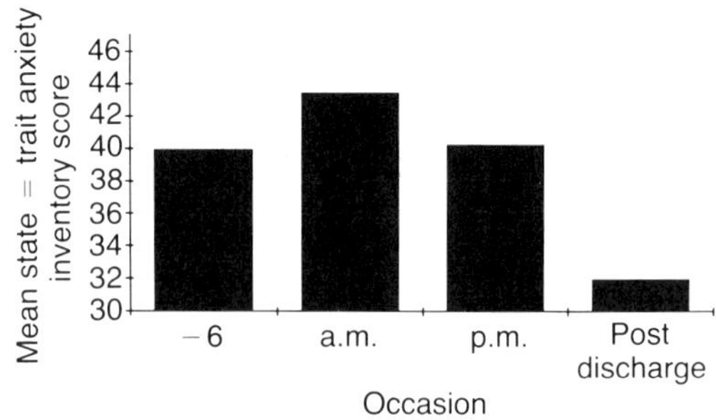

Fig. 10-1. Mean State-Trait Anxiety Inventory Scores measured 6 days prior to surgery (−6), on the morning of admission (AM), in the hospital on the evening of admission (PM), and at home in the week following discharge (postdischarge). These patients stayed in the hospital more than 1 day after surgery. Note that anxiety was elevated on all three occasions prior to surgery. (From Johnston,[4] with permission.)

In an unpublished study restricted to outpatients at the University of Chicago Division of the Biological Sciences, Pritzker School of Medicine scheduled to undergo lithotripsy, 41 patients aged 21 to 71 years completed the POMS questionnaire as a measure of anxiety, both in the clinic when the decision was made to undergo lithotripsy and again in the preoperative holding area while the patient was not premedicated, approximately 1 hour before entering the operating room. As in our previous study, the average anxiety score of patients did not change from the outpatient clinic to 1 hour prior to surgery; anxiety levels both in the clinic and 1 hour before surgery were greater than those reported in individuals not subjected to stress and were approximately the same as levels for volunteers prior to public speaking. Thus, controlling anxiety is a high priority to surgery, and the level of anxiety is not different between inpatients and outpatients.

Prophylaxis Against Anxiety

Before specific medications to reduce anxiety are considered, it is important to realize that certain nonpharmacologic techniques can also be effective. The purpose of the preoperative visit is not only to assess fitness and preparation for surgery but also to calm the patient. In their classic study, Egbert et al. found that a preoperative visit by an anesthesiologist was more effective than a barbiturate in decreasing anxiety.[1] The value of a preoperative visit has been confirmed by other investigators. For example, patients who are given maximally informative preparatory booklets prior to their surgery have less anxiety than those given minimally informative booklets or routine care.[5] Preoperative assurance from hospital nonanesthesia staff as well as the use of booklets have been shown to reduce preoperative anxiety; however, a booklet containing information was less effective than a visit.[6] Audiovisual instructions have also been successful in reducing preoperative anxiety; patients receiving such instructions required significantly less narcotic analgesia in the first 24 hours after surgery than a control group.[7]

Relaxation training is another anxiety-reducing technique that may benefit patients who are to undergo surgery.[8] Using this technique, a subject focuses attention on a positive or neutral theme and passively ignores distracting thoughts. Doing so has been shown to decrease oxygen consumption and lower blood pressure in both unmedicated and premedicated patients with hypertension.[9] Patients with ischemic heart disease and premature ventricular contractions (PVCs) who practiced the relaxation response had a reduced frequency of PVCs, especially during sleep.[10] Although used to help hospitalized patients having difficulty with sleep,[11] relaxation response has had only limited use in patients who are to undergo surgery. In one study, relaxation training was given to ambulatory patients scheduled to undergo excision of a skin cancer without general anesthesia.[12] Relaxation response was elicited 20 minutes per day until the day of surgery; the control group read for 20 minutes each day. Patients who were taught the relaxation response subjectively felt that their anxiety was highest before entering the study; control patients experienced their highest anxiety during surgery and when facing the biopsy results. However, anxiety levels as assessed by the State-Trait Anxiety Inventory were not different immediately before or after surgery in either the control or the study group. Unlike drugs, which can exert their effect relatively quickly, these nonpharmacologic techniques of relieving anxiety are best started at least 24 hours before the surgical procedure. Since more and more outpatient surgery clinics set up preoperative visits with an anesthesiologist at least 24 hours prior to a procedure, the use of these nonpharmacologic methods will probably increase.

Anxiety and the Elderly

Elderly patients who undergo surgery in outpatient facilities may be just as anxious as their younger counterparts. The treatment of this anxiety is not only humanistic, but it may also have a significant effect on outcome after surgery. There is virtually no data on the existence and relief of anxiety in elderly outpatients, although some information is available for inpatients. In one retrospective investigation, the relationship between psychiatric symptoms and age, sex, and degree of hypercalcemia was examined in 441 patients operated on for primary hyperparathyroidism in Uppsala from 1956 to 1979.[13] A follow-up with a mailed questionnaire was completed in 1983, 4 to 27 years postoperatively. Psychiatric symptoms were found in 23 percent of the patients (102 of 441); after symptoms related to the degree of hypercalcemia were factored out, psychiatric symptoms were more common and more severe among older patients. The most common symptoms were depression and anxiety, which occurred in 78 patients. In another study of elderly patients (average age, 74 years) undergoing extraction of senile cataract, anxiety the day or weekend before surgery did not change when compared with the level of anxiety 1 week postoperatively.[14] No other data specifically examine changes in anxiety from before surgery to after surgery in the elderly.

Pharmacologic Methods of Anxiety Relief

Midazolam (Versed)

Midazolam is a water-soluble benzodiazepine with an initial distribution halflife of 7.2 minutes and an elimination halflife of 2.5 hours (range, 2.1 to 3.4 hours)[15] (Fig. 10-2). Its metabolites have negligible soporific effects,[16] and it does not produce thrombosis or thrombophlebitis in humans after injection.[17,18]

Midazolam's effectiveness as a sedative in patients undergoing dental procedures or general surgery has been demonstrated in several studies using blinded observers,[19–21] patient self-report measures,[22,23] and a range of doses administered by various routes (e.g., 7.5 to 10 mg or 0.115 mg/kg IV, 15 mg PO, 0.07 mg/kg IM). Its effectiveness as an anxiolytic in patients undergoing dental procedures, oral surgery, orthopaedic surgery, day case surgery, and bronchoscopy has also been demonstrated using blinded observers,[21–25] patient self-report measures,[21,26,27] and a range of doses administered by various routes (e.g., 15 mg PO, 0.1 to 0.14 mg/kg IV, 0.07 mg/kg IM). In one study, anxiety reduction after midazolam 15 mg PO was demonstrated by visual analogue scale, but not by the State-Trait Anxiety Inventory.[27] In another study, when midazolam was given in a dose of 7.5 mg PO, subjective anxiety scores, measured by a visual analogue scale, were not different from control; a significant reduction in anxiety was present after the administration of 15 mg PO.[21]

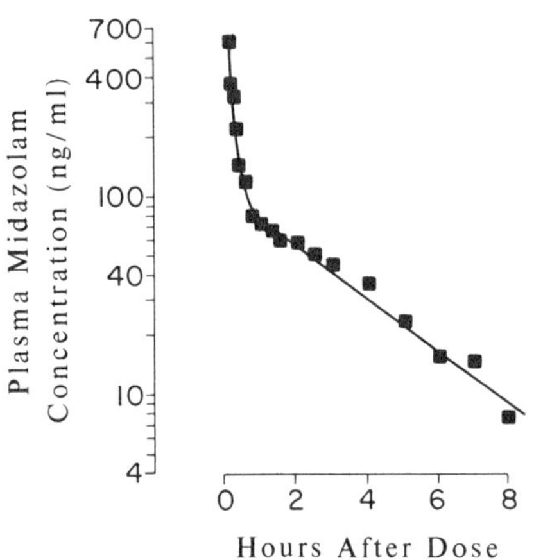

Fig. 10-2. Plasma midazolam concentrations following intravenous administration of midazolam to a patient. In this patient, the elimination half-life was 2.3 hours. (From Greenblatt et al.,[15] with permission.)

Nausea is occasionally reported after the administration of benzodiazepines such as midazolam.[28] This finding, however, has not been confirmed in other studies. For example, in one study, 60 women scheduled for abortion received an average of either 0.36 mg/kg midazolam or 6.43 mg/kg thiopental for induction (dose determined according to loss of lid reflex).[29] None of 31 patients who received midazolam had nausea or vomiting after the procedure compared with 2 of 29 patients who received thiopental. In a similar study of patients who received either 0.2 mg/kg midazolam or 3 mg/kg thiopental for induction of anesthesia for operative cases 90 minutes in length, none of 23 patients experienced nausea after midazolam compared with 2 of 26 patients who received thiopental.[30] Interestingly, reversal of midazolam-induced sedation with the benzodiazepine antagonist flumazenil may be associated with increased nausea. For example, in one double-blind study of 100 patients undergoing induced abortion under midazolam anesthesia, patients who received flumazenil (Ro 15-1788) had a higher incidence of nausea and/or vomiting in the recovery room (16 percent) compared with patients who received placebo (4 percent).[31] In another study, physostigmine and glycopyrrolate reversal of midazolam-induced sedation was associated with nausea in 5 of 8 volunteers and/or with vomiting in three.[32]

For elderly individuals, midazolam has been described in the literature more as a hypnotic than a sedative-anxiolytic. In one study, 12 young (mean age, 28 years) and

12 elderly (mean age, 72 years) subjects received a single oral dose of midazolam (15 mg), nitrazepam (5 mg), or placebo in a double-blind, crossover comparison.[33] On psychomotor tests, including critical flicker fusion, motor reaction time, and central reaction time, although the elderly overall performed at a consistently lower level than the young, there was no difference between the age groups in relative response to either medication.

In many endoscopy units, midazolam has replaced diazepam as the intravenous sedative of choice. One study examined the dose of intravenous midazolam used to produce adequate sedation prior to upper gastrointestinal endoscopy in 800 consecutive patients.[34] The dose of midazolam required for sedation decreased markedly with age in both male (r = .787) and female (r = .768) patients. In a similar study of elderly patients undergoing gastroscopy, midazolam was given intravenously to 40 patients in doses of 0.07 mg/kg for sedation prior to esophagogastroduodenoscopy.[35] Less effective in the young, this dose was very effective as a sedative in elderly patients based on time to sedation, adequacy of sedation, and absence of gagging during the procedure. Midazolam does not decrease the gag reflex; the psychological component that contributes to gagging is presumably lessened.

Midazolam has been used as an induction agent in general anesthesia for the elderly (refer to Ch. 15). In one study of 23 elderly patients, the time required for induction after midazolam 0.15 mg/kg IV was rather long compared to the time required after thiopental, and a clinically significant (>30 percent) but transient decrease in blood pressure occurred in 9 of 23 patients.[36] A marked amnesic effect was observed, especially when diazepam was used for premedication. In another study, larger doses of midazolam (0.3 mg/kg) were used for induction in unpremedicated young (<50 years of age) and elderly (>50 years of age) patients.[37] An inverse correlation occurred between the age of the patients and time elapsed before loss of consciousness. Greater reliability of effect and significantly shorter induction time were noted in patients more than 50 years of age than in younger patients.

Diazepam (Valium and Generic Forms)

Diazepam has been used extensively in the past, but its popularity in outpatient surgery has been diminished by the availability of other shorter-reacting, water-soluble anxiolytics. For intravenous injection, diazepam is solubilized with propylene glycol, which results in pain on injection as well as a high incidence of thrombophlebitis. When 10 mg diazepam was injected into the largest available vein, 23 percent of patients developed thrombosis or thrombophlebitis 2 to 3 days after injection, and 39 percent of patients developed thrombosis or thrombophlebitis 7 to 10 days after injection.[38] Injection into large antecubital veins was followed by a significantly lower incidence of thrombosis than that which occurred when injection was made into smaller vessels. Sequelae were more common in older patients (Fig. 10-3). In the United States, however, diazepam is also

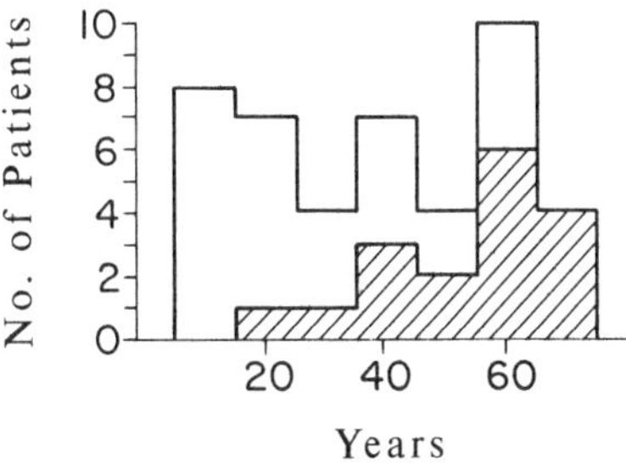

Fig. 10-3. Incidence of venous thrombosis 7 to 10 days after intravenous injection of 10 mg diazepam, related to age of patients. Bars indicate total number of patients for each age; hatched bars indicate number of patients who developed thrombosis. (From Hegarty et al.,[38] with permission.)

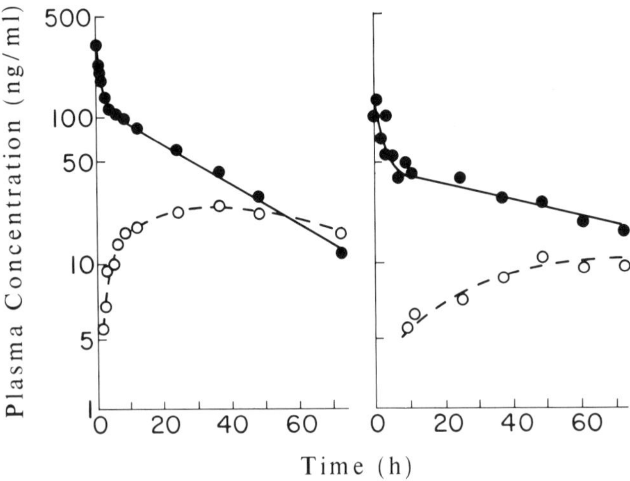

Fig. 10-4. Plasma concentration-time profiles of diazepam and desmethyldiazepam after intravenous injection of 0.1 mg/kg. The left panel shows a normal 20-year-old; the right panel shows a normal 67-year-old. The solid lines refer to diazepam and the dashed lines to desmethyldiazepam. The excretion halflife of diazepam for the younger individual is 21.6 hours and for the older individual is 51.9 hours. (From Klotz et al.,[39] with permission.)

available in tablet form, but midazolam is not.

When diazepam is injected intravenously, plasma levels show a smooth biexponential decline, with a distribution halflife of 0.5–1 hour and an excretion of halflife of 32.9 ± 8.8 hours (mean ± SD)[39] (Fig. 10-4). The major metabolite in plasma, desmethyldiazepam, can be detected after 2 hours and only declines after 36 hours. This metabolite has pharmacologic properties that are similar to its parent drug, which may account for diazepam's apparent long action.[40] Food ingestion also has an effect on diazepam pharmacokinetics. When patients ingested either mineral water and an egg, hamburger with milk, or rusks and mineral water 5 hours after administration of diazepam, serum diazepam levels were significantly higher in both groups that ingested food.[41] These serum levels were associated with the subjective recurrence of fatigue.

Diazepam is an effective anxiolytic. In one study of outpatients in which premedication with diazepam 0.25 mg/kg PO was compared with placebo, diazepam decreased preoperative discomfort and apprehension significantly.[42] The patients in this study were discharged on time regardless of whether they received diazepam or a placebo, although discharge was not attempted until the evening after surgery. When diazepam is given orally, a period of at least 1 hour must elapse before it takes effect. This time lag makes it difficult to premedicate patients "on call." Once the drug is given, though, it is effective for several hours. In the previously mentioned study, for example, premedication given early in the morning remained effective for up to 6 hours. Diazepam potency for sedation seems to be about one-half to one-fourth that of midazolam (Fig. 10-5). In one study, midazolam in a dose of 0.05 to 0.15 mg/kg IV produced sedation similar to that produced by diazepam in a dose of 0.1 to 0.3 mg/kg IV.[43]

The elimination halflife of diazepam is longer in elderly than in young subjects (Fig. 10-4). The halflife ($t_{1/2\beta}$) after both intravenous and oral administration increases

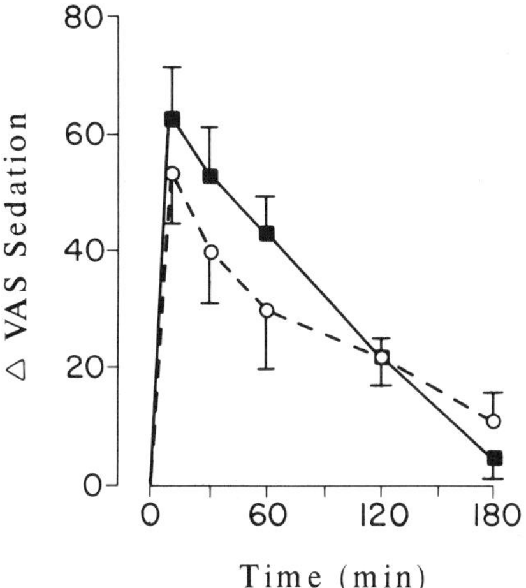

Fig. 10-5. Mean change in the subjective visual analogue scale for sedation for diazepam (open circles) and midazolam (dark squares). Sedation was initially greater after 5 mg midazolam compared with 10 mg diazepam. However, after 80 minutes, sedation with diazepam was comparable to midazolam. (From Galletly et al.,[78] with permission.)

from 20 hours at 20 years of age to about 90 hours at 80 years of age, with a correlation coefficient ($t_{1/2\beta}$ to age) of 0.83.[44] This prolongation of $t_{1/2\beta}$ is thought to be primarily dependent on an increase in the initial distribution volume of the drug. Plasma concentration alone, however, does not affect activity of this drug. At equal plasma doses, the central nervous system of elderly patients is increasingly sensitive to the depressant effects of diazepam. For example, in patients undergoing cardioversion, there is a negative correlation between age and dose of drug required before the patient fails to respond to vocal stimuli.[45] In patients undergoing gastroscopy, the dose of diazepam required to produce adequate sedation diminished with increasing age.[46] Metabolism of desmethyldiazepam is also affected by age. In the elderly, the initial presence and peak values were observed later and the metabolite was present in lower concentrations.[44]

Lorazepam (Ativan and Generic Forms)

As a sedative, lorazepam is approximately four times as potent as diazepam on a milligram for milligram basis. Its duration of action is also approximately three to four times greater than that of equivalent doses of diazepam. After an intravenous dose, the mean ± SE elimination halflife ($t_{1/2\beta}$) for the parent compound is 15.7 ± 1.7 hours.[47] Lorazepam causes fewer venous sequelae after intravenous injection than diazepam, although these sequelae are present in 15 percent of patients 7 to 10 days after injection (compared with 39 percent for diazepam).[38] An oral dose of 2.5 mg lorazepam produces as much drowsiness as 10 mg diazepam.[48] However, the onset and duration of action is much longer than that of diazepam. Even with intravenous injection, there is an unexplained delay of 40 minutes before peak drug effect; the drug continues to be effective 4.5 hours after intravenous injection.[49] Although its long duration of action and prolonged onset of action make lorazepam unsuitable for use immediately before an operation, it could be used for anxious patients seen by a surgeon or an anesthesiologist at least one day prior to an operation, so that it can be given several hours or even the night before an outpatient procedure. Unfortunately, it is such a potent amnestic agent that outpatients may not remember why they came to the surgical center.

Triazolam (Halcion)

Triazolam, used extensively as a hypnotic, has a plasma halflife of 2.3 hours.[50] Because of its relatively short halflife, it may also prove useful as a preoperative anxiolytic. In one study, 90 patients undergoing minor gynecologic surgery received either triazolam 0.25 mg, diazepam 10 mg, or placebo 2 hours prior to anesthesia.[51] Diazepam and triazolam both produced sedation, although according to a linear analogue scale, only diazepam reduced anxiety. In another study, 58 female patients who underwent laparoscopy received either triazolam 0.25 mg, lorazepam 2 mg, or placebo orally.[52] A test comprising a list of adjectives was used to assess anxiety and showed that both triazolam and lorazepam, but not placebo, were associated with significant anxiety reduction. Oral triazolam can be an effective sedative-anxiolytic for outpatients undergoing ambulatory surgery in certain situations because its elimination halflife is shorter than that of diazepam.

Drawbacks in the Pharmacologic Treatment of Anxiety Relief

Death after parenteral administration of sedative-anxiolytic medication received much attention recently when the Public Citizen Health Research Group, a Washington-based nonprofit organization that fights for consumer protection against unsafe food and drugs, filed a petition with the Food and Drug Administration (FDA) to sharply restrict the use of midazolam because it had been associated with 40 deaths in 2 years.[53] A congressional investigation into FDA approval of midazolam showed that the drug was linked to serious side effects and deaths and faulted the FDA with failure to gather all available data before clearing the drug.[54] Many of the deaths cited as being caused by the drug, in fact, have been in elderly patients undergoing endoscopy where patient vital signs were poorly supervised, or in elderly debilitated patients, also inadequately monitored, where the drug was administered for sedation (with or without narcotics) because a general anesthetic was thought to be "too risky." Clinical experience has resulted in reduced total dosage recommendations, although it has always been recommended that the drug be *titrated* in small incremental, 1–2 mg IV, bolus doses. Originally, the drug was approved for use in adults for intravenous sedation in doses of 0.1 to 0.15 mg/kg with a maximum dose of 0.2 mg/kg; the recommended dose for elderly patients was 0.07 to 0.10 mg/kg.[55] The following year, the dose recommendation for intravenous sedation was lowered to 0.1 mg/kg.[56] Most recently, a total dose of no greater than 5 mg has been recommended (Versed product information sheet, issued May 1988). Initially, the potency of midazolam was thought to be approximately two times that of diazepam; however, more recent clinical experience indicates that its potency ratio is closer to three to four times that of diazepam.[43,57]

The benzodiazepines, both individually and in combination with other drugs (particularly narcotics), can cause hypotension. In normal volunteers, midazolam 0.15 mg/kg reduced systolic pressure 5 percent and diastolic pressure 10 percent; this effect persisted for at least 20 minutes.[58] The decrease in blood pressure with midazolam 0.05 mg/kg is similar to that caused by diazepam 0.15 mg/kg.[59] In patients with heart disease, hypotension can be more profound.[60] For example, patients who were to undergo coronary artery bypass grafting received either midazolam 0.2 mg/kg or diazepam 0.5 mg/kg IV.[60] Generally, both groups were hemodynamically stable, although systolic blood pressure in those who received midazolam decreased 34 percent at the fifth minute after induction compared with an 18 percent decrease in those who received diazepam, and 9 of 20 patients receiving midazolam experienced apnea compared with none of the patients who received diazepam.

Hypotension with the benzodiazepines can be more profound when combined with narcotic analgesics. In one report, four patients experienced severe hypotension with sufentanil as an induction agent 30 minutes after intravenous lorazepam 2 to 5 mg.[61] A similar case of severe hypotension with sufentanil was described after 5 mg intramuscular midazolam.[62] Administering midazolam and fentanyl produces similar results.[63] After induction of anesthesia for coronary artery bypass grafting, mean arterial pressure decreased 17 percent in patients given 10 μg/kg fentanyl and then 0.25 mg/kg midazolam intravenously.[63] In another study, after induction of anesthesia that included 75 μg/kg fentanyl, mean arterial pressure decreased 24 percent and 32 percent after 0.075 mg/kg and 0.15 mg/kg midazolam, respectively; the lowest mean arterial pressure after the higher midazolam dose was 45 mmHg, and 10 of 12 patients had mean pressures lower than 70 mmHg.[64] The decrease in pressure after fentanyl was greater in the second study because midazolam was injected sooner after fentanyl.

Baroreflex control of heart rate is blunted with the benzodiazepines. The pressor baroreflex slope declined after either diazepam 0.4 mg/kg or midazolam 0.3 mg/kg with maximal changes (45 percent diazepam and 43 percent midazolam) when the plasma concentration of drugs was highest.[65] This loss of baroreflex control, however, is not as great as that with halogenated agents.[66]

Three cases of ventricular irritability have been reported after preoperative sedation with midazolam. In one of the three, the patient had an abnormal echocardiogram.[67] In several other studies of patients with coronary artery disease and midazolam (see above), no ventricular irritability was reported.

The benzodiazepines are also associated with respiratory depression. Intravenous midazolam was given to 100 patients during endoscopy: initial baseline oxygen saturation of 95 percent decreased to 92 percent after midazolam and to 89 percent during endoscopy; in 7 percent of these patients, the level decreased below 80 percent.[68] Response to CO_2 is also blunted following IV bolus doses of benzodiazepines. Ventilatory and mouth occlusion pressure responses to CO_2 were measured in healthy volunteers after 0.3 mg/kg diazepam or 0.15 mg/kg midazolam: ventilatory response curves were flatter than those of control groups.[69] This decrement is not as severe as that after narcotics in which the ventilatory response curves are also shifted to the right.[70] Ventilatory depression with midazolam is much more profound in patients with chronic obstructive pulmonary disease (COPD). In one study, patients with COPD received 0.2 mg/kg midazolam IV over 15 seconds. Within 15 minutes, the slope of the CO_2 response curve returned to 33 percent of control in patients with COPD compared with a return to 75 percent of control in normal patients; sedation was similar for the two groups.[71]

Fatigue associated with preoperative anxiolytics may conceivably put patients at risk of personal injury and consequently may delay discharge of patients who are scheduled to go home on the day of their surgery. Even in instances in which no surgery has taken place, fatigue has been a dramatic factor in unfortunate accidents. The Three Mile Island incident, the crash of a United Air Lines flight over Salt Lake City, and the death of Libby Zion are examples that have attracted media attention to the catastrophic relationship between fatigue and human error.[72–74] A patient who has undergone ambulatory surgery will not, in all likelihood, be involved in the extreme examples cited, but no epidemiologic study has yet been undertaken to show the relationship between the lingering effects of anesthetics and accidents. In general, the benzodiazepines do influence recovery from anesthesia, and it is important that this interaction is understood. When patients are premedicated with anxiolytics, it is important to consider whether these anxiolytics significantly prolong the effect of anesthetics.[75]

Recovery from anesthesia is initially slower after anxiolytics are administered preoperatively. Studies performed in nonpatient subjects have shown that longer excretion rates of anxiolytics are associated with longer depression of psychomotor fuction. However, with the exception of lorazepam, which has much longer effects, there is no difference in discharge times when patients who have received premedicant anxiolytics are compared with those who have not.

In a study of nonpatient subjects who received either diazepam 0.3 mg/kg or saline, perceptual speed was impaired for 5 hours and body sway was impaired for as long as 7 hours after drug administration.[76] In a similar study, which included 0.15 mg/kg diazepam, reaction times and coordination were impaired up to 2 hours after drug administration.[77] In volunteers who received either midazolam 5 mg or diazepam 10 mg, results of various psychomotor tests, including letter deletion, visual reaction time, addition, and seven-digit recall, initially showed that midazolam was more than two times as potent as diazepam.[78] After 3 hours, this effect showed signs of reversal, with subjects in the midazolam group beginning to improve beyond those of the diazepam group (Fig. 10-5).

Clearly, volunteer studies in nonpatients demonstrate the prolonged effects of the benzodiazepines. The clinical significance of these findings, however, is not as clear, especially since the effects of other anesthetics and surgery are not included. For example, when 15 mg midazolam was administered to patients undergoing an excisional breast biopsy, approximately 4 hours after surgery or 6 hours after drug administration, performance was similar to baseline.[79] In a study of patients undergoing minor outpatient procedures, patients who received 15 mg midazolam demonstrated decreased scores on the digit substitution test up to 2 hours after receiving midazolam; the changes after 7.5 mg were less marked.[21] Unfortunately, patients were not studied for longer than 2 hours.

Recovery in outpatients who have received either midazolam or diazepam has not been as dramatically different as might be expected. In outpatients who underwent bronchoscopy and received either local anesthesia and diazepam 0.2 mg/kg intravenously or midazolam 0.05 or 0.10 mg/kg intravenously, performance, measured by a visualization test, aiming test, and perceptual speed test, was no different between the two groups; 2 hours after sedation, performance was similar to that before sedation.[80] However, 17 percent of patients receiving midazolam 0.1 mg/kg were unable to walk a straight line 2 hours after injection, although patients who received midazolam 0.05 mg/kg or diazepam 0.10 mg/kg could. In another study, sedation during recovery, discharge times, and postoperative Trieger test scores were similar for patients receiving 0.1 to 0.3 mg/kg diazepam or 0.05 to 0.15 mg/kg midazolam.[43] In a third study of patients undergoing ambulatory gynecologic surgery, after either intravenous midazolam 0.07 mg/kg or diazepam 0.15 mg/kg, with administration of fentanyl 1.5 μg/kg followed by etomidate for induction and maintenance of anesthesia, there was no difference in recovery Trieger test scores at 30 minutes and 3 hours, recall of previous operative events, or recall of pain on injection of etomidate.[81]

Because of its long duration of action, lorazepam has been avoided by some for outpatient ambulatory surgery. In one study in which 4 mg lorazepam was administered intravenously 6 hours before anesthesia, 70 to 80 percent of patients experienced amnesia lasting as long as 4 hours after administration; after 2 mg intravenous, amnesia was present in 50 percent with a latency period of 30 minutes and a duration of action of 30 minutes.[82] In another study, 58 female patients undergoing laparoscopy received either triazolam 0.25 mg, lorazepam 2 mg, or placebo as oral premedication.[52] Two hours after their operations, more patients who received lorazepam scored lower than the median value on a paper and pencil psychomotor test (15 of 18) than those who received triazolam (6 of 18) or placebo (6 of 18).

The results of psychomotor performance after anesthesia must be interpreted carefully. A necessary limitation to interpretation of any study is the nature of the tasks and their relationship to actual functioning. For example, does a delay in visual reaction time mean that a patient is truly more likely to have an automobile accident? A further limitation is that patients may perceive psychomotor tests as trivial and irrelevant, and give them little attention; conversely, they may view the tests as a contest and expend more effort on them than they might on normal daily routines. In either case, the tests may not represent a true measure of patients' ability to function once they leave the hospital. Finally, even though psychomotor performance may be affected by certain drug techniques, patients usually do not stay in the hospital because they are too sleepy: nausea is frequently the reason for a longer hospital stay. For example, in one study, ambulatory patients received either midazolam 5 mg or placebo IM and then fentanyl 100 μg, oxymorphone 1 mg, or placebo immediately prior to induction; various measures of recovery were not different between groups, although patients who had nausea or vomiting had prolonged times to discharge.[75] This problem of nausea and premedicants will be more extensively discussed below.

In addition to the possibility of prolonged recovery, the potential for amnesia after premedication is also a concern. In one anecdotal report, several patients who intravenously received 2 mg of midazolam in the preoperative waiting area reported later that they did not remember meeting their surgeon or anesthesiologist before the operation and wondered if in fact both were present for it.[83] This is alarming, although more controlled studies have failed to show evidence of retrograde amnesia. In one study, for example, all 20 volunteers remembered the card and number shown to them before an injection of 0.15 mg/kg midazolam.[58] In another study, amnesia was tested by showing patients six photographs (equally divided between commonplace objects and objects relevant to dentistry) before premedication and then again in the operating room before the start of the surgical procedure (extraction of third molar teeth with sedation).[27] Patients received either midazolam 15 mg orally or diazepam 10 mg intravenously at equivalent times with appropriate controls. Recall before and after drug administration was similar for patients receiving either drug; however, on the average, patients had recall of approximately 4.5 fewer photographs after premedication than before ($P < .001$). In a similar study, recall for perioperative events was much lower when greater doses of either intravenous midazolam (0.15 mg/kg versus 0.05 mg/kg) or diazepam (0.3 mg/kg versus 0.1 mg/kg) were given; amnesia for patients given intravenous diazepam 0.2 mg/kg was similar to amnesia in patients given intravenous midazolam 0.1 mg/kg.[43] In another study, 2.8 percent of patients who received intramuscular midazolam 0.1 mg/kg recalled the induction of anesthesia for dilatation and curettage compared with 42 percent of patients who received placebo ($P < .0001$).[84] It is interesting that so many patients who received placebo did not have recall for induction.

Recommendations

If the patient may benefit from preoperative medication, either because of an expressed desire or because anxiety seems present despite attempts at comforting, diazepam oral 5 or 10 mg is administered at 6:00 A.M. on the day of surgery. If surgery is scheduled for 1:00 P.M. or later, the drug

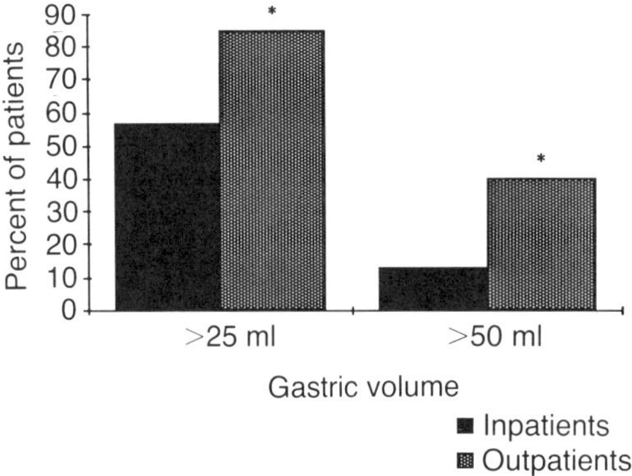

Fig. 10-6. Mean gastric volume and pH of inpatients and outpatients. The asterisk (*) indicates $P < .025$. (From Ong et al.,[92] with permission.)

should be ingested at 8:00 A.M. on the day of surgery. In those patients seen for the first time in the preoperative holding area who seem in need of preoperative medication, again either because they express that desire or because they seem anxious despite attempts at comforting, or for those patients who have received oral diazepam and who are still anxious midazolam 0.05 mg/kg intravenous is highly effective.

THE RISK OF ASPIRATION IN OUTPATIENTS

Patients who undergo ambulatory surgery may be at risk for aspiration. A patient is at risk for pulmonary damage secondary to aspiration of stomach contents if at least 25 ml of a solution with pH ≤2.5 is aspirated.[85] In addition, patients who aspirate volumes as low as 0.3 ml/kg with a pH of 1.0 have a very high mortality rate.[86] Various studies of gastric pH and volume in outpatients have shown that unpremedicated outpatients are at a significant risk for aspiration of acidic stomach contents: mean pH has been found to vary from 1.86 to 2.34, mean gastric volumes have ranged from 25.6 to 45.48 cc, and the percent of patients with residual volumes ≥25 ml and pH ≤2.5 has ranged from 36 percent to 56 percent.[87–91] In fact, there is conflicting evidence that outpatients may be at a greater risk for aspiration than inpatients. In one study, gastric volume and pH were compared in 21 inpatients and 21 outpatients.[92] Average pH did not vary, but outpatients had greater gastric volumes than inpatients (Fig. 10-6). Four of the outpatients had gastric volumes over 95 cc with pH < 2.0, values that are dramatic and much higher than values seen in outpatients in the other studies mentioned above. In a similar study of 25 inpatients and 25 outpatients, no difference was seen in gastric volumes, pH, or number of patients at risk of aspiration.[89]

Certain classes of patients, like those with hiatal hernia or those who are morbidly obese, may be particularly at risk for aspiration. In one study, 85 percent of obese patients had gastric pH <2.5 and 86 percent had more than 25 ml volume in the stomach; 75 percent had both increased volume and pH <2.5.[93] These patients may also be more prone to morbidity from aspiration because of management difficulties caused by their obesity.

Smokers are similarly prone to morbidity from aspiration. In a study of smokers versus nonsmokers undergoing outpatient surgery, the average gastric volume ± SD in nonsmokers was 8.6 ± 5.6 ml, and in those patients who had smoked on the day of the operation it was 18.8 ± 10.8 ml.[94] Four of the 19 smokers had more than 25 ml of gastric juice with a pH of 2.0 or less. Although smoking itself may not have resulted in increased gastric acidity, there is some association between increased anxiety—the reason some smokers may smoke—and increased gastric acidity.[95] For example, in one study, gastric pH measurements taken from two patients during psychotherapy indicated that hydrochloric acid secretion increased during periods of anxiety.[96] In a review of their own work as well as that of others, Gray and Ramsey showed examples of the way various stress factors, such as burns, surgery, fractures, and emotion, are associated with increased gastric acidity.[97]

Pregnancy may also increase the risk of aspiration, although patients presenting for surgery during the first trimester have not been at increased risk. In a study of gastric volume in early pregnancy, nonpregnant patients undergoing minor gynecologic procedures under general anesthesia were compared with pregnant patients undergoing therapeutic abortion during the first 20 weeks of pregnancy.[98] There were no differences in the number of patients with gastric volume >25 ml; in nonpregnant patients, mean gastric pH ($\pm$SEM) was lower (1.7 ± 0.3 nonpregnant versus 2.4 ± 0.2 pregnant) and a greater number of them had a pH < 2.5 (19 of 20 nonpregnant versus 43 of 62 pregnant).

Length of Fast and the Risk of Aspiration

In an effort to decrease the incidence of aspiration, patients are routinely asked to fast for at least 6 hours prior to surgery. However, patients taking other medication may do so with a sip of water at least 2 hours prior to a procedure. In one study of 40 patients in which one group, given diazepam by mouth with 50 ml of water, was compared with a similar group, given diazepam IM, stomach contents were less (median volume, 20 ml intramuscular group versus 1.5 oral group) and pH was higher (median pH 1.8 intramuscular group versus 2.4 oral group) in the patients given diazepam orally.[99] In a study examining the effect of 100 cc water 2 hours before surgery without a pill but with an intramuscular premedicant (meperidine and promethazine), volume and pH, although variable, were no different if water or no water was ingested.[100] In a similar study, the incidence of gastric volume >25 ml and pH <2.5 was no different if patients ingested orange juice or coffee 2 to 3 hours before surgery or fasted overnight; not unexpectedly, more patients who had coffee or orange juice felt less hungry and less thirsty than the group who fasted.[101] In another study, patients who received tea or coffee with milk and one slice of buttered toast on the morning of surgery had no difference in gastric contents than a similar group of patients who fasted.[102] In that study, the time between breakfast and surgery in the nonfasted group ranged from 2 to 4 hours, with the shortest interval being 105 minutes; in the case with an interval of 105 minutes, 5 ml of gastric contents with a pH 4.1 was aspirated. An 18-gauge tube was used to aspirate stomach contents so it is possible that large fragments of food could not have been aspirated. In another study of outpatients, bromosulfophthalein (BSP) was used to measure residual gastric volume in patients who received BSP in 10 ml water with a placebo and then either 150 ml water or no further fluid.[103] Patients who received 150 ml of water had a significantly lower residual gastric volume than those who did not (mean $\pm$ SD, 20.6 ± 14.1 ml for those who received 150 ml water versus 29.9 ± 18.2 ml for those who received no water); pH did not vary between groups. If 150 mg ranitidine is ingested orally at the same time that 150 ml water is ingested, gastric volume will decrease further (mean $\pm$ SD, 17.6 ± 14.5 cc without ranitidine to 8.3 ± 7.3 cc with ranitidine); pH will also increase (1.75 ± 0.94 to 5.52 ± 1.79).[104]

Pharmacologic Methods to Decrease Gastric Volume and Increase Gastric pH

H_2 Receptor Antagonists

Cimetidine and ranitidine are reversible competitive antagonists of the action of histamine on H_2 receptors, and as such, inhibit gastric secretion in response to acetylcholine, histamine, or gastrin. They inhibit the production of gastric juice and they reduce hydrogen ion concentration. Ranitidine is four to six times as potent as cimetidine, and elimination halflives are similar for each drug (2 to 3 hours): since ranitidine is often administered at half the dose of cimetidine, its effectiveness in this dose ratio is relatively longer (8 to 12 hours).[105] Many studies have shown that H_2 receptor antagonists increase gastric pH and decrease gastric volume. In one study of outpatients undergoing therapeutic abortion in the first trimester of pregnancy, cimetidine 400 mg or ranitidine 150 mg, given 90 to 120 minutes before scheduled surgery, increased gastric pH and reduced mean gastric volume[106] (Fig. 10-7). The average ± SEM gastric pH was 1.06 ± 0.1 in the unpremedicated patients; the average ± gastric volume was 22.1 ± 1.5 ml. The average ± SEM pH increased significantly after either cimetidine (5.0 ± 0.4) or ranitidine (5.2 ± 0.3); similarly, gastric volumes decreased after either cimetidine (13.2 ± 2.4 ml) or ranitidine (11.1 ± 1.5 ml). Average gastric pH and volume were superior to control for patients who received either cimetidine or ranitidine, and the patients in each group who had both a pH ≤2.5 and a volume ≥25 ml are as follows: 4 of 33 patients with cimetidine, none of 33 patients with ranitidine, and 23 of 66 patients with placebo.

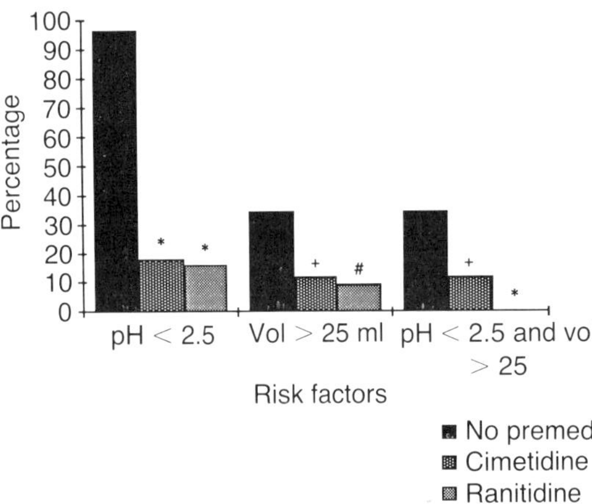

Fig. 10-7. Effectiveness of cimetidine and ranitidine in reducing the risk of aspiration in outpatients. * $P < .001$ versus no premedication. # $P < .02$ versus no premedication. + $P < .05$ versus no premedication. (From Stock et al.,[106] with permission.)

Cimetidine inhibits drug metabolism through its impairment of cytochrome P-450 biotransformations. Drugs, like diazepam, that are dependent on the cytochrome P-450 microsomal enzyme system, will show a potentiation of action when taken with cimetidine.[107] This potentiation occurs after as little as one day of therapy with cimetidine and one injection of diazepam. Lorazepam, not transformed through the cytochrome P-450 microsomal enzyme system, is conjugated with glucuronic acid and is not potentiated when administered with cimetidine.[108] Cimetidine also decreases blood flow in the liver acutely by 25 percent during fasting and by 33 percent after chronic administration so that drugs such as propranolol, whose hepatic elimination depends on blood flow in the liver, will be eliminated from the body more slowly when cimetidine is also administered.[109] Hence, pulse rates at rest are markedly slower after propranolol and cimetidine than after the same dose of propranolol alone. Other drug interactions with cimetidine (recommendations for therapy are given in parentheses) include the following: oral anticoagulants, e.g., warfarin (monitor coagulation parameters); theophylline (decrease maintenance dosage by 50 percent but do not change loading dose); phenytoin and carbamazepine (reduce maintenance dosage by 33 percent), and lidocaine (reduce maintenance dosage by 50 percent).[110] Bupivacaine clearance is also reduced after cimetidine.[111] Ranitidine, unlike cimetidine, has a much weaker effect on cytochrome P-450, and in most studies its effect on drug interactions is not statistically significant.[112]

Famotidine and nizatidine, two new H_2 receptor antagonists, are similar to cimetidine and ranitidine. Famotidine is approximately 7.5 times more potent than ranitidine and 20 times more potent than cimetidine on an equimolar basis; famotidine 20 mg bid or 40 mg at bedtime is as effective as standard doses of cimetidine and ranitidine for healing duodenal ulcers.[113] Nizatidine is three times more potent than cimetidine.[114] Both nizatidine and famotidine are similar to ranitidine in that they do not bind to cytochrome P-450 and hence do not interfere with hepatic metabolisms of various drugs.[115] For example, in humans, cimetidine inhibited the hepatic elimination of diazepam by about 45 percent, whereas ranitidine, nizatidine, and famotidine did not affect the pharmacokinetics of diazepam. To date, there has been no published data about outpatients who have undergone surgery with either famotidine or nizatidine.

H_2 Receptor Antagonists in the Elderly

Many physicians seem unaware of the potential side effects of the H_2 receptor antagonists in the elderly outpatient. When cimetidine was used as one of the tracers in a study of 1,797 prescriptions filled for elderly outpatients (mean age, 72 years) through a national pharmacy service, physicians generally failed to adjust drug doses either for advancing age or body weight.[116] Those patients receiving the highest doses were also the oldest, those most at risk for complications from these drugs.

Transient mental confusion is one complication of this class of drugs, particularly in the elderly patient. One study reported 36 cases of mental confusion after cimetidine.[117] The syndrome typically begins within 48 hours of the first dose. On occasion, alterations in mental function follow an acute deterioration of renal or hepatic function. Mental confusion may include restlessness, disorientation, agitation, hallucinations, focal twitching, seizures, unresponsiveness, and apnea. This syndrome is associated with trough concentrations greater than 2.0 μg/ml. Confusion after ranitidine has been described, although it is much more unusual.[118,119]

Cimetidine is predominantly excreted unchanged in the urine. A greater proportion of ranitidine is eliminated by hepatic metabolism, with a significant proportion eliminated by presystemic metabolism. In the young rat, the liver contributes approximately 30 percent to the clearance of cimetidine, whereas in the aged rat, all clearance is renal.[120] This absence of the hepatic component of excretion in the elderly rat resulted in a decreased overall systemic clearance of the drug. Ranitidine clearance is also prolonged in elderly humans by 50 percent after a single intravenous or oral dose and by approximately 30 percent after chronic dosing.[121,122] The inhibition of drug metabolism that is caused by cimetidine is similar in both the young and old.[123]

Sodium Citrate

The soluble antacids, such as sodium citrate or Bicitra (Willen Drug Co., Baltimore, MD), have recently become popular. Hypoxia and lung pathology are not as severe if these soluble antacids are aspirated.[124] Although gastric pH increases, gastric volume can also increase after administration of these soluble antacids. In one study, outpatients received either 15 ml or 30 ml Bicitra orally.[88] Eighty-eight percent of patients in the control group had a gastric pH ≤ 2.5, and 36 percent had a gastric content volume ≥ 25 ml with pH ≥ 2.5. Bicitra, 15 ml and 30 ml orally, increased mean gastric pH and decreased the proportion of patients with a gastric pH ≤ 2.5 to 32 and 16 percent, respectively. However, the proportion of patients with a gastric volume ≥25 ml increased from 36 percent in the control group to 56 percent after 15 ml Bicitra and to 84 percent after 30 ml Bicitra.

Metoclopramide

Metoclopramide is a dopamine antagonist which increases lower esophageal sphincter pressure, speeds gastric emptying time, and has antiemetic properties.[125] In a study of outpatients scheduled for surgery who received either intravenous metoclopramide 10 mg or a control substance, gastric volume (mean ± SEM) was reduced with metoclopramide (15.6 ± 2.6 ml versus 32.7 ± 7.6 ml); the proportion of patients with a gastric volume ≥25 ml was also reduced with metoclopramide (20 percent versus 36 percent).[88] In a study of outpatients undergoing tubal ligation, gastric fluid volume in the control group was 83.9 ± 2.3 ml; in the patients pretreated with metoclopramide 10 mg, gastric fluid volume was 11.1 ± 0.63 ml.[126] Metoclopramide is also useful in combination with other drugs for even greater reductions in gastric volume. When intravenous metoclopramide 10 mg was included with either 15 ml or 30 ml Bicitra, the proportion of patients with a gastric volume ≥25 ml decreased from 56 percent and 84 percent to 28 percent and 36 percent, respectively.[88] Similarly, in another study, gastric fluid volume (mean ± SEM) in patients receiving cimetidine was 51 ± 2.33 ml; in those treated with both cimetidine and metoclopramide, gastric fluid volume was 12.05 ± 0.79 ml.[126] Gastric pH was better treated with cimetidine than with metoclopramide, although none of the patients treated with both metoclopramide and cimetidine had a gastric fluid pH <2.5.

Metoclopramide is also an effective antiemetic.[127] A beneficial side effect of administering metoclopramide preoperatively may be less nausea and vomiting postoperatively as well as intraoperatively for patients who undergo regional anesthesia. Its duration of action is relatively brief, however, and conflicting views are expressed in the literature. For example, in one study of patients undergoing a fentanyl, N_2O, succinylcholine anesthetic for therapeutic abortion, use of metoclopramide 10 mg and droperidol 1.25 mg was compared; both droperidol and metoclopramide did not decrease postoperative nausea and vomiting.[128] However, patients who received metoclopramide sat up, walked, and were discharged earlier than control patients, although the reason for this was unclear; discharge time from the recovery room after droperidol was similar to that for patients who received placebo, although more patients who received droperidol complained of dizziness at home compared with patients receiving metoclopramide or placebo. Similarly, postoperative nausea and vomiting were not decreased in patients who received 10 to 20 mg metoclopramide prior to minor gynecologic surgery with a methohexitone, N_2O anesthetic.[129] However, in another study, metoclopramide, given in a dose of 0.15 mg/kg at the time of umbilical cord clamping, reduced the incidence of intraoperative postdelivery nausea (12 percent for metoclopramide versus 36 percent for placebo) and vomiting (0 percent for metoclopramide versus 15 percent for placebo) during epidural anesthesia with fentanyl supplementation for elective cesarean section.[130] The results were similar in two other separate studies of women undergoing ambulatory gynecologic procedures. Of 101 women under mask anesthesia, those who received metoclopramide 10 mg had significantly less postoperative nausea and vomiting (4 of 48) than a similar control group (9 of 53).[131] In the second study, of 199 women who received either intravenous droperidol 2.5 mg or metoclopramide 10 mg before induction of anesthesia (fentanyl, thiopentone, etomidate, and nitrous oxide by facemask), the incidence of nausea or vomiting decreased significantly (to 21 percent after droperidol and to 26 percent after metoclopramide) in comparison to that of the untreated group (placebo, 47 percent).[132]

Anticholinergics

Anticholinergics have been shown to have little prophylactic effect against the factors that contribute to the acid aspiration syndrome. For example, in one study of outpatients undergoing surgery, glycopyrrolate given in doses of 4 to 5 μg/kg intramuscularly 45 to 90 minutes before induction of anesthesia failed to increase gastric pH or to reduce gastric volume.[89] Administered with metoclopramide, anticholinergics cause little change in lower esophageal sphincter tone, unlike metoclopramide alone, which increases barrier pressure.[133]

Recommendations

Sodium citrate and metoclopramide, or an H_2 receptor antagonist, can be administered to patients who are at risk for acid aspiration, e.g., patients with hiatal hernia, the morbidly obese, and those who are pregnant. The idea of feeding patients clear liquids as little as 2 hours before surgery seems attractive, although it has not been widely accepted by practicing anesthesiologists.

NARCOTIC (OPIOID) ANALGESICS

Narcotics can be administered as preoperative medicants to decrease preoperative anxiety, to increase preoperative sedation, and to decrease pain. They may also be administered as a supplement during general anesthesia (refer to Ch. 13).

The effect of narcotics on anxiety relief is controversial. Fentanyl has been particularly fashionable because compared with meperidine or morphine, its duration of action is relatively short. Fentanyl has been shown to decrease anxiety,[134] to be no better than control,[135,136] to be less effective than midazolam,[137] and to be useful with diazepam.[135,138] In the majority of studies that have examined the relationship between fentanyl and anxiety, either there have been no controls or only a single dose of the drug was used.

Narcotics slow gastric emptying time and, hence, might result in an increase in gastric volume. In one study, patients received either an opioid (meperidine) and an anticholinergic, or a benzodiazepine.[102] There was a trend, although not a significant one, toward larger volumes in the stomach after narcotic premedication. Decreased respiratory drive and even apnea may also result after narcotic administration.

Narcotic premedicants may also cause postoperative nausea which can prolong recovery time. One study of 420 patients undergoing dilatation and curettage compared patients given morphine 10 mg, and those given meperidine 50 mg with atropine 0.6 mg 60 to 90 minutes before their surgery.[139] Incidence of vomiting was greater if patients received morphine (49 percent) than if they received meperidine (36 percent) or atropine alone (29 percent); the incidence of nausea and vomiting was greatest with morphine (67 percent), less with meperidine (51 percent), and least with atropine alone (46 percent). In another study, patients received varying doses of morphine (up to 10 mg) with or without varying doses of atropine (up to 1.2 mg).[140] Vomiting episodes increased as the morphine dose increased; atropine caused vomiting to decrease. Conversely, in a study of premedication with meperidine 1 mg/kg and atropine in patients undergoing a therapeutic abortion, vomiting rates were not increased if meperidine was administered.[141]

When midazolam, morphine-scopolamine, and placebo premedicants were compared in 193 female patients, nausea as well as prolonged recovery occurred more in the morphine-scopolamine groups than in the midazolam and placebo groups.[84] In a randomized cross-over study of 19 patients undergoing ambulatory oral surgery, subcutaneous morphine-scopolamine (mean dose of morphine, 0.13 mg/kg) resulted in the more frequent occurrence of postoperative nausea (five patients) than rectal diazepam (mean dose, 0.57 mg/kg; no patients).[142]

In various studies, two different narcotics have been compared without placebo, and both drugs led to elevated levels of postoperative nausea. For example, in one study of 40 patients scheduled for termination of pregnancy who received either nalbuphine 0.25 mg/kg or fentanyl 1.5 μg/kg immediately before induction of anesthesia, the mean scores on a nausea scale were not different between groups.[143] In another study, 36 female patients received either butorphanol 40 μg/kg or fentanyl 2 μg/kg just prior to the induction of anesthesia; the incidence of postoperative nausea was quite high in both groups (55 to 61 percent).[144] In a study of patients presenting for midtrimester therapeutic abortion by dilatation and extraction, patients received either fentanyl or alfentanil infusion or bolus; the incidence of nausea was 52 to 68 percent and the incidence of vomiting was 30 to 60 percent, despite the fact that all of the patients had been pretreated with intravenous droperidol 0.625 mg.[145] In another study in which either fentanyl or alfentanil was used for pelvic laparoscopy, both groups of females had over a 40 percent incidence of postoperative nausea.[146]

A narcotic is not recommended as a preoperative medicant for an outpatient unless the patient is in pain preoperatively. Occasionally, both a benzodiazepine and a narcotic can be administered.

Anticholinergics

In outpatients, routine premedication with anticholinergics is uncommon and probably unnecessary. In procedures involving intraoral examinations or instrumentation with bronchoscopes, the antisialagogue effect of anticholinergics can be useful. If topical anesthetics are to be used, salivation may dilute the anesthetic and the antisialagogues may prevent this. Conversely, the dry mouth produced by these drugs is very uncomfortable. Patients awaiting anesthesia who are relatively fluid-deprived as well as anxious may have a dry mouth without the use of the anticholinergics. One study found this to be true in 26 to 50 percent of patients 1 hour after receiving placebo on the day of operation.[147]

Anticholinergics are relatively similar in terms of their ability to decrease salivation. Glycopyrrolate 0.2 mg was compared in a double-blind study with atropine 0.6 mg or scopolamine 0.4 mg.[148] The antisialagogue actions of all three drugs were similar. Glycopyrrolate produced less tachycardia, pyrexia, and blurred vision than atropine, and its sedative effect was less than that of scopolamine. In another study, 1.0 mg atropine, 0.5 mg hyoscine, and 0.2 mg glycopyrrolate were compared; again, the antisialagogue actions of all three drugs were similar.[149] In a third study, significant dryness resulted between 60 and 90 minutes after atropine administered either orally or intramuscularly; similarly, glycopyrrolate produced significant dryness at 60 minutes after either 0.2 or 0.4 mg IM.[150]

PROPHYLAXIS AGAINST POSTOPERATIVE NAUSEA AND VOMITING

Postoperative nausea, with or without vomiting, leads the list in many outpatient surgery centers, including our own, as the most common complication after outpatient surgery. An ambulatory surgery center in Phoenix reported that postoperative nausea and vomiting were the most common complications in their recovery room: nausea occurred in 30 percent and emesis in 20 percent of their patients.[151] The problem is quite pervasive and will also be discussed in Chapter 18. Studies show that females have more nausea and vomiting postoperatively than males. In one study of 554 patients given a variety of premedicants and an ether nitrous oxide anesthetic, females had a higher incidence of nausea (81 percent) than males (43 percent).[152] In a similar study of 300 patients, females also had more postoperative nausea and vomiting than males (females, 55 percent versus males, 23 percent).[153] Age in no way influenced a patient's emetic symptoms in these two studies. In a study of 2,528 patients, females again had a higher incidence of vomiting than males, particularly after age 20, but vomiting decreased in both sexes with increasing age.[154] For example, in patients 10 to 19 years of age, the incidence of postoperative vomiting was 44.8 percent in males and 47.9 percent in females; however, in patients more than 40 years of age, the incidence of vomiting was 13.8 percent in males and 27.8 percent in females. Pregnant ambulatory patients have an increased incidence of preoperative nausea. In one study comparing 66 patients scheduled for first trimester abortion with 66 patients scheduled for minor gynecologic surgery, 38 percent of the patients scheduled for abortion had preoperative nausea and vomiting compared with 8 percent of the nonpregnant patients.[155]

It is imperative that the premedicants that are administered do not exacerbate the problem of postoperative nausea and vomiting. The use of narcotics as premedicants, as already discussed, may increase postoperative nausea. Conversely, drugs such as metoclopramide may help alleviate it. Two drugs, droperidol and transdermal scopolamine, which have shown particular promise in the ambulatory surgery setting, deserve review here. Other drugs, including prochlorperazine (Compazine and others), perphenazine (Trilafon and others), benzquinamide (Emete-con), promazine (Sparine), and trimethobenzamide (Tigan and others) are frequently used in the outpatient recovery room and can be used prophylactically as preoperative medicants; however, they have not been studied much in a controlled fashion in the ambulatory setting.

Droperidol

Droperidol has had variable success as an antiemetic in patients undergoing ambulatory surgery. Lower doses seem to be more effective. In addition, recovery in ambulatory patients who receive the drug may be problematic.[175] The effects of low doses of droperidol (0.25 mg and 0.5 mg) and placebo, administered immediately after induction, were studied in patients who received prostaglandin for the termination of pregnancy.[156] Preoperative nausea (49 percent) and vomiting (29 percent) were similar in all groups. Preoperatively and postoperatively, the incidence of nausea and vomiting was unchanged in the placebo group. Although droperidol was effective in significantly reducing postoperative nausea (from 48 percent to 21 percent, lower dose; from 49 percent to 19 percent, higher dose), vomiting was significantly reduced only in the group that received the lower dose of droperidol (from 27 percent to 10 percent). Recovery times were not different for the three groups studied. In a study of 100 patients undergoing ambulatory oral surgery, droperidol 0.014 mg/kg or saline was administered intravenously 5 minutes after intubation.[157] The incidence of nausea and vomiting overall were 18 percent and 7 percent, respectively, in the droperidol group compared with 27 percent and 11 percent, respectively, in the saline group—a change not statistically significant. At 6 to 12 hours after anesthesia, slightly more patients given droperidol were nauseated than those given saline. In addition, the time to orientation was similar in both groups. More patients given saline could walk a straight line at 30 minutes after anesthesia, but this number was not significantly different at 60 minutes. Perceptual speed was better at both 30 and 60 minutes in patients who received saline. In a different study, droperidol 1.25 mg and droperidol 0.25 mg were compared with placebo in patients undergoing ambulatory dental surgery.[158] The lower dose of droperidol reduced nausea (35 percent, placebo group; 10 percent, low-dose droperidol group) without delaying recovery times (time to opening eyes on command). The higher dose of droperidol did not reduce nausea and prolonged recovery time significantly (2 minute increase); discharge times, however, were not different.

For decreasing the incidence of nausea and vomiting, the relative effectiveness of droperidol, compared with metoclopramide, is highly variable. In one study comparing droperidol 1.25 mg with metoclopramide 10 mg, droperidol did not decrease nausea and vomiting, and recovery times were similar.[128] Conversely, in another study, both droperidol 2.5 mg and metoclopramide 10 mg decreased the incidence of nausea or vomiting; patients treated with either drug were no more sedated than those given placebo, although, interestingly, patients receiving droperidol had significantly less complaints of postoperative pain than patients who received metoclopramide.[132]

Transdermal Scopolamine

Scopolamine has been effective in preventing motion sickness. However, when it is administered orally or parenterally, its duration of action is short and the incidence of side effects is relatively high. A transdermal delivery system for the drug has been developed that circumvents these problems. When a patch is applied behind the ear, it is effective for up to 72 hours and the levels of scopolamine achieved in the blood are quite low. In one study, using a modified radioreceptor assay, scopolamine was detected in 4 of 12 volunteers given the drug transdermally.[159] In those four, peak plasma concentrations were obtained after 8 hours and were relatively stable after that time. Side effects include dry mouth, drowsiness, blurred vision, and mydriasis. Because it produces dry mouth, transdermal scopolamine has been used in treating patients with sialorrhea and drooling, or those having surgery for oral, laryngeal, and pharyngeal lesions.[160]

In one study using volunteers, motion sickness was provoked by having subjects in a slowly rotating room execute head movements outside of the room's plane of rotation.[161] Transdermal scopolamine produced a 63 percent reduction in motion-induced symptoms compared with 75 percent for oral scopolamine and 86 percent for a combination of promethazine and ephedrine. In another study of 96 female patients scheduled for ambulatory surgery, patients were randomly selected to receive either transdermal scopolamine 45 to 60 minutes before the induction of anesthesia, intravenous droperidol 1.25 mg 5 minutes before the end of surgery, or placebo.[162] Sedation was greater after droperidol, but nausea over the following 24 hours was less with both transdermal scopolamine or droperidol. Actual vomiting on the ward, however, did not differ between the groups. In addition, visual disturbances were more frequent after transdermal scopolamine. In another study comparing transdermal scopolamine and placebo in 40 patients undergoing minor gynecologic surgery, patients receiving transdermal scopolamine the evening before surgery had significantly less nausea (45 percent) than those receiving placebo (75 percent).[163] Perhaps the earlier application of the scopolamine patch provided for a more rapid achievement of a therapeutic plasma concentration. Additional information about this drug can be found in a review by Clissold and Heel.[164] Further investigation of transdermal scopolamine is warranted in the ambulatory surgery setting.

Recommendations

It is advisable to consider prophylactic drug treatment for nausea only for patients who have had a prior history of severe nausea and vomiting after anesthesia, or for those who get nauseated easily, e.g., they get car sickness frequently. For patients who are seen 24 hours prior to the procedure, transdermal scopolamine can be administered with instructions to apply the patch the night before surgery. Otherwise, droperidol 0.25 mg can be given in the operating room immediately before induction of anesthesia.

PROPHYLACTIC ANTIBIOTICS

Surgical wounds are either clean, potentially contaminated (e.g., in procedures in which a bronchus, the gastrointestinal (GI) tract, or the oral-pharyngeal tract are entered), contaminated, or dirty.[165] In clean wounds, bacterial contamination is generally small and the major source of infection is the patient's skin, the operating room environment, or the surgical team. In contaminated procedures where there is either gross contamination or active infection, the amount of infection is related to the inoculum that soils the wound. Prophylactic antibiotics have minimal use for operations that are clean or that present little risk of sepsis. They may be useful, however, in decreasing the incidence of wound infections for trauma or burn surgery; for surgery in areas that are infected, heavily contaminated, or that have an impoverished blood supply or considerable tissue destruction; for operations that are long; for surgery in cases in which active infection is present but remote from the operative site; and for surgery in individuals who are obese, diabetic, elderly, malnourished, immunosupressed, or taking steroids.[166,167] Antibiotic usage must not be taken lightly: some individuals can develop hypersensitivity phenomenon, and antibiotic usage may contribute to antibiotic resistance of indigenous hospital flora.

Prophylactic antibiotic administration is most effective when given at the time of, or immediately prior to, exposure to possible pathogens. In one animal study, antibiotics given before bacterial contamination significantly decreased the magnitude of cutaneous infection compared with that found in control; antibiotics given 3 to 5 hours after bacterial inoculation were ineffective.[168] In a similar study, as the time interval between bacterial injection to produce dermal lesions and antibiotic administration increased, antibiotic effect decreased until 3 hours after lesion induction, when the lesion produced was no different in size than that in the control.[169]

The cephalosporins are well-suited for use as prophylactic antibiotics because of their wide spectrum of effectiveness and because they need not be supplemented by other antibiotics. They are, in fact, probably the most commonly used prophylactic antibiotic for surgery. For example, in a retrospective study of 5,288 patients in Pennsylvania in 1974, the cephalosporins were the most common antibiotic administered prophylactically.[170] Many studies have shown that antibiotics are more effective than placebo when used prophylactically prior to surgery. No study, however, has shown that one cephalosporin is more effective than another.[171] A study to demonstrate a difference, for a clean operation with an infection rate of 2 percent, would require more than 2,000 patients to show a

50 percent decrease in infection rate at the $P < 0.05$ level, and the number of patients enrolled in such studies is usually much smaller.

Antimicrobial prophylaxis is also useful in preventing endocarditis in patients with valvular heart disease, prosthetic heart valves, and other cardiac abnormalities in procedures that are associated with transient bacteremia.[172] Patients with mitral valve prolapse are also at an increased risk of developing endocarditis.[173] Streptococci from the mouth, enterococci from the GI or genitourinary tract, and staphylococci from the skin can cause endocarditis, and antimicrobials used for endocarditis prophylaxis are directed toward these organisms. Endotracheal intubation is not an indication for antibiotic prophylaxis unless it is associated with other procedures in which prophylaxis is indicated.[174] Recommendations for endocarditis prophylaxis in adults are listed in Table 10-1.

SUMMARY

Premedication to relieve anxiety may seem desirable but has not been universally accepted in outpatient surgery because of the desire not to delay "home readiness" and because of the side effects of preme-

Table 10-1. Recommended Antibiotic Regimens for Patients in Whom Endocarditis Prophylaxis is Indicated[174]

	Before procedure[a]	After first dose[b]
Dental procedures[c]		
Standard therapy (choose A or B)		
A. Penicillin V	2.0 g PO 1 hr	1.0 g PO 6 hr
B. Aqueous penicillin G	2 × 10^6 units IV or IM 30–60 min	1 × 10^6 units IV or IM 6 hr
Penicillin-allergic standard therapy		
Erythromycin	1.0 g PO 1 hr	500 mg PO 6 hr
Maximal therapy (choose A and B; C may be substituted for parenteral regimen [A and B] after the first dose)		
A. Ampicillin	1.0–2.0 g IV or IM 30 min	1.0–2.0 g IV or IM 8 hr
B. Gentamicin	1.5 mg/kg IV or IM 30 min	1.5 mg/kg IV or IM 8 hr
C. Penicillin V		1.0 g PO 6 hr
Penicillin-allergic maximal therapy		
Vancomycin	1.0 g IV slowly over 1 hr starting 1 hr before	Not necessary
Gastrointestinal/genitourinary procedures[d]		
Standard therapy (choose A and B)		
A. Ampicillin	2.0 g IV or IM 30–60 min	2.0 g IV or IM 8 hr
B. Gentamicin	1.5 mg/kg IV or IM 8 hr	1.5 mg/kg IV or IM 8 hr
Penicillin-allergic standard therapy (choose A and B)		
A. Vancomycin	1.0 g IV slowly over 1 hr starting 1 hr before	1.0 g IV (slowly over 1 hr) 8–12 hr
B. Gentamicin	1.5 mg/kg IV or IM 1 hr	1.5 mg/kg IV or IM 8–12 hr
Low-risk therapy		
Amoxicillin	3.0 g PO 1 hr	1.5 g PO 6 hr

[a] The dose and time the dose should be administered before the procedure.

[b] The dose and time of the second dose in relation to the first dose.

[c] Standard therapy for dental procedures is indicated for all procedures that cause gingival bleeding and oral/respiratory tract surgery. Maximal therapy for dental procedures is indicated for patients at particularly high risk, e.g., those with prosthetic heart valves or surgically constructed systemic-pulmonary shunts.

[d] Low-risk therapy for gastrointestinal/genitourinary procedures is indicated for procedures such as liver biopsy, upper gastrointestinal endoscopy or proctosigmoidoscopy without biopsy, barium enema, uncomplicated vaginal delivery, and brief bladder catheterization with sterile urine.

dicant drugs. However, control of anxiety in the very anxious patient would seem, at the very least, to be humane. In addition, the appropriate titration of drug does not seem to prolong hospital stay. Prophylaxis for every outpatient against acid aspiration pneumonitis is controversial. Drugs are available to increase gastric pH and decrease gastric volume; however, there are no controlled studies of outpatients showing that these drugs actually decrease the incidence of aspiration and/or the morbidity associated with it, and these medications are not without side effects of their own. Nausea is a problem that can prolong the ambulatory patient's stay in the hospital; for this reason, drugs must be avoided that contribute to nausea, and drug therapy that can help to alleviate the problem should be considered. Preoperative antibiotics are useful for certain kinds of outpatient surgery. Among prophylactic antibiotics, the cephalosporins are currently the most frequently used prior to outpatient surgery.

REFERENCES

1. Egbert LD, Battit GE, Turndorf H, Beecher HK: The value of the preoperative visit by an anesthetist. JAMA 185:553, 1963
2. McNair DM, Lorr M, Droppleman LF: Profile of Mood States. Educational and Industrial Testing Service, San Diego, 1971
3. Lichtor JL, Johanson CE, Mhoon D, et al: Preoperative anxiety: does anxiety level the afternoon before surgery predict anxiety level just before surgery? Anesthesiology 67:595, 1987
4. Johnston M: Anxiety in surgical patients. Psychol Med 10:145, 1980
5. Wallace LM: Psychological preparation as a method of reducing the stress of surgery. J Human Stress 10:62, 1984
6. Leigh JM, Walker J, Janaganathan P: Effect of preoperative anaesthetic visit on anxiety. Br Med J 2:987, 1977
7. Weis OF, Sriwatanakul K, Weintraub M, Lasagna L: Reduction of anxiety and postoperative analgesic requirements by audiovisual instruction. Lancet 1:43, 1983
8. Benson H, Beary JF, Carol MP: The relaxation response. Psychiatry 37:37, 1974
9. Benson H: Systemic hypertension and the relaxation response. N Engl J Med 296:1152, 1977
10. Benson H, Alexander S, Feldman CL: Decreased premature ventricular contractions through use of the relaxation response in patients with stable ischaemic heart-disease. Lancet 2:380, 1975
11. Berlin RM: Management of insomnia in hospitalized patients. Ann Intern Med 100:398, 1984
12. Domar AD, Noe JM, Benson H: The preoperative use of the relaxation response with ambulatory surgery patients. J Human Stress 13:101, 1987
13. Joborn C, Hetta J, Palmér M, et al: Psychiatric symptomatology in patients with primary hyperparathyroidism. Ups J Med Sci 91:77, 1986
14. Karhunen U, Jönn G: A comparison of memory function following local and general anesthesia for extraction of senile cataract. Acta Anaesthesiol Scand 26:291, 1982
15. Greenblatt DJ, Locniskar A, Ochs HR, Lauven PM: Automated gas chromatography for studies of midazolam pharmacokinetics. Anesthesiology 55:176, 1981
16. Dundee JW: New I.V. anaesthetics. Br J Anaesth 51:641, 1979
17. Dundee JW, Samuel IO, Toner W, Howard PJ: Midazolam: a water-soluble benzodiazepine. Anaesthesia 35:454, 1980
18. Pagano RR, Graham CW, Galligan M, et al: Histopathology of veins after intravenous lorazepam and RO21-3981. Can Anaesth Soc J 25:50, 1978
19. Clark MS, Silverstone LM, Coke JM, Hicks J: Midazolam, diazepam, and placebo as intravenous sedatives for dental surgery. Oral Surg Oral Med Oral Pathol 63:127, 1987
20. Barclay JK, Hunter KM, McMillan W: Midazolam and diazepam compared as sedatives for outpatient surgery under local analgesia. Oral Surg Oral Med Oral Pathol 59:349, 1985
21. Raybould D, Bradshaw EG: Premedication

for day case surgery. A study of oral midazolam. Anaesthesia 42:591, 1987
22. Driessen JJ, Smets MJW, Goey LS, Booij LHDJ: Comparison of diazepam and midazolam as oral premedicants for bronchoscopy under local anesthesia. Acta Anaesthesiol Belg 33:99, 1982
23. van Wijhe M, de Voogt-Frenkel E, Stijnen T: Midazolam versus fentanyl/droperidol and placebo as intramuscular premedicant. Acta Anaesthesiol Scand 29:409, 1985
24. van der Bijl P, Roelofse JA, de v. Joubert JJ, Breytenbach HS: Intravenous midazolam in oral surgery. Int J Oral Maxillofac Surg 16:325, 1987
25. Barker I, Butchart DGM, Gibson J, et al: I.V. sedation for conservative dentistry. A comparison of midazolam and diazepam. Br J Anaesth 58:371, 1986
26. Vinik HR, Reves JG, Wright D: Premedication with intramuscular midazolam: a prospective randomized double-blind controlled study. Anesth Analg 61:933, 1982
27. O'Boyle CA, Harris D, Barry H, et al: Comparison of midazolam by mouth and diazepam I.V. in outpatient oral surgery. Br J Anaesth 59:746, 1987
28. Feldmeier C, Kapp W: Comparative clinical studies with midazolam, oxazepam and placebo. Br J Clin Pharmacol 16:suppl 1;151S, 1983
29. Berggren L, Eriksson I: Midazolam for induction of anaesthesia in outpatients: a comparison with thiopentone. Acta Anaesthesiol Scand 25:492, 1981
30. Reves JG, Vinik R, Hirschfield AM, et al: Midazolam compared with thiopentone as a hypnotic component in balanced anaesthesia: a randomized, double-blind study. Can Anaesth Soc J 26:42, 1979
31. Wolff J, Carl P, Clausen TG, Mikkelsen BO: Ro 15-1788 for postoperative recovery. A randomized clinical trial in patients undergoing minor surgical procedures under midazolam anaesthesia. Anaesthesia 41:1001, 1986
32. Alexander CM, Gross JB: Sedative doses of midazolam depress hypoxic ventilatory responses in humans. Anesth Analg 67:377, 1988
33. Castleden CM, Allen JG, Altman J, St. John-Smith P: A comparison of oral midazolam, nitrazepam and placebo in young and elderly subjects. Eur J Clin Pharmacol 32:253, 1987
34. Bell GD, Spickett GP, Reeve PA, et al: Intravenous midazolam for upper gastrointestinal endoscopy: a study of 800 consecutive cases relating dose to age and sex of patients. Br J Clin Pharmacol 23:241, 1987
35. Brophy T, Dundee JW, Heazelwood V, et al: Midazolam, a water-soluble benzodiazepine, for gastroscopy. Anaesth Intensive Care 10:344, 1982
36. Kanto J, Aaltonen L, Himberg JJ, Hovi-Viander M: Midazolam as an intravenous induction agent in the elderly: a clinical and pharmacokinetic study. Anesth Analg 65:15, 1986
37. Dundee JW, Halliday NJ, Loughran PG, Harper KW: The influence of age on the onset of anaesthesia with midazolam. Anaesthesia 40:441, 1985
38. Hegarty JE, Dundee JW: Sequelae after the intravenous injection of three benzodiazepines—diazepam, lorazepam and flunitrazepam. Br Med J 2:1384, 1977
39. Klotz U, Antonin KH, Bieck PR: Pharmacokinetics and plasma binding of diazepam in man, dog, rabbit, guinea pig and rat. J Pharmacol Exp Ther 199:67, 1976
40. Randall LO, Scheckel CL, Banziger RF: Pharmacology of the metabolites of chlordiazepoxide and diazepam. Curr Ther Res 7:590, 1965
41. Linnoila M, Korttila K, Mattila MJ: Effect of food and repeated injections on serum diazepam levels. Acta Pharmacol Toxicol 36:181, 1975
42. Jakobsen H, Hertz JB, Johansen JR, et al: Premedication before day surgery. A double-blind comparison of diazepam and placebo. Br J Anaesth 57:300, 1985
43. White PF, Vasconez LO, Mathes SA, et al: Comparison of midazolam and diazepam for sedation during plastic surgery. Plast Reconstr Surg 81:703, 1988
44. Klotz U, Avant GR, Hoyumpa A, et al: The effects of age and liver disease on the disposition and elimination of diazepam in adult man. J Clin Invest 55:347, 1975
45. Reidenberg MM, Levy M, Warner H, et al: Relationship between diazepam dose,

plasma level, age, and central nervous system depression. Clin Pharmacol Ther 23:371, 1978
46. Giles HG, MacLeod SM, Wright JR, Sellers EM: Influence of age and previous use on diazepam dosage required for endoscopy. Can Med Assoc J 118:513, 1978
47. Greenblatt DJ, Shader RI, Franke K, et al: Pharmacokinetics and bioavailability of intravenous, intramuscular, and oral lorazepam in humans. J Pharm Sci 68:57, 1979
48. Dundee JW, McGowan WAW, Lilburn JK, et al: Comparison of the actions of diazepam and lorazepam. Br J Anaesth 51:439, 1979
49. Dundee JW, Lilburn JK, Nair SG, George KA: Studies of drugs given before anaesthesia. XXVI: lorazepam. Br J Anaesth 49:1047, 1977
50. Eberts FS, Jr., Philopoulos Y, Reineke LM, Vliek RW: Triazolam disposition. Clin Pharmacol Ther 29:81, 1981
51. Pinnock CA, Fell D, Hunt PCW, et al: A comparison of triazolam and diazepam as premedication agents for minor gynaecological surgery. Anaesthesia 40:324, 1985
52. Thomas D, Tipping T, Halifax R, et al: Triazolam premedication: a comparison with lorazepam and placebo in gynaecological patients. Anaesthesia 41:692, 1986
53. U.S. is asked to sharply limit use of sedative. New York Times, Sec 1, p 37, February 14, 1988
54. Leary WE: House report faults F.D.A. approval of sedative. New York Times, Sec C p 11, October 18, 1988
55. Physicians' Desk Reference, 41st ed. Medical Economics Co., Oradell, New Jersey, p. 1685
56. Physicians' Desk Reference, 42nd ed. Medical Economics Co., Oradell, New Jersey, p. 1754
57. Khanderia U, Pandit SK: Use of midazolam hydrochloride in anesthesia. Clin Pharm 6:533, 1987
58. Forster A, Gardaz JP, Suter PM, Gemperle M: I.V. midazolam as an induction agent for anaesthesia: a study in volunteers. Br J Anaesth 52:907, 1980
59. Sunzel M, Paalzow L, Berggren L, Eriksson I: Respiratory and cardiovascular effects in relation to plasma levels of midazolam and diazepam. Br J Clin Pharmacol 25:561, 1988
60. Samuelson PN, Reves JG, Kouchoukos NT, et al: Hemodynamic responses to anesthetic induction with midazolam or diazepam in patients with ischemic heart disease. Anesth Analg 60:802, 1981
61. Spiess BD, Sathoff RH, El-Ganzouri ARS, Ivankovich AD: High-dose sufentanil: four cases of sudden hypotension on induction. Anesth Analg 65:703, 1986
62. West JM, Estrada S, Heerdt M: Sudden hypotension associated with midazolam and sufentanil. Anesth Analg 66:693, 1987 (letter)
63. Massaut J, d'Hollander A, Barvais L, Dubois-Primo J: Haemodynamic effects of midazolam in the anaesthetized patient with coronary artery disease. Acta Anaesthesiol Scand 27:299, 1983
64. Heikkilä H, Jalonen J, Arola M, et al: Midazolam as adjunct to high-dose fentanyl anaesthesia for coronary artery bypass grafting operation. Acta Anaesthesiol Scand 28:683, 1984
65. Marty J, Gauzit R, Lefevre P, et al: Effects of diazepam and midazolam on baroreflex control of heart rate and on sympathetic activity in humans. Anesth Analg 65:113, 1986
66. Kotrly KJ, Ebert TJ, Vucins E, et al: Baroreceptor reflex control of heart rate during isoflurane anesthesia in humans. Anesthesiology 60:173, 1984
67. Arcos GJ: Midazolam-induced ventricular irritability. Anesthesiology 67:612, 1987 (letter)
68. Bell GD, Reeve PA, Moshiri M, et al: Intravenous midazolam: a study of the degree of oxygen desaturation occurring during upper gastrointestinal endoscopy. Br J Clin Pharmacol 23:703, 1987
69. Forster A, Gardaz JP, Suter PM, Gemperle M: Respiratory depression by midazolam and diazepam. Anesthesiology 53:494, 1980
70. Knill R, Cosgrove JF, Olley PM, Levison H: Components of respiratory depression after narcotic premedication in adolescents. Can Anaesth Soc J 23:449, 1976
71. Gross JB, Zebrowski ME, Carel WD, et al: Time course of ventilatory depression after

thiopental and midazolam in normal subjects and in patients with chronic obstructive pulmonary disease. Anesthesiology 58:540, 1983

72. Asch DA, Parker RM: The Libby Zion case. One step forward or two steps backward? N Engl J Med 318:771, 1988
73. Price WJ, Holley DC: The last minutes of flight 2860: an analysis of crew shift work scheduling. p. 287. In Reinberg A, Vieux N, Andlauer P (eds): Night and Shift Work. Biological and Social Aspects. Pergamon Press, Oxford, 1981
74. Ehret CF: New approaches to chronohygiene for the shift worker in the nuclear power industry. p. 263. In Reinberg A, Vieux N, Andlauer P (eds): Night and Shift Work. Biological and Social Aspects. Pergamon Press, Oxford, 1981
75. Shafer A, White PF, Urquhart ML, Doze VA: Outpatient premedication: use of midazolam and opioid analgesics. Anesthesiology 71:495, 1989
76. Korttila K, Ghoneim MM, Jacobs L, Lakes RS: Evaluation of instrumented force platform as a test to measure residual effects of anesthetics. Anesthesiology 55:625, 1981
77. Korttila K, Linnoila M: Recovery and skills related to driving after intravenous sedation: dose-response relationship with diazepam. Br J Anaesth 47:457, 1975
78. Galletly D, Forrest P, Purdie G: Comparison of the recovery characteristics of diazepam and midazolam. Br J Anaesth 60:520, 1988
79. Nightingale JJ, Norman J: A comparison of midazolam and temazepam for premedication of day case patients. Anaesthesia 43:111, 1988
80. Korttila K, Tarkkanen J: Comparison of diazepam and midazolam for sedation during local anaesthesia for bronchoscopy. Br J Anaesth 57:581, 1985
81. Clyburn P, Kay NH, McKenzie PJ: Effects of diazepam and midazolam on recovery from anaesthesia in outpatients. Br J Anaesth 58:872, 1986
82. Pandit SK, Heisterkamp DV, Cohen PJ: Further studies of the anti-recall effect of lorazepam: a dose-time-effect relationship. Anesthesiology 45:495, 1976
83. Philip BK: Hazards of amnesia after midazolam in ambulatory surgical patients. Anesth Analg 66:97, 1987 (letter)
84. Raeder JC, Breivik H: Premedication with midazolam in out-patient general anaesthesia. A comparison with morphine-scopolamine and placebo. Acta Anaesthesiol Scand 31:509, 1987
85. Roberts RB, Shirley MA: Reducing the risk of acid aspiration during cesarean section. Anesth Analg 53:859, 1974
86. James CF, Modell JH, Gibbs CP, et al: Pulmonary aspiration-effects of volume and pH in the rat. Anesth Analg 63:665, 1984
87. Manchikanti L, Canella MG, Hohlbein LJ, Colliver JA: Assessment of effect of various modes of premedication on acid aspiration risk factors in outpatient surgery. Anesth Analg 66:81, 1987
88. Manchikanti L, Grow JB, Colliver JA, et al: Bicitra® (sodium citrate) and metoclopramide in outpatient anesthesia for prophylaxis against aspiration pneumonitis. Anesthesiology 63:378, 1985
89. Manchikanti L, Roush JR: Effect of preanesthetic glycopyrrolate and cimetidine on gastric fluid pH and volume in outpatients. Anesth Analg 63:40, 1984
90. Pandit SK, Kothary SP, Pandit UA, Mirakhur RK: Premedication with cimetidine and metoclopramide. Effect on the risk factors of acid aspiration. Anaesthesia 41:486, 1986
91. Manchikanti L, Colliver JA, Roush JR, Canella MG: Evaluation of ranitidine as an oral antacid in outpatient anesthesia. South Med J 78:818, 1985
92. Ong BY, Palahniuk RJ, Cumming M: Gastric volume and pH in out-patients. Can Anaesth Soc J 25:36, 1978
93. Vaughan RW, Bauer S, Wise L: Volume and pH of gastric juice in obese patients. Anesthesiology 43:686, 1975
94. Wright DJ, Pandya A: Smoking and gastric juice volume in outpatients. Can Anaesth Soc J 26:328, 1979
95. Spielberger CD, Jacobs GA: Personality and smoking behavior. J Pers Assess 46:396, 1982
96. Mahl GF, Karpe R: Emotions and hydrochloric acid secretion during psychoanalytic hours. Psychosom Med 15:312, 1953
97. Gray SJ, Ramsey CG: Adrenal influences upon the stomach and the gastric responses

to stress. Recent Prog Horm Res 13:583, 1957

98. Wyner J, Cohen SE: Gastric volume in early pregnancy: effect of metoclopramide. Anesthesiology 57:209, 1982
99. Hjortsø E, Mondorf T: Does oral premedication increase the risk of gastric aspiration? Acta Anaesthesiol Scand 26:505, 1982
100. McGrady EM, Macdonald AG: Effect of the preoperative administration of water on gastric volume and pH. Br J Anaesth 60:803, 1988
101. Hutchinson A, Maltby JR, Reid CRG: Gastric fluid volume and pH in elective inpatients. Part I: coffee or orange juice versus overnight fast. Can J Anaesth 35:12, 1988
102. Miller M, Wishart HY, Nimmo WS: Gastric contents at induction of anaesthesia. Is a 4-hour fast necessary? Br J Anaesthesia 55:1185, 1983
103. Sutherland AD, Maltby JR, Sale JP, Reid CRG: The effect of pre-operative oral fluid and ranitidine on gastric fluid volume and pH. Can J Anaesth 34:117, 1987
104. Maltby JR, Sutherland AD, Sale JP, Shaffer EA: Preoperative oral fluids: is a five-hour fast justified prior to elective surgery? Anesth Analg 65:1112, 1986
105. Douglas WW: Histamine and 5-hydroxytryptamine (serotonin) and their antagonists. p. 624. In Gilman AG, Goodman LS, Rall TW, Mural F (eds): The Pharmacological Basis of Therapeutics. 7th Ed. Macmillan, New York, 1985
106. Stock JGL, Sutherland AD: The role of H_2 receptor antagonist premedication in pregnant day care patients. Can Anaesth Soc J 32:463, 1985
107. Klotz U, Reimann I: Delayed clearance of diazepam due to cimetidine. N Engl J Med 302:1012, 1980
108. Patwardhan RV, Yarborough GW, Desmond PV, et al: Cimetidine spares the glucuronidation of lorazepam and oxazepam. Gastroenterology 79:912, 1980
109. Feely J, Wilkinson GR, Wood AJJ: Reduction of liver blood flow and propranolol metabolism by cimetidine. N Engl J Med 304:692, 1981
110. Sedman AJ: Cimetidine-drug interactions. Am J Med 76:109, 1984
111. Noble DW, Smith KJ, Dundas CR: Effects of H-2 antagonists on the elimination of bupivacaine. Br J Anaesth 59:735, 1987
112. Smith SR, Kendall MJ: Ranitidine versus cimetidine. A comparison of their potential to cause clinically important drug interactions. Clin Pharmacokinet 15:44, 1988
113. Berardi RR, Tankanow RM, Nostrant TT: Comparison of famotidine with cimetidine and ranitidine. Clin Pharm 7:271, 1988
114. Callaghan JT, Bergstrom RF, Rubin A, et al: A pharmacokinetic profile of nizatidine in man. Scand J Gastroenterol [Suppl] 136:9, 1987
115. Pasanen M, Arvela P, Pelkonen O, et al: Effect of five structurally diverse H_2-receptor antagonists on drug metabolism. Biochem Pharmacol 35:4457, 1986
116. Campion EW, Avorn J, Reder VA, Olins NJ: Overmedication of the low-weight elderly. Arch Intern Med 147:945, 1987
117. Schentag JJ, Cerra FB, Calleri G, et al: Pharmacokinetic and clinical studies in patients with cimetidine-associated mental confusion. Lancet 1:177, 1979
118. Silverstone PH: Ranitidine and mental confusion. Lancet 1:1071, 1984 (letter)
119. Epstein CM: Ranitidine and mental confusion. Lancet 1:1071, 1984 (letter)
120. Henderson GI, Speeg KV, Jr., Roberts RK, et al: Effect of aging on hepatic elimination of cimetidine and subsequent interaction of aging and cimetidine on aminopyrine metabolism. Biochem Pharmacol 37:2667, 1988
121. Young CJ, Daneshmend TK, Roberts CJ: Effects of cirrhosis and ageing on the elimination and bioavailability of ranitidine. Gut 23:819, 1982
122. Greene DS, Szego PL, Anslow JA, Hooper JW: The effect of age on ranitidine pharmacokinetics. Clin Pharmacol Ther 39:300, 1986
123. Divoll M, Greenblatt DJ, Abernethy DR, Shader RI: Cimetidine impairs clearance of antipyrine and desmethyldiazepam in the elderly. J Am Geriatr Soc 30:684, 1982
124. Eyler SW, Cullen BF, Murphy ME, Welch WD: Antacid aspiration in rabbits: a comparison of Mylanta and Bicitra. Anesth Analg 61:288, 1982
125. Albibi R, McCallum RW: Metoclopramide: pharmacology and clinical application. Ann Intern Med 98:86, 1983

126. Rao TLK, Madhavareddy S, Chinthagada M, El-Etr AA: Metoclopramide and cimetidine to reduce gastric fluid pH and volume. Anesth Analg 63:1014, 1984
127. Proctor JD, Chremos AN, Evans EF, Wasserman AJ: An apomorphine-induced vomiting model for antiemetic studies in man. J Clin Pharmacol 18:95, 1978
128. Cohen SE, Woods WA, Wyner J: Antiemetic efficacy of droperidol and metoclopramide. Anesthesiology 60:67, 1984
129. Dundee JW, Clarke RSJ, Howard PJ: Studies of drugs given before anaesthesia. XXIII: metoclopramide. Br J Anaesth 46:509, 1974
130. Chestnut DH, Vandewalker GE, Owen CL, et al: Administration of metoclopramide for prevention of nausea and vomiting during epidural anesthesia for elective cesarean section. Anesthesiology 66:563, 1987
131. Miller CD, Anderson WG: Silent regurgitation in day case gynaecological patients. Anaesthesia 43:321, 1988
132. Madej TH, Simpson KH: Comparison of the use of domperidone, droperidol and metoclopramide in the prevention of nausea and vomiting following gynaecological surgery in day cases. Br J Anaesth 58:879, 1986
133. Fell D, Cotton BR, Smith G: IM atropine and regurgitation. Br J Anaesth 55:256, 1983 (letter)
134. Conner JT, Herr G, Katz RL, et al: Droperidol, fentanyl and morphine for i.v. surgical premedication. Br J Anaesth 50:463, 1978
135. Dionne RA: Differential pharmacology of drugs used for intravenous premedication. J Dent Res 63:842, 1984
136. Morrison JD: Studies of drugs given before anaesthesia. XXII: phenoperidine and fentanyl, alone and in combination with droperidol. Br J Anaesth 42:1119, 1970
137. Van de Velde A, Camu F, Claeys MA: Midazolam for intramuscular premedication: dose-effect relationships compared to diazepam, fentanyl and fentanyl-droperidol in a placebo controlled study. Acta Anaesthesiol Belg 37:127, 1986
138. Scamman FL, Klein SL, Choi WW: Conscious sedation for procedures under local or topical anesthesia. Ann Otol Rhinol Laryngol 94:21, 1985
139. Dundee JW, Kirwan MJ, Clarke RSJ: Anaesthesia and premedication as factors in postoperative vomiting. Acta Anaesthesiol Scand 9:223, 1965
140. Riding JE: Post-operative vomiting. Proc R Soc Med 53:671, 1960
141. Clark AJM, Hurtig JB: Premedication with meperidine and atropine does not prolong recovery to street fitness after out-patient surgery. Can Anaesth Soc J 28:390, 1981
142. Lundgren S: Comparison of rectal diazepam and subcutaneous morphine-scopolamine administration for outpatient sedation in minor oral surgery. Acta Anaesthesiol Scand 29:674, 1985
143. Bone ME, Dowson S, Smith G: A comparison of nalbuphine with fentanyl for postoperative pain relief following termination of pregnancy under day care anaesthesia. Anaesthesia 43:194, 1988
144. Pandit SK, Kothary SP, Pandit UA, Mathai MK: Comparison of fentanyl and butorphanol for outpatient anaesthesia. Can J Anaesth 34:130, 1987
145. White PF, Coe V, Shafer A, Sung ML: Comparison of alfentanil with fentanyl for outpatient anesthesia. Anesthesiology 64:99, 1986
146. Brown EM, Kunjappan VE, Alexander GD: Fentanyl/alfentanil for pelvic laparoscopy. Can Anaesth Soc J 31:251, 1984
147. Forrest WH, Jr., Brown CR, Brown BW: Subjective responses to six common preoperative medications. Anesthesiology 47:241, 1977
148. Sengupta A, Gupta PK, Pandey K: Investigation of glycopyrrolate as a premedicant drug. Br J Anaesth 52:513, 1980
149. Mirakhur RK, Reid J, Elliott J: Volume and pH of gastric contents following anticholinergic premedication. Anaesthesia 34:453, 1979
150. Mirakhur RK, Dundee JW, Connolly JDR: Studies of drugs given before anaesthesia. XVII: anticholinergic premedicants. Br J Anaesth 51:339, 1979
151. Dawson B, Reed WA: Anaesthesia for day-care surgery: a symposium (III). Anaes-

thesia for adult surgical out-patients. Can Anaesth Soc J 27:409, 1980
152. Knapp MR, Beecher HK: Postanesthetic nausea, vomiting, and retching. Evaluation of the antiemetic drugs dimenhydrinate (Dramamine), chlorpromazine, and pentobarbital sodium. JAMA 160:376, 1956
153. Howat DDC: Anti-emetic drugs in anaesthesia. A double blind trial of two phenothiazine derivatives. Anaesthesia 15:289, 1960
154. Burtles R, Peckett BW: Postoperative vomiting. Some factors affecting its incidence. Br J Anaesth 29:114, 1957
155. Sutherland AD, Stock JG, Davies JM: Effects of preoperative fasting on morbidity and gastric contents in patients undergoing day-stay surgery. Br J Anaesth 58:876, 1986
156. Millar JM, Hall PJ: Nausea and vomiting after prostaglandins in day case termination of pregnancy. The efficacy of low dose droperidol. Anaesthesia 42:613, 1987
157. Valanne J, Korttila K: Effect of a small dose of droperidol on nausea, vomiting and recovery after outpatient enflurane anaesthesia. Acta Anaesthesiol Scand 29:359, 1985
158. O'Donovan N, Shaw J: Nausea and vomiting in day-case dental anaesthesia. The use of low-dose droperidol. Anaesthesia 39:1172, 1984
159. Muir C, Metcalfe R: A comparison of plasma levels of hyoscine after oral and transdermal administration. J Pharm Biomed Anal 1:363, 1983
160. Talmi YP, Finkelstein Y, Zohar Y, Laurian N: Reduction of salivary flow with Scopoderm TTS. Ann Otol Rhinol Laryngol 97:128, 1988
161. Graybiel A, Knepton J, Shaw J: Prevention of experimental motion sickness by scopolamine absorbed through the skin. Aviat Space Environ Med 47:1096, 1976
162. Tigerstedt I, Salmela L, Aromaa U: Double-blind comparison of transdermal scopolamine, droperidol and placebo against postoperative nausea and vomiting. Acta Anaesthesiol Scand 32:454, 1988
163. Tolksdorf W, Meisel R, Müller P, Bender HJ: Transdermales scopolamin (TTS-Scopolamin) zur prophylaxe postoperativer übelkeit und erbrechen. Anaesthesist 34:656, 1985
164. Clissold SP, Heel RC: Transdermal hyoscine (scopolamine). A preliminary review of its pharmacodynamic properties and therapeutic efficacy. Drugs 29:189, 1985
165. Postoperative wound infections: the influence of ultraviolet irradiation of the operating room and of various other factors. National Academy of Sciences, National Research Council, Division of Medical Sciences, Ad Hoc Committee on Trauma. Ann Surg 160:suppl. 2, 1, 1964
166. Nichols RL: Use of prophylactic antibiotics in surgical practice. Am J Med 70:686, 1981
167. Hunt TK: Surgical wound infections: an overview. Am J Med 70:712, 1981
168. Miles AA, Miles EM, Burke J: The value and duration of defence reactions of the skin to the primary lodgement of bacteria. Br J Exp Pathol 38:79, 1957
169. Burke JF: The effective period of preventive antibiotic action in experimental incisions and dermal lesions. Surgery 50:161, 1961
170. Shapiro M, Townsend TR, Rosner B, Kass EH: Use of antimicrobial drugs in general hospitals. N Engl J Med 301:351, 1979
171. Kaiser AB: Overview of cephalosporin prophylaxis. Am J Surg 155:52, 1988 (suppl.)
172. Prevention of bacterial endocarditis. Med Lett 26:3, 1983
173. Clemens JD, Horwitz RI, Jaffe CC, et al: A controlled evaluation of the risk of bacterial endocarditis in persons with mitral-valve prolapse. N Engl J Med 307:776, 1982
174. Shulman ST, Amren DP, Bisno AL, et al: Prevention of bacterial endocarditis. Committee report, American Heart Association. Circulation 70:1123A, 1984
175. Melnick B, Sawyer R, Karambelkar D, et al: Delayed side effects of droperidol after ambulatory general anesthesia. Anesth Analg 69:748, 1989

11

Monitoring Techniques

Casey D. Blitt

Monitoring improves the administration of anesthesia with regard to effectiveness of drugs and techniques and recognition of adverse effects. Monitoring also allows early recognition of potentially life-threatening complications so that timely therapeutic intervention can avert disastrous consequences. Esophageal intubation, anesthesia circuit disconnection, errors in gas supply or flow, and anesthetic overdose are among the complications for which monitoring can provide early detection. Because of its ability to signal potential disasters, monitoring becomes an important patient safety consideration.

Monitoring is essentially data collection, and the information gathered alerts the anesthesiologist how to best manage the patient. Data may be collected manually, sensorially, or automatically. Although all of these methods are useful, automatic methods provide continual input and free the anesthesiologist from repetitive tasks, thereby allowing more time for making decisions. It must be noted, however, that automatic data collection has its drawbacks; occasionally there are false alarms, incorrect data display, and suboptimal performance. Consequently, monitoring modalities with redundancy or backup features are desirable to assure that adequate input can be received even if one system fails.

WHAT NEEDS MONITORING

Two broad areas in anesthesia requiring monitoring are easily identifiable: the anesthetic delivery system (machine, gas flows, ventilator, vaporizer, etc.) and the effect of the anesthetic on the patient. There is clearly an overlap of these areas. The effects of anesthesia on the patient may be categorized by organ system or by individual monitoring modalities.

It is my intent to discuss monitoring primarily by systems, with the exception of some modalities that affect so many systems that they must be discussed separately.

Monitoring the patient undergoing surgery and anesthesia on an ambulatory basis should be essentially no different than monitoring that would performed on the same patient if admitted to the hospital. The nature of surgical procedures performed in the ambulatory setting is such that some of the more invasive monitoring modalities, particularly those involving the cardiovascular system, are used infrequently. By such modalities, we refer to intra-arterial catheters, pulmonary artery catheters, and central vascular catheters.

ORGAN SYSTEMS

Central Nervous System

Operations using electroencephalographic monitoring, somatosensory evoked potentials, or monitoring of intracranial pressure are not likely to be utilized in the outpatient setting. Thus, the primary monitor for the central nervous system (CNS) is one that assesses depth of anesthesia. There is no uniformly applicable or consistently reliable measure of anesthetic depth. Lack of movement in response to a surgical stimulus (in the patient who has not received neuromuscular blocking drugs) is the best clinical indicator of anesthetic-induced CNS depression. We have developed a habit of using the autonomic nervous system to "mirror" anesthetic depth. The measurement of inspired and end-tidal anesthetic concentrations can allow us to use the ED_{50} (minimum alveolar concentration [MAC]) and ED_{95} to estimate adequate anesthesia. Measurement of lower esophageal contractility as a guide to the depth or adequacy of anesthesia could be used in intubated patients in the outpatient setting.[1] The ultimate usefulness and cost-effectiveness of this modality in outpatient anesthesia remains to be determined.

Cardiovascular System

Mechanical devices are appealing, but the senses of touch, hearing, and vision can be important in monitoring the cardiovascular system, particularly in the outpatient setting. Pulse palpation, capillary refill, color of the blood, and heart sounds may all be examined using the senses or the senses combined with simple instruments, such as a precordial or esophageal stethoscope. These modalities are quite subjective and virtually impossible to quantitate, with the exception of heart rate. In critical situations, the senses may be of value only to determine the presence or absence of a pulse or heart beat. In an era of mechanical devices, sensory modalities are most useful as backup systems for more sophisticated and quantitative monitoring devices. Precordial or esophageal stethoscopes should not necessarily be discarded, but pulse oximetry and capnography are much more important monitoring devices. Vigilance by machines should not replace vigilance by the anesthesiologist.

Blood Pressure

Blood pressure may be measured noninvasively by palpation, auscultation, or the oscillometric method. The palpation method derives systolic blood pressure only. The oscillometric method is used in most automatic blood pressure measuring devices.[2,3] The obvious advantage of automatic determination of blood pressure is that it allows measurements to be taken no matter what other tasks the anesthesiologist is performing.

An automatic blood pressure device should be available at every anesthetizing location. In addition, a recorder that can be attached to the automatic blood pressure device to produce a written record is an important consideration. The written record allows the information to be transferred at a later time to the anesthesia record, or it may be included as part of the permanent record if desired. The written blood pressure record is invaluable, as it represents "what actually happens" and serves as an "in-flight recorder" should a disaster occur.

Complications resulting from noninvasive blood pressure devices have been reported in the anesthesia literature. For example, nerve damage was reported secondary to continuous inflation of an automatic blood pressure cuff.[4] Petechiae secondary to pinching of the skin by the automatic blood pressure cuff also occur, but appear to be of no clinical significance.

A noninvasive, beat-to-beat blood pressure measurement device (FINAP) is in advanced stages of testing and development.[5] The finger blood pressure has been shown to reflect systemic arterial pressure accurately, but there are certain instances in which the modality is not effective. Beat-to-beat blood pressure measurement in such a noninvasive fashion may prove to be desirable in the ambulatory setting.

Electrical Activity of the Heart

Monitoring the electrical activity of the heart is routine anesthetic practice and constitutes one of the standards of monitoring care. The cost is moderate, the operation of equipment is not complicated, and the risk to patients is small. The use of the ECG is primarily for recognition of cardiac dysrhythmias, alterations in myocardial oxygen supply/demand balance, and electrical changes caused by electrolyte abnormalities. Standard leads I or II are best for dysrhythmia determination and a modified V_5 lead configuration is best for ischemia determination.[6] Equipping instruments for monitoring ECG activity with recording devices so that a written record of a tracing can be obtained is recommended. This is very important for documentation as well as for recognition of complex dysrhythmias and other abnormalities in the ECG.

Pulmonary System and Airway

Monitoring the adequacy of gas exchange in anesthetized patients is absolutely critical if hypoxia or hypercapnea is to be avoided. Hearing, vision, and touch can all be used to monitor the respiratory system and airway. Ausculation of breath sounds, visual inspection of chest excursion, visual observation of reservoir bag movement (spontaneous ventilation), the feel of the reservoir bag, and observation of blood color can all be examined using the senses, either alone or in combination with a stethoscope. However, these modalities are very subjective and make it difficult to quantitate pulmonary function. Auscultation of both lung fields in the midaxillary line as well as auscultation of the stomach to confirm tracheal placement of an endotracheal tube are exceptions to this rule.[7] Even auscultation, however, may fail to detect esophageal intubation or main stem bronchus placement.[8] The use of the senses as respiratory monitors is most effective as a backup system to more sophisticated and quantitative monitors.

Constituents of the Anesthetic Circuit

Monitoring all of the constituents of the anesthetic circuit represents the state of the art in indirect pulmonary and airway monitoring. The information may be obtained via a multiplexed mass spectrometer system or individual "stand alone" units.[9,10] Ideally, we should monitor all constituents of the anesthetic circuit, including oxygen, carbon dioxide, and nitrogen, as well as the anesthetic gases, which include nitrous oxide and the halogenated hydrocarbons.

The mass spectrometer is capable of sensing the individual masses of elements or molecules in a mixture of unknown composition and reporting the makeup of that mixture broken down into its individual parts.[9,10] Typically, gases are sampled from a side port on an elbow inserted between the endotracheal tube or mask and the Y piece of a circle system. An electric beam accelerates the gas ions in a high voltage field through a slit that creates a narrow ion beam. This beam passes through a magnetic field that deflects the heavier ions less, thus creating a spectrum of ions according to molecular weight. Each gas species is collected on a metal plate, from which the current is amplified as a measure of concentration of that gas.

Most "stand alone" gas analyzers operate on the principle of nondispersive infrared absorption.[9,10] Instruments are currently available to measure and display carbon dioxide, oxygen, nitrous oxide, and the halogenated hydrocarbons. The stand alone infrared gas analysis systems cannot measure nitrogen. Measuring the concentrations of those gas constituents of the anesthetic circuit can provide the following information[9,10]: An oxygen reading can verify fractional inspired oxygen concentration from flow meters, track end-tidal oxygen values during closed circuit anesthesia, and help evaluate oxygen uptake. Carbon dioxide measurements can verify that the endotracheal tube has been placed in the trachea, and can verify the adequacy of ventilation. A nitrogen reading can verify a leak-free anesthesia delivery system, monitor nitrogen washout during induction, and aid in detection of air emboli. A reading of nitrous oxide can verify inspired concentrations from flow meters, help evaluate uptake of nitrous oxide during anesthesia, and monitor washout during emergence and recovery. A reading for halogenated anesthetics can verify the inspired concentration of anesthetic being used, ascertain appropriate calibration of vaporizers, evaluate anesthetic washout during recovery, and evaluate uptake (end-tidal concentration) during anesthesia.

In one cost analysis, it was determined that discrete gas analyzers were less expensive than a multiplexed system when the number of locations to monitor was fewer than six.[10] This same evaluation stated that an average case cost of gas analysis (in 1985) was between $2 to $3 per anesthetic. Irrespective of anesthetic and respiratory gas monitoring, it is mandatory to monitor oxygen delivery by the anesthetic delivery apparatus. Gaseous oxygen may be analyzed by either paramagnetic analyzers or polarographic oxygen electrodes.[9] These devices have a relatively slow response time and function to indicate mean concentrations. Almost all of the oxygen analyzers now used on anesthesia machines use polarographic electrodes. The electrode contains a liquid electrolyte solution that must be replaced periodically. The electrode itself, as well as the batteries, requires occasional replacement.

Airway Pressure

Airway pressures should be measured with a pressure gauge preferably incorporated into the anesthesia machine breathing circuit.[7] Alarms should sound when a pressure that is too high or too low is encountered. Low circuit pressure alarms are mandatory if mechanical ventilation is used to allow early detection of anesthetic disconnections.

End-Tidal Gases

The ability to measure the volume of gas moving in and out of the patient's lungs with each breath (e.g., ventimeters) is critical to the safe administration of anesthesia. Devices that are currently available are primarily flow sensors and are available only with circle systems.[7] Although problems of inertia, friction, collection of moisture, and foreign material have been reported, ventimeters are invaluable and should be mandatorily incorporated into all anesthetic circuits. This modality will allow tidal volume as well as minute volume measurements.

End-tidal carbon dioxide allows us to assess alveolar ventilation in patients with relatively normal circulation and lung function.[7] It approximates arterial carbon dioxide with a small arterial-to-alveolar gradient. End-tidal carbon dioxide may be measured by infrared analysis or via a mass spectrometer system. Monitoring end-tidal carbon dioxide helps to determine optimal minute ventilation; alerts the anesthesiologist to conditions of no breathing that may be related to ventilator malfunction, circuit disconnect, or airway obstruction; and allows the detection of inspired carbon dioxide concentrations that may be due to exhausted soda lime. A critical function of end-tidal carbon dioxide measurement allows the identification of an esophageal intubation.[7,8] End-tidal carbon dioxide is virtually infallible in detecting esophageal intubation when endotracheal tube placement is in doubt. The measurement of end-tidal carbon dioxide (known as capnography) should be done for all patients receiving general anesthesia. It is highly desirable that the instrument measuring the end-tidal carbon dioxide is able to display a carbon dioxide wave form.[10] The carbon dioxide wave form is capable of providing a great deal of information, and can be analyzed for five basic characteristics: height, frequency, rhythm, baseline, and shape.[11] There is only one normal shape (Fig. 11-1). The height depends on the end-tidal carbon dioxide value, the frequency depends on respiratory rate, the rhythm depends on the state of the respiratory center or on the function of the ventilator, and the baseline should be at zero.

Certain basic rules regarding capnography are easily identified. A sudden decrease in carbon dioxide to zero or a very low level indicates a technical disturbance or defect, such as a kinked endotracheal tube, a defective carbon dioxide analyzer, a circuit disconnection, or a defective ventilator.

A sudden change in baseline that may or may not be combined with changes in the plateau level usually indicates a calibration error, an exhausted carbon dioxide absorber, or water condensation in the carbon dioxide analyzer. A sudden decrease in carbon dioxide value (but not to zero) with either spontaneous or mechanical ventilation indicates leakage in the respiratory system (low airway pressure) or obstruction (high airway pressure). An exponential decrease in carbon dioxide within 1 or 2 minutes indicates a sudden disturbance in lung circulation or ventilation that may occur with circulatory arrest, pulmonary embolism, sudden hypotension, or sudden hyperventilation.

A gradual increase in carbon dioxide in either spontaneous or mechanical ventilation indicates hypoventilation, absorption

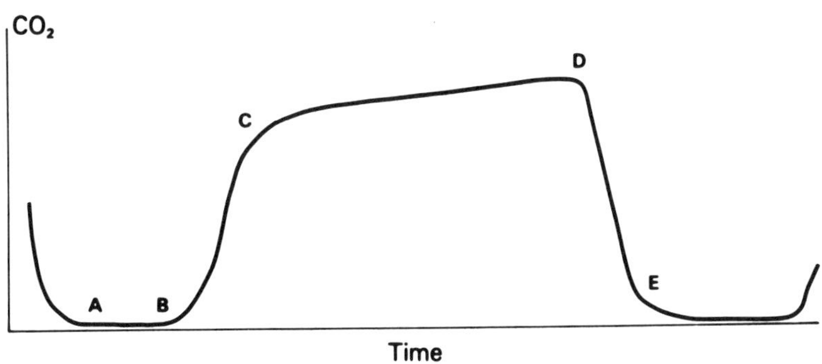

Fig. 11-1. The normal capnogram. A, beginning of exhalation; AB, anatomic dead space gas being exhaled; BC, the ascending limb representing increasing concentration of carbon dioxide from increasingly distal airways; CD, alveolar plateau containing mixed alveolar gases; D, end-tidal carbon dioxide; DE, the descending limb and the inspiratory phase of respiration showing rapidly decreasing carbon dioxide concentration as fresh gas is inhaled. (From Swedlow,[10] with permission.)

of carbon dioxide from an external source (such as the peritoneal cavity during laparoscopy), or rapidly increasing body temperature (such as may occur in malignant hyperthermia). A sudden increase in carbon dioxide during either spontaneous or mechanical ventilation may be due to the injection of sodium bicarbonate, a sudden release of a vascular occlusion tourniquet, or a sudden increase in pulmonary blood flow. A gradual upshift of the carbon dioxide baseline and topline usually indicates defective carbon dioxide absorption, a calibration or technical error in the carbon dioxide analyzer, or increasing deadspace resulting in rebreathing. Gradual lowering of the end-tidal carbon dioxide (in which the curve retains it normal shape, but the height of the plateau gradually drops) usually occurs in a mechanically ventilated patient and is caused by gradual hyperventilation, decreasing body temperature, or decreasing body or lung perfusion.

Thus, capnography is capable of defining problems relating to gas supply to the patient as well as respiratory, circulatory, and CNS effects on respiration. Three of the more common abnormalities in capnograph wave forms and their causes are illustrated in Figure 11-2.

The Neuromuscular Junction

Monitoring the neuromuscular junction with a nerve stimulator has proven to be useful during anesthesia involving the use of neuromuscular blocking drugs.[12] These devices permit administration of muscle re-

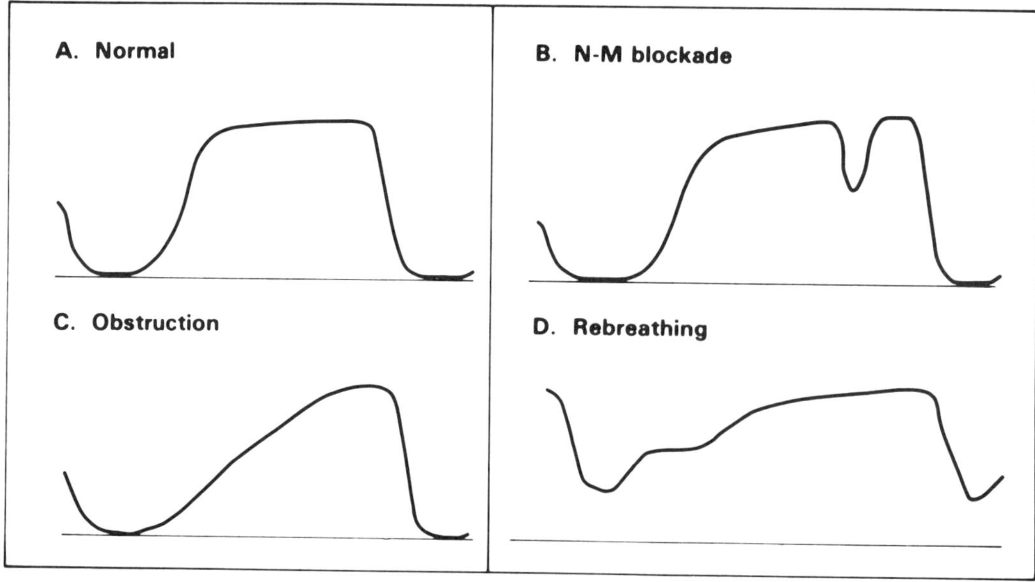

Fig. 11-2. **(A)** Normal capnogram. **(B)** Partial neuromuscular blockade with spontaneous diaphragmatic movement is seen which results in a cleft due to the inrush of carbon dioxide-free gas as the diaphragm contracts. It may be the first clinical sign that neuromuscular function is returning. **(C)** Prolonged exhalation secondary to a partially kinked endotracheal tube or small airway obstruction. The alveolar plateau is absent. This indicates that the lung units do not drain their carbon dioxide-rich gas in a time-coordinated manner. **(D)** Rebreathing can occur in various circumstances, such as faulty valves, exhausted carbon dioxide absorber, or inadequate fresh gas flow in a Mapleson D type circuit. (From Swedlow,[10] with permission.)

laxants such that optimal surgical relaxation is achieved while permitting timely drug reversal either spontaneously or with antagonists. Prior to the development of nerve stimulators, anesthesiologists used other clinical indices of adequate ventilation and skeletal muscle strength. These included tongue protrusion, grip strength, vital capacity, tidal volume, inspiratory force, and the ability to lift the head for 5 seconds. Most of these clinical indices require a cooperative patient and are inappropriate while surgery is in progress. The most satisfactory and reliable method of monitoring neuromuscular function, especially during surgery, is the stimulation of an appropriate nerve and the observation of the evoked response in the skeletal muscle supplied by the nerve. Most frequently, the ulnar nerve-adductor pollicis muscle system of the thumb is used.

The four commonly used patterns of stimulation for monitoring neuromuscular blockade are single twitch, train of four, tetanus, and post-tetanic. In the clinical situation, these responses are evaluated visually or by touch. The train of four is a more sensitive monitor of neuromuscular blockade than the single twitch response. Although the nerve stimulator assesses reversal of neuromuscular blockade, skeletal muscle function also should be determined by clinical tests at the end of an anesthetic.

Should a peripheral nerve stimulator be used on every anesthetized patient who receives muscle relaxants in the outpatient setting? This question is not easy to answer. The recent introduction of the intermediate-acting nondepolarizing neuromuscular blocking drugs has made the peripheral nerve stimulator somewhat superfluous at times. Additionally, succinylcholine, a short-acting depolarizing neuromuscular blocker, is frequently used in the outpatient setting. It is my opinion that a peripheral nerve stimulator need not be used routinely in the ambulatory surgical setting, but should be available at every anesthetizing location to help assess the degree of neuromuscular blockade when such a consideration becomes important.

MULTISYSTEM MONITORING

Oxygenation

Adequate oxygenation in anesthetized patients depends on a complex interaction of both pulmonary and cardiovascular systems. The ability to measure arterial oxygenation is critical to prevent such disasters as hypoxic encephalopathy. Assessment of oxygenation can be accomplished by direct measurement of arterial blood gases, transcutaneous oxygen measurement, and pulse oximetry. This discussion will focus on pulse oximetry.

Oxygen saturation of hemoglobin can be accurately determined by light reflected from or passed through the skin and subcutaneous vessels. The light absorbance differences between reduced hemoglobin and oxyhemoglobin may be described quantitatively by the molecular extinction coefficients in Beer's law. Pulse oximetry functions by positioning any pulsating arterial vascular bed between a light source (with two waves of different length) and a detector. The pulsating vascular bed expands and relaxes, thereby creating a change in the light path which modifies the amount of light detected. The detected pulse or waveform is produced solely from arterial blood, and beat-to-beat continuous calculation of arterial hemoglobin saturation is accomplished. The technology uses a light source generated by two light-emitting diodes with wave lengths at approximately 660 and 940 nm. A photodiode is mounted in a receptacle that is placed somewhere on the body, usually on a finger or toe. Heating or other arterialization techniques are not necessary. Circuit control, saturation calculation, and readout are managed by a computer. Calibration is not required. Any event that significantly reduces vascular pulsation will reduce the ability of the instrument to obtain and process the signal and thereby calculate oxygen saturation.[13,14]

Hypothermia, hypotension, and infusion of vasoconstrictor drugs can limit the usefulness of this monitoring modality. Abnormal hemoglobin, such as carboxyhemoglobin, sulfhemoglobin, and methemoglobin, can cause errors in measurement.[13,14] In addition, errors in measurement can occur in patients receiving intravascular administration of certain dyes, such as indocyanine green, methylene blue, and indigo carmine.[15] Instrumentation that involves the production of wave lengths of light similar to those produced by the pulse oximeter can also interfere with function of the instrument. The most common interference is from the infrared heating lamp.[16] Motion and electrocautery can also hamper the proper functioning of the instrument. When using pulse oximetry, it is important to remember the relationship of hemoglobin oxygen saturation to arterial oxygen tension. This is described by the oxyhemoglobin dissociation curve (see Fig. 4-12), and correlations between arterial oxygen saturation (SO_2) and partial pressures are given in Table 11-1.

Pulse oximetry has been proven to be quite valuable since its introduction in 1983 and has achieved widespread acceptance. Pulse oximetry is noninvasive, easy to use, and relatively inexpensive. It should be used on every anesthetized patient. With the widespread availability of pulse oxim-

Table 11-1. Correlation Between Arterial Oxygen Saturation and Partial Pressure

	PaO_2 (mmHg) pH Levels								
SO_2	6.80	7.00	7.20	7.30	7.40	7.50	7.60	7.80	8.00
99	271	225	188	171	156	143	130	108	90
98	194	161	134	122	111	101	92	77	64
97	161	133	111	101	92	84	77	64	53
96	142	118	98	89	82	74	68	56	47
95	130	108	90	82	74	68	62	52	43
94	121	100	84	76	69	63	58	48	40
93	114	95	79	72	66	60	55	45	38
92	109	90	75	68	62	57	52	43	36
91	104	87	72	66	60	55	50	41	34
90	100	83	69	63	58	53	48	40	33
88	94	78	65	59	54	49	45	37	31
86	89	74	61	56	51	47	42	35	29
84	85	70	58	53	49	44	40	34	28
82	81	67	56	51	47	42	39	32	27
80	78	65	54	49	45	41	37	31	26
78	75	62	52	47	43	39	36	30	25
76	72	60	50	45	41	38	34	29	24
74	69	58	48	44	40	36	33	28	23
72	67	56	46	42	39	35	32	27	22
70	65	54	45	41	37	34	31	26	21
68	63	52	43	40	36	33	30	25	21
66	61	50	42	38	35	32	29	24	20
64	59	49	41	37	34	31	28	23	19
62	57	47	39	36	33	30	27	23	19
60	55	46	38	35	32	29	26	22	18
55	51	42	35	32	29	27	24	20	17
50	47	39	32	29	27	24	22	19	15
45	43	35	30	27	25	22	20	17	14
40	39	33	27	25	22	21	19	16	13
35	36	30	25	22	20	19	17	14	12

etry and capnography, arterial blood gas analysis has become less important. In addition, arterial blood gas analysis is not available in many outpatient facilities. Transcutaneous oxygen and carbon dioxide measurements are less reliable than pulse oximetry and capnography, respectively. With further technologic improvements, transcutaneous gas analysis could become extremely useful in the outpatient setting.

Temperature

Anesthesiologists should monitor temperature and strive to maintain it within normal values, because abnormal temperature can adversely impact numerous organ systems. Hypothermia is the most common temperature disorder resulting from anesthesia and surgery. Approximately 60 percent of patients have temperatures less than 36°C (96.8°F) on admission to the recovery room.[17] Factors that contribute to decreased patient temperature during anesthesia and surgery include the following: (1) the operating room is cold, (2) the patient's body is excessively exposed in the operating room environment, and body cavities may be exposed to cold irrigating solutions, (3) the patient receives nonwarmed intravenous solutions, (4) body heat is required to warm the cool, dry inspired (anesthetic) gases, (5) anesthesia reduces body metabolism (i.e., heat production), (6) anesthesia causes vasodilatation (i.e., increased heat loss), and (7) anesthesia interferes with thermoregulatory mechanisms in the hypothalamus.

Shivering, which increases tissue oxygen consumption as much as 400 to 500 percent,[17] and increased metabolism are used by the awakening patient to restore normothermia. Because the response to hypothermia and rewarming can be hazardous to patients with pre-existing diseases (e.g., coronary artery disease), prevention of hypothermia is preferred.

Causes of intraoperative hyperthermia include infection, hyperthyroidism, excessive external warming, and malignant hyperthermia. Malignant hyperthermia is a life-threatening disease that may be diagnosed (albeit somewhat late) by temperature monitoring.

The thermistor and the thermocouple are commonly used for measuring temperatures.[17] Numerous sites for monitoring temperature have been described; the most commonly used are rectal, nasopharyngeal, esophageal, and tympanic membrane locations. Although there are studies that support the tympanic membrane site as the best index of core temperature, a significant objection to its use is the possibility of tympanic membrane perforation.[17] Rectal, bladder, esophageal, and nasopharyngeal temperatures most closely correlate with tympanic membrane and core temperatures.[17] These sites are recommended rather than risking trauma to the tympanic membrane. Other monitoring sites that have been used are the forehead and axilla.

Liquid crystal thermometers in the form of an adhesive strip can be affixed to the patient's skin; changes in the color of the liquid crystals reflect changes in temperature. While these devices have been found to correlate very poorly with other temperature monitors, they can be used to indicate trends during brief outpatient procedures.

Standards for Monitoring

Should temperature monitoring be routine or should the availability of temperature monitoring be the standard of care? These are difficult questions to answer; however, medical judgment, good medical practice, and personal preference all become factors. It is my opinion that the ability to measure temperature should be available at every anesthetizing location in the outpatient setting and should be used whenever the anesthesiologist's clinical judgment deems it necessary.

Even if there are little data to prove conclusively that monitors are beneficial, it is clear that certain minimum monitoring standards must be set. Several groups have adopted minimum standards.[18,19] All require the physical presence of qualified anesthesia personnel in the room where the anesthetic is being administered. This implies that all the modern mechanical monitoring devices cannot take the place of a vigilant anesthesiologist. It also reflects the fact that monitors are of value only if someone is present to observe the information that the monitors obtain.

Standards are the most cost-effective and dramatic way to reduce the number of malpractice claims. Anesthesiology practice standards instituted in Massachusetts have resulted in a substantial decrease in legal action relating to hypoxic injury in that state. The standards in Massachusetts require the mandatory use of pulse oximeters and capnography, and the use of these monitoring modalities has led to reduced anesthesia malpractice premiums. For obvious reasons, physicians, not insurance companies or other interested parties, should be the ones to develop standards.

In the absence of state-accepted standards, anesthesiologists can follow recommended guidelines to assure optimal patient care. Before administering an anesthetic, the anesthesiologist should undertake a thorough ''preflight'' check of anesthesia apparatus, as endorsed by the American Society of Anesthesiologists.[20] Once the preflight check list and the presence of qualified personnel criteria have been satisfied, the following list of monitors, in this author's opinion, serves as an absolute minimum requirement for patients having general anesthesia in the outpatient setting: (1) pulse oximeter, (2) capnography (CO_2 monitoring), (3) automatic blood pressure mea-

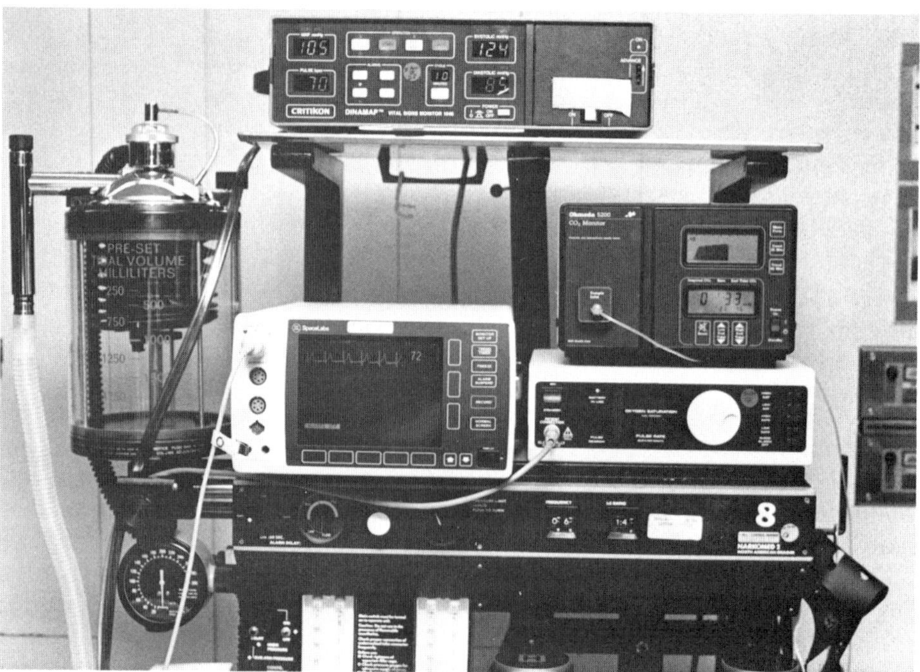

Fig. 11-3. A typical monitoring array used in the ambulatory surgical setting. Clockwise from the top: automatic oscillometric blood pressure monitor, infrared CO_2 monitor, pulse oximeter, ECG, and temperature monitor.

surement, (4) oscilloscopic ECG, (5) expiratory gas flow meter (ventimeter or equivalent) if circle system is being used, (6) airway pressure monitor, (7) circuit low-pressure alarm if mechanical ventilation is used, (8) oxygen analyzer with low-concentration alarm, and (9) availability of temperature monitor.

For patients undergoing regional anesthesia, the following monitors should be minimum requirements: (1) oxygen source with a means for providing artificial ventilation, (2) pulse oximeter, (3) automatic blood pressure measurement, (4) oscilliscopic ECG, and (5) temperature monitor.

For limited procedures in the outpatient setting (i.e., those in which neither general anesthesia nor regional anesthesia is performed), the following monitoring modalities should be the minimum standard: (1) oscilloscopic ECG, (2) pulse oximeter, and (3) automatic blood pressure measurement. A typical monitoring array for an outpatient anesthetic setting is shown in Figure 11-3.

RECORDKEEPING SYSTEMS

Computers are used for signal processing, data manipulation, and display in such monitoring devices as automatic blood pressure devices and pulse oximeters. Computers show great promise for producing an automated anesthesia record system,[21] and preliminary systems are now in place to perform this task. However, the following problems need to be addressed before an automated anesthesia system is a reality for the majority of practicing anesthesiologists: (1) there must be a voice activation or minimal data entry requirement, (2) there must be a capability for adding comments in real time, (3) a variety of devices must be interfaced, (4) data entry must be artifact-free, and (5) anesthesiologists and lawyers must understand that artifacts can occur and that if brief episodes of hypotension (or even hypoxemia) are seen, these do not necessarily contribute to poor patient outcome.

It has been shown that there is a significant difference when a written record is compared with automated data collection.[22] For the short term, however, conventional recordkeeping systems, particularly in the ambulatory surgery setting, will continue to prevail.

SUMMARY

With the development of solid-state electronics and miniature devices, many monitors have appeared in recent years. Growth will continue to occur. However, if monitors are to be cost-effective, they must be durable and capable of being updated periodically to keep abreast of changes in the field. This means, of necessity, monitoring devices should be software driven, with software programs that can be changed or updated when necessary. When choosing a monitoring device, these factors should be important considerations. Interfacing of various pieces of monitoring equipment, even when produced by the same manufacturer, has become frustrating and needs to be addressed, especially by equipment manufacturers. Anesthesiologists look forward to a completely centralized monitoring array without a spaghetti-like tangle of wires, hoses, and power cords. Alarms must be readily identifiable as to their source. In general, the anesthetic workplace needs to be improved and standardized so as to minimize the occurrence of human error.

By improving monitoring in the outpatient operating room, we essentially are shifting potential anesthesia problems, particularly hypoxia, to the recovery room. With this in mind, monitoring capabilities for *early recognition of hypoxia in the recovery room* must be available. This means all patients in the recovery room setting should have a pulse oximeter available to monitor their respiratory status.

Regardless of biases, training, or age, we must realize that monitors have become a permanent part of the anesthesiologist's battery of equipment, and it is important that they are used effectively. Monitoring is a means to achieve an end; that end is to make anesthesia as safe as possible.

REFERENCES

1. Evans JM, Davies WL, Wise CC: Lower esophageal contractility: a new monitor of anesthesia. Lancet 1:1151, 1984
2. Maier WR: Noninvasive blood pressure monitoring. p. 81. In Blitt CD (ed): Monitoring in Anesthesia and Critical Care Medicine. 2nd Ed. Churchill Livingstone, New York, 1990
3. Geddes LA, Voel ZM, Combs C, et al: Characterization of the oscillometric method for measuring indirect blood pressure. Ann Biomed Eng 10:271, 1982
4. Sy WP: Ulnar nerve palsy related to use of automatically cycled blood pressure cuff. Anesth Analg 60:687, 1981
5. Smith NT, Wesseling KH, DeWitt B: Evaluation of two prototype devices producing noninvasive, pulsatile, calibrated blood pressure measurement from a finger. J Clin Monit 1:17, 1985
6. Stevenson RL, Rogers MC: Electrocardiographic monitoring and dysrhythmia analysis. p. 135. In Blitt CD (ed): Monitoring in Anesthesia and Critical Care Medicine. 2nd Ed. Churchill Livingstone, New York, 1990
7. Fairley HB: Respiratory monitoring. p. 339. In Blitt CD (ed): Monitoring in Anesthesia and Critical Care Medicine. 2nd Ed. Churchill Livingstone, New York, 1990
8. Birmingham PK, Cheney FW, Ward RJ: Esophageal intubation: a review of detection techniques. Anesth Analg 65:886, 1986
9. Severinghaus JW: Monitoring anesthetic and respiratory gases. p. 265. In Blitt CD (ed): Monitoring in Anesthesia and Critical Care Medicine. 1st Ed. Churchill Livingstone, New York, 1985
10. Swedlow DB: Mass spectrometers and respiratory gas monitoring. p. 205. In Barash PG (ed): American Society of Anesthesiologists Annual Refresher Courses. JB Lippincott, Philadelphia, 1985
11. Smalhout B: A Quick Guide to Capnography and Its Use in Differential Diagnosis. Hewlett-Packard, Andover, MA, 1983
12. Crowley MP, Savarese JJ, Ali HH: Monitoring the neuromuscular junction. p. 635. In Blitt CD (ed): Monitoring in Anesthesia and Critical Care Medicine. 2nd Ed. Churchill Livingstone, New York, 1990
13. Yelderman M, New W: Evaluation of pulse oximetry. Anesthesiology 59:349, 1983
14. Sendak JM, Harris AP, Donham RT: Accuracy of pulse oximetry during severe arterial oxygen desaturation. Anesthesiology 65:A133, 1986
15. Scheller MS, Unger RJ, Kelner MJ: Effects of intravenously administered dyes on pulse oximetry readings. Anesthesiology 65:550, 1986
16. Brooks TD, Paulus DA, Winkle WE: Infrared heat lamps interfere with pulse oximeters. Anesthesiology 61:630, 1984
17. Cork RC: Temperature monitoring. p. 557. In Blitt CD (ed): Monitoring in Anesthesia and Critical Care Medicine. 2nd Ed. Churchill Livingstone, New York, 1990
18. Eichorn JH, Cooper JB, Cullen DJ, et al: Standards for patient monitoring during anesthesia at Harvard Medical School. JAMA 256:1017, 1986
19. Standards for basic intraoperative monitoring. In American Society of Anesthesiologists Newsletter. American Society of Anesthesiologists, Chicago, 1986
20. Anesthesia apparatus checkout recommendations. In American Society of Anesthesiologists Newsletter. American Society of Anesthesiologists, Chicago, 1986
21. Saunders RJ: Computers in anesthesiology. p. 651. In Blitt CD (ed): Monitoring in Anesthesia and Critical Care Medicine. 2nd Ed. Churchill Livingstone, New York, 1990
22. Logas WG, McCarthy RJ, Narbone RF, et al: Analysis of the accuracy of the anesthetic record. Anesth Analg 66:S107, 1987

12

Monitored Anesthesia Care

John Zelcer
Paul F. White

While there is a growing body of literature on optimal monitoring requirements for general and regional anesthesia, there is little clinically useful information regarding recommended guidelines and minimum requirements for providing monitored anesthesia care (MAC). In view of the increasing number of operative procedures being performed on outpatients in which MAC is the anesthetic technique of choice, it is surprising how little information has been published in the medical literature regarding techniques for MAC. Given the wide spectrum of patients (e.g., American Society of Anesthesiologists [ASA] physical status I through IV), surgical procedures, and pharmacologic agents used, it is obvious that there is a need for additional clinical investigations of monitoring and sedation practices during MAC.

This chapter reviews the basic objectives of MAC and discusses the rational use of monitoring devices and sedative-analgesic medications during MAC cases in the ambulatory surgery setting. In addition to describing specific intraoperative and postoperative monitoring requirements, we discuss monitoring requirements for certain specialized outpatient procedures (e.g., radiation therapy, extracorporeal shockwave lithotripsy [ESWL]/Lithostar [Sieman's Medical Systems, Italy]). Finally, an understanding of the pharmacologic and physiologic effects of the commonly used sedative-hypnotic, anxiolytic, and analgesic drugs is important in order to achieve optimal surgical conditions as well as acceptable patient outcome while providing MAC.

DEFINITION OF MONITORED ANESTHESIA CARE

The ASA refers to MAC as "instances in which an anesthesiologist has been called upon to provide specific anesthesia services to a particular patient undergoing a planned procedure, in connection with which a patient receives local anesthesia or, in some cases, no anesthesia at all. In such a case, the anesthesiologist is providing specific services to the patient and is in control of his or her non-surgical medical care, including the responsibility of monitoring his or her vital signs, and is available to administer anesthetics or provide other medical care as appropriate."[1]

It is also a policy of the ASA that all institutional regulations pertaining to anesthesia services should be observed, and that all the usual services performed by the anesthesiologist should be furnished, including (1) the usual noninvasive cardiocirculatory and respiratory monitoring, (2) the administration of oxygen when indicated, and (3) the intravenous administration of sedatives, anxiolytics, antiemetics, analgesics, β-blockers, vasopressors, bronchodilators, antihypertensives, or other pharmacologic therapy.

Furthermore, the ASA Monitoring Standards specifically include MAC in the Standard for Basic Intra-operative Monitoring. These policies imply the same level of care for MAC as is required for all other anesthetic procedures.

ROLE OF MONITORED ANESTHESIA CARE IN THE PRACTICE OF ANESTHESIA

The incidence of MAC as the anesthetic technique of choice varies among institutions, but is usually between 10 and 20 percent of all outpatient procedures. Monitored anesthesia care is being increasingly used for many outpatient surgical procedures (e.g., cosmetic surgery, cataracts, cystoscopy, placement of "deep" lines, vascular shunts). Inguinal herniorrhaphy[2] and laparoscopic sterilization procedures[3] are also being performed more frequently under local anesthesia. In fact, local infiltration and peripheral nerve block techniques account for 40 to 50 percent of all nongeneral anesthetics administered in this country (unpublished data, Dr. K. L. Allenstein, Madison, Wisconsin). However, many patients are reluctant to undergo local infiltration (or nerve block) anesthesia without supplemental medication because of concerns about pain and awareness during surgery.[4]

In most situations, the primary objective in providing MAC is to assist our surgical colleagues in providing for patient comfort and safety during operations under local anesthesia. This objective can be achieved by careful monitoring of the patient's vital signs and by providing anxiolysis, analgesia, amnesia, and sedation without compromising cardiorespiratory function or delaying recovery. The drugs administered by the anesthesiologist to achieve the desired surgical conditions include a wide variety of centrally active injectable and inhaled adjuvants.[5,6] In fact, sedative-analgesic drugs may be the sole agents for procedures such as bronchoscopy, upper or lower gastrointestinal endoscopy, and in vitro fertilization procedures.[7] The spectrum of adjuvant therapy used during MAC includes benzodiazepines,[4,8] opioid (narcotic) and nonopioid analgesics,[9] subanesthetic doses of barbiturates, etomidate and propofol,[10–12] ketamine,[4,13] inhalational agents,[6] and nitrous oxide.[14] Drug administration may be pre-, intra-, or postoperative, with anesthetic drugs from two or more drug groups often being combined.[4,9,15] A wide variety of routes of administration (e.g., oral, parenteral, rectal) have also been used in patients receiving MAC.

There is an ever-present risk of synergistic interactions between sedative and analgesic drugs with respect to respiratory and cardiovascular depression. The potential for compromising the respiratory system due to depression of esophageal and laryngeal reflexes,[14] upper airway obstruction,[10] and depression of hypercarbic[16] and hypoxic[17] ventilatory responses has been described during sedation anesthesia. Interestingly, when sedative drugs are administered by carefully titrated infusions (versus large intermittent bolus doses), the respiratory depressant effects can be minimized.[18] Unwanted cardiovascular problems (e.g., hypotension, hypertension, drug-induced arrhythmias) can also be avoided by using careful drug administration techniques. Thus, there is a need for specific and diligent monitoring to assess the efficacy of adjunctive drugs and to minimize their potentially deleterious side effects.

USE OF SEDATIVE-ANALGESIC DRUGS DURING MONITORED ANESTHESIA CARE

Sedation is frequently desirable during local anesthesia to produce amnesia and analgesia and to enhance patient comfort during the operation. Forms of adjuvant therapy range from oral premedication to produce mild sedation to a subhypnotic state which approaches general anesthesia. Benzodiazepines are useful for producing amnesia, anxiolysis, and sedation. However, large doses of diazepam (0.3 mg/kg IV) impair driving skills for at least 10 hours and may prolong recovery to a greater extent than patients undergoing general anesthesia.[19,20] Temazepam 20 to 40 mg orally is an effective alternative to parenteral benzodiazepines for sedation during outpatient endoscopy or oral surgery.[21,22]

Midazolam, a rapid and short-acting parenteral benzodiazepine, should be administered by careful intravenous titration to achieve the desired clinical effect because of the marked interpatient pharmacodynamic variability. The effects of aging and pre-existing medical conditions in enhancing the patient's sensitivity to midazolam should also be considered when these drugs are used for sedation during local anesthesia. With respect to its sedative effects, midazolam appears to be two to four times more potent than diazepam (Fig. 12-1).[4] In most studies, midazolam has been reported to produce more profound perioperative amnesia and sedation when compared with diazepam. Although midazolam has a short elimination halflife (2 to 4 hours), objective measures of recovery have failed to demonstrate a more rapid return to baseline function (versus diazepam).[23–26]

Analgesic medication is frequently combined with a benzodiazepine to improve patient comfort during local anesthesia. Concomitant use of potent opioid analgesics (e.g., fentanyl 1.5 μg/kg IV) can cause profound ventilatory depression,[27] resulting in significant hypoxemia in healthy outpatients when administered after midazolam or diazepam.[9] Therefore, supplemental oxygen is recommended when benzodiazepine-opioid combinations are used.

An advantage of ketamine-induced analgesia is the lack of clinically significant respiratory depression when used in conjunction with benzodiazepines.[4,13] For outpatient plastic surgery, midazolam 0.05 to 0.1 mg/kg IV (infused over 3 to 5 minutes) followed by ketamine 0.25 to 0.5 mg/kg IV produced excellent sedation, amnesia, and analgesia during the injection of local anesthetic solutions.[4] Similar conditions can be achieved with 30 to 50 percent nitrous oxide or a low concentration of enflurane (i.e., 0.5 percent).[6] With inhalational techniques, care must be taken to avoid excessively deep sedation (anesthesia) and its potential complications of excitement, respiratory and cardiovascular depression, and aspiration. Moreover, perioperative side effects (e.g., coughing), concern over operating room pollution, and the availability of improved medications for intravenous sedation have limited the more widespread use of these techniques.

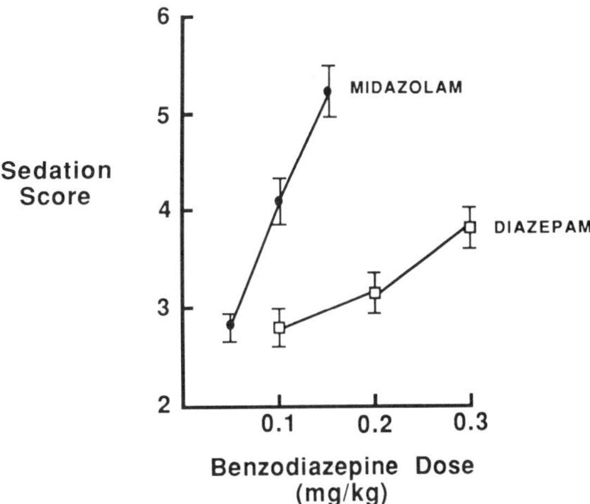

Fig. 12-1. Dose-response curves for the level of sedation as a function of midazolam or diazepam dose. A score of 2 indicates minimal sedation, while a score of 6 equals unconscious (hypnotic) state. (From White et al.,[4] with permission.)

Intravenous sedative-hypnotics have been infused in subhypnotic doses (e.g., thiopental 3 to 6 mg/min IV or methohexital 1 to 2 mg/min IV) to produce varying degrees of sedation.[10–12] Propofol has a pharmacodynamic-kinetic profile which is ideally suited to administration by continuous infusion because of its rapid onset of action,

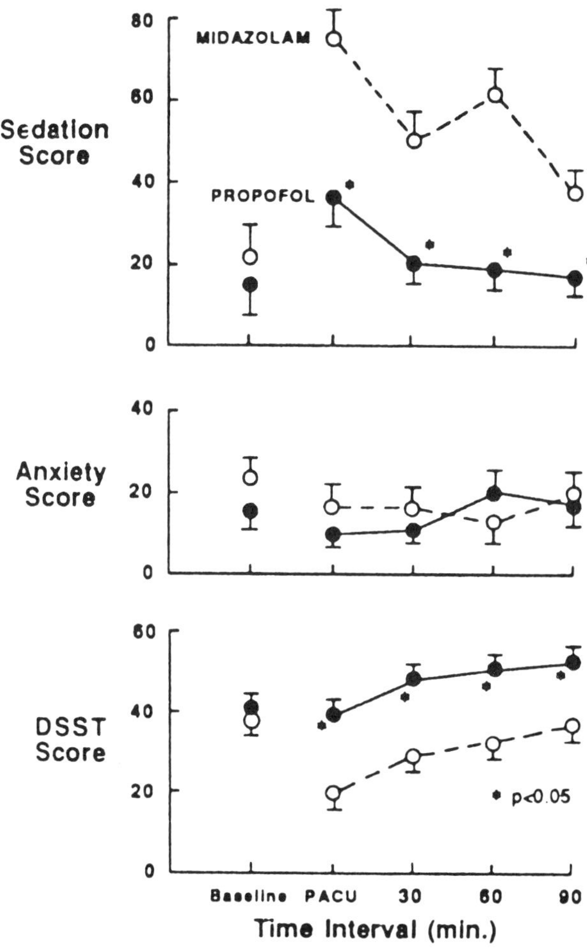

Fig. 12-2. Comparison of preoperative (baseline) and postoperative sedation, anxiety, and digit-symbol substitution test (DSST) scores in patients receiving midazolam (○----○) or propofol (●———●) during local or regional anesthesia (From Negus and White,[12] with permission).

short duration of effect, and minimal side effects.[11] In a recent comparative study, use of a propofol infusion to produce intraoperative sedation during local and regional anesthesia was associated with a more rapid recovery than midazolam (Fig. 12-2).[12] However, midazolam did provide more effective intraoperative amnesia and less discomfort during injection. As suggested earlier, the doses of anxiolytic, sedative-hypnotic, and analgesic medications (Table 12-1) should be carefully titrated to minimize cardiorespiratory depression and allow for a rapid recovery after surgery. The availability of specific antagonist drugs (e.g., flumazenil) may prove extremely valuable in reversing residual sedation and amnesia after MAC.[28,29]

DEFINING LEVELS OF SEDATION DURING MONITORED ANESTHESIA CARE

The American Dental Association Council on Dental Education has proposed specific definitions for sedation and analgesia during local anesthesia (Table 12-2).[30] In considering the different levels of sedation, it is important to emphasize that patients under "conscious sedation" must be ca-

Table 12-1. Classification of Parenteral Sedative and Analgesic Drugs Used During Monitored Anesthesia Care in the Outpatient Setting

Drug	Usual adult dose
Analgesics	
Alfentanil (Alfenta)	0.5–1.0 mg
Fentanyl (Sublimaze)	50–150 μg
Hydromorphone (Dilaudid)	0.5–2.0 mg
Meperidine (Demerol)	30–100 mg
Morphine sulfate	3–10 mg
Nalbuphine (Nubain)	5–15 mg
Oxymorphone (Numorphan)	0.5–2.0 mg
Sufentanil (Sufenta)	5–15 μg
Sedative-anxiolytic	
Diazepam (Valium)	5–15 mg
Hydroxyzine (Vistaril)	25–100 mg
Lorazepam (Ativan)	1–2 mg
Midazolam (Versed)	2.5–7.5 mg
Propofol (Diprivan)	25–75 mg
Thiopental (Pentothal)	50–150 mg
Sedative-analgesic	
Butorphanol (Stadol)	1–2 mg
Ketamine (Ketalar)	20–40 mg

pable of rational response to commands and be able to maintain airway patency (Table 12-3).[31] Since conscious sedation clearly lies on a dose-dependent continuum leading from minimal sedation to general anesthesia, the critical factor is that the sedation produced does not alter cardiac, respiratory, and reflex functions to the extent of requiring external support.[31–33] The objectives of conscious sedation as outlined by Scamman et al.[33] are listed below.

1. The first objective is to relieve anxiety and produce amnesia. These goals are accomplished by means of good preoperative communication and instruction, low levels of visual and auditory stimuli in the operating room, and by keeping the patient warm and covered.

Table 12-2. Definitions Proposed by the American Dental Association Council on Dental Education

Analgesia	Diminution or elimination of pain in the conscious patient
Local anesthesia	Elimination of sensation and motor activity in one part of the body by the topical application or regional (peripheral) injection of local anesthetics
Conscious sedation	Depressed level of consciousness which allows the patient the ability to independently and continuously maintain an airway and respond appropriately to physical stimulation and verbal command
Deep sedation (hypnosis)	Controlled state of depressed consciousness accompanied by partial or complete loss of protective reflexes, including the ability to independently maintain an airway and respond purposefully to physical stimulation or verbal command

(From McCarthy et al.,[30] with permission.)

Table 12-3. Conscious Sedation Versus Deep Sedation Techniques for Outpatient Surgery

Conscious sedation	Deep (unconscious) sedation
Mood altered	Patient unconsciousness
Patient cooperative	Patient unable to cooperate
Protective reflexes intact	Protective reflexes obtunded
Vital signs stable	Vital signs labile
Local anesthesia provides analgesia	Pain eliminated centrally
Amnesia may be present	Amnesia always present
Short recovery room stay	Occasional prolonged recovery room stay or overnight admission required
Low risk of complications	Higher risk of complications
Postoperative complications infrequent	Postoperative complications reported in 25–75 percent of cases
Uncooperative or mentally handicapped patient cannot always be managed	Useful in managing difficult or mentally handicapped patients

(Modified from Kallar et al.,[31] with permission.)

2. The second objective is to provide relief from pain and other noxious stimuli. Opioid analgesics are given to supplement local or topical anesthetics and to block pain sensations remote from the operative site.

3. The final objective is to achieve adequate sedation with minimal risk. Sedative medication should not interfere with the patient's ability to communicate verbally, and the usual monitoring devices and emergency systems must be available.

MONITORING AND PATIENT OUTCOME

There is the expectation that all forms of anesthesia for good-risk patients undergoing routine procedures should have zero mortality and minimal morbidity. Vigilance and improved monitoring techniques are crucial aids toward achieving this goal.[34] One of the major limiting factors in the rational selection of monitors is the lack of appropriate morbidity (outcome) data from general, regional, and local (MAC) anesthetic procedures regarding the effectiveness of particular monitoring practices in minimizing adverse outcome.[35]

In a comprehensive survey of the anesthesia literature,[36] Pace was unable to find a single study that specifically evaluated outcome as a function of choice of monitoring during anesthesia. However, Pierce reported that closed claims analysis of anesthesia morbidity and mortality strongly suggested that a large percentage of anesthesia accidents resulting in severe brain damage or death were preventable by the use of currently available monitoring techniques.[37] In a study that focused on respiratory mishaps during anesthesia,[38] it was found that inadequate ventilation was the most common cause of these events and the investigators concluded that 69 percent of respiratory claims may have been prevented with better monitoring (e.g., pulse oximetry).

The incidence of serious complications associated with sedation anesthesia was reported in a British study which examined morbidity and mortality in dental anesthesia services for the years 1970 through 1979.[39] There were 100 deaths associated with an estimated total of 15 million anesthetic administrations, giving an overall incidence rate of approximately 1 in 152,000. Two-thirds of these occurred in dental offices and hospital-based outpatient clinics. One-third of the deaths occurred in association with predominantly sedation anesthesia, and were more likely to occur at the hands of operator-anesthetists (e.g., oral surgeons). The most common precipitating causes were respiratory obstruction, hypoxia, or cardiovascular collapse related to arrhythmias, bradycardia, or nonsupine positioning. Apart from the obvious human tragedy, hypoxic events are also among the most highly compensated injuries in medical claims.[40]

Interestingly, there is an unpublished report (FASA Special Study I, Federated Ambulatory Surgery Association, Alexandria, Virginia, 1985) describing higher overall complication rates after ambulatory surgery with combined local and sedation anesthesia techniques (1:106) than with either general (1:120), regional (1:277), or local anesthesia alone (1:268). The length of the operative procedure was also an important factor in determining morbidity after ambulatory surgery. For procedures lasting less than 1 hour, the incidence of perioperative complications was 1:155; this ratio increased in a linear fashion to 1:35 for procedures lasting longer than 3 hours. Since the release of midazolam in the United States in 1986, the Food and Drug Administration (FDA) has received reports of at least 66 deaths associated with its use outside the operating room. Most of these individuals were receiving midazolam for conscious sedation, and the usual cause of death was respiratory and/or cardiovascular depression.[41] While no data has been reported on the monitoring practices in these cases, many were upper or lower gastrointestinal endoscopy procedures in patients premedicated with an opioid analgesic. In general, the sedative medication was administered by a nurse or the operating endoscopist with little or no monitoring. These procedures are often performed in a darkened environment where clinical monitoring (e.g., skin coloration) is of limited value. Pulse oximetry is extremely valuable in this situation because significant decreases in oxygen saturation are known to occur.[42]

Since procedures scheduled for MAC are usually considered to be "minor operations," many private and academic institutions will delegate the responsibility for patient care to their most inexperienced personnel. Some experts have suggested that avoiding adverse outcome from anesthesia may be more dependent on the way in which monitoring is performed rather than the particular array of monitors chosen.[39] In considering the optimal monitoring standards during MAC, important factors are the drugs used, the desired state of consciousness, and the value and limitations of specific modes of monitoring.

MONITORING STANDARDS

There has been significant activity at state, federal, and international levels to establish minimum (or basic) safety monitoring standards.* There is clear guidance with respect to minimum requirements for both personnel and equipment (with specific mention of MAC) in the recommendations by the ASA which were adopted in October 1986.[1] These include carefully phrased caveats which make allowance for the judgment of the individual anesthesiologist, as well as for extenuating circumstances.

Emphasis on accident prevention is an essential element in the establishment of standards for patient monitoring.[43] Safety monitoring, defined as "accident prevention monitoring" and arising as a direct consequence of human factor issues (e.g., vigilance, ergonomics, and errors of judgment), has as much importance in MAC as in other anesthetic practices.[44] As with other types of anesthesia, the optimal level of care during MAC is achieved by meticulous attention to detail.[45] This is particularly important when multiple sedative-analgesic drugs are being used and when caring for patients with clinical or laboratory findings which reflect poor cardiovascular, respiratory, or other major system reserves. The first and essential element stated in all standards manuals is the presence of qualified anesthesia personnel in the operating room throughout the conduct of the anesthetic. The ASA has specified that patient oxygenation, ventilation, circulation, and temperature be continually evaluated (where continual is defined as "repeated regularly and frequently in steady succession").[46] The phrasing of the ASA recommendations which is relevant to anesthesiologists providing MAC includes the following.

1. Oxygenation: during *all* anesthetics, adequate illumination and exposure of the patient is necessary to assess color. While qualitative clinical signs may be adequate, there are quantitative methods whose use is encouraged (e.g., pulse oximetry).
2. Ventilation: during monitored anesthesia care, the adequacy of ventilation shall be evaluated, at least, by continual observation of qualitative clinical signs (e.g., respiratory rate).
3. Circulation: every patient receiving anesthesia shall have the ECG continuously displayed from the beginning of anesthesia until preparing to leave the anesthetizing location.

* Examples of these include the Standards for Basic Intra-operative Monitoring established by the ASA (1986); the Guidelines to the Practice of Anesthesia as Recommended by the Canadian Anaesthetist's Society (1987); and the Standards on Monitoring During Anesthesia devised by the faculty of Anaesthetists of the Royal Australasian College of Surgeons (1988).

4. Body temperature: a means to continuously measure the patient's temperature shall be readily available.

Some of these requirements may be waived by the responsible anesthesiologist under extenuating circumstances; however, it is recommended that when this is done, it should be so stated in a note in the patient's medical record. It should also be mentioned that these are recommendations for *minimum* monitoring standards and may be inadequate in some situations. The judgment of the physician as to the appropriate selection and usage of any devices should be based on requirements dictated by the patient's medical condition, the anesthetic and analgesic agents used, and the surgical procedure itself.

SPECIFIC MONITORING REQUIREMENTS

What constitutes the minimum objective information from which the anesthesiologist can reliably deduce a patient's true physiologic state? The choice of monitoring devices, particularly when the emphasis is on patient safety, requires concomitant attention to quality control, safety procedures, risk recognition, decision making, and other efforts to reduce human error.[34] Furthermore, desirable characteristics of monitoring mechanisms used during outpatient MAC include that they be effective, noninvasive, manageable, and economic.[47,48]

The rationale for using noninvasive monitors is that most surgical procedures for which MAC is used involve minimal physiologic trespass (even for patients with significant systemic disease). With recent developments in computer microchip applications, information that previously could only be derived by invasive techniques is now being increasingly acquired by noninvasive devices.[49] Consideration must be given to the fact that many devices have practical limitations with respect to accuracy (e.g., capnography), interference from the electrocautery (e.g., pulse oximeters) and fragility (e.g., oxygen analyzers), as well as issues of appropriate usage (e.g., special ECG lead configurations for detecting myocardial ischemia). Finally, there is the increasingly important issue of the cost-benefit ratio and the potential for patient injury from the monitoring device itself.[50]

Since one of the most controversial issues during MAC is the rational use of pharmacologic agents, monitoring must include an ongoing evaluation of both the desired effects and side effects of all drugs (including those administered by the surgeon), the influence of the patient's position and the surgical procedure, as well as the psychological wellbeing of the patient. In addition to the eyes and ears of the observer, the senses of touch, temperature, pressure, and smell may all play important roles in evaluating the patient's physical and mental wellbeing during MAC.[45,50] Many monitoring devices are merely mechanical extensions of these senses and may create a barrier between the patient and the anesthesiologist. Vandam points out that monitoring is an extension of the physical examination, and that by keeping in close contact with the patient (e.g., feeling the pulse, observing respirations, watching the operative field, and using other senses to detect unusual events), anesthesiologists can improve the quality of monitoring during all types of anesthesia.[51]

Global Patient Monitoring

MAC provides a unique opportunity for the anesthesiologist and patient to discuss the effectiveness of the therapeutic modalities being used (e.g., local anesthesia, adjunctive sedative-analgesic therapy). In order to be effective, the anesthesiologist must remain in close verbal and/or tactile contact with the patient, particularly when centrally active drugs which can produce cardiorespiratory depression are being administered. It is useful to explain to the patient at the time of the preoperative visit that feedback will be encouraged during the procedure (e.g., in preparation for the surgical stimulus), as this will be helpful in achieving the desired level of comfort and safety. Development of good rapport with the patient facilitates both the evaluation process and intraoperative management of the case.

The age and physical status of the patient is a useful guide in evaluating system reserves and in determining their sensitivity to the sedative-analgesic drugs used during MAC.[52] Other important issues include past experiences with general, regional, and local anesthesia, preoperative anxiety level, previous problems with local anesthetics and sedative-analgesic medications, and history of postoperative complications (e.g., dizziness, lethargy, nausea, and vomiting). Apart from the desirable aim of satisfactory patient acceptance, there are practical issues to be considered, such as delayed discharge from the ambulatory surgery facility because of nausea and vomiting secondary to narcotic analgesic administration or excessive drowsiness after benzodiazepine-induced sedation.

Patient positioning and anticipating the physiologic impact of postural changes (e.g., Trendelenburg or reverse Trendelenburg),[53] as well as avoidance of nerve damage due to pressure (e.g., ulnar nerve compression) or abnormal position (i.e., brachial plexus palsy secondary to shoulder abduction) are crucial. Although safe positioning can be assured by maintaining contact with the patient, sedatives and analgesics may obscure progressive discomfort, and it is recommended that the anesthesiologist check the patient's position before and at least once during the procedure.

Respiratory Function Monitoring

Hypoxemia has been well-documented during sedation anesthesia, particularly when combinations of sedatives and narcotics are used.[9,27,29,54–56] Recently, Bailey et al. reported that while sedative doses of midazolam alone did not produce hypoxemia or apnea, midazolam increased the incidence of hypoxemia produced by fentanyl when they were administered in combination.[27] Similarly, although apnea was not produced by analgesic doses of fentanyl alone, it occurred frequently when the benzodiazepine-opioid analgesic combination was administered. Common etiologies of compromised respiratory function include direct depression of central respiratory drive, depression of ventilatory responses to hypoxia and hypercarbia, decreases in the tone of oropharyngeal and head and neck musculature resulting in upper airway obstruction, and reduction of respiratory muscle tone leading to decreased ventilatory effort and increased ventilation-perfusion mismatching. Local anesthetics, narcotic analgesics, sedative-anxiolytics, and inhalational supplements can effect these mechanisms. When combinations of drugs which cause respiratory depression, obtundation of protective reflexes, alterations in the state of consciousness, and/or interference with lower esophageal sphincter function are administered, the risks of respiratory depression and pulmonary aspiration will be increased. Since varying degrees of respiratory depression are expected during MAC when it is supplemental with sedative-analgesic combinations (Fig. 12-3), it is prudent to administer supplemental oxygen. A simple, inexpensive, disposable O_2 delivery system involving the use of an intranasal cannulae and capnograph can provide the anesthetist with a useful respiratory monitor (Fig. 12-4).

Clinical Assessment

Specific monitoring must begin with clinical observation of the respiratory pattern, rate, and tidal volume. The anesthesiologist must be alert to signs of partial or complete airway obstruction, hypoventilation, and

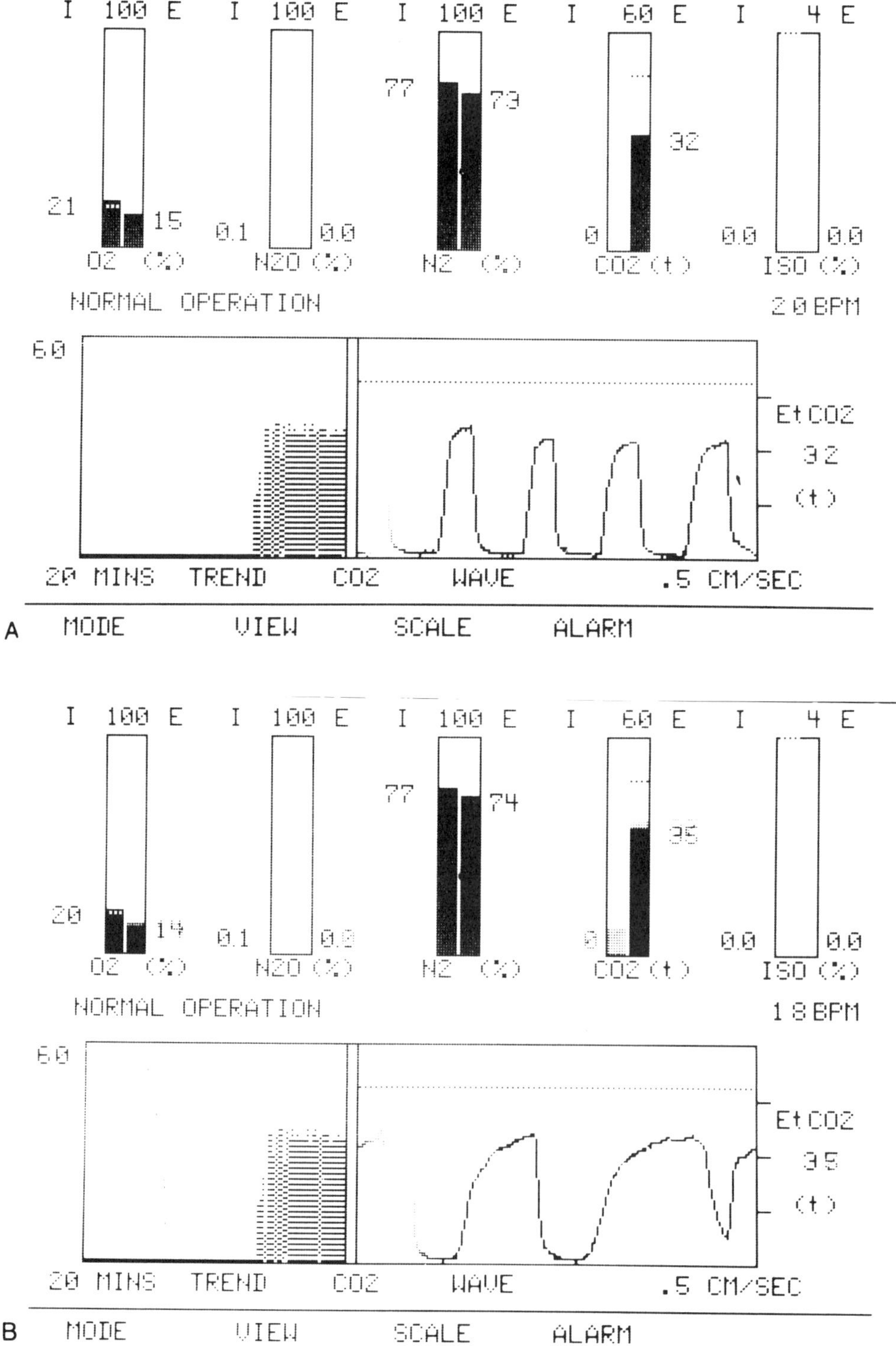

Fig. 12-3. (**A**) Ohmeda 600 multiple gas monitor capnograph tracing during MAC in a patient receiving midazolam infusion 0.05 to 0.1 mg/min IV for sedation. (**B**) Following supplementation with an opioid analgesic (fentanyl 25 μg IV), a marked slowing of the respiratory rate and increase in end-expiratory carbon dioxide concentration was noted.

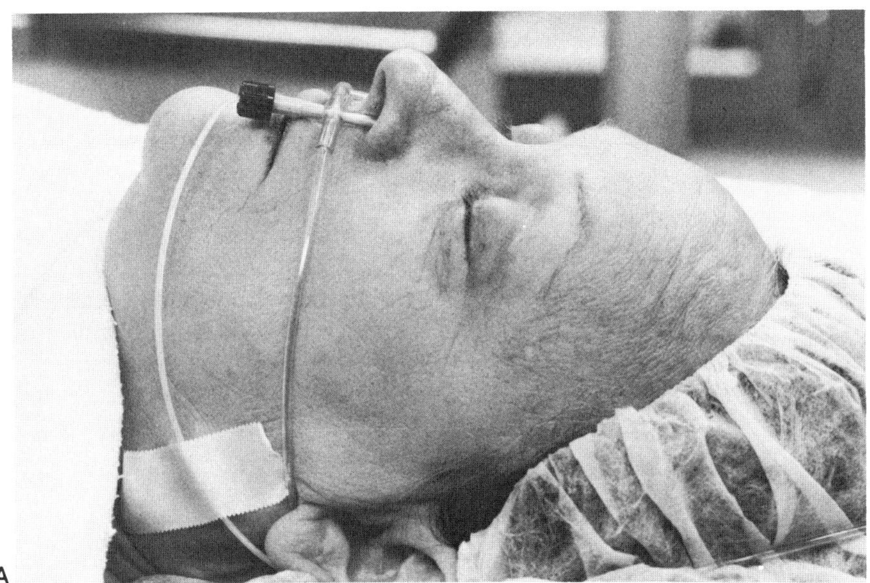

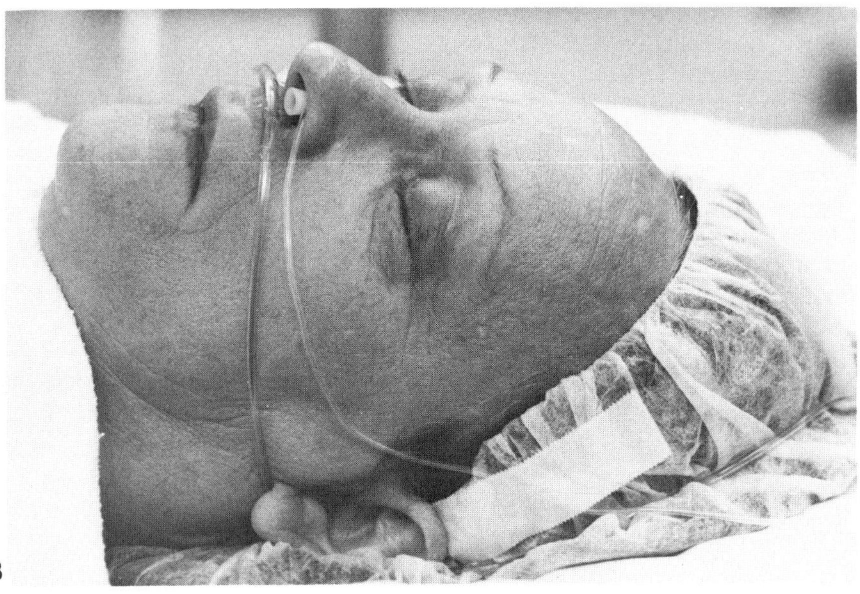

Fig. 12-4. Oxygen delivery via nasal prongs during MAC, with sedation produced by a midazolam infusion 0.05 to 0.1 mg/min IV. A 14-gauge IV cannulae was inserted into one of the nasal prongs (**A**) and a nasal adapter set (Datex, Instrumentarium Corp., Helsinki, Finland) was used to monitor end-expiratory carbon dioxide (**B**).

regurgitation. Careful observation of thoracic and abdominal respiratory excursions, timing the respiratory rate, palpation for movement of air at the mouth, and/or observing cyclical condensation of exhaled vapor on the inner wall of a facemask are basics of respiratory assessment. Changes in vital signs are often late manifestations of inadequate ventilation. Furthermore, preoccupation and distraction can interfere with the early recognition of inadequate ventilation.[57]

Stethoscopy

The simplest device to assist in monitoring ventilation is the precordial, paralaryngeal, or pretracheal stethoscope. In MAC, a heavy metal, open-sided receiver connected to a monaural stethoscope is still considered the technique of choice.[58] A benefit of this nonelectronic device is that heart tones and breath sounds are well-conducted at times when electronic devices experience temporary interference. In addition, subtle signs of patient discomfort (e.g., breath-holding, phonation) or incipient airway obstruction may be detected earlier and an untoward outcome avoided. A disadvantage of this technique is that breath sounds may appear adequate even when tidal volumes are small. Electronic amplified stethoscopes can provide for louder, clearer breath sounds and heart tones, and are subject to less interference with general communication in the operating room.[59] Disadvantages of electronic devices include annoying amplification of noise from surgical instruments or electrosurgical interference, as well as the possibility that the anesthesiologist may fail to detect absence of breath sounds.

Pulse Oximetry

Many anesthesiologists consider pulse oximetry monitoring mandatory for most anesthetic procedures, including MAC. When using sedation techniques, pulse oximetry permits better titration of respiratory depressant drugs and earlier intervention (e.g., verbal and tactile stimulation) and oxygen supplementation. However, there have been reported inaccuracies with pulse oximetry monitoring during profound desaturation,[60] interference due to nail polish and exogenous dyes,[61,62] with compromised tissue perfusion,[63] or if intense ambient light reaches the sensor.[64] Some of these potential problems (e.g., nail polish) are easily avoided.[65] In practice, pulse oximetry is an easy to use, sensitive, reliable, noninvasive measure of oxygen saturation that is capable of providing an early warning of impending desaturation prior to the development of clinical signs of hypoxemia.[66] Among the patient and operative risk factors for developing hypoxemia, the most frequently reported predisposing conditions during ambulatory gynecologic surgery are obesity, advanced age, and lithotomy position.[67]

Carbon Dioxide Monitoring

Expired carbon dioxide (CO_2) sampling can be obtained during MAC by using nasal cannulae or facemasks as support for the CO_2 sampling tube.[68,69] A stable, discernible capnograph tracing (Fig. 12-3) has been demonstrated to be readily achievable in the majority of patients having transcannula CO_2 sampling, with an acceptable correlation between end-expiratory and arterial CO_2 tension readings.[70] However, problems with these devices include displacement and false sampling, as well as delays in alarm responses. Thus, while they may assist in providing us with an indication of the degree of respiratory depression (or airway obstruction), they should not be relied on for accurate measurement of end-tidal CO_2 values.

Circulatory Monitoring

The cardiovascular system is a sensitive indicator of the patient's physiologic state. Apart from reflecting the effectiveness of administered drugs in blocking the adverse effects of noxious stimuli, close monitoring of circulatory responses provides early warning signs of undesirable side effects. Circulatory stimulation can be due to patient anxiety, inadequate analgesia, or drugs (e.g., ketamine, epinephrine, cocaine). Cardiovascular depression may be due to direct myocardial depression (β-blockers, inhaled agents) or peripheral vasodilation (local anesthetics, benzodiazepines, butyrophenones, antihypertensive therapy), while indirect causes include reflex bradycardia (e.g., anxiety-provoked, carotid sinus pressure). These responses will be more critical in patients with significant cardiovascular disease or other limitations in organ reserves, and may be modified by chronic or concomitant drug therapy.

Clinical Assessment

Assessment of cardiovascular function should include regular evaluation of peripheral perfusion by observation of skin color and capillary refill in the nail beds and mucous membranes. Brisk refill indicates good cardiac output and adequate tissue perfusion.

Pulse Monitoring

The important characteristics of the pulse are quality, rate, and regularity. Even when sophisticated noninvasive monitors are being used, it is valuable to periodically feel a peripheral pulse to determine its quality. Potential inaccuracies with all automated monitoring devices make it important to maintain this simple clinical skill (i.e., palpation). Precordial stethoscopes are a second adjunct which can be used to confirm the pulse rate and regularity, and are particularly helpful in the presence of electrosurgical interference. Pulse oximeters display pulse rate and provide an audible pulse tone in addition to oxygen saturation. Although some oximeters display pulse amplitude, these tracings may be artificially enhanced and therefore should not be relied on as indicators of pulse strength or tissue perfusion.[63]

Blood Pressure Monitoring

Blood pressure may be determined by manual estimation using a sphygmomanometer or an automated ultrasonic (Doppler) or oscillotonometric device. All methods have potential inaccuracies,[71] and patient injuries have been reported with these automated indirect methods. In addition, routine use of automated blood pressure devices have been alleged to have a negative impact on the vigilance of anesthesia residents.[72] Blood pressure alone may be a poor indicator of cardiac output in certain patient populations. For example, if myocardial oxygen consumption (MVO_2) exceeds maximum oxygen delivery in patients with coronary artery disease, myocardial ischemia can occur despite an adequate blood pressure. While the rate-pressure product is not an absolute reflection of MVO_2, it is easily derived and may be used as a guide to recommended limits of cardiovascular challenge.[73,74]

Electrocardiography

When the ECG is correctly configured and calibrated, it can provide valuable information regarding heart rate, disturbances of conduction and cardiac rhythm, as well as myocardial ischemia. In view of the potential for myocardial depression, hypoxia, and drug-induced arrhythmias (e.g., epinephrine, cocaine, local anesthetic agents), an argument can be made for mandatory ECG monitoring during MAC.[75] Detection of left ventricular and anterior ischemia will usually be seen on leads V_4 or V_5, while inferior ischemia can be observed by monitoring leads II, III, or AVF. However, right ventricular and posterior ischemia is difficult to detect using standard leads.[76] Most ECG monitors used in the operating room provide only three leads for monitoring, in which case the CM_5 configuration has been shown to be the most sensitive method for detecting S-T segment changes associated with left ventricular ischemia. Although the limited sensitivity and specificity of the ECG as an index of inadequate myocardial perfusion is clearly recognized, it will continue to be used for this purpose until more accurate, noninvasive devices for measuring cardiac performance are available. Since myocardial ischemia is unlikely in healthy outpatients undergoing MAC,[77] some investigators argue that the ECG need not be used for "routine anesthesia" and that a pulse monitor (e.g., oximeter) and precordial stethoscope will detect dysrhythmias.[76] While there is no hard evidence to support improved outcome with ECG monitoring, it seems prudent to establish a preanesthetic baseline with the particular configuration being used so that any change in appearance can be compared with this tracing. The primary role of ECG monitoring during MAC is to serve as a detector of arrhythmias and a warning of myocardial ischemia; thus, it is an important adjunct to cardiovascular assessment by blood pressure measurement and stethoscopy.[75]

Temperature Monitoring

One of the most frequently stated reasons for monitoring body temperature is to detect malignant hyperthermia, a serious though rare complication of anesthesia. Yet, the most likely temperature derangement during MAC is inadvertent hypothermia. Heat loss during surgery is enhanced by factors such as airconditioned operating rooms, poorly insulated patient coverings, the surgical requirement for extensive surface exposure, and evaporation of antiseptic solution. Reduced heat production occurs as a result of limitation of patient activity, as well as drug-induced decreases in resting muscle tone. Temperature monitoring during MAC has practical limitations since tympanic membrane, nasopharyngeal, and rectal temperature probes are often impractical and uncomfortable. As an alternative, axillary temperature is a reasonable reflection of muscle temperature. Although surface temperature is a poor indicator of core body temperature, there is evidence that surface warmth (e.g., radiant heat) can minimize postanesthetic shivering.[78] Patients receiving regional anesthesia experience similar rates of shivering to those having general anesthesia; however, the duration of hypothermia is longer and rate of temperature rise in the first hour of their recovery room stay is slower.[79] The main focus of temperature monitoring should be to prevent hypothermia and the resultant shivering, which can be uncomfortable and may cause increased oxygen consumption, interference with surgery, and increased pain at the operative site.

Central Nervous System

Careful evaluation of the central nervous system (CNS) is a mainstay in assessing the efficacy of MAC, particularly in evaluating whether the adjunctive drugs used have achieved the desired degree of analgesia, sedation, anxiolysis, and overall patient comfort. Stimulation of the CNS as a result of drug overdosage (e.g., ketamine, local anesthetic toxicity), hypoxia, pain or discomfort, and fear can produce agitation and/or confusion. Excessive CNS depression (e.g., failure to respond to verbal or tactile stimulation) is usually due to sedative overdosage or drug interactions (e.g., midazolam-fentanyl), but may also be secondary to respiratory insufficiency and hypoxia. Many short-acting sedative-hypnotics (e.g., thiopental) have long elimination halflives and can accumulate with repeated dosing or continuous infusion techniques. Other sedative medications have long-acting metabolites (e.g., desmethyldiazepam) which can act synergistically with other drugs (e.g., opioid analgesics) to cause prolonged effects. In patients with evidence of increased intracranial pressure (ICP), respiratory depressant drugs should be administered with *extreme* caution since an increase in end-tidal CO_2 will increase cerebral blood flow and ICP.

Recovery Room Monitoring After Monitored Anesthesia Care

The principal aims in recovery room monitoring are to assess the residual effects of drugs administered intraoperatively and to determine when the patient is fit for discharge, which in ambulatory surgery implies "home readiness." One important difference between the recovery period and the operative phase is that the patient recovering from local anesthesia may not be experiencing the same degree of pain as patients emerging from general anesthesia, thereby increasing the potential for late manifestations of drug-induced side effects (e.g., respiratory depression). The overall incidence of recovery room morbidity varies from 18 to 30 percent,[80–82] and includes airway obstruction, hypoventilation, hypotension or hypertension, arrhythmias, inadequate analgesia, nausea and vomiting, and postanesthetic shivering. Recovery room monitoring following MAC is a natural extension of intraoperative monitoring, with particular emphasis on respiratory adequacy, cardiovascular stability, and return to baseline cerebral functioning. This requires regular clinical evaluation, as well as the use of pulse oximetry, blood pressure, and temperature monitoring. Adequate staffing, good patient supervision, and allowance for adequate recovery time are all essential components of safe recovery following MAC.[83]

Monitored Anesthesia Care Outside the Operating Room

Diagnostic Radiologic Procedures and Radiotherapy in Children

These procedures are characterized by the requirement for sedation with or without analgesia and by significant limitations with respect to patient access for short periods of time. Specific monitoring issues in this setting must make allowance for the possibility that the anesthesiologist may be required to observe the patient from a separate room. Patient assessment may also be compromised by excessive noise and poor lighting. Monitors which will provide relevant information in these cases include pulse oximetry, automated blood pressure and heart rate device, ECG, and remote stethoscopy.[59] Special non-ferrous (plastic) connectors and props are required on monitoring equipment during magnetic resonance imaging (MRI).[84] The sedative medications that are used for these procedures include barbiturates (e.g., thiopental 2 to 4 mg/kg IV, methohexital 15 to 30 mg/kg rectally), midazolam 0.15 to 0.3 mg/kg IM, ketamine 3 to 6 mg/kg IM or 0.5 to 1.0 mg/kg IV, or inhalational agents (e.g., halothane 0.25 to 0.75 percent, enflurane 0.5 to 1 percent). Since these patients are rarely intubated, atropine is frequently administered as an adjuvant to minimize secretions and respiratory complications (e.g., coughing, laryngospasm). As in all pediatric cases, marked sensitivity of cardiovascular reflexes and rapid depletion of pulmonary oxygen reserves with hypoventilation emphasize the need for careful monitoring of cardiovascular and respiratory function.

Similarly, postoperative monitoring should pay particular attention to airway patency and reflexes, normal ventilation, and level of consciousness.

Extracorporeal Shockwave Lithotripsy

Extracorporeal shockwave lithotripsy has all but replaced open surgery for the treatment of renal and upper urinary tract calculi. While the majority of ESWL machines use water submersion to prevent deflection of the energy waves at an air-tissue interface, new generation devices (e.g., Lithostar) will allow treatment without body immersion and are currently being used for disintegration of calculi in other locations (e.g., the gallbladder). With the newer (dry) ESWL devices, intravenous sedation-analgesia techniques are highly effective.[84] The preferred anesthetic technique in most ESWL submersion units is continuous epidural anesthesia with varying degrees of sedation.[85,86] Local anesthesia (intercostal nerve blocks)[87] techniques and deep sedation-analgesic techniques (Monk TG, White PF, unpublished data) have also been used.[87] The primary role of adjunctive (intravenous) medication is to minimize anxiety and prevent inadvertent patient movement in order to keep the stone in the target focus. Intravenous midazolam has become the drug of choice in this situation. Monitoring is based on the need to evaluate the cardiovascular or respiratory effects of the local anesthetic and sedative-analgesic drugs. Other monitoring concerns relate to the requirement for ECG synchronization in order to prevent shockwave-induced cardiac arrhythmias, monitoring restrictions imposed by body immersion and patient positioning, and the safety problems induced by working in a dimly lit and extremely noisy environment. Use of a headset to provide background music can be extremely helpful in this situation (Thompson GF, personal communication). Specific monitors therefore must include an ECG, automated blood pressure device, and pulse oximeter.[85] Common problems encountered include hypotension (from the local anesthetic-induced sympathetic blockade), hypoventilation (due to sedative-analgesic drugs and residual neural blockade), upper airway obstruction, and occasional arrhythmias. Finally, it is important to remember that an overriding consideration is appropriate electrical isolation and safety, and that only those devices which meet the ESWL manufacturer's guidelines should be used.

LIMITATIONS OF MONITORING

While the emphasis in this chapter has been on the appropriate usage of various monitoring devices, it is also important to critically examine the information these devices provide. There are obvious limitations of all monitoring methods, and it is therefore important to maintain a degree of skepticism in evaluating whether the monitored data accurately reflects the patient's true physiologic state. Many factors effecting the accuracy of pulse oximeters,[88] noninvasive blood pressure measuring devices,[71] and ECG monitors[76] have been described in the anesthesia literature. Calkins has drawn attention to the appreciable risk to the patient because of the extensive dependence on equipment per se, and especially the complex triad of anesthesiologist, equipment, and patient.[89] The present plethora of monitor designs, information presentation, and alarms is an ergonomic nightmare which may actually serve to enhance the potential for human error.[90]

The final common pathway for all monitored information is the CNS of the anesthesiologist caring for the patient. Essential characteristics of this vital element in the monitoring triad is that the anesthesiologist must be present in the operating room, and must be diligent, knowledgeable, alert, and actively "involved" in the conduct of the anesthetic. There are significant limitations with respect to human performance; not surprisingly, human error is a major contributor to negative outcomes following anesthetic mishaps.[91] Nevertheless, Cooper believes that the ultimate safety feature in anesthesia is a trained, vigilant anesthesiologist, and any technical solution that diminishes the patient-physician relationship is a step in the wrong direction.[92]

SUMMARY

The optimal conduct of MAC is dependent on knowing as much as possible about the true physiologic state of the patient, including the past record and present trend. Certain derived information will contribute to the accuracy and quality of this assessment. The selection and management of appropriate monitors to assist in this objective is of obvious importance. However, emphasis on issues related to quality assurance, patient safety procedures, risk recognition, and efforts to reduce human error are crucial to the success of any MAC technique. In any individual case, the choice of monitoring and sedation techniques should be based on the balanced judgment of the responsible anesthesiologist, taking into account the specific medical, surgical, and anesthetic requirements of the individual patient rather than any general recommendations. In MAC, achievement of optimal results is dependent on the knowledge, vigilance, experience, and general wariness of a responsible and qualified anesthesiologist.

REFERENCES

1. Position on Monitored Anesthesia Care. The American Society of Anesthesiologists, Park Ridge, IL, 1986
2. Ryan JA, Adye BA, Jolly PC, Mulroy MF: Outpatient inguinal herniorrhaphy with both regional and local anesthesia. Am J Surg 148:313, 1984
3. Wheeless CR: Outpatient laparoscope sterilization under local anesthesia. Obstet Gynecol 39:767, 1972
4. White PF, Vasconez LO, Mathes SA, et al: Comparison of midazolam and diazepam for sedation during plastic surgery. Plastic Reconstr Surg 81:703, 1988
5. White PF, Shafer A: Clinical pharmacology and uses of injectable anesthetic and analgesic drugs in outpatient anesthesia. p. 37. In Wetchler BV (ed): Problems in Anesthesia. JB Lippincott, Philadelphia, 1988
6. Philip BK: Supplemental medication for ambulatory procedures under regional anesthesia. Anesth Analg 64:117, 1985
7. Zelcer J, Tyers MR, White PF: Comparison of alfentanil and fentanyl as adjuvants to propofol. Anesthesiology 71:A28, 1989
8. Al-Khudhairi D, Whitwam JG, McCloy RF: Midazolam and diazepam for gastroscopy. Anesthesia 37:1002, 1982
9. Tucker MR, Ochs MW, White RP: Arterial blood gas levels after midazolam or diazepam administered with or without fentanyl as an intravenous sedative for outpatient surgical procedures. J Oral Maxillofac Surg 44:688, 1986
10. Urquhart ML, White PF: Comparison of sedative infusion techniques for sedation during regional anesthesia—methohexital, etomidate and midazolam. Anesth Analg 68:249, 1989
11. Mackenzie N, Grant IS: Propofol for intravenous sedation. Anesthesia 42:3, 1987
12. Negus JB, White PF: Use of sedative infusions during local and regional anesthesia—a comparison of midazolam and propofol. Anesthesiology 69:A711, 1988
13. White PF, Way WL, Trevor AJ: Ketamine: its pharmacology and therapeutic uses. Anesthesiology 56:119, 1982
14. Nishino T, Takizawa K, Yokokawa N, Hiraga K: Depression of swallowing reflex during sedation and/or relative analgesia produced by inhalation of 50% nitrous oxide in oxygen. Anesthesiology 67:995, 1987
15. Colon GA, Gilbert N: Lorazepam (Ativan) and fentanyl (Sublimaze) for outpatient office plastic surgical anesthesia. Plastic Reconstr Surg 78:486, 1986

16. Takasaki M: Ventilation and ventilatory response to carbon dioxide during caudal anesthesia with lidocaine or bupivacaine in sedated children. Acta Anaesthesiol Scand 32:218, 1988
17. Alexander CM, Gross JB: Sedative doses of midazolam depress hypoxic ventilatory responses in humans. Anesth Analg 67:377, 1988
18. Mora CT, Torjman M, DiGiorgio K: Sedative and ventilatory effects of midazolam and flumazenil. Anesthesiology 67:A534, 1987
19. Korttila K, Linnoila M: Recovery and skills related to driving after intravenous sedation: dose-response relationship with diazepam. Br J Anaesth 47:457, 1975
20. Gale GD: Recovery from methohexitone, halothane and diazepam. Br J Anaesth 48: 691, 1976
21. Douglas JG, Nimmo WS, Wanless R, et al: Sedation for upper gastro-intestinal endoscopy: a comparison of oral temazepam and i.v. diazepam. Br J Anaesth 52:811, 1980
22. O'Boyle CA, Harris D, Barry H: Sedation in outpatient oral surgery: comparison of temazepam by mouth and diazepam i.v. Br J Anaesth 58:378, 1986
23. Berggren L, Eriksson I, Mollenholt P, Wickbom G: Sedation for fibreoptic gastroscopy: a comparative study of midazolam and diazepam. Br J Anaesth 55:298, 1983
24. Magni VC, Frost A, Leung JWC, Cotton PB: A randomized comparison of midazolam and diazepam for sedation in upper gastrointestinal endoscopy. Br J Anaesth 55: 1095, 1983
25. Korttila K, Tarkkanen J: Comparison of diazepam and midazolam for sedation during local anesthesia for bronchoscopy. Br J Anaesth 57:581, 1985
26. Barker I, Butchart DGM, Gibson J, et al: I.V. sedation for conservative dentistry: a comparison of midazolam and diazepam. Br J Anaesth 58:371, 1986
27. Bailey PL, Moll JWB, Pace NL, et al: Respiratory effects of midazolam and fentanyl: potent interaction producing hypoxemia and apnea. Anesthesiology 69:A813, 1988
28. White PF, Shafer A, Boyle WA, et al: Benzodiazepine antagonism does not provoke a stress response. Anesthesiology 70:636, 1989
29. Mora CT, Torjman M, White PF: Effects of diazepam and flumazenil on sedation and hypoxic ventilatory response. Anesth Analg 68:473, 1989
30. McCarthy FM, Solomon AL, Jastak JT, et al: Conscious sedation: benefits and risks. J Am Dental Assoc 109:546, 1984
31. Kallar SK, Dunwiddie WC: Conscious sedation. p. 93. In Wetchler BV (ed): Problems in Anesthesia. JB Lippincott, Philadelphia, 1988
32. Shane SM: p. 1. Conscious Sedation for Ambulatory Surgery. University Park Press, Baltimore, 1983
33. Scamman FL, Klein SL, Choi WW: Conscious sedation for procedures under local or topical anesthesia. Ann Otol Rhinol Laryngol 94:21, 1985
34. Bendixen HH: Foreword: the tasks of the anesthesiologist. p. xi. In Saidman LJ, Smith NT (eds): Monitoring in Anesthesia. Butterworth, Boston, 1984
35. Wilson ME: The study of morbid events. p. 109. In Lunn JN (ed): Quality of Care in Anaesthetic Practice. The Pitman Press, Bath, 1984
36. Pace NL: But what does monitoring do to patient outcome? (editorial) Int J Clin Monit Comput 1:197, 1985
37. Pierce EC: Monitoring instruments have significantly reduced anesthetic mishaps. J Clin Monit 4:111, 1988
38. Caplan RA, Posner K, Ward RW, Cheney FW: Respiratory mishaps: principal areas of risk and implications for anaesthetic care. Anesthesiology 67:A469, 1987
39. Coplans MP, Curson I: Deaths associated by dentistry. Br Dental J 153:357, 1982
40. McKay WPS, Noble WH: Critical incidents detected by pulse oximetry during anesthesia. Can J Anesth 35:265, 1988
41. Editorial: Midazolam—is antagonism justified? Lancet 140, 1988
42. Bell GD, Spickett GP, Reeve PA, et al: Intravenous midazolam for upper gastrointestinal endoscopy: a study of 800 consecutive cases relating dose to age and sex of patient. Br J Clin Pharmacol 23:703, 1987
43. Eichhorn JH, Cooper JB, Cullen DJ, et al: Standards for patient monitoring during anesthesia at Harvard Medical School. JAMA 256:1017, 1986
44. Cooper JB, Newbower RS, Long CD,

McPeek B: Preventable anesthesia mishaps: a study of human factors. Anesthesiology 49:399, 1978
45. Moyers J: Monitoring instruments are no substitute for careful clinical observation. J Clin Monit 4:107, 1988
46. Standards for Basic Intraoperative Monitoring. American Society of Anesthesiologists, Park Ridge, IL, 1986
47. Philip JH, Raemer DB: Selecting the optimal anesthesia monitoring array. Med Instrum 19:122, 1985
48. Whitcher C, Ream A, Parsons D, et al: Anesthetic mishaps and the cost of monitoring: a proposed standard for monitoring equipment. J Clin Monit 4:5, 1988
49. Hug CC, Jr.: Monitoring. p. 411. In Miller RD (ed): Anesthesia. 2nd Ed. Churchill Livingstone, New York, 1986
50. Hamilton WK: We monitor too much. J Clin Monit 2:264, 1986
51. Vandam LD: The senses as monitors. p. 9. In Blitt CD (ed): Monitoring in Anesthesia and Critical Care Medicine. 2nd Ed. Churchill Livingstone, New York, 1990
52. White PF: Anesthetic techniques for the elderly outpatient. Int Anesthesiol Clin 26: 105, 1986
53. Wilcox S, Vandam LD: Alas, poor Trendelenburg and his position! A critique of its uses and effectiveness. Anesth Analg 67: 574, 1988
54. Huang TT, Rejaie I, Lewis SR: Relative hypoxemia during rhytidoplasty. Plastic Reconstr Surg 58:32, 1976
55. McNabb TG, Goldwyn RM: Blood gas and hemodynamic effects of sedatives and analgesics when used as a supplement to local anesthesia in plastic surgery. Plastic Reconstr Surg 58:37, 1976
56. Singer R, Thomas PE: Pulse oximeter in the ambulatory aesthetic surgical facility. Plastic Reconstr Surg 82:111, 1988
57. Newbower RS, Cooper JB, Long CD: Failure analysis—the human element. In Gravenstein JS (ed): Essential Non-invasive Monitoring in Anesthesia. Grune & Stratton, Orlando, FL, 1980
58. Blitt CD: Precordial and esophageal stethoscopes. p. 29. In Blitt CD (ed): Monitoring in Anesthesia and Critical Care Medicine. 2nd Ed. Churchill Livingstone, New York, 1990
59. Philip JH, Raemer DB: An electronic stethoscope is judged better than conventional stethoscopes for anesthesia monitoring. J Clin Monit 2:151, 1986
60. Severinghaus JW, Naifeh KH: Accuracy of response of six pulse oximeters to profound hypoxia. Anesthesiology 67:551, 1987
61. Cote CJ, Goldstein EA, Fuchsman WH, Hoaglin DC: The effect of nail polish on pulse oximetry. Anesth Analg 67:683, 1988
62. Scheller MS, Ungar RJ, Kelner MJ: Effects of intravenously administered dyes on pulse oximeter readings. Anesthesiology 65:550, 1986
63. Lawson D, Norley I, Korbon G, et al: Blood flow limits and pulse oximeter signal detection. Anesthesiology 67:599, 1987
64. Brooks TD, Paulus DA, Winkle WE: Infrared heat lamps interfere with pulse oximeters. Anesthesiology 61:630, 1984
65. White PF, Boyle WA: Oximetry and nail polish. Anesth Analg 68:546, 1989
66. Cohen DE, Downes JJ, Raphaely RC: What difference does pulse oximetry make? Anesthesiology 68:181, 1988
67. Raemer DB, Warren DL, Morris R, et al: Hypoxemia during ambulatory gynecologic surgery as evaluated by the pulse oximeter. J Clin Monit 3:244, 1987
68. Goldman JM: A simple, easy and inexpensive method for monitoring $ETCO_2$ through nasal cannulae. Anesthesiology 67:606, 1987
69. Pressman MA: A simple method of measuring $ETCO_2$ during MAC and major regional anesthesia. Anesth Analg 67:905, 1988
70. Louwsma DL, Silverman DG. Reproducibility of end tidal CO_2 by nasal cannula. Anesthesiology 69:A268, 1988
71. Runciman WB, Ilsley AH, Rutten AJ: Systemic arterial blood pressure. Anaesth Intensive Care 16:54, 1988
72. Kay J, Neal M: Effect of automatic blood pressure devices on vigilance of anesthesia residents. J Clin Monit 2:148, 1986
73. Jones RM, Knight PR, Hill AB: Rate pressure product. Anesthesia 35:1010, 1980
74. Reitan JA, Barash PG: Noninvasive monitoring. p. 117. In Saidman LJ, Smith NT (eds): Monitoring in Anesthesia. Butterworth, Boston, 1984
75. Blitt CD: Monitoring for outpatient anesthesia. p. 685. In Blitt CD (ed): Monitoring in Anesthesia and Critical Care Medicine.

1st Ed. Churchill Livingstone, New York, 1985
76. Tyers MR, Russell WJ, Runciman WB: Electrocardiographic monitoring in anesthesia. Anaesth Intensive Care 16:66, 1988
77. Gravenstein JS, Paulus DA (eds): Clinical Monitoring Practice. JB Lippincott, New York, 1987, p. 30
78. Lipton JM, Giesecke AH: Body temperature and shivering in the perioperative patient. Semin Anesth 7:3, 1988
79. Vaughan RW, Vaughan MS: Temperature: our most neglected perioperative monitor, Semin Anesth 7:38, 1988
80. Van der Walt JH, Mackay P: Patient safety in the recovery room. Anaesth Intensive Care 16:77, 1988
81. Zelcer J, Wells DG: Anaesthetic-related recovery room complications. Anaesth Intensive Care 15:168, 1987
82. Cullen DJ: The recovery room. Semin Anesth I:333, 1982
83. Faculty of Anaesthetists, Royal Australasian College of Surgeons: Guidelines for the care of patients recovering from anesthesia. Policy Statement (2-83), p. 4, 1983
84. Schelling G, Weber W, Sackmann M, Peter K: Pain control during extracorporeal shockwave lithotripsy of gallstone by titrated alfentanil. Anesthesiology 70:122, 1989
85. Abbott MA, Samuel JR, Webb DR, et al: Anesthesia for extracorporeal shock wave lithotripsy. Anaesthesia 40:1065, 1985
86. Silbert BS, Kluger R, Dixon GCE, Berg J: Anesthesia for extracorporeal shock wave lithotripsy at the Victorian Lithotripsy Service—the first 300 patients. Anaesth Intensive Care 16:310, 1988
87. Malhotra V, Long CW, Meister MJ: Intercostal blocks with local infiltration anesthesia for extracorporeal shock wave lithotripsy. Anesth Analg 66:85, 1987
88. Griffiths DM, Ilsley AH, Runciman WB: Pulse meters and pulse oximeters. Anaesth Intensive Care 16:49, 1988
89. Calkins JM: Monitoring the anesthetic delivery system. p. 615. In Blitt CD (ed): Monitoring in Anesthesia and Critical Care Medicine. 2nd Ed. Churchill Livingstone, New York, 1990
90. Kestin IG, Miller BR, Lockhart CH: Auditory alarms during anesthesia monitoring. Anesthesiology 69:106, 1988
91. Cooper JB, Newbower RS, Kitz RJ: An analysis of major errors and equipment failures in anesthetic management: considerations for prevention and detection. Anesthesiology 60:34, 1984
92. Cooper JB: Anesthesia can be safer: the role of engineering and technology. Med Instrum 19:105, 1985

13

Local Anesthesia and Sedation Techniques

Beverly K. Philip

Patients who undergo ambulatory surgery desire a rapid recovery in order to resume their normal activities. The anesthetic care of ambulatory patients can help attain this goal by providing the minimal anesthesia needed to satisfy the physical and emotional requirements of the particular operation. Local anesthetic techniques enhanced with supplemental sedation can often meet that objective. This chapter discusses the local anesthetic agents used for ambulatory surgical patients and reviews their mechanism of action and physiologic disposition. Local anesthetic techniques are also described, including three areas of current and potential interest to anesthesiologists: infiltration anesthesia, retrobulbar anesthesia, and intravenous regional anesthesia. The chapter concludes with a discussion of supplemental medications for local and regional anesthesia, with emphasis on considerations relevant to the adult ambulatory surgical patient.

LOCAL ANESTHETIC AGENTS

Localized anesthesia may be produced by a variety of means, including mechanical trauma, low temperature, anoxia, and chemical irritants. Clinically, only substances that produce a transient and completely reversible blockade of nerve function are used. These substances fall into two major chemical classes, the amino-esters and the amino-amides.[1]

The chemical identification of cocaine as a benzoic acid ester led to the synthesis of the amino-esters, a series of compounds that are benzoic acid ester derivatives. Benzocaine (ethyl 4-aminobenzoate) was identified by Ritsert in 1890. Poor water solubility limits the drug's usefulness as an injectable local anesthetic, but benzocaine is an effective topical anesthetic and remains widely used in nonprescription medications for dermal abrasions, sunburn, and mucous membrane anesthesia. Procaine, synthesized by Einhorn and Brown in 1905, is an ester of para-aminobenzoic acid (2-diethylaminoethyl 4-aminobenzoate). This compound is water soluble and remains useful for infiltration procedures and peripheral nerve blockade. Two other benzoic acid-derivative anesthetics are still clinically used. Tetracaine (2-methylaminoethyl 4-butylaminobenzoate) is used with ambulatory patients primarily for topical anesthesia of the mucous membranes and conjunctivae; inpatient applications also include spinal anesthesia. Chloroprocaine (2-diethylaminoethyl 4-amino-2-chlorobenzoate), the least toxic of the amino-esters, is used for infiltration and nerve blockade as well as for epidural anesthesia.

The first amino-amide to be synthesized

was lidocaine, which was developed by Löfgren in 1943. Lidocaine is an amide derivative of diethylamino acetic acid (2-ethylaminoacet-2,6-xylidide). This drug differs from the previously released para-aminobenzoic acid ester derivatives by being essentially free of sensitizing reactions, and it soon replaced procaine in standard clinical practice. Lidocaine remains widely used in ambulatory anesthesia for topical anesthesia, infiltration, and peripheral nerve blockade, as well as for epidural and spinal anesthesia. The amino-amide prilocaine (2-propylamino-2′-propionotoluidide) offers the advantage of lower systemic toxicity due to a slower rate of absorption, greater tissue distribution, and increased hepatic metabolism.[2] For this reason, there has been a resurgence of interest in prilocaine 0.5 percent for use in intravenous regional anesthesia.[3]

Mepivacaine (1-methyl-2′,6′-hexahydropicolinylxylidide) has clinical properties similar to lidocaine except that it lacks topical anesthetic activity. Bupivacaine (1-butyl-2′,6′-hexahydropicolinylxylidide) is a homologue of mepivacaine having greater potency than its parent drug and longer duration of action. Bupivacaine is used in ambulatory anesthesia for local or nerve block infiltration to provide prolonged postoperative sensory analgesia; use in other applications, such as ambulatory epidural or spinal anesthesia, is restricted by the excessive recovery time required. Etidocaine (2-N-ethylpropylamino-2′,6′-butyroxylidide) is more potent and longer acting than the related drug lidocaine, but since etidocaine produces marked motor blockade, it has limited use in the ambulatory setting. Suggested doses of local anesthesia agents for infiltration can be found in Table 13-1.

Compounds that demonstate clinical utility as local anesthetic agents have a common chemical arrangement consisting of an aromatic portion, an intermediate chain, and an amine portion. Chemical structure is related to the biologic activity of the compounds. The amine portion is associated with hydrophilic properties, and the aromatic end is associated with lipophilicity. Changes in the amine or aromatic portion will alter a compound's lipid/water partition coefficient and its protein-binding characteristics. Within either of the anesthetic structural groups, changes in the physicochemical properties result in changes in biologic activity, specifically in potency and duration of action. An increase in molecular weight (up to a maximum weight) will tend to result in an increase in anesthetic potency. Alterations in chemical structure within each structural group also result in changes in the rate of degradation and, therefore, in the intrinsic toxicity of the

Table 13-1. Recommended Doses of Local Anesthetic Agents

		Plain solutions		Epinephrine-containing solutions	
Agent	Concentration (%)	Maximum adult dose (mg)	Maximum dose (mg/kg)	Maximum adult dose (mg)	Maximum dose (mg/kg)
Short duration					
Procaine	1–2	800	11	1,000	14
Chloroprocaine					
Moderate duration					
Lidocaine	0.5–1	300	4	500	7
Mepivacaine	0.5–1	300	4	500	7
Prilocaine	0.5–1	500	7	600	8
Long duration					
Bupivacaine	0.25–0.5	175	2.5	225	3

compounds. Different degradation products may have different in vivo effects. The structural differences between lidocaine and prilocaine result in the formation of o-toluidine as a prilocaine metabolite, rather than 2,6-xylidine. O-toluidine is responsible for the production of methemoglobin, which is seen after administration of high doses of prilocaine.

The chemical differences between the amino-ester and amino-amide groups have clinical significance. The groups differ in their mode of metabolism and in their allergic potential. Metabolism of the amino-esters occurs primarily due to hydrolysis by the plasma enzyme pseudocholinesterase. Patients who are unable to produce an adequate quantity of normal pseudocholinesterase enzyme show a decreased tolerance to ester-type local anesthetics, which causes prolongation of action and increased risk of toxicity.[4] Amide local anesthetic compounds undergo enzymatic breakdown primarily in the liver. Patients with liver disease and decreased hepatic microsomal function may show reduced tolerance to amide-type local anesthestic drugs. Metabolism of the amino-ester group anesthetics results in the (re-)formation of para-aminobenzoic acid. It is this compound that is responsible for the allergic reactions seen in a small percentage of the population. The amino-amides are not metabolized to para-aminobenzoic acid, and allergic reactions are rare.[5] There is no reported evidence of cross-sensitivity between the structurally dissimilar amino-ester and amino-amide groups.

Mechanism of Action

The excitation process in peripheral nerves is a multistep phenomenon. During nerve inactivity, a resting potential of approximately −60 to −90 mV exists across the nerve membrane. When excitation occurs, the cell membrane becomes more permeable to sodium ions. The initial phase of depolarization due to the influx of sodium ions results in the electrical potential within the cell becoming progressively less negative. When the threshold potential of approximately −50 to −60 mV is reached, the potential difference between the interior and the exterior surface of the cell membrane permits a maximum increase in permeability to sodium ions. This rapid phase of depolarization, associated with an extremely rapid influx of sodium ions into the axoplasm, results in the cell interior becoming positively charged to approximately +40 mV at the peak of the action potential. At the end of depolarization, the membrane permeability to sodium ion decreases, and high potassium permeability is restored. Potassium flows out of the cell, and repolarization of the membrane occurs. The electrical potential within the cell becomes progressively more negative until the resting potential is again reached and the original electrochemical equilibrium has been restored. Under normal conditions, the entire process of depolarization occurs within 1 msec.

Local anesthetic agents act primarily by interfering with the excitation-conduction process in the nerve membrane. Their specific point of interference in this electrophysiologic process has been investigated, and a decrease in the rate of the depolarization phase has been observed, particularly the phase of slow depolarization.[1] When depolarization is not sufficient to reach the threshold potential, a propagated action potential cannot develop. The anesthetic-receptor combination results in blockade of the sodium channel and, therefore, decreased sodium permeability. In summary, the primary action of local anesthetic agents consists of a reduction in nerve cell membrane permeability to sodium ions, a subsequent decrease in the rate of rise of the depolarization phase of the action potential, and a failure of a propagated action potential to develop, which causes conduction blockade.

A local anesthetic receptor site at the sodium channel has been postulated, and several nonclinical local anesthetic compounds have been shown to act at sites on the external and internal surfaces of the sodium channel.[1] Although the cationic forms of many anesthetics are believed to be the forms active at the sodium channel receptor site, other compounds exist as uncharged molecules at physiologic pH and still exert anesthetic activity. These compounds, such as benzocaine and benzyl alcohol, are believed to act by membrane expansion. Compounds which are highly lipid soluble can penetrate the lipid portion of the cell membrane more readily, causing a conformational change in the membrane. It is the resultant decrease in the diameter of the sodium channel that results in the inhibition of sodium conductance and in neural blockade. Most of the clinically useful local anesthetic agents can exist in both a charged and an uncharged form, namely, procaine, lidocaine, mepivacaine, prilocaine, bupivacaine, and etidocaine. These agents therefore act by both a receptor mechanism and a receptor-independent mechanism at the cationic receptor site and as a physicochemical disturbance within the nerve membrane.

Active Forms

Most of the clinically useful local anesthetic agents are available as salts, most commonly as the hydrochloride. In solution, the salts exist both as uncharged molecules of the anesthetic base (B) and as positively charged cations (BH^+). The relative proportion between the uncharged and charged forms depends on the pK_a of the specific chemical compound and the pH of the solution, according to the equation $pK_a = pH - \log (B/BH^+)$. Since the pK_a is constant, the relative proportion of free base and charged cation depends on the pH of the solution. As the pH is decreased and the hydrogen ion concentration is increased, relatively more cation will be present than free base. As the pH is increased and the hydrogen ion concentration is decreased, relatively more of the local anesthetic will exist as free base. Both the charged and uncharged forms are involved in producing neural block.[1] The uncharged base form is responsible for diffusion through the neural sheath. The charged cation binds to the receptor site at the cell membrane and is the active form responsible for the electrophysiologic process of conduction blockade.

The local anesthetics are weak bases with a pK_a of approximately 7.7 to 9.1 and are poorly water soluble. They are usually marketed as acidic solutions of pH ≤ 6.5, which increases their water solubility and shelf stability. However, at this decreased pH the charged form predominates, and the drug is less able to enter the nerve sheath. The clinical result of the predominance of cationic form is a prolonged onset of action, which is a potential hindrance in the ambulatory setting. However, onset can be shortened by increasing the pH of the local anesthetic solution. This is easily done by the addition of sodium bicarbonate in the form of 1 mEq/10 ml lidocaine, mepivacaine, or chloroprocaine; or 0.1 mEq/20 ml bupivacaine[6] (McKay, unpublished data). These alkalinized solutions lack shelf stability and must be prepared shortly before use.

When added to local anesthetic drugs, carbon dioxide can decrease the onset time and potentiate the block.[7] This is partly due to action at the local anesthetic membrane receptor site, where a decrease in pH results in an increased formation of active cation. Nonionizable local anesthetics are not potentiated by CO_2. Carbon dioxide has also been shown to increase the degree of block independent of solution pH.[7] The addition of CO_2 can be accomplished either by aerating with CO_2 gas or by using carbonated local anesthetic salts.[8] Reports are not unanimous,[3] but carbonated solutions of local anesthetics have been shown to decrease clinical onset time for brachial plexus and epidural blocks.[7,9,10]

Physiologic Disposition

The activity and toxicity of local anesthetic drugs are influenced by their physiologic disposition. These factors include their systemic absorption, distribution, metabolism, and excretion. The major determinants of drug absorption are the site of injection, the dose administered, the presence of an added vasoconstrictor, and the pharmacologic profile of the particular agent. In general, the highest lidocaine anesthetic blood level is obtained after intercostal nerve block.[11,12] Caudal, lumbar epidural, brachial plexus, and sciatic-femoral injections produce blood anesthetic levels of decreasing magnitude, while subcutaneous injections for local infiltration produce the lowest levels (Fig. 13-1). The high concentration seen following intercostal blockade is probably due to deposition of the local anesthetic over multiple vessels and large vascular surface area, which allows a greater rate and degree of absorption. The potential for systemic toxicity after any given dose is therefore greater at a site permitting faster absorption and increased blood levels. Anesthetic blood levels have been compared after brachial plexus block and intravenous regional anesthesia of the upper limb.[13] The venous level of lidocaine measured following tourniquet release in intravenous technique (1.5 ± 0.2 μg/ml) was significantly lower than the peak level measured after plexus block (2.5 ± 0.5 μg/ml). The intraarticular injection of 100 mg bupivacaine for analgesia after knee arthroscopy produced peak concentrations of 0.48 ± 0.20 μg/ml at 43.4 ± 23.1 minutes.[14]

The topical administration of local anesthetics to different sites also results in differing blood levels and therefore differing potential for toxicity. In general, the greatest absorption occurs after intratracheal instillation.[15] The intratracheal spray formu-

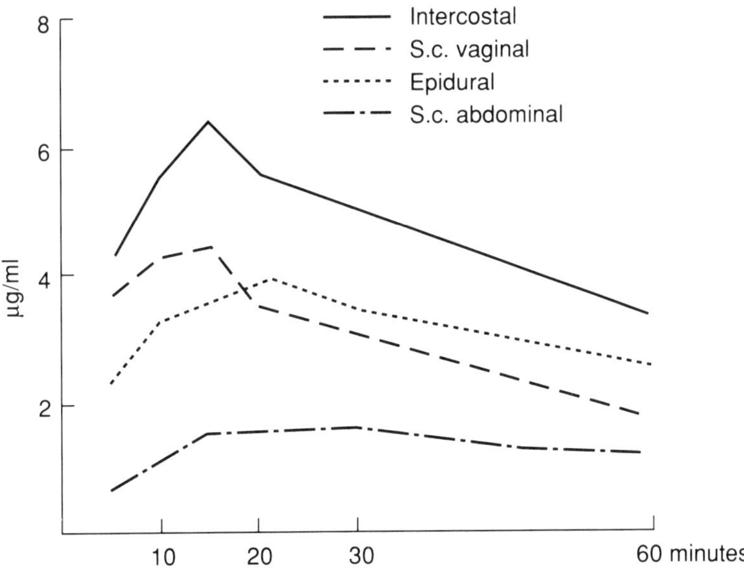

Fig. 13-1. Plasma lidocaine levels after injection of 20 ml of 2 percent lidocaine at different sites. (From Scott et al.,[11] with permission.)

lation causes a wide dispersion and rapid uptake of anesthetic. There is less absorption after administration into the nose or urinary bladder. These differences are related to the vascularity of the administration site and to the particular pharmaceutical preparation used. The use of ointments or gels for mucous membrane anesthesia would result in delayed vascular absorption and lower potential for toxicity.

At any site, the blood level of local anesthetic is a function of the total dose of drug administered, and not the specific concentration or volume used. There tends to be a linear relationship between dose of drug and peak blood level. Depending on the site of administration, a peak anesthetic blood level of 0.5 to 2.0 μg/ml is achieved for each 100 mg of lidocaine or mepivacaine given. The addition of a vasoconstrictor decreases the rate of absorption irrespective of the site of administration, which reduces the potential for systemic toxicity. Epinephrine in a concentration of 5 μg/ml (1:200,000) significantly reduces the peak blood levels for lidocaine and mepivacaine[11,12]; less influence is seen on peak levels of prilocaine, bupivacaine, or etidocaine. The specific drug also influences the rate of absorption. Vascular absorption is more rapid for lidocaine and mepivacaine than for other agents, a phenomenon related to the former drugs' relatively lower lipid solubility and tendency to cause vasodilation. In contrast, tetracaine is absorbed rapidly after intratracheal instillation at a rate comparable to intravenous absorption and with comparable toxicity.

The blood level of local anesthetic agents following absorption from the site of administration is a function of both the rate of distribution from vascular to tissue compartments and the rate of elimination. The initial rapid phase of redistribution is related to uptake by highly perfused tissues. The secondary slower phase reflects distribution to more poorly perfused tissues as well as elimination via metabolic and excretory pathways. In general, an increased rate of tissue redistribution appears to correlate with lower protein binding and increased lipid solubility characteristics of the anesthetic agent. The rate of redistribution of prilocaine is significantly faster than that for lidocaine or mepivacaine, whose rates are similar.

The metabolism of local anesthetic compounds is governed by their chemical structure.[1] The amino-esters are primarily hydrolyzed by plasma pseudocholinesterase. The rate of hydrolysis varies among the agents in this class. Chloroprocaine undergoes the fastest hydrolysis and has the shortest duration of action and the least toxicity. Tetracaine undergoes the slowest hydrolysis among the amino-esters and has the longest duration of action and the most toxicity. Procaine is intermediate in effects. The amino-amides are primarily metabolized in the liver. Prilocaine, in addition, undergoes some metabolism in the kidney. A similar correlation between rate of metabolism and toxicity occurs with this class of local anesthetics as well. Prilocaine, which undergoes the most rapid metabolism, is the least toxic. Drug uptake and metabolism are also influenced by the physiologic status of the patient. The rate of disappearance of lidocaine from the blood has been shown to be prolonged in patients with impaired myocardial contractility and subsequent decreased tissue perfusion, and in hepatectomized patients during liver transplantation.

Local anesthetic drugs are excreted primarily in metabolized form, most often via the kidney. In the ester class of local anesthetic agents, less than 2 percent of a procaine dose is excreted in the urine as unchanged drug. Approximately 90 percent of the primary procaine metabolite, para-aminobenzoic acid, is found in the urine. Similarly, only small amounts of unchanged chloroprocaine and tetracaine are excreted by the kidney. In the amide class of drugs, the same is generally true. For lidocaine, less than 10 percent of intravenously administered drug is found unchanged, and approximately 80 percent is found as various metabolites in the urine. The renal clearance of prilocaine is higher than lidocaine as a result of decreased protein binding.

INFILTRATION ANESTHESIA

Local anesthesia is provided by surgeons, and sometimes by anesthesiologists, for many procedures. Outpatient herniorrhaphy can be performed under ilioinguinal/iliohypogastric field block,[16] circumcision under dorsal penile nerve block,[17] dental procedures under block of appropriate branches of the mandibular and maxillary divisions of the trigeminal nerve,[18] extracorporeal shock wave lithotripsy under intercostal nerve blocks and local infiltration,[19] and laparoscopy under peritoneal lavage anesthesia.[20] For many procedures, the operative site can be infiltrated with 0.25 percent bupivacaine in conjunction with general or major regional anesthetics to provide prolonged postoperative pain relief. Plastic surgical operations performed under local anesthesia include facelifts, mammoplasties, abdominoplasties, and other liposuction surgery.[21] For plastic surgery, large volumes of local anesthetic agent may be needed to infiltrate the large and often vascular operative areas; consequently, potential problems of drug overdose and toxicity may arise.

Two classes of drugs are administered during local infiltration, and toxicity may develop with either. The first is the local anesthetic agent. The maximum dose recommended for a single administration of plain lidocaine is 4 mg/kg; when used with added epinephrine, as is more usual, the recommended dose is 7 mg/kg.[5] Plasma levels have been measured after the subcutaneous abdominal injection of 20 ml 2 percent lidocaine.[11] Peak levels occurred at approximately 15 minutes and were 1.95 ± 0.23 μg/ml. By 1 hour postinjection, blood levels were approximately 1.1 μg/ml. More vascular areas, such as the face, would be expected to produce higher plasma concentrations. Levels of 4 μg/ml lidocaine have been associated with the threshold for toxic symptoms.[22]

A concentration of 0.5 percent lidocaine with epinephrine is usually injected for sensory analgesia. Considering the maximal allowable dose (Table 13-1), a volume of 98 ml would be permitted for an adult weighing 70 kg. However, the volume of solution needed to provide anesthesia for such procedures as facelift, mammoplasty, and abdominoplasty has been reported to be as high as 300 ml[23] to 1,200 ml.[24] To avoid toxicity with these volumes, surgeons have evaluated the use of lower concentrations of local anesthetic. Buffington et al.[23] reported excellent clinical results with 0.26 percent lidocaine in a series of 1,316 patients. Klein[24] used 0.1 percent lidocaine, infiltrating a mean total of 1,250 ml or 1,250 mg (range, 825 to 3,100 mg) into subcutaneous fat over a 1- to 5-hour period. The mean dose of lidocaine was 18.4 mg/kg body weight, and the mean dose per unit time was 8.5 mg/kg/hr. Venous blood samples were taken 1 hour after completion of injection. Lidocaine levels averaged 0.34 μg/ml, with the highest level at 0.61 μg/ml. No symptoms of toxicity were observed.

The other class of injected agents that can cause toxicity is the vasoconstrictors. Vasoconstrictors, most often epinephrine, are added to local anesthetic solutions to be used as infiltration anesthesia to reduce blood loss. Plasma levels of catecholamine have been measured after the injection of 21 ml of 1:200,000 epinephrine in 0.5 percent lidocaine for rhinoplasty[25] (Fig. 13-2). There was a 566 percent increase in plasma epinephrine levels (to 4.1 pmol/ml) 2 minutes after injection. "Considerable tachycardia" was reported, but not further specified. By 5 minutes after injection, the

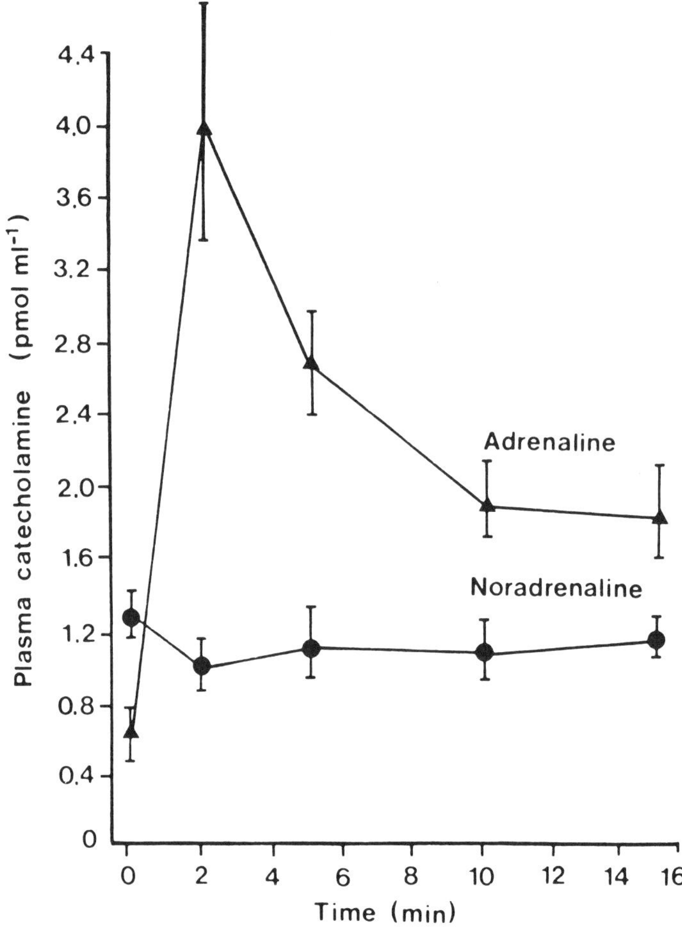

Fig. 13-2. Plasma catecholamine concentrations after the infiltration of 0.5 percent lidocaine with epinephrine (adrenaline) 1:200,000 for rhinoplasty. (From Cotton et al.,[25] with permission.)

plasma epinephrine concentration had declined to 2.4 pmol/ml and by 15 minutes it had decreased to 1.3 pmol/ml. This can be compared with a level of 1.2 pmol/ml reported in response to endotracheal intubation.[26] Plasma norepinephrine concentrations were also measured during rhinoplasty[25] and did not change during the study period; this indicates that the observed epinephrine was of exogenous origin. A 30 percent increase in cardiac output has also been reported after the intraoral injection of 5.4 ml of lidocaine with 1:100,000 epinephrine.[27]

Practitioners have tried to limit the potential for toxicity by using more dilute epinephrine concentrations. Decreasing the epinephrine concentration from 1:200,000 to 1:400,000 resulted in no change in vasoconstrictor efficacy, measured as blood loss after liposuction.[28] Epinephrine concentrations of 1:1,000,000[24] and 1:1,666,666[23] have also been used, resulting in retention of clinically satisfactory hemostasis. Other nonsympathomimetic vasoconstrictors have not gained clinical popularity.[1] Toxicity from absorbed epinephrine is seen as hypertension and tachycardia. If significant hypertension develops, increments of propranolol (0.25 to 0.5 mg) or labetolol (5 to 10 mg) may be used for treatment. Clonidine, a centrally acting α_2-agonist with antihypertensive and sedative properties, may also be given preoperatively in a dose of 5 μg/kg (approximately 0.3 mg PO).[29]

Another concern related to the infiltration of local anesthetics is the pain associated with the injection itself. Attempts to anesthetize the skin without a needle injection have been handicapped by the poor diffusion of local anesthetic through intact skin.[30] A topically active emulsion consisting of 5 percent lidocaine base and 5 percent prilocaine base has been developed that circumvents this problem. Known as EMLA (eutectic mixture of local anesthetics), the combination has been shown to contain droplets of 80 percent active local anesthetics.[30] When applied prior to venipuncture, EMLA produces a significant decrease in subjective and observed pain in children[30] and adults.[31] The analgesia is comparable to that produced by intradermal infiltration of 0.2 ml of 1 percent lidocaine using 28- to 30-gauge needles.[32,33] However, the onset of analgesia produced by this compound is slow, requiring an application time of 60 minutes prior to needle puncture.[34,35] It has also been observed that EMLA is more effective for skin penetration on the dorsum of the hand and in the antecubital area than on the lower arm.[35] Other practical considerations include the need for an occlusive dressing, and a residual skin greasiness which may interfere with tape application.[32] EMLA does produce effective skin analgesia, but the time constraints, in particular, will limit its use for the adult ambulatory patient.

The pain associated with local anesthetic injection can also be altered by the choice of agent used. Morris et al.,[36] using a 26-gauge needle, compared discomfort from the injection of normal saline and five local anesthetics. In order of most to least painful, the anesthetics were 1 percent etidocaine, 0.5 percent bupivacaine, 1 percent mepivacaine, 2 percent chloroprocaine, and 1 percent lidocaine. Etidocaine was significantly more painful than all other agents, and normal saline without preservative was ranked below mepivacaine. The differences in perceived discomfort between agents could not be related to pH, pK_a, osmolality, or the presence of additives; higher lipid solubility was observed to parallel more pain. Another study compared three local anesthetics commonly used for infiltration and rated them also in decreasing order of pain on injection: 1 percent lidocaine with epinephrine 1:100,000, 1 percent lidocaine plain, and 1 percent procaine.[37]

The pain of skin infiltration when using lidocaine can be reduced by additive substances. One such substance is sodium bicarbonate.[38] The addition of bicarbonate to a final concentration of 0.1 mEq/ml anesthetic is effective for 1 percent lidocaine with or without commercially added epinephrine. Presumably, the mechanism of lessened pain in this case is the increased alkalinity of the solutions: pH is changed from 6.49 to 7.38 for plain 1 percent lidocaine before and after bicarbonate, and from pH 4.05 to 7.37 for lidocaine with epinephrine. Both of the pH-adjusted lidocaine solutions were judged less painful than normal saline. Normal saline alone does not provide local skin analgesia when injected. Another approach to reducing the pain of lidocaine infiltration is the inclusion of benzyl alcohol. Benzyl alcohol is a local anesthetic in its own right and, in a 0.9 percent concentration, it is routinely found as the bacteriostatic compound in sodium chloride multidose vials. Normal saline with 0.9 percent benzyl alcohol was judged less painful than 1 percent procaine or 1 percent lidocaine.[39] Local analgesia for pinprick lasts approximately 2 minutes. Normal saline with benzyl alcohol appears to be the least uncomfortable of the injectable agents for brief skin anesthesia.

RETROBULBAR ANESTHESIA

Local anesthesia for ophthalmic surgery is only occasionally performed by anesthesiologists. However, many ophthalmic procedures are being done, and knowledge of the appropriate blocks represents an opportunity for expansion of the anesthesiologist's practice. The technical aspects of ophthalmic anesthesia are well-described in *Anesthesia for Ophthalmology*[40] and other textbooks.

The choice of an appropriate local anesthetic agent depends primarily on the duration of surgical anesthesia that is needed. A concentration of 2 percent lidocaine can provide approximately 1 to 2 hours of retrobulbar anesthesia.[41,42] The addition of epinephrine 1:100,000 to lidocaine will increase the duration of the anesthesia to approximately 3 hours,[43] but there is possible risk of retinal artery spasm with retrobulbar placement of epinephrine.[44] Consequently, intrinsically longer-acting local anesthetic agents are often chosen for potentially lengthier procedures.[45] Longer postoperative analgesia is also a beneficial result of using longer-acting agents.

A solution of 0.5 percent bupivacaine for retrobulbar anesthesia can provide approximately 3 to 5 hours of sensory blockade and 6 to 10 hours of motor blockade.[46,47] However, incomplete akinesia of the globe has been reported at this concentration, and onset of anesthesia with bupivacaine is slower than with lidocaine. A concentration of 0.75 percent bupivacaine provides complete retrobulbar motor blockade and 8 to 12 hours of anesthesia,[48] although onset of anesthesia is still slower than with lidocaine. The problem of slow block onset can be addressed by combining 0.75 percent bupivacaine with 2 percent lidocaine (or 2 percent mepivacaine). A concentration of 1 percent etidocaine has an onset similar to that of 2 percent lidocaine (approximately 3 minutes)[43] and a duration of retrobulbar block of 5 hours or more. Rarely, less-than-complete sensory anesthesia occurs.

Hyaluronidase is a substance that depolymerizes hyaluronic acid, the "ground substance" of mesenchymal tissue. Historically, it has been added to all local anesthetic solutions for retrobulbar anesthesia to improve the quality of blockade by spreading the anesthetic. Onset time may also be shortened. The role of hyaluronidase in retrobulbar anesthetic solutions has been re-evaluated by Nicoll et al.[49] The addition of hyaluronidase to either 0.5 percent bupivacaine or 0.5 percent bupivacaine/2 percent lidocaine did produce total akinesia in a significantly greater number of patients (Fig. 13-3). Duration of action remained adequate despite the potential for faster anesthetic uptake and removal. The effectiveness of hyaluronidase has not been consistently demonstrated for use with other somatic blocks; its effectiveness with retrobulbar blockade may be related to increased interstitial pressure produced by the limited bony orbit and by the postblock application of a pressure balloon. Increased systemic toxicity caused by increased absorption of local anesthetic is a potential, but not reported, complication of the use of hyaluronidase. Allergic reactions have been rarely reported.

Complications associated with retrobulbar blockade may be attributed either to the local anesthetic used or to direct trauma from the needle injection itself. Complications from local anesthetic agents do not usually result from absolute overdose, since only a small volume of drug is used (2 to 5 ml). Nonetheless, unintentional intravenous injection of even small amounts of anesthetic can cause typical central nervous system and cardiovascular toxic symptoms.[5] In addition, there is a unique pattern of toxic symptoms that may be seen after retrobulbar blockade, consisting of the sudden onset of respiratory depression, apnea, and loss of consciousness.[50,51] Convulsions or cardiovascular collapse occur rarely. The time lapse from administration of anesthesia to onset of these symptoms has averaged 8 minutes (range, 2 to 40 minutes) and has occurred in some form in 0.27 percent of 6,000 studied patients.[50] The presumed mechanism for these events is the

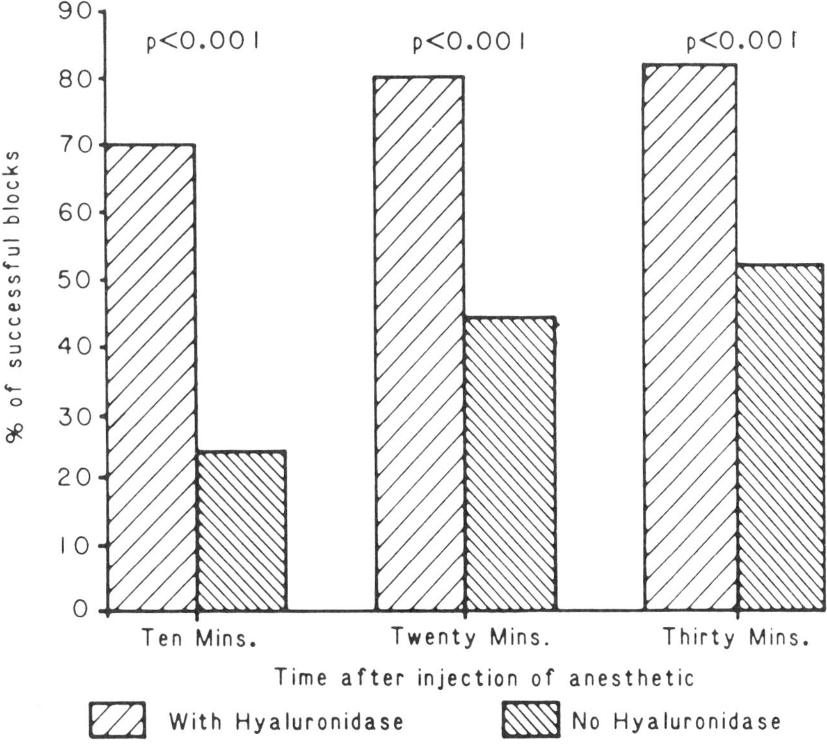

Fig. 13-3. Frequency of complete akinesia after a single retrobulbar injection of local anesthetic with or without hyaluronidase. (From Nicoll et al.,[49] with permission.)

subdural injection of local anesthetic into the brain via the optic nerve sheath or superior orbital fissure. Intra-arterial anesthetic injection with retrograde flow also remains a possibility. Transient contralateral vision loss and akinesia may occur by a similar mechanism.

Injection of local anesthetic into the retrobulbar space can trigger the oculocardiac reflex. The afferent limb of this arc is the ophthalmic division of the trigeminal nerve via the ciliary ganglion, and the efferent limb is the vagus nerve.[52] Ectopic rhythms develop, and a profound slowing of the heart rate occasionally occurs and can proceed to sinus arrest. Arrhythmias are generally common during ophthalmic anesthesia and surgery, particularly surgery on the extraocular muscles. However, the unpredictable onset and severity of the oculocardiac reflex mandate heart rate monitoring as well as the presence of personnel and equipment to provide cardiopulmonary resuscitation during all intraorbital blocks. Initial treatment consists of intravenous atropine and occasionally precordial pressure to enable the atropine to reach the central circulation. Prophylactic intramuscular anticholinergic is ineffective. Routine prophylaxis with intravenous atropine is not recommended because of the resulting tachyarrhythmias that can be deleterious in the elderly population.[53] Anxiety-generated vasovagal reactions also occur.

Traumatic complications of retrobulbar blockade include retrobulbar hemorrhage, retinal artery occlusion, and scleral perforation. Retrobulbar hemorrhage occurs in up to 5 percent of blocks done with a sharp needle, but the incidencc approaches zero when the specialized blunted needle is used.[54] Retrobulbar hemorrhage may develop from a small, slow venous leak or from a significant arterial laceration. Signs of a significant retrobulbar hemorrhage include rapid orbital swelling, marked proptosis with immobility of the globe, and blood staining of the lids and conjunctiva.[41] Visual decrement or loss can occur after significant hemorrhage and may be related to increased intraorbital pressure on the ophthalmic artery, causing ischemic damage to the optic nerve or retina. Retinal artery occlusion, another potential traumatic complication, may be the result of vessel laceration and hemorrhage within the arterial sheath. This complication is seen more often in patients with underlying hematologic or vascular diseases. Epinephrine in the anesthetic solution has also been implicated as a causative factor[44]; injection of a combined lidocaine/epinephrine solution has been observed to cause a 50 percent decrease in ophthalmic artery pulse pressure. The complication of scleral perforation has been reported to occur in 3 of 4,000 cases.[55] Visual loss can occur following scleral perforation as a result of intraocular hemorrhage and retinal detachment. The injection of lidocaine into the vitreous has been reported not to cause injury.[41] In order to minimize these traumatic complications of retrobulbar anesthesia, a careful approach must be used. Needle insertion and drug injection should be performed slowly and gently, and a blunt, a 3.5 to 4.0-cm Atkinson needle is recommended.

The peribulbar approach to ophthalmic anesthesia has been suggested as a means to avoid traumatic injury.[56] With that technique, local anesthetic is deposited outside the muscle cone and, therefore, further from the globe and optic nerve and artery. Lid akinesia and anesthesia may be obtained with the same injections. Another potential advantage is reduced visual impairment during the effect of the block. However, a higher rate of incomplete anesthesia or akinesia has been reported, and onset of this block is slower than with the retrobulbar technique.[56] Minor complications, such as periorbital ecchymosis, do occur. Major complications may be reduced but not prevented; perforation of the globe has been reported with the peribulbar technique.[57]

INTRAVENOUS REGIONAL ANESTHESIA

Intravenous regional anesthesia (IVRA), also known as the Bier block,[58] is an intravascular infiltration technique commonly used by anesthesiologists for procedures involving the distal extremities. It is simple to perform and provides good surgical anesthesia with rapid onset.

This technique probably produces its anesthetic effects at two sites of action. The initial analgesia is produced by diffusion of local anesthetic from the veins to the small nerves or nerve endings.[59,60] For the upper extremity, the pattern of anesthesia onset after dilute lidocaine IVRA is related to the anatomic distribution of the peripheral nerves in the forearm, although the sequence of motor or sensory loss is variable.[61] The nerve endings as a site of action are also supported by investigations which isolated the local anesthetic from the hand.[62] Tourniquets were inflated on the upper arm and the wrist; injection of anesthetic and radioisotope into veins between the tourniquets demonstrated that no radioisotope was detected and no analgesia was obtained distal to the wrist tourniquet. Other investigations indicate that IVRA is also produced by a second mechanism. Conduction block of the nerve trunks occurs at the site of maximum drug concentration, primarily around the elbow.[63,64] Ischemic changes in the tourniquet-compressed extremity may play a role in contributing to or accentuating local anesthetic-induced blockade.[65]

Regional anesthesia by the intravenous route can be provided for the upper extremity with a padded tourniquet on the upper arm or wrist. The double tourniquet introduced by Hoyle[66] is often used on the upper arm to allow inflation of the distal cuff onto anesthetized tissue, thereby prolonging patient comfort. Intravenous regional anesthesia may also be provided for the lower extremity by placing a tourniquet on the calf muscle.[67,68] Extra padding is needed on the lower leg to avoid compression of the superficial peroneal nerve at the fibular neck. Because of the large mass of tissue, it is considerably more difficult to obtain good anesthesia for the entire lower extremity by placing a tourniquet on the thigh; in addition, such tourniquet placement is associated with an increased incidence of systemic toxicity.[68,69]

The technique for producing IVRA consists of exsanguination of the extremity, inflation of a pneumatic tourniquet, and the intravenous injection of a local anesthetic agent. Exsanguination of the extremity is usually accomplished by elevating the extremity briefly, then wrapping it with an Esmarch bandage from the tips of the digits to the edge of the tourniquet.[5] Inadequate exsanguination of the fingertips and hand (or toes and foot) will leave a significant residuum of blood, which will dilute the local anesthetic and reduce the effectiveness of the block in that area. When IVRA is used for a fracture or an otherwise injured extremity, an Esmarch wrap may not be well-tolerated. In that case, a longer period of elevation and gravity drainage (5 to 10 minutes) or a pneumatic splint may be used to accomplish the exsanguination.[70]

The location and type of intravenous access for the instillation of local anesthetic should also be considered. Intravenous access close to the operative site may permit faster diffusion of relatively undiluted local anesthetic and therefore may produce a more complete block.[71] The antecubital fossa should be avoided as an injection site as high injection pressures at this site may force anesthetic under the inflated tourniquet and predispose toward systemic toxic reactions.[70] A small-gauge catheter is entirely adequate for drug injection. This catheter can be occluded by an obturator or injection-site cap during exsanguination of the limb. Although use of a scalp-vein

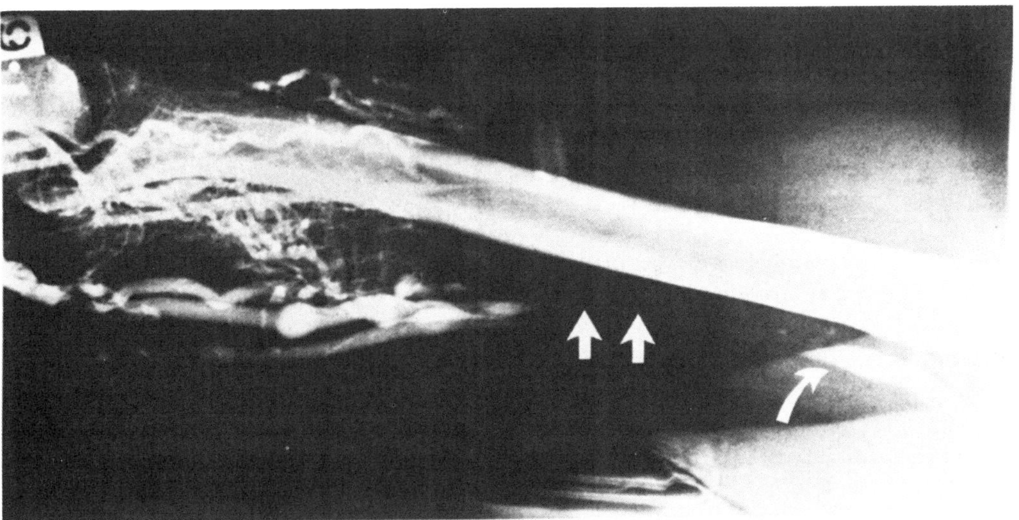

Fig. 13-4. Phlebography after injection of contrast material into an exsanguinated, 300 mmHg tourniquet-compressed upper extremity. Note the filled axillary vein proximal to the cuff (curved arrow, right) and a continuous line of contrast medium on the medial side of the humerus (two straight arrows). (From Rosenberg et al.,[73] with permission.)

needle has also been recommended,[71] the same investigator also reports that dislodgement of the steel needle during exsanguination is his most common cause of technique failure.

Perhaps the most critical element to the success of intravenous regional anesthesia is the tourniquet. Proper functioning of the tourniquet and its inflation system must be checked before use. If the tourniquet fails during the block, the intravenous local anesthetic will be released into the systemic circulation; analgesia will be lost and a systemic toxic reaction may occur. It has, however, been evident that leakage of local anesthetic can occur despite an apparently correctly functioning tourniquet[72] (Fig. 13-4). Causes of these leaks have included systemic hypertension, calcified peripheral vessels, intraosseous circulation, and obesity.[70,74,75] The potential for local anesthetic leakage around the cuff on an obese extremity is exacerbated by the commonly used double tourniquet. Each section of the double tourniquet must be narrower, and the pressure transmitted by a 5- to 6-cm cuff section may not be adequate to occlude the deeply underlying vessels.[74,75] Another potential cause of local anesthetic leak is an excessive rate of local anesthetic injection, causing intravascular pressures to transiently exceed cuff occlusive pressure.[76] Grice et al.[74] evaluated factors which avoided elevated venous pressures and which thereby reduced the possibility of anesthetic solution leakage. They studied venous pressure tracings distal to the tourniquet as well as proximal leakage of xenon-133 labeled saline, and were able to identify the following conditions which improved safety: injection into a distal rather than proximal vein, slow rate of injection (over 90 seconds, or approximately 0.5 ml/sec), prior exsanguination with an Esmarch bandage, and a tourniquet pressure of at least 300 mmHg. For hypertensive systolic blood pressures, an estimated tourniquet pressure of systolic pressure plus 100 mmHg may be used.

Timing of the tourniquet release at the end of the procedure can also help reduce the incidence of systemic anesthetic toxicity. Peak drug levels after tourniquet release have been found to be inversely proportional to tourniquet time (Fig. 13-5), with an initial release of approximately 30 percent of the drug followed by gradual washout of the remainder.[77] An initial inflation period of 15 to 30 minutes is recommended to allow adequate tissue fixation of the drug. Intermittent release of the tourniquet cuff after the procedure is also suggested. Cyclic deflation slows the time to maximum blood anesthetic concentration.[78] Peak anesthetic levels occur within 30 seconds of cuff release[77]; cyclic deflation and inflation should therefore occur at 10 to 15-second intervals to minimize peak levels.[69]

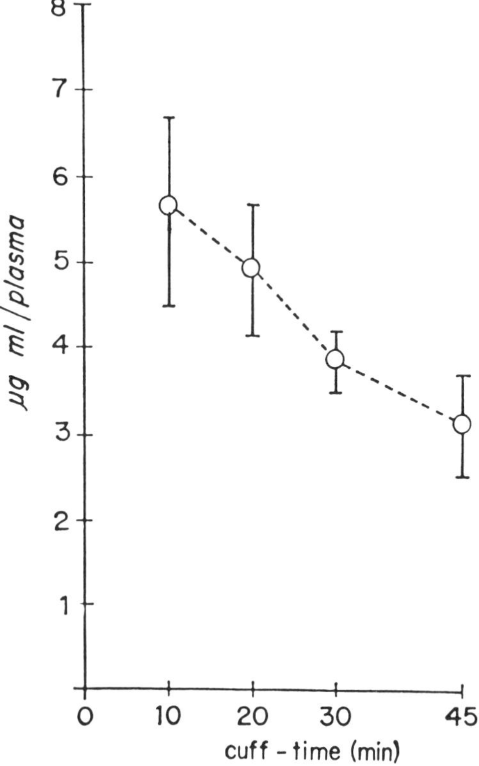

Fig. 13-5. Relationship between tourniquet cuff time and plasma levels of 1 percent lidocaine at a minute after cuff release. (Adapted from Tucker and Boas,[77] with permission.)

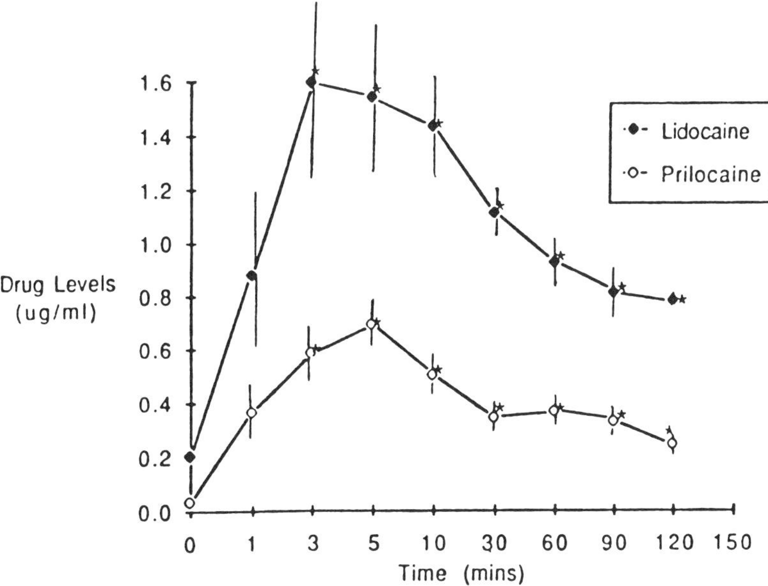

Fig. 13-6. Whole blood drug levels following tourniquet deflation, comparing prilocaine and lidocaine. (From Bader et al.,[81] with permission.)

The choice of local anesthetic agent for IVRA has been the subject of considerable discussion. Lidocaine is the drug most commonly used in a dose of 3 mg/kg: 40 ml of 0.5 percent for the upper extremity or 75 to 100 ml of 0.25 percent to 0.33 percent for the lower extremity.[79] A dosage of 40 ml of 0.5 percent prilocaine for the upper extremity is also consistently effective.[80] Methemoglobin may be produced by the prilocaine metabolite o-toluidine, but clinically significant methemoglobin levels are not seen after the doses of prilocaine used for IVRA.[81] Maximum anesthetic blood levels after IVRA are lower with prilocaine than with equal doses of lidocaine, because of the former's rapid tissue redistribution and accelerated hepatic metabolism[81] (Fig. 13-6). This potential for less systemic toxicity recommends more widespread use of prilocaine for IVRA. Chloroprocaine also has the potential for low systemic toxicity, but it can cause phlebitis and therefore should not be used.[82] Bupivacaine has the advantage of prolonged analgesia, from 7 to 12 hours, after tourniquet release.[83] However, there have been many reports of serious systemic toxicity,[84] including cardiac arrest, that have required prolonged resuscitation despite an intact tourniquet.[73] In the United Kingdom, there have been several deaths associated with bupivacaine IVRA.[85] Drug toxicity has not been the only factor implicated in these catastrophes. Skill and technique are at issue, since nonanesthetists inadequately trained in overdose resuscitation usually have been involved.[86,87] In the United States and the United Kingdom, bupivacaine is not presently recommended for IVRA. Dosages of 40 ml of 0.5 percent ketamine appear to produce intravenous analgesia, but in a series of 14 patients, each one lost consciousness for 10 minutes after tourniquet release.[88]

SUPPLEMENTAL MEDICATION FOR AMBULATORY LOCAL AND REGIONAL ANESTHESIA

Supplemental medication for ambulatory local and regional anesthesia serves two major functions.[89] One is to provide drug-

Table 13-2. Selected Drugs for Supplemental Medication

Class	Drug	Suggested dose
Sedative-anxiolytics	Diazepam	0.05–0.15 mg/kg
	Midazolam	0.03–0.15 mg/kg
	Droperidol	5–17 μg/kg
Analgesics	Fentanyl	1–3 μg/kg
	Alfentanil	5–20 μg/kg
	Butorphanol	7–28 μg/kg
Inhalation analgesia	Enflurane	0.5%
	Nitrous oxide	30–50%

(Adapted from Philip,[89] with permission.)

induced tranquility (sedation) and relaxation (anxiolysis) during the surgical procedure. The other is to provide additional analgesia for the minor discomforts that occur even with a successful local anesthetic block. Supplemental sedative-anxiolytic and analgesic drugs can greatly increase the ambulatory patient's satisfaction with local anesthetic techniques. Drugs chosen for supplementation should have an appropriately short onset and duration of action, few side effects, and a minimal likelihood of adverse reactions developing after discharge. They must be given in appropriate doses, preferably by the intravenous route. It should also be emphasized that verbal reassurance is an effective supplementation for ambulatory local and regional procedures. A list of selected drugs for supplemental medication may be found in Table 13-2.

Sedative-Anxiolytics

Benzodiazepines

Diazepam is the first of the benzodiazepines used for supplemental sedation. Sedation appears within 2 to 3 minutes of intravenous administration.[90] Diazepam is rapidly cleared from plasma, with a distribution halflife of approximately 1 hour.[91] However, the total dose of intravenous diazepam should be limited to avoid prolonged effects. Ataxia and dizziness sufficient to delay discharge are present in 8 percent and 16 percent of subjects, respectively, 1 hour after administration of 10 mg of diazepam. After 20 mg, these causes of delayed discharge are present in 40 percent and 30 percent of subjects. Intravenous diazepam also causes respiratory depression[92] which coincides with drowsiness. To avoid overmedication of the ambulatory patient, diazepam should be used in 2.5-mg increments at 2 to 3-minute intervals. Individual response is widely variable, and drug dosage must be reduced in the elderly.[94]

After a period of early recovery, drowsiness and an increase in plasma concentration have been reported at 6 to 8 hours, probably due to enterohepatic recirculation.[90] Diazepam undergoes metabolism in the liver, with an elimination halflife of 24 to 48 hours in adult subjects and one of even longer duration in the elderly.[94,95] Diazepam metabolites, notably desmethyldiazepam, are also pharmacologically active. After intravenous diazepam administration, plasma levels of desmethyldiazepam increase over 48 hours.[90] Diazepam should not be considered a drug with short duration of action, and ambulatory patients should be cautioned that they may feel tired for a day or more after its administration.

The major drawback of diazepam administered intravenously for supplemental sedation is local pain and phlebitis. Because diazepam is insoluble in water, it is formulated in organic solvents including propylene glycol and ethyl alcohol (Valium, Roche Laboratories, Nutley, NJ). The incidence of venous sequelae after diazepam is greater when injected into smaller veins and increases with time: 23 percent after 2 to 3 days and 39 percent after 7 to 10 days.[96] Also, a faster rate of injection is associated with a higher incidence of immediate pain.[97]

Diazepam is particularly useful with local anesthesia because it increases the seizure threshold for local anesthetic drugs.[98] This should not, however, be construed as reason to exceed the permissible dose of local anesthetic.[84]

Diazepam given intravenously may be used to produce brief amnesia in the ambulatory patient, for the placement of the local anesthetic or for the operative procedure. However, the doses that may be needed are excessive for the ambulatory patient. Doses of 5 and 10 mg IV diazepam were required to produce a lack of recall lasting approximately 30 minutes in 50 percent and 90 percent of patients, respectively.[99] A more rapid rate of diazepam injection generates amnesia more frequently.[97] Retrograde amnesia after administration of intravenous diazepam has been variably reported.[100,101]

Lorazepam is a benzodiazepine that causes significant sedation and amnesia, but the duration of these effects is long,[102,103] and its use is not recommended for supplementation of ambulatory patients.[104] Short-acting benzodiazepines, such as triazolam,[105] can be used as oral premedicants for ambulatory local procedures.

Midazolam is a newer benzodiazepine that is water-soluble and causes minimal venous irritation.[106] It is at least twice as potent as diazepam.[107] Amnesia appears to be produced more consistently with this benzodiazepine; anterograde amnesia lasting 20 to 40 minutes has been reported in 90 to 96 percent of patients after receiving 5 mg IV midazolam. It should, however, be emphasized that some patients become distressed when they cannot recall perioperative events,[108] particularly those patients who choose local and regional anesthesia to remain aware of their surroundings. The potential for amnesia should, therefore, be discussed with the patient in advance.

The administration of 5 mg midazolam generates sedation and anxiolysis appearing within 1 to 2 minutes.[109] Motor performance recovers in 34 minutes, and subjects are awake and walking unaided at 73 minutes.[107,110] Midazolam plasma levels demonstrate a redistribution halflife of approximately 15 minutes and an elimination halflife of 2 to 3 hours, with no evidence of enterohepatic recirculation and recurrence of drowsiness.[111] Metabolites have low hypnotic activity.[112] Large doses of midazolam will, however, result in prolonged drowsiness.[113] Also, administration of inappropriately large doses of midazolam can result in excessive adverse effects, particularly respiratory depression. Cardiorespiratory arrests have been reported, particularly in the elderly during endoscopic procedures. To supplement ambulatory anesthesia, midazolam should be given in small 1 to 2-mg increments and time should be allowed for it to take effect. With this benzodiazepine, too, there is considerable variation in individual dose response.

Midazolam can also be administered by infusion to provide sedation and amnesia for local procedures. Correlation between plasma levels of midazolam and clinical endpoints has been made (Fig. 13-7). A midazolam concentration of 300 ng/ml has been found to provide adequate sedation during total intravenous anesthesia for surgical procedures.[112] At midazolam concentrations between 150 and 200 ng/ml, patients were arousable and became able to respond verbally; at concentrations between 100 and 150 ng/ml, patients appeared drowsy. Amnesia was present at concentrations above 100 ng/ml, and sedation persisted until concentrations declined below 75 ng/ml.[113] Concomitant narcotic (alfentanil) produced more sedation at the same midazolam concentrations.

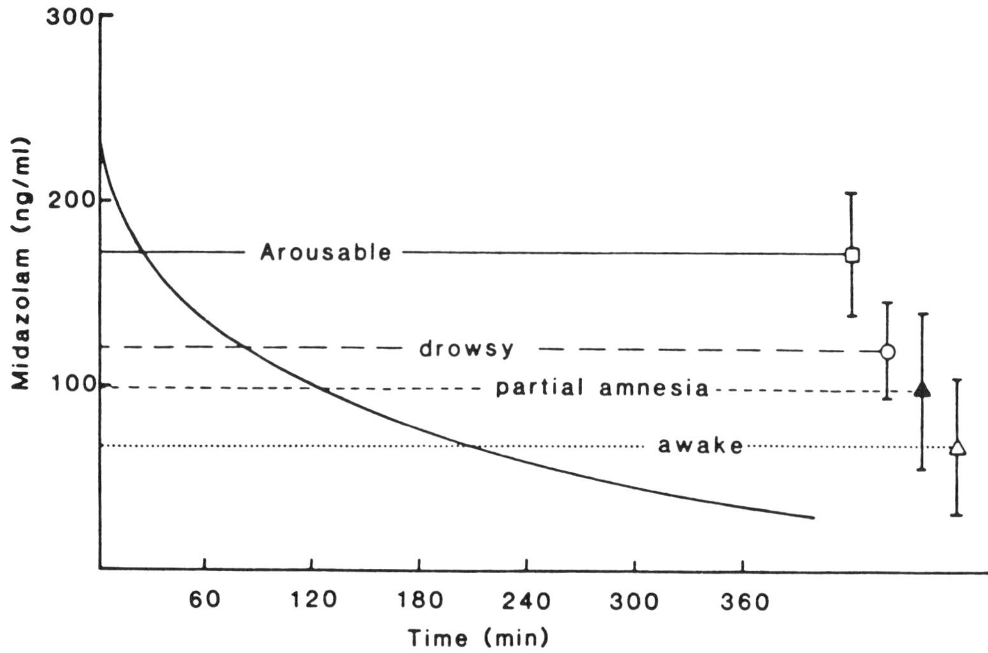

Fig. 13-7. A postinfusion concentration-time profile of mean plasma midazolam concentrations associated with various pharmacodynamic endpoints. (From Persson et al.,[113] with permission.)

If midazolam is to be used by continuous infusion, care must be taken to provide only that amount of midazolam needed to produce the desired level of sedation or amnesia, and to terminate the infusion at an appropriate time, in order to avoid excessive sedation after the procedure and prolonged recovery times. When giving midazolam by infusion to supplement local procedures, a satisfactory level of sedation should be achieved first by titrating a loading dose using incremental boluses or rapid infusion. A maintenance infusion rate of 0.04 to 0.10 mg/kg/hr, sufficient to continue the desired level of sedation, may then be given. Supplemental narcotics may be given concurrently, but they increase the potential for significant respiratory depression. Both loading and maintenance doses are reduced in the elderly.

Midazolam has been compared with diazepam for supplementation of ambulatory regional anesthesia.[114] Dixon et al. gave a midazolam, 0.10 mg/kg, or diazepam, 0.18 mg/kg, to patients having spinal, epidural, or brachial plexus blocks.[115] The degree of intraoperative sedation is similar after either sedative using these moderate doses. However, when residual sedation is evaluated after 2 hours' recovery, 80 percent of the patients who receive midazolam are awake. After the same period of recovery from diazepam, only 67 percent of patients are awake. Amnesic effectiveness under these conditions can also be compared.[115] Fifty percent of patients who receive 0.10 mg/kg midazolam remember nothing of their operation, but only 18 percent of patients who receive 0.18 mg/kg diazepam are completely amnesic. Midazolam does provide relatively more rapid recovery and more effective amnesia than diazepam when used to supplement regional anesthesia for ambulatory dental[115,116] and endoscopic[117,118] procedures.

Various benzodiazepine antagonists have been tried. Nonspecific antagonists such as naloxone (0.4 mg), physostigmine (1 to 2 mg), and aminophylline (1 mg/kg) have inconsistent success and significant side effects, and their routine use for the ambulatory patient is not recommended. A specific benzodiazepine antagonist, flumazenil (RO 15-1788), has been developed and is awaiting licensure in the United States. Flumazenil competitively displaces benzodiazepines at the specific benzodiazepine-GABA-chloride channel receptor complex.[119] Flumazenil can prevent or abolish (when given before or after) all centrally mediated benzodiazepine effects. It has no agonist activity and minimal side effects, such as recurrence of anxiety, at the dose used to reverse excess postoperative benzodiazepine effect, 0.2 to 1.0 mg.[119,120–124] Effect begins 1 minute after intravenous injection,[123] making possible the titration of the degree of reversal. The elimination halflife of flumazenil is approximately 1 hour; the potential for resedation by the original benzodiazepine therefore exists and has been observed.[125] Caution will be needed to avoid the premature discharge of ambulatory patients.[126]

Droperidol

Droperidol has been used for many years as a supplement to surgical and diagnostic procedures. This butyrophenone derivative produces sedation and a sense of detachment. Amnesia is minimal.[127] Droperidol does not significantly affect respiration, although wide individual variation of response occurs.[128] Droperidol is used for its sedative and particularly for its antiemetic properties.[129,130] Doses of 0.005 to 0.017 mg/kg, or 0.625 to 1.25 mg in adults, given by the intravenous or intramuscular route significantly reduce the incidence of postoperative vomiting.[131–133] Significant side effects are not reported at these doses. Higher doses produce increased side effects, such as excessive sedation, extrapyramidal symptoms, anxiety, and prolonged sedation, and should not be used for ambulatory patients.

Analgesics

Fentanyl

Fentanyl is a potent narcotic widely used to supplement ambulatory procedures. After intravenous administration, subjective response to fentanyl begins within 2 minutes and lasts 45 to 60 minutes.[134] Study of plasma fentanyl kinetics shows that termination of effect is due to redistribution into blood and peripheral tissues, with a redistribution halflife of 13.4 minutes.[134] Increments of 25 to 50 μg fentanyl may be given intravenously, beginning with an initial dose totalling 50 to 200 μg (1 to 3 μg/kg) and followed by additional doses after 30 to 60 minutes, to achieve desired analgesia. Continuous infusion of fentanyl has also been used.[135] The elderly require reduced drug doses.

Although fentanyl is an appropriate narcotic for ambulatory procedures, its use is not without problems. Fentanyl causes marked respiratory depression comparable in magnitude and duration to that seen after morphine.[136] There is also evidence of a recurrence of respiratory depression, accompanied by decreases in PaO_2 and pH and increase in $PaCO_2$.[137,138] The clinician should be aware that somnolence, respiratory depression requiring ventilatory support, and respiratory arrest have occurred 0.5 to 4 hours after apparent recovery from fentanyl administration.[139] The addition of droperidol, given as Innovar (Janssen Pharmaceutica Inc., Piscataway, NJ), does not alter the respiratory depression caused by fentanyl.[137] Rigidity after fentanyl[140,141] has not been reported in the awake sedated ambulatory patient.

Naloxone has been used to reverse narcotic side effects, primarily respiratory depression. Naloxone, however, has sequelae of its own. Unless carefully titrated, it can eliminate analgesia. Hypertension, pulmonary edema, ventricular arrhythmias, and cardiac arrest in healthy, young patients have been reported after 0.08 to 0.4 mg naloxone.[142,143] The routine "prophylactic" use of naloxone after narcotic supplementation cannot be recommended.

Alfentanil

The needs of outpatient anesthesia have prompted the search for new short-acting narcotic analgesics. Alfentanil[144,145] is a fentanyl analog with approximately one-fifth the potency and one-third the duration of action of the older drug. Clinically, alfentanil produces more sedation and briefer respiratory depression, but induces more rigidity and more hypotension at equal analgesic doses. The pharmacokinetic characteristics of alfentanil include a rapid redistribution halflife of 11.6 minutes, and an elimination halflife of 94 minutes,[146] which is considerably shorter than that of fentanyl (219 minutes[134]). Termination of alfentanil effect after a single dose is due more to total body clearance than redistribution; alfentanil has less lipid solubility and a smaller volume of distribution than fentanyl, allowing more of the alfentanil to be available for hepatic clearance.[147,148] Clearance is lower in the obese, in patients with liver dysfunction, and in patients with variant cytochrome P-450 isozyme.[149] Continued administration of alfentanil, in large or repeated doses, may result in prolongation of therapeutic and depressant effects. Clinical recovery has been consistently rapid if appropriate doses are used.[90,151–153]

Delayed respiratory depression requiring reintubation and mechanical ventilation has been reported with alfentanil. This respiratory depression has occurred concurrent with resedation, at approximately 45 minutes after the termination of long but appropriately titrated infusions of alfentanil during general anesthesia.[153,154] Plasma alfentanil level during the apneic event in one patient, was 87 ng/ml, which is below the ceiling level usually associated with resumption of spontaneous ventilation (99 to 240 ng/ml[155]), but blood gas determinations showed evidence of a period of hypoventilation. A decrease in the level of stimulation required to maintain consciousness and respiratory effort has been implicated. The occurrence of a secondary increase in plasma alfentanil level has not been reported.

The pharmacokinetics of alfentanil suggest that it may be best used by continuous infusion for the supplementation of ambulatory procedures. Greater stability of clinical effect and quicker recovery can result.[92] To administer alfentanil by infusion, a simple in-line burette may be used, but a calibrated syringe pump, such as the Bard Alfenta infuser (Harvard Mini-Infuser 900, C.R. Bard MedSystems, North Reading, MA), provides the advantage of less intraoperative calculation of doses. After incremental bolus dose(s) of 5 μg/kg, an infusion rate of 0.25 to 0.5 μg/kg/min may be used to continue narcotic supplementation. It is important to continually titrate the infusion rate to patient response in order to avoid relative overdose and side effects.

Other Opioids

New narcotics have been synthesized in an attempt to achieve analgesia with fewer side effects. Two such drugs that have potential for use as anesthetic supplementation in the ambulatory setting are the agonist-antagonists butorphanol and nalbuphine. These drugs are active at the κ opioid receptor and are characterized by antagonist activity at the classic opioid μ receptor. Butorphanol is approximately five times as potent as morphine, while nalbuphine is considered to have a potency equal to that of morphine. These narcotics cause limited respiratory depression; with continued drug administration, only minimal increases occur after the equivalent of 10 mg morphine. Butorphanol has a subjectively pleasant, sedative effect. Onset of action for both drugs is within 2 minutes after intravenous administration, but their duration of action is long, similar to morphine. Reduced doses of these agonist-antagonist narcotics must be used to supplement ambulatory procedures.[156–159] Other κ receptor agonists are also under investigation.[160]

Inhalation Analgesia

Subanesthetic concentrations of anesthetic gases and vapors provide analgesia and sedation that can be used to supplement local anesthesia. Inhalation analgesia is particularly useful for minor surgery on closed-space infections, which are difficult to block with local anesthetic.[161] Most inhalation anesthetic agents have been used. In practice, halothane use is limited by the incidence of cardiac dysrhythmias[162] and the possibility of halothane-related hepatotoxicity. Isoflurane has a pungent odor and can cause respiratory tract irritation, two conditions that reduce acceptance of that drug.[163] Methoxyflurane is effective for inhalation analgesia when given intermittently at concentrations of 0.2 to 0.5 percent (1.2 to 3.1 minimum alveolar concentration [MAC]),[164] but its use is not recommended for ambulatory patients due to the possibility of renal damage. Agents currently in use for ambulatory inhalation analgesia are nitrous oxide and enflurane.

During enflurane inhalation, psychomotor function is impaired at end-tidal concentrations greater than 0.09 MAC (0.2 percent inspired).[165] At 0.24 MAC enflurane (0.53 percent inspired), sufficient drowsiness sometimes develops to preclude completing the tests. Dose-related amnesia is also seen. Similar concentrations, approximately 0.5 percent inspired enflurane or 40 percent inspired nitrous oxide, have been reported to achieve maximal analgesia without loss of consciousness in obstetric patients.[166]

Nitrous oxide is the most widely used agent for inhalation analgesia. Concentrations of 10 to 60 percent in oxygen are used, with wide variability in individual response. The quality of analgesia that is provided can be improved by administering the drug in less stressful surroundings.[167] Onset of analgesia is rapid, as is termination of the effect once administration ceases. Psychomotor testing during the inhalation of 30 percent end-tidal nitrous oxide shows maximal impairment by 7 minutes.[168] Impairment of driving skills has been demonstrated 30 minutes after administration ceases.[169] Any ambulatory patient who receives nitrous oxide sedation must have appropriate postanesthetic supervision.

Outside of the operating room, inhalational analgesia and sedation are sometimes provided by patient-controlled systems. Inhalers are available that will deliver 0.3 to 0.9 percent methoxyflurane in air[158] or 50 percent nitrous oxide in oxygen, either premixed[170] or from tandem cylinders.[160] These inhaling devices need patient cooperation to maintain a tight mouthpiece or mask seal in order to receive anesthetic, but this safety feature can be circumvented by propping the inhaler on a pillow.[164] Patient-controlled devices such as these are intended to be safe enough to use without an anesthesiologist present. However, the patient receiving self-administered inhalation analgesia still requires a trained individual in constant attendance; this attendant must terminate or decrease the anesthetic if drowsiness, confusion, or excitement develops.

The inhalation of nitrous oxide is associated with side effects. Lichtenthal et al.[171] reported that concentrations of over 30 percent sometimes caused excitement. Stewart et al.,[172] evaluating 50 percent nitrous oxide in oxygen, reported a 20.6 percent incidence of minor side effects including nausea or vomiting (5.7 percent), dizziness or lightheadedness (10.3 percent), excitement (3.7 percent), and numbness (0.3 percent). These investigators did not include as complications the drowsiness or light sleep exhibited by 7.6 percent of patients. Oversedation can, however, eliminate one of the advantages of inhalation analgesia: the preservation of airway reflexes. The swallowing response to fluid in the pharynx, which leads to reflex closure of the glottis, is impaired in patients breathing 50 percent nitrous oxide in oxygen.[173]

SUMMARY

The local anesthetic agents which may be used for outpatients fall into two major chemical classes: the amino-esters and the amino-amides. The differing structures of these two groups are associated with differences in their biologic activity and mode of metabolism and, therefore, their toxicity. Activity and toxicity are also influenced by the drugs' physiologic disposition (absorption, distribution, metabolism, and excretion). The agents in common use for ambulatory surgical patients are the short- and intermediate-acting drugs in both chemical groups, as well as the long-acting amide bupivacaine for prolonged postoperative analgesia.

Safe use of the local anesthetic agents for infiltration anesthesia requires knowledge of their potential toxicities, which may arise from the agent itself or from an added vasoconstrictor. In order to infiltrate the large areas that may be needed, very dilute solutions have been advocated and used successfully. Another concern is the pain of the injection itself. An effective, topically-active emulsion (EMLA) has been developed, but it requires prolonged preinjection application (60–90 min). The local anesthetic agents used for infiltration cause different levels of discomfort when injected, with etidocaine being the most painful and lidocaine and procaine the least painful. Addition of sodium bicarbonate to lidocaine has been shown to reduce discomfort with both plain and epinephrine-containing solutions.

For retrobulbar anesthesia, the duration of surgical anesthesia that is desired dictates the choice of local anesthetic agent. Longer-acting agents will provide postoperative analgesia as well; the slower onset of bupivacaine can be shortened by combining it with lidocaine. Hyaluronidase is usually added to enhance the quality of blockade, and improved akinesia has been demonstrated. Complications from retrobulbar blockade may arise from several sources, including incorrect placement of the anesthetic agent, which can gain entry into blood vessels or into the central nervous system directly. Stimulation of the oculocardiac reflex may cause profound bradycardia. Direct trauma from the block needle can be minimized by careful technique.

Intravenous regional anesthesia is produced at a combination of sites of action. Diffusion of local anesthetic from the veins to the nerves, as well as conduction block at the site of maximal drug concentration, are involved. Attention to technical details of tourniquet preparation and exsanguination will improve success. Leakage of local anesthetic can occur if the tourniquet fails, but also if the cuff is improperly sized or inadequately pressurized, or if the anesthetic is injected so that intravascular pressures exceed cuff occlusive pressures. Such leakage may cause a systemic toxic reaction in addition to loss of analgesia. Lidocaine is the only agent currently available for use with intravenous regional anesthesia, although prilocaine is efficacious and has a reduced potential for toxicity.

Supplemental medications are often given with local and regional anesthesia to improve patient acceptance. Verbal reassurance is a valuable adjunctive technique. When drugs are chosen, consideration for both sedation and analgesia is necessary.

Supplemental drugs for the ambulatory patient should have an appropriate duration of action and minimal side effects, and the intravenous route is preferable. Among the sedative-anxiolytics, useful agents include diazepam and midazolam; among the analgesics, useful agents include fentanyl, alfentanil, and butorphanol. Continuous infusions may be used for the administration of midazolam and alfentanil. Inhalation analgesia with subanesthetic concentratons of nitrous oxide or enflurane is also effective.

REFERENCES

1. Covino BG, Vassallo HG: Local Anesthetics. Mechanisms of Action and Clinical Use. Grune & Stratton, Orlando, FL, 1976
2. Wildsmith JAW: Prilocaine—an underutilized local anesthetic. Reg Anesth 10:155, 1985
3. Arthur GR, Covino BG: What's new in local anesthetics? Anesthesiol Clin North Am 6:357, 1988
4. Smith AR, Hur D, Resano F: Grand mal seizures after 2-chloroprocaine epidural anesthesia in a patient with plasma cholinesterase deficiency. Anesth Analg 66:677, 1987
5. Philip BK, Covino BG: Local and regional anesthesia. p. 225. In Wetchler BV (ed): Anesthesia for Ambulatory Surgery. JB Lippincott, Philadelphia, 1985
6. Crews JC, Clark RB: Effect of alkalinization on the pH of local anesthetic solutions. Anesth Analg 66:1203, 1987
7. Bokesch PM, Raymond SA, Strichartz GR: Dependence of lidocaine potency on pH and pCO_2. Anesth Analg 66:9, 1987
8. Gissen AJ, Covino BG, Gregus J: Differential sensitivity of fast and slow fibers in mammalian nerve IV. Effect of carbonation of local anesthetics. Reg Anesth 10:68, 1985
9. Nickel PM, Bromage PR, Sherrill DL: Comparison of hydrochloride and carbonated salts of lidocaine for epidural analgesia. Reg Anesth 11:62, 1986
10. Sukhani R, Winnie AP: Clinical pharmacokinetics of carbonated local anesthetics II: interscalene brachial block model. Anesth Analg 66:1245, 1987
11. Scott DB, Jebson PJR, Braid DP, et al: Factors affecting plasma levels of lignocaine and prilocaine. Br J Anaesth 44:1040, 1972
12. Tucker GT, Moore DC, Bridenbaugh PO, et al: Systemic absorption of mepivacaine in commonly used regional block procedures. Anesthesiology 37:277, 1972
13. Mazze RI, Dunbar RW: Plasma lidocaine concentrations after caudal, lumbar epidural, axillary block, and intravenous regional anesthesia. Anesthesiology 27:574, 1966
14. Katz JA, Kaeding CS, Hill JR, Henthorn TK: The pharmacokinetics of bupivacaine when injected intra-articularly after knee arthroscopy. Anesth Analg 67:872, 1988
15. Adriani J, Campbell D: Fatalities following topical application of local anesthetics to mucous membranes. JAMA 162:1527, 1956
16. Flanagan L, Bascom JU: Herniorrhaphies performed on outpatients under local anesthesia. Surg Gynecol Obstet 153:557, 1981
17. Vater M, Wandless J: Caudal or dorsal nerve block? A comparison of two local anaesthetic techniques for postoperative analgesia following day case circumcision. Acta Anaesthesiol Scand 29:175, 1985
18. Wilson IH, Richmond MN, Strike PW: Regional analgesia with bupivacaine in dental anaesthesia. Br J Anaesth 58:401, 1985
19. Malhotra V, Long CW, Meister MJ: Intercostal blocks with local infiltration anesthesia for extracorporeal shock wave lithotripsy. Anesth Analg 66:85, 1987
20. Deeb RJ, Viechnicki MB: Laparoscopic tubal ligation under peritoneal lavage anesthesia. Reg Anesth 10:24, 1985
21. Newman J, Dolsky RL: Evaluation of 5458 cases of lipo-suction surgery. Am J Cosm Surg 1:25, 1984
22. Philip BK: Complications of regional anesthesia for obstetrics. Reg Anesth 8:17, 1983
23. Buffington CW, Buehler PK, Glauber DT, et al: A new system of infiltration anesthesia and sedation for plastic surgery. Plast Reconstr Surg 74:671, 1984
24. Klein JA: The tumescent technique for lipo-suction surgery. Am J Coms Surg 4:263, 1987
25. Cotton BR, Henderson HP, Achola KJ,

Smith G: Changes in plasma catecholamine concentrations following infiltration with large volumes of local anaesthetic solution containing adrenaline. Br J Anaesth 58:593, 1986

26. Derbyshire DR, Smith G: Sympathoadrenal responses to anaesthesia and surgery. Br J Anaesth 56:725, 1984
27. Dionne RA, Goldstein DS, Wirdzek PR: Effects of diazepam premedication and epinephrine-containing local anesthetic on cardiovascular and plasma catecholamine responses to oral surgery. Anesth Analg 63:640, 1984
28. Dolsky RL, Fetzek J, Anderson R: Evaluation of blood loss during lipo-suction surgery. Am J Cosm Surg 4:257, 1987
29. Ghignone M, Noe C, Calvillo O, Quintin L: Anesthesia for ophthalmic surgery in the elderly: the effects of clonidine on intraocular pressure, perioperative hemodynamics, and anesthetic requirement. Anesthesiology 68:707, 1988
30. Hallen B, Uppfeldt A: Does lidocaine-prilocaine cream permit painfree insertion of IV catheters in children? Anesthesiology 57:340, 1982.
31. Hallen B, Carlsson P, Uppfeldt A: Clinical study of a lignocaine-prilocaine cream to relieve the pain of venepuncture. Br J Anaesth 57:326, 1985
32. Soliman IE, Broadman LM, Hannallah RS, McGill WA: Comparison of the analgesic effects of EMLA to intradermal lidocaine infiltration prior to venous cannulation in unpremedicated children. Anesthesiology 68:804, 1988
33. Arendt-Nielsen L, Bjerring P: Laser-induced pain for evaluation of local analgesia: a comparison of topical application (EMLA) and local injection (lidocaine). Anesth Analg 67:115, 1988
34. Hallen B, Olsson GL, Uppfeldt A: Painfree venepuncture. Effect of timing of application of local anaesthetic cream. Anaesthesia 39:969, 1984
35. Evers H, von Dardel O, Juhlin L, et al: Dermal effects of compositions based on the eutectic mixture of lignocaine and prilocaine. Br J Anaesth 57:997, 1985
36. Morris R, McKay W, Mushlin P: Comparison of pain associated with intradermal and subcutaneous infiltration with various local anesthetic solutions. Anesth Analg 66:1180, 1987
37. Morris RW, Whish DKM: A controlled trial of pain on skin infiltration with local anesthetics. Anaesth Intensive Care 12:113, 1984.
38. McKay W, Morris R, Mushlin P: Sodium bicarbonate attenuates pain on skin infiltration with lidocaine, with or without epinephrine. Anesth Analg 66:572, 1987
39. Wightman MA, Vaughn RW: Comparison of compounds for intradermal anesthesia. Anesthesiology 45:687, 1976
40. Bruce RA, McGoldrick KE, Oppenheimer P: Anesthesia for Ophthalmology. Aesculapius Publishing, Birmingham, 1982
41. Feibel RM: Current concepts in retrobulbar anesthesia. Surv Ophthalmol 30:102, 1985
42. Wittpenn JR, Rapoza P, Sternberg P, et al: Respiratory arrest following retrobulbar anesthesia. Ophthalmology 93:867, 1986
43. Smith PH, Kim JW: Etidocaine used for retrobulbar block: a comparison with lidocaine. Ophthalmic Surg 11:268, 1980
44. Horven I: Ophthalmic artery pressure during retrobulbar anesthesia. Acta Ophthalmol 56:574, 1978
45. Holecamp TLR, Arribas NP, Boniuk I: Bupivacaine anesthesia in retinal detachment surgery. Arch Ophthalmol 97:109, 1979
46. Laaka V, Nikki P, Tarkkanen A: Comparison of bupivacaine with and without adrenalin and mepivacaine with adrenalin in intraocular surgery. Acta Ophthalmol 50:229, 1972
47. Carolan JA, Cerasoli JR, Houle TV: Bupivacaine in retrobulbar anesthesia. Ann Ophthalmol 6:843, 1974
48. Gills JP, Rudisill JE: Bupivacaine in cataract surgery. Ophthalmic Surg 5:67, 1974
49. Nicoll JMV, Treuren B, Acharya PA, et al: Retrobulbar anesthesia: the role of hyaluronidase. Anesth Analg 65:1324, 1986
50. Nicoll JMV, Acharya PA, Ahlen K, et al: Central nervous complications after 6000 retrobulbar blocks. Anesth Analg 66:1298, 1987
51. Chang JL, Gonzalea-Abola E, Larson CE, Lobes L: Brainstem anesthesia following

retrobulbar blockade. Anesthesiology 61:789, 1984

52. McGoldrick KE: Current concepts in anesthesia for ophthalmic surgery. Anesthesiol Rev 7:7, 1980
53. Meyers EF: Problems during eye surgery under local anesthesia. Is standby necessary? Anesthesiol Rev 6:23, 1979
54. Gifford H: Discussion: the effect of retrobulbar injections of procaine on the optic nerve. Trans Am Acad Ophthalmol Otolaryngol 59:356, 1955
55. Ramsay RC, Knobloch WH: Ocular perforation following retrobulbar anesthesia for retinal detachment surgery. Am J Ophthalmol 86:61, 1978
56. Davis DB, Mandel MR: Posterior peribulbar anesthesia: an alternative to retrobulbar anesthesia. J Cataract Refract Surg 12:182, 1986
57. Kimble JA, Morris RE, Witherspoon CD, Feist RM: Globe perforation from peribulbar injection. Arch Ophthalmol 5:749, 1987
58. Bier A: Ueber einem neuen Weg Localanaesthesia an den Gliedmassen zu erzeugen. Arch Klin Chir 86:1007, 1908
59. Miles DW, James J, Clark DE, Whitwam JG: Site of action of "intravenous regional anaesthesia." J Neurol Neurosurg Psychiatry 27:574, 1964
60. Fleming SA, Veiga-Pires JA, McCutcheon RM, Emanuel CI: A demonstration of the site of action of intravenous lignocaine. Can Anaesth Soc J 13:21, 1966
61. Urban BJ, McKain CW: Onset and progression of intravenous regional anesthesia with dilute lidocaine. Anesth Analg 61:834, 1982
62. Lillie PE, Glynn CJ, Fenwick DG: Site of action of intravenous regional anesthesia. Anesthesiology 61:507, 1984
63. Raj PP, Garcia CE, Burleson JW, Jenkins MT: The site of action of intravenous regional anesthesia. Anesth Analg 51:776, 1972
64. Shanks CA, McLeod JG: Nerve conduction in regional intravenous analgesia using 1 per cent lignocaine. Br J Anaesth 42:1060, 1970
65. Rosenberg PH, Heavner JE: Multiple and complementary mechanisms produce analgesia during intravenous regional anesthesia. Anesthesiology 62:840, 1985
66. Hoyle JR: Tourniquet for intravenous regional analgesia. Anaesthesia 19:294, 1964
67. Nussbaum LM, Hamelberg W: Intravenous regional anesthesia for surgery on the foot and ankle. Anesthesiology 64:91, 1986
68. Davies JAH, Walford AJ: Intravenous regional anaesthesia for foot surgery. Acta Anaesthesiol Scand 30:145, 1986
69. Valli HK, Rosenberg PH, Hekali R: Comparison of lidocaine and prilocaine for intravenous regional anesthesia of the whole lower extremity. Reg Anesth 12:128, 1987
70. Goold JE: Intravenous regional anaesthesia. Br J Hosp Med 33:335, 1985
71. Colbern EC: The Bier block for intravenous regional anesthesia. Anesth Analg 49:935, 1970
72. Davies JAH, Wilkey AD, Hall ID: Bupivacaine leak past inflated tourniquets during intravenous regional analgesia. Anaesthesia 39:996, 1984
73. Rosenberg PH, Kalso EA, Tuorminen MK, Linden HB: Acute bupivacaine toxicity as a result of venous leakage under the tourniquet cuff during a Bier block. Anesthesiology 58:95, 1983
74. Grice SC, Morell RC, Balestrieri FJ, et al: Intravenous regional anesthesia: evaluation and prevention of leakage under the tourniquet. Anesthesiology 65:316, 1986
75. Ogden PN: Failure of regional analgesia using a double cuff tourniquet. Anaesthesia 39:456, 1984
76. Duggan J, McKeown DW, Scott DB: Venous pressures in intravenous regional anesthesia. Reg Anesth 9:68, 1984
77. Tucker GT, Boas RA: Pharmacokinetic aspects of intravenous regional anesthesia. Anesthesiology 34:538, 1971
78. Sukhani R, Garcia CJ, Winnie Ap, Rodvold KA: Arterial blood levels of lidocaine after intravenous regional anesthesia: cyclic versus single deflation of tourniquet. Reg Anesth 11:49, 1986 (abstr)
79. Brown EM, Smiler BG, Wenokur ME: Intravenous regional anesthesia for sequential operations on two extremities. Anesthesiology 35:223, 1971
80. McKeown DW, Meiklejohn B, Scott DB: Bupivacaine and prilocaine in intravenous

regional anaesthesia. Anaesthesia 39:150, 1984

81. Bader AM, Concepcion M, Hurley RJ, Arthur GR: Comparison of lidocaine and prilocaine for intravenous regional anesthesia. Anesthesiology 69:409, 1988
82. Harris WH, Slater EM, Bell HM: Regional anesthesia by the intravenous route. JAMA 194:1273, 1965
83. Porta MC, Hajman CM, Meis M, et al: Anesthese loco-regionale intra-veineuse à la bupivacaine à 0.5%. Cah Anesthesiol 32:669, 1984
84. Kalso E, Rosenberg PH: Bupivacaine and intravenous regional anaesthesia—a matter of controversy. Ann Chir Gynaecol 73:190, 1984
85. Heath ML: Deaths from intravenous regional block. Br Med J 285:913, 1982
86. Reynolds F: Editorial: bupivacaine and intravenous regional anaesthesia. Anaesthesia 39:105, 1984
87. Moore DC: Bupivacaine toxicity and Bier block: the drug, the technique, or the anesthetist. Anesthesiology 61:782, 1984
88. Amiot JF, Bouju P, Palacci JH, Balliner E: Intravenous regional anaesthesia with ketamine. Anaesthesia 40:899, 1985
89. Philip BK: Supplemental medication for ambulatory procedures under regional anesthesia. Anesth Analg 64:1117, 1985
90. Baird ES, Hailey DM: Delayed recovery from a sedative: correlation of the plasma levels of diazepam with clinical effects after oral and intravenous administration. Br J Anaesth 144:803, 1972
91. Klotz U, Antonin KH, Bieck PR: Pharmacokinetics and plasma binding of diazepam in man, dog, rabbit, guinea pig and rat. J Pharmacol Exp Ther 199:67, 1976
92. White PF, Coe V, Shafer A, Sung ML: Comparison of alfentanil with fentanyl for outpatient anesthesia. Anesthesiology 64:99, 1986
93. Gross JB, Smith L, Smith TC: Time course of ventilatory response to carbon dioxide after intravenous diazepam. Anesthesiology 57:18, 1982
94. Mandelli M, Tognoni G, Garattini S: Clinical pharmacokinetics of diazepam. Clin Pharmacokinet 3:72, 1978
95. Klotz U, Avant GR, Hoyumpa A, et al: The effects of age and liver disease on the disposition and elimination of diazepam in adult man. J Clin Invest 55:347, 1975
96. Hegarty JE, Dundee JW: Sequelae after the intravenous injection of three benzodiazepines—diazepam, lorazepam, and flunitrazepam. Br Med J 2:1384, 1977
97. Korttila K, Mattila MJ, Linnoila M: Prolonged recovery after diazepam sedation: the influence of food, charcoal ingestion and the injection rate on the effects of intravenous diazepam. Br J Anaesth 48:333, 1976
98. DeJong RH, Heavner JE: Diazepam prevents local anesthetic seizures. Anesthesiology 34:523, 1971
99. Dundee JW, Pandit SK: Anterograde amnesic effects of pethidine, hyoscine and diazepam in adults. Br J Pharmacol 44:140, 1972
100. Clarke RSJ: New drugs—boon or bane? Premedication and intravenous induction agents. Can Anaesth Soc J 30:166, 1983
101. Cox HD, Deshon GE, Mittemeyer BT, et al: Ataralgesia in outpatient urology. Urology 9:164, 1977
102. Pandit SK, Heisterkamp DV, Cohen PJ: Further studies of the anti-recall effect of lorazepam: a dose-time–effect relationship. Anesthesiology 45:495, 1976
103. Swerdlow BN, Holley FO: Intravenous anaesthetic agents. Pharmacokinetic-pharmacodynamic relationships. Clin Pharmacokinet 12:79, 1987
104. Dundee JW, McGowan WAW, Lilburn JK, et al: Comparison of the actions of diazepam and lorazepam. Br J Anaesth 51:439, 1979
105. Riefkohl R, Kosanin R: Experience with triazolam as a preoperative sedative for outpatient surgery under local anesthesia. Anesthetic Plast Surg 8;155, 1984
106. Reves JG, Fragen RJ, Vinik HR, Greenblatt DJ: Midazolam: pharmacology and uses. Anesthesiology 62:310, 1985
107. Dundee JW, Samuel IO, Toner W, Howard PJ: Midazolam: a water-soluble benzodiazepine. Anaesthesia 35:454, 1980
108. Philip BK: Hazards of amnesia after midazolam in ambulatory surgical patients. Anesth Analg 66:97, 1987
109. Connor JT, Katz RL, Pagano RR, Graham

GW: RO 21-3981 for intravenous surgical premedication and induction of anesthesia. Anesth Analg 57:1, 1978

110. Gamble JAS, Kawar P, Dundee JW, et al: Evaluation of midazolam as an intravenous induction agent. Anaesthesia 36:868, 1981
111. Davis PJ, Cook DR: Clinical pharmacokinetics of the newer intravenous anaesthetic agents. Clin Pharmacokinet 11:18, 1986
112. Persson P, Nilsson A, Hartvig P, Tamsen A: Pharmacokinetics of midazolam in total I.V. anaesthesia. Br J Anaesth 59:548, 1987
113. Persson MP, Nilsson A, Hartvig P: Relation of sedation and amnesia to plasma concentrations of midazolam in surgical patients. Clin Pharmacol Ther 43:324, 1988
114. McClure JH, Brown DT, Wildsmith JAW: Comparison of the i.v. administration of midazolam and diazepam as sedation during spinal anaesthesia. Br J Anaesth 55:1089, 1983
115. Dixon J, Power SJ, Grundy EM, et al: Sedation for local anaesthesia. Comparison of intravenous midazolam and diazepam. Anaesthesia 39:372, 1984
116. Aun C, Flynn PJ, Richards J, Major E: A comparison of midazolam and diazepam for intravenous sedation in dentistry. Anaesthesia 39:589, 1984
117. Rosenbaum NL: The use of midazolam for intravenous sedation in general dental practice. Br Dent J 158:139, 1985
118. Sainpy D, Boileau S, Vicari F: Etude comparative du midazolam et du diazepam intraveineux comme agents de sedation en endoscopie digestive. Ann Fr Anesth Reanim 3:177, 1984
119. Berggren L, Eriksson I, Mollenholt P, Wickbom G: Sedation for fiberoptic gastroscopy: a comparative study of midazolam and diazepam. Br J Anaesth 55:289, 1983
120. Klotz U, Kanto J: Pharmacokinetics and clinical use of flumazenil (RO 15-1788). Clin Pharmacokinet 14:1, 1988
121. Kirkegaard L, Knudson L, Jensen S, Kruse A: Antagonism of benzodiazepine sedation in outpatients undergoing gastroscopy. Anaesthesia 41:1184, 1986
122. Riishede L, Krogh B, Nielsen JL, et al: Reversal of flunitrazepam sedation with flumazenil. Acta Anaesthesiol Scand 32:433, 1988
123. White PF, Shafer A, Boyle WA, et al: Benzodiazepine antagonism does not provoke a stress response. Anesthesiology 70:636, 1989
124. Rodrigo MRC, Rosenquist JB: The effect of RO 15-1788 (Anexate) on conscious sedation produced with midazolam. Anaesth Intensive Care 15:185, 1987
125. Ricou B, Forster A, Bruckner A, et al: Clinical evaluation of a specific benzodiazepine antagonist (RO 15-1788). Br J Anaesth 58:1005, 1986
126. Philip BK, Hauch MA, Mallampati SR, Simpson TH: Flumazenil for reversal of sedation after midazolam-induced ambulatory general anesthesia. Anesthesiology 71:A301, 1989
127. Editorial: Midazolam—is antagonism justified? Lancet 2:140, 1988
128. Korttila K, Linnoila M: Skills related to driving after intravenous diazepam, flunitrazepam or droperidol. Br J Anaesth 46:961, 1974
129. Prokocimer P, Delavault E, Rey F, et al: Effects of droperidol on respiratory drive in humans. Anesthesiology 59:113, 1983
130. Janssen PAJ, Niemeggers CJE, Schellekens KHL, et al: The pharmacology of dehydrobenzperidol, a new potent and short acting neurolept agent chemically related to haloperidol. Arzneimittelforschung 13:205, 1963
131. Winning TJ, Brock-Utne JG, Downing JW: Nausea and vomiting after anesthesia and minor surgery. Anesth Analg 56:674, 1977
132. Korttila K, Kauste A, Auvinen J: Comparison of domperidone, droperidol, and metoclopramide in the prevention and treatment of nausea and vomiting after balanced general anesthesia. Anesth Analg 58:396, 1979
133. Rita L, Goodarzi M, Seleny F: Effect of low dose droperidol on postoperative vomiting in children. Can Anaesth Soc J 28:259, 1981
134. Wetchler BV, Collins IS, Jacob L: Antiemetic effects of droperidol on the ambulatory surgery patient. Anesthesiol Rev 9:23, 1982

135. McClain DA, Hug CC: Intravenous fentanyl kinetics. Clin Pharmacol Ther 28:106, 1980
136. White PF: Use of continuous infusion versus intermittent bolus administration of fentanyl or ketamine during outpatient anesthesia. Anesthesiology 59:294, 1983
137. Rigg JRA, Goldsmith CH: Recovery of ventilatory response to carbon dioxide after thiopentone, morphine and fentanyl in man. Can Anaesth Soc J 23:370, 1976
138. Becker LD, Paulson BA, Miller RD, et al: Biphasic respiratory depression after fentanyl-droperidol or fentanyl alone used to supplement nitrous oxide anesthesia. Anesthesiology 44:291, 1976
139. Stoeckel H, Schuttler J, Magnussen H, Hengstmann JH: Plasma fentanyl concentrations and the occurrence of respiratory depression in volunteers. Br J Anaesth 54:1087, 1982
140. Adams AP, Pybus DA: Delayed respiratory depression after use of fentanyl during anesthesia. Br Med J 1:278, 1978
141. Christian CM, Waller JL, Moldenhauer CC: Postoperative rigidity following fentanyl anesthesia. Anesthesiology 58:275, 1983
142. Scamman FL: Fentanyl-02-N20 rigidity and pulmonary compliance. Anesth Analg 62:332, 1983
143. Andree RA: Sudden death following naloxone administration. Anesth Analg 59:782, 1980
144. Partridge BL, Ward CF: Pulmonary edema following low-dose naloxone administration. Anesthesiology 65:709, 1986
145. Kay B: Alfentanil. Br J Anaesth 54:1011, 1982
146. Niemegeers CJE, Janssen PAJ: Alfentanil (R 39209), a particularly short-acting morphine-like narcotic for intravenous use in anaesthesia. Drug Devel Res 1:83, 1981
147. Bovill JG, Sebel PS, Blackburn CL, Heykants J: The pharmacokinetics of alfentanil (R39209): a new opioid analgesic. Anesthesiology 57:439, 1982
148. Reitz JA: Alfentanil in anesthesia and analgesia. Drug Intell Clin Pharm 20:335, 1986
149. Hull CJ: The pharmacokinetics of alfentanil in man. Br J Anaesth 55:157S, 1983
150. Shafer A, Sung ML, White PF: Pharmacokinetics and pharmacodynamics of alfentanil infusions during general anesthesia. Anesth Analg 65:1021, 1986
151. Sinclair ME, Cooper GM. Alfentanil and recovery. Anaesthesia 38:435, 1983
152. Collins KM, Plantevin OM: Use of alfentanil in short anaesthetic procedures. J R Soc Med 78:456, 1985
153. Sanders RS, Sinclair ME, Sear JW: Alfentanil in short procedures. Anaesthesia 39:1202, 1984
154. Mahla ME, White SE, Moneta MD: Delayed respiratory depression after alfentanil. Anesthesiology 69:593, 1988
155. Jaffe RS, Coalson D: Recurrent respiratory depression after alfentanil administration. Anesthesiology 70:151, 1989
156. Ausems ME, Hug CC, Stanski DR: Plasma concentrations of alfentanil required to supplement nitrous oxide anesthesia for general surgery. Anesthesiology 65:362, 1986
157. Pandit SK, Kothary SP, Pandit UA, Mathai MK: Comparison of fentanyl and butorphanol for outpatient anaesthesia. Can Anaesth Soc J 34:130, 1987
158. Garfield JM, Garfield FB, Philip BK, et al: A comparison of clinical and psychological effects of fentanyl and nalbuphine in ambulatory gynecologic patients. Anesth Analg 66:1303, 1987
159. Lind LJ, Mushlin PS: Sedation, analgesia, and anesthesia for radiologic procedures. Cardiovasc Intervent Radiol 10:247, 1987
160. Philip BK, Freiberger D, Gibbs R, et al: Butorphanol compared with fentanyl for ambulatory general anesthesia. Proceedings of the Society for Ambulatory Anesthesia, San Antonio, 1989 (abstr)
161. Althaus JS, DiFazio CA, Moscicki JC, VonVoigtlander PF: Enhancement of anesthetic effect of halothane by spiradoline, a selective k-agonist. Anesth Analg 67:823, 1988
162. Flomenbaum N, Gallagher EJ, Eagen K, Jacobsen S: Self-administered nitrous oxide: an adjunct analgesic. JACEP 8:95, 1979
163. Willatts DG, Harrison AR, Groom JF, Crowther A: Cardiac arrhythmias during outpatient dental anaesthesia: comparison

of halothane with enflurane. Br J Anaesth 55:399, 1983

164. Tracey JA, Holland AJC, Unger L: Morbidity in minor gynaecological surgery: a comparison of halothane, enflurane, and isoflurane. Br J Anaesth 54:1213, 1982
165. Cohen SE: Inhalation analgesia and anesthesia for vaginal delivery. p. 121. In Shnider SM, Levinson G (eds): Anesthesia for Obstetrics. Williams & Wilkins, Baltimore, 1979
166. Cooke TL, Smith M, Winter PM, et al: Effect of subanesthetic concentrations of enflurane and halothane on human behavior. Anesth Analg 57:434, 1978
167. Abboud TK, Shnider SM, Wright RG, et al: Enflurane analgesia in obstetrics. Anesth Analg 60:133, 1981
168. Dworkin SF, Schubert MM, Chen ACN, Clark DW: Analgesic effects of nitrous oxide with controlled painful stimuli. JADA 107:581, 1983
169. Korttila K, Ghoneim MM, Jacobs L, et al: Time course of mental and psychomotor effects of 30 percent nitrous oxide during inhalation and recovery. Anesthestiology 44:220, 1981
170. Davidson KW, Kahn RF: Nitrous oxide analgesia for outpatient procedures. Am Fam Physician 31:209, 1985
171. Lichtenthal P, Philip J, Sloss LJ, et al: Administration of nitrous oxide in normal subjects. Chest 72:316, 1977
172. Stewart RD, Paris PM, Stoy WA, Cannon G: Patient-controlled inhalational analgesia in prehospital care: a study of side-effects and feasibility. Crit Care Med 11:851, 1983
173. Nishino T, Takizawa K, Yokokawa N, Hirago K: Depression of the swallowing reflex during sedation and/or relative analgesia produced by inhalation of 50% nitrous oxide in oxygen. Anesthesiology 67:995, 1987

14

Regional Anesthesia for Adult Outpatients

Michael F. Mulroy

Regional anesthesia for outpatient surgery has many advocates. Its purported advantages include postprocedural analgesia and reduced nausea and vomiting. However, these potential advantages must be evaluated against the need for additional time and expertise to perform regional techniques. This chapter reviews arguments for and against regional anesthesia, and discusses the modifications of drug selection and technique that are required in the outpatient setting. Finally, the use of specific techniques is also discussed.

REGIONAL VERSUS GENERAL ANESTHESIA: ADVANTAGES AND DISADVANTAGES

The increasing use of outpatient anesthesia has been well-documented in preceding chapters. Unfortunately, insufficient data have been offered to help identify ideal anesthetic techniques. Regional anesthesia has been advocated for outpatients in preference to general anesthesia for several alleged advantages: (1) less nausea and vomiting, (2) greater potential for postoperative analgesia, (3) reduced risk of aspiration pneumonitis, (4) shortened recovery time, (5) reduced recovery nursing requirements, and (6) enhanced ability to communicate with an alert patient intraoperatively and postoperatively.[1,2] If true, these advantages would cause regional anesthesia to be preferred because, as reported by Meridy, nausea and vomiting after general anesthesia are the most common anesthetic-related causes of unplanned hospital admission.[3] Nausea and a general feeling of "hangover" are the most commonly reported side effects in outpatients receiving systemic anesthesia.[4] Although there are many reports in the current literature which document these side effects and compare various general anesthetic techniques, there are few well-structured comparisons of regional and general anesthesia.

In reviewing the role of regional anesthesia in outpatients, what is found is a series of anecdotal reports of the advantages of specific applications. Ryan et al. have described the use of spinal or epidural anesthesia to facilitate outpatient inguinal herniorrhaphy.[5] Their technique utilizes local wound infiltration with a long-acting local anesthetic at the end of herniorrhaphy performed under a short-acting regional technique. They claim an early return of motor and bladder function, less nausea and vomiting, and prolonged sensory anesthesia, which allow early discharge. Although they compared outpatients to a comparable inpatient population, their study did not assess patients treated with general or local anesthesia alone. Both Hinkle and Hannallah et al. have confirmed that similar local anesthetic infiltration techniques in the pediatric population will reduce narcotic requirement and speed recovery,[6,7] but, again, regional techniques alone were not compared with general anesthesia.

Burke has reported the use of spinal anesthesia for outpatient laparoscopy in over 1,000 cases and claims a high degree of patient satisfaction and rapid discharge.[8] Similarly, Bridenbaugh and Soderstrom reported the use of epidural anesthesia for outpatient laparoscopy.[9] Neither of these two reports offers comparative data for a general anesthesia patient group. Beskin and Baxter have likewise extolled the virtues of regional anesthesia for foot surgery.[2] They claim that the use of ankle blocks has increased their capacity to perform outpatient foot surgery and has improved their patients' cooperation and acceptance, but they present no objective data on which to base these conclusions.

One study that does compare a regional technique to general anesthesia is the application by Patel and colleagues of the "three-in-one" leg block for outpatient knee arthroscopy.[10] Sixty patients having regional block of the femoral, lateral femoral cutaneous, and obturator nerves were compared with 30 patients having general anesthesia with nitrous oxide and narcotics. The recovery time for the regional anesthesia group was shorter than that of the general anesthetic group (56 minutes versus 95 minutes), and the incidence of postoperative pain was much less with regional anesthesia. Only two patients receiving regional anesthesia had postoperative nausea and vomiting. These investigators also claimed that patients were sufficiently alert to view the arthroscopy findings on a television monitor during the procedure. Unfortunately, comparative studies such as that of Patel et al. are not common. Further reporting of experience with regional techniques and comparison to general anesthesia will be needed to document the advantages of regional anesthesia in outpatients.

Promoting Regional Anesthesia

Because of the lack of data concerning its use, the additional time required for its induction, and the potential lack of patient acceptance, regional anesthesia is applied in a limited fashion in the outpatient setting. Successful application depends first on the anesthesiologist's level of comfort and expertise with specific regional blocks. The time pressures of an outpatient unit frequently require that blocks be performed expeditiously and with a high rate of success. The anesthesiologist who has mastered regional techniques in the inpatient operating room can introduce them to the outpatient setting by initially choosing the most appropriate patients and procedures. A careful documentation of improvement in patient recovery times and levels of alertness can help impress on the surgeon the potential advantages of regional anesthesia. Usually, the primary obstacle in outpatient anesthesia is convincing the surgeon that the investment of a few additional minutes at the beginning of a case represents a substantial improvement in the patient's acceptance of the overall outpatient experience. This requires patience and persistence on the part of the anesthesiologist, but it can be well worth the effort.

Modifications in Technique

The performance of regional techniques on outpatients requires some changes from standard inpatient procedures. First of all, the selection of drugs requires greater individualization. For inpatient anesthesia, the longest-acting local anesthetic agent is frequently chosen to provide the longest duration of postprocedural analgesia. For outpatients, the duration of block may potentially limit discharge, especially if anesthesia of the lower extremities is involved. Shorter acting local anesthetics must be used, ideally with the duration tailored to the total anticipated duration of the surgical procedure (Table 14-1). This is particularly true of spinal or epidural blockade. The longer-acting agents, such as bupivacaine or tetracaine, have little place in outpatient anesthesia. The anticipated duration of shorter-acting agents, such as chloroprocaine and lidocaine, are listed in Table 14-1. In general, the duration of chloroprocaine (approximately 75 minutes for two-segment regression of a lumbar epidural block) is ideal for most outpatient procedures performed under epidural anesthesia (Fig. 14-1). In cases in which the anticipated duration of surgery is unclear, the use of continuous (catheter) techniques may be more appropriate than the selection of a longer-acting drug whose duration of action may prove to be excessive.

For subarachnoid anesthesia, lidocaine is currently the most popular drug in the outpatient setting, although experience is showing that its duration may be longer than previously appreciated.[11] Procaine, with its shorter duration, may prove to be more appropriate for ambulatory anesthesia. In assessing any local anesthetic drug for appropriate use in axial blockade, the total duration of sensory blockade may be more important than the more traditional (and easier to quantitate) two-segment regression in determining anesthetic duration. The critical aspect here is that the choice of drug must be tailored to the anticipated duration of surgery in order to minimize recovery and discharge time.

For peripheral nerve block of the arm or foot, extended duration is not usually a problem and is in fact one of the objectives sought. In such cases, the longer-acting drugs, such as bupivacaine, may have a role. Prolonged anesthesia from excessively long blockade may produce anxiety in some patients when it persists after hospital discharge, and it may mask important signs of cast compression of the extremity. An intermediate duration drug may be more appropriate for peripheral nerve blockade in outpatients.

The choice of technique and details of performance of regional anesthesia must also be modified for ambulatory patients. The ideal outpatient regional techniques are those which involve the most rapid onset and the least likely chance of complications. For this reason, intravenous regional anes-

Table 14-1. Choice of Local Anesthetic Drugs

	Application			
Local anesthetic	Spinal	Epidural	Peripheral nerve block	Duration
Procaine	5% (hyperbaric) 2% (hypobaric)	NA	NR	45–90 min
2-Chloroprocaine	NA	2% 3% (motor block)	NR	45–90 min
Lidocaine	5% (hyperbaric) 1.5–2% (isobaric)	1.5% 2% (motor block)	0.5–1%	60–120 min
Mepivacaine	NA	1%[a] 1.5% (motor block)	1%	2–6 hr peripherally
Bupivacaine	0.75% (hyperbaric)[b] 0.5% (isobaric)	0.5%[b]	0.25–0.5%	4–24 hr peripherally
Etidocaine	NR	1.5%[b]		
Tetracaine	1% (hyperbaric)[b]	NA	NR	3–5 hr

[a] Possibly too long for outpatient use.
[b] Probably too long for outpatient use.
NA = not available.
NR = not recommended.

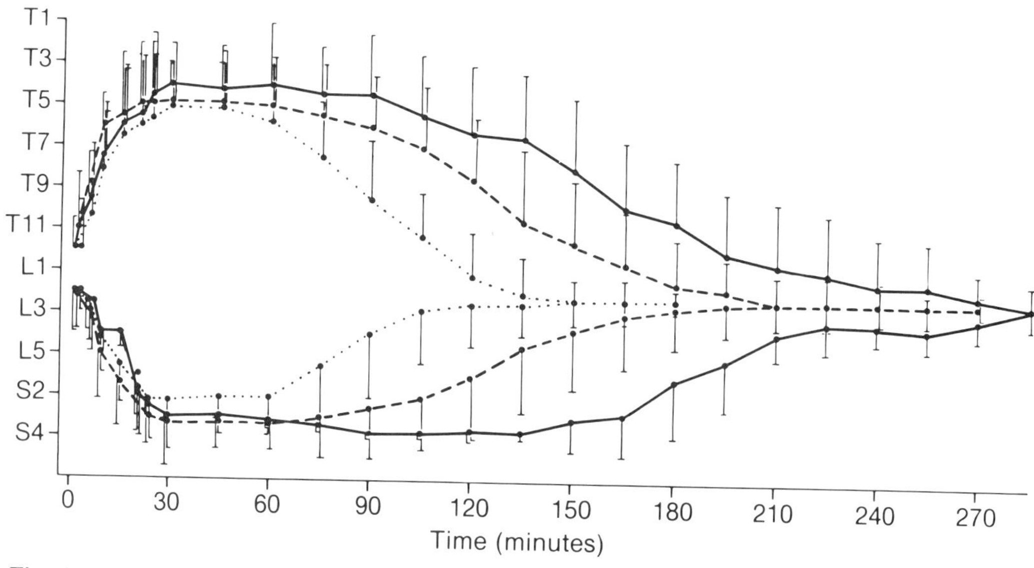

Fig. 14-1. Duration of epidural local anesthestics. The extent and duration of sensory blockade (± SD) after injection of 20 cc of local anesthetic solution with 1:200,000 epinephrine is shown for three local anesthetics used for outpatient extracorporeal shock wave lithotripsy. The average time to discharge from the hospital was 269 ± 63 minutes for 2-chloroprocaine (·····), 284 ± 62 minutes for lidocaine (— — — —), and 357 ± 71 minutes for mepivacaine (——). (From Kopacz and Mulroy,[38] with permission.)

thesia and spinal anesthesia are highly desirable in the outpatient setting. Specific steps must be taken to reduce the time required for regional anesthesia. Consequently, the presence of additional personnel to facilitate room turnover and performance of blocks is highly desirable, and the use of a separate induction room will allow the performance of a block while the operating room is being cleaned, or while the previous case is being completed. The most important time-saving aspect, however, is education of the patient prior to the day of surgery. This is best obtained by the use of a preoperative visit in an anesthesiologist's office or in a preoperative screening clinic. At this time, the patient can be instructed in the advantages of regional anesthesia and how the regional technique is performed. This saves considerable time on the day of surgery.

Patient screening is important in applying regional anesthesia in the outpatient setting. Some patients are clearly not candidates for regional technique because of a morbid fear of needle insertion or, more commonly, a nonspecific anxiety about any degree of alertness in the operating room. The young healthy outpatient population is frequently interested in observing and participating in the surgical procedure. Yet, there are many patients whose level of anxiety is such that heavy sedation is required for them to tolerate any procedure under regional techniques. Some sedation is desirable for most patients, and the appropriate agents and dosages have been described in Chapters 12 and 13. Excessive doses may produce prolonged somnolence with benzodiazepines or an increased incidence of nausea and vomiting with narcotics, and these side effects will negate much of the potential advantage of a regional technique. The patient who demonstrates a need for this level of sedation is a poor candidate for a regional technique and may best be treated with general anesthesia.

Likewise, the patient who is uncooperative because of age or mental disability is not an appropriate candidate for regional technique. Finally, those patients who, because of body habitus (either deformity or profound obesity), are difficult challenges for the regional anesthetist are probably not appropriate candidates for the performance of regional blocks. Appropriate selection will improve the success rate of regional techniques and preserve their advantages in the outpatient setting.

It should also be noted that patients scheduled for regional anesthesia need to be treated according to the same standards as those who are expected to undergo general anesthesia. Specifically, the history/physical, laboratory data, fasting state, and postprocedural care are the same for both regional and general anesthesia patients. The use of a regional technique cannot guarantee the absence of vomiting and aspiration, nor will it guarantee that the patient will be sufficiently alert to require no postoperative accompaniment.

Safety Aspects

The safety standards for performance of regional anesthesia are the same as those for general anesthesia. Appropriate resuscitation equipment must be available in any location where regional techniques are performed, including specialized induction rooms. Specifically, provision for oxygenation and cardiac resuscitation are necessary. Patients undergoing regional anesthesia techniques must be monitored closely for the development of signs of systemic toxicity. This requires special attention to the mental status of the patient, since no electronic device currently available can monitor increasing blood levels of local anesthetic drugs. The only signs that are available are the subtle changes in mental alertness and the development of the classic subjective signs of systemic local anesthetic toxicity. A blood pressure cuff and an ECG are very useful supplemental monitors in regional techniques, since many procedures involve some change in arterial pressure or pulse rate. The use of a mechanical pulse monitor is essential if large volumes of local anesthetic are injected which require monitoring the pulse rate changes produced by an epinephrine-containing test dose. There has been recent concern over the cardiotoxicity of the longer-acting amide local anesthetic agents. This is not a frequent problem, since these drugs are rarely appropriate in the outpatient setting.

SPECIFIC BLOCKS

Spinal Anesthesia

Of all the regional anesthetic techniques for outpatients, spinal blockade is the fastest, most predictable, and most reliable that can be used. It can be used in approximately 50 percent of outpatient surgical procedures (Table 14-2). The anatomy is easily perceived in all but the most obese patients, and the procedure itself is readily performed in experienced hands. The onset of the anesthesia is almost immediate, and the delay needed for surgical preparation and draping is usually sufficient to guarantee adequate anesthesia for most procedures. In general, the dose response is highly predictable, and the duration can be adjusted to the anticipated duration of surgery by the selection of the appropriate drug. The very small doses of local anesthetic required for subarachnoid blockade eliminate the chance of systemic toxicity with this technique. Spinal anesthesia, covering effectively half of the body, provides adequate surgical conditions for lower abdominal, groin, pelvic, lower extremity, and perineal surgery. The ability to provide sacral anesthesia makes it superior to epidural techniques.

The choice of local anesthetic for outpatient spinal anesthesia is probably best restricted to procaine or lidocaine. The use of tetracaine and bupivacaine may be associated with a 6 to 8 hour recovery room

Table 14-2. Application of Techniques to Specific Operations

Region/typical procedures	Applicable techniques		
	Spinal	Epidural	Regional
Head and neck			Local infiltration ? Superficial cervical plexus block
Arm			
Below elbow-superficial			Intravenous regional, local
Carpel tunnel			
Cyst removal			
Periosteal surgery			Axillary block
Colles fracture			
Arthrodesis of finger			
Above elbow			Interscalene block
Epicondylar stripping			? Supraclavicular block
Trunk	Possibly	Possibly	Local infiltration Intercostal blocks
Lower abdominal			
Laparoscopy	Yes	Yes	? Local
Herniorrhaphy	Yes	Yes	Yes
Lower extremity			
Arthroscopy of knee	Yes	Yes	Sciatic/femoral/lateral femoral cutaneous, "3-in-1"
Foot surgery Bunionectomy	Yes	Possibly consider caudal	Sciatic/femoral/lateral femoral cutaneous Popliteal fossa block Local
Perineal Hemorrhoidectomy, vaginal biopsy	Yes	Caudal	? Local

stay, with an increased potential for unplanned overnight admission. Although procaine lost popularity as a spinal anesthetic in previous decades because of its short duration, this very property may foster a renewed interest in the drug in the outpatient setting. Procaine is marketed commercially in a 10 percent solution, which, when mixed with an equal volume of cerebrospinal fluid, becomes a hyperbaric solution. The solution is more hyperbaric when mixed with 10 percent dextrose. Procaine is not recommended for use in a final concentration of more than 5 percent. Epinephrine will prolong procaine's duration from 45 to 60 minutes to 60 to 90 minutes. Accurate dosage information in the outpatient setting is missing, but an approximate 30 to 50 percent increase in total milligram dosage over the equivalent dose of lidocaine is required.

Lidocaine is a more familiar agent and is marketed in a 5 percent solution already prepared in a hyperbaric 7.5 percent dextrose solution. The 2 percent preservative-free preparation will act as a hypobaric solution. The duration appears to be approximately 60 minutes for lower abdominal anesthesia, but Moore et al. reported analgesia lasting at least 120 minutes for knee arthroscopy when lidocaine with epinephrine was used for spinal blockade.[11] Although Chambers et al. reported that epinephrine does not have a statistically significant effect in prolonging the duration of lidocaine spinal anesthesia,[12] it does have a positive affect on the quality of blockade produced when added to subarachnoid local anesthetic drugs. Smith and colleagues reported that the incidence of inadequate or patchy blocks during tetracaine and lidocaine anesthesia is increased if epinephrine is omitted.[13] It seems reasonable to continue to add epinephrine to lidocaine solutions for the outpatient and to rely on the substitution of procaine rather than the elimination of epinephrine if a shorter duration is desired with spinal anesthesia.

In terms of specific techniques for spinal anesthesia, all of the positions and approaches traditionally used for inpatients are applicable to the outpatient setting. The classic lateral decubitus position is most commonly used, although the sitting position can readily be used for hyperbaric injections for leg or perineal surgery. The jack-knife position, used in perianal surgery, is an ideal situation for the injection of hypobaric local anesthetic solution, which can be administered to the patient in the prone position with the surgical table already flexed to place the sacral part of the spinal canal uppermost.

The two main drawbacks in applying spinal anesthesia in the outpatient setting are the presence of autonomic blockade and the potential for postdural puncture headache. Autonomic blockade is an inevitable side effect of subarachnoid anesthesia and occurs with even the lowest concentrations of anesthetic agent. A high level of spinal anesthesia is associated with sufficient sympathetic blockade to produce a decrease in blood pressure, which usually responds readily to standard therapy. An infusion of 500 cc of crystalloid solution should be given in anticipation of vasodilatation in the lower extremities. Supplemental oxygen and careful monitoring of block level and blood pressure are necessary. Attention has recently focused on the incidence of sudden bradycardia associated with high spinal anesthesia.[14] The patient population at risk for this complication is young healthy patients undergoing minor ambulatory surgical procedures (e.g., arthroscopy, dilatation and curettage) in an outpatient unit. Careful monitoring is required and, ideally, this complication can be avoided by the use of the lowest block level acceptable for the intended surgery.

A more common problem associated with the autonomic blockade is concern over urinary retention following spinal anesthesia. Pflug et al. have shown that autonomic function will have returned to baseline when motor function in the lower extremity, proprioception of the big toe, and sensory function in the perianal region have returned to normal.[15] Axelsson and colleagues have shown that return of full detrusor tone may require 1 to 2 hours longer,[16] and it is not surprising that there is an incidence of inability to void in the short-stay unit, particularly in male patients. This may be related to overdistention of the bladder, but no study has confirmed any correlation of this problem with the amount of intraoperative fluid administered. The one factor that does appear to contribute to urinary retention is the duration of sympathetic block. In an obstetrical population, Bridenbaugh showed that the incidence of bladder catheterization was directly related to the duration of local anesthetic used for epidural anesthesia for cesarean section.[17] Ryan et al. have also shown that long-acting spinal anesthesia for hernia repair is associated with a 30 percent incidence of catheterization, compared with a 6 percent incidence in outpatient herniorrhaphies performed with short-acting spinal or epidural anesthesia.[5] It appears that urinary retention should be an infrequent problem with the short-duration spinal anesthetics used in outpatients; however, it will occur, particularly in association with groin or perineal procedures. In such procedures, pain at the incisional site associated with attempts at voiding may be a contributing factor to urinary retention, and generous use of local anesthetic wound infiltration may help to reduce problems with urination. Many surgeons feel that the inability to void is an indication for overnight admission and the insertion of an indwelling Foley catheter. Further study is needed to find if simple drainage of the bladder with an "in and out" catheterization prior to discharge would be satisfactory in an outpatient population.

The concern about postspinal headache is another deterrent to the use of spinal anesthesia in the outpatient setting. The overall incidence of postspinal headache was reported as 10 percent by Vandam and Dripps in their classic report of 10,000 spinal anesthetics.[18] Using their experience and data on causative factors, this incidence can be reduced to 1 percent or less in hospitalized patients through meticulous selection of patients, needles, and technique. Because classic postdural puncture headache occurs only when the patient assumes the upright position, it has been assumed that the risk is greater in ambulatory patients. Thus, there has been a reluctance in many institutions to use spinal anesthesia on outpatients who ambulate in the immediate postoperative period. The reluctance to apply spinal anesthesia to outpatients has been fostered by the report of Flaaten and Raeder,[19] who described a 37 percent incidence of headaches in 51 young healthy patients having vasectomies under spinal anesthesia with a 25-gauge needle. Their report has stirred controversy,[20] one of the debatable issues being their conclusion that spinal anesthesia is not appropriate for outpatients. They selected a group of patients who, under most circumstances, would be inappropriate candidates for spinal anesthesia in that their subjects were young men having a relatively trivial surgical procedure (vasectomy). The spinal anesthetic was performed with no benefit of local anesthesia. It is not surprising that their patients expressed a considerable degree of dissatisfaction with the anesthesia, nor that a large number of them complained of headache. It is noteworthy that only two of these patients actually required therapy with epidural blood patch to cure their headaches.

Other investigators have suggested that there really is no increased incidence of headache in ambulatory patients. Vandam and Dripps remarked that there was no substantiation for the traditional bedrest required of patients following spinal anesthesia.[18] Jones reported that 1,134 patients in his institution were allocated to random durations of bedrest following lumbar puncture. There was no correlation between the duration of recumbency and the incidence of headache.[21] Carbaat and van Crevel looked specifically at 100 patients receiving diagnostic lumbar puncture with 17-gauge needles, half of whom were retained in the hospital overnight in the supine position and half of whom were discharged as outpatients.[22] The incidence of headache was exactly the same in the two groups, although the bedridden group had a delay in the onset of headache symptoms of 24 hours. Thornberry and Thomas recently reported a similar study of 80 obstetric patients who had spinal anesthesia and who were allocated to either 24 hours of bedrest or early ambulation. Surprisingly, their incidence of headache was actually higher in the bedridden group, and the incidence of "severe" headache was significantly increased (20 percent versus 2 percent).[23]

The experience of other investigators suggests that the problem of postdural puncture headache is not at disproportionately high risk in the outpatient. Burke has reported an incidence of less than 5 percent headache in a series of over 1,000 laparoscopies,[8] and this patient population would be regarded at high risk of headaches according to the previous data of Vandam and Dripps.[18] Perz and colleagues at the University of Vermont have given a preliminary report of their experience in 228 outpatients receiving spinal anesthesia,[24] with an incidence of headache of 11 percent; this is not different from the reported incidence in inpatients. In my own institution, Neal and Bridenbaugh report an approximately 7 percent incidence of headache in outpatients.[25] It does appear that there is a finite risk of headache when performing spinal anesthesia on outpatients and that all possible steps should be taken to minimize this risk and to weigh the advantages of spinal anesthesia against the complications associated with a positional headache.

The major problem with outpatient spinal headaches is the potential hindrance to the patient's resumption of normal activity. Even though a postdural spinal headache might be an acceptable complication for an inpatient who anticipates 3 to 4 days' hospitalization and bedrest, this complication can be a serious setback for a young active patient anticipating a rapid return to work or to resumption of household responsibilities. Patients need to be informed that there is risk of headache, and every possible measure should be taken to reduce the potential for this complication as well as to treat it aggressively if it does occur. Appropriate steps in reducing the incidence include careful selection of patients. Younger patients (under 40 years of age) have a higher incidence of headaches, and there may be slightly greater potential for headache in women. A patient in this age group, particularly a woman, who has an urgent need to return to full ambulatory function within 24 hours after a procedure may not be an ideal candidate for an outpatient spinal anesthetic.

The technique itself can be modified to reduce the chance of headache. Primarily, this involves the use of small-gauge needles, preferably with the rounded Greene "pencil-point" or Whitacre sideport, which appear to reduce the incidence of persistent dural leakage by splitting the dural fibers rather than cutting them.[25] Insertion of the needle with the bevel parallel to the dural fibers is also reported to substantially reduce the incidence of postspinal leakage.[26] Adequate hydration and the avoidance of straining or lifting may also reduce the incidence of this complication.

If a patient does receive a spinal anesthetic, careful follow-up by phone 24 to 48 hours postsurgery is needed to ascertain whether the patient has developed disabling symptoms of headache. If headache does develop, treatment should be tailored to the patient's social condition. If the patient can tolerate the headache and can maintain bedrest at home, this may be the best therapy for the first 24 hours. If the headache is severe or the patient needs prompt resolution of symptoms in order to resume normal routine, the patient should be brought back to the hospital for an immediate epidural blood patch. The details of therapeutic treatment are well-documented,[27] and headaches occurring in outpatients should be treated in the same manner as those of inpatients.

In summary, spinal anesthesia is one of the most useful techniques in outpatient regional anesthesia. The advantages are ease of administration, rapid onset of action, and high reliability and predictability. These advantages must be considered along with the disadvantages of possible urinary retention and postspinal headache. If the incidence of these side effects in a specific clinical setting does not differ widely from the 2 percent probability of unplanned overnight hospital admission following outpatient general anesthesia, the choice of technique becomes a matter of preference.

Epidural Anesthesia

Because of concern about spinal headaches in the outpatient population, many anesthesiologists prefer to use peridural anesthesia, either through the lumbar approach or through caudal injection, for the ambulatory patient. In the absence of dural puncture, there is no chance of postdural headache. Unfortunately, even in the best hands, there is a small but measurable risk of unintentional dural puncture by the needle or the catheter during the performance of lumbar epidural or caudal anesthesia. The probability of puncture is decreased by the operator's level of expertise, but the potential risk remains. Unfortunately, if dural puncture does occur with the 17- or 19-gauge needles commonly used for peridural blocks, the chance of headache exceeds 50 percent in younger patients (under 35 years of age). It is probably appropriate to advise patients that the chance of headache is less with epidural block than with spinal anesthesia, but all factors must be weighed in assessing that risk.

Epidural anesthesia offers some distinct advantages over subarachnoid blockade. The onset of anesthesia is more gradual and often less threatening to young patients, and the presence of segmental blockade allows the extent of anesthesia to be tailored to the actual surgical field. The "density" of blockade may also be adjusted by choosing higher or lower concentrations of local anesthetic drug, depending on the requirements for motor relaxation for a given surgical procedure.

The advantages of peridural blockade must be weighed against several factors that compare negatively with spinal anesthesia. First, the onset of blockade is slower than with the spinal technique, and 15 to 20 minutes are frequently required to attain adequate surgical anesthesia. Consequently, either the surgeon must wait for the onset of the blockade in the operating room, or an induction room must be provided outside the operating room where the patient can receive the block and wait for the onset of anesthesia. Epidural anesthesia is also hampered by slightly decreased reliability, particularly because of the wide variation in dose response in younger patients. Bromage has shown that age is probably the single most important determinant of epidural anesthetic dosage and that young patients require significantly higher doses than are commonly used in the older surgical candidates or in the parturient (Fig. 14-2).[28] This high-dose requirement plus the inherent variability of response make the prediction of appropriate dose difficult in the characteristically young patient currently treated in outpatient facilities.

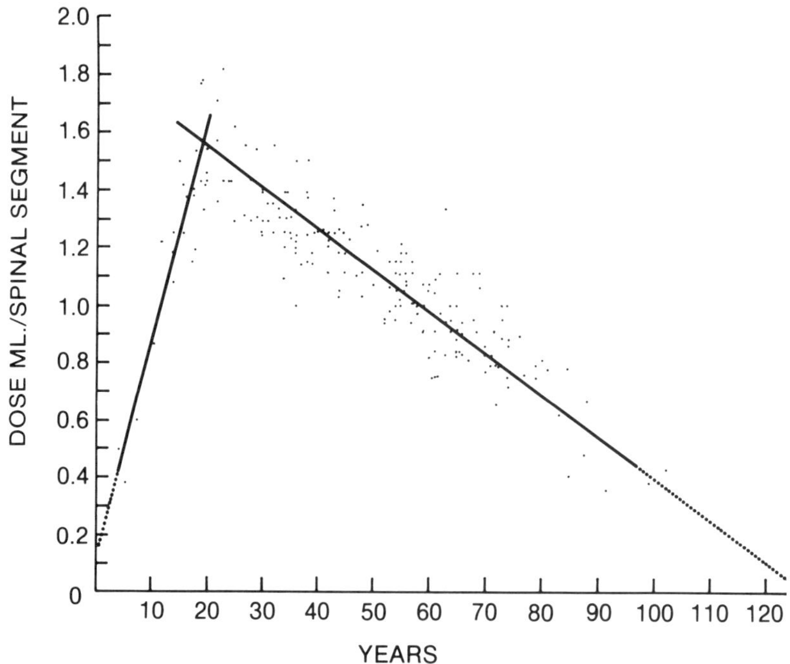

Fig. 14-2. Effect of age on epidural dosage. The dose requirement for epidural lidocaine (2 percent with epinephrine 1:200,000) decreases with age; young patients (as commonly seen for ambulatory surgery) have the highest dose requirement and typically require 25 to 40 percent more than their elderly inpatient counterparts. (From Bromage,[28] with permission.)

This high-dose requirement is the source of an additional disadvantage of peridural blockade, specifically, the increased risk of local anesthetic toxicity. Dosages approaching the maximum recommended milligram dosage for many of the short-acting drugs are frequently required to produce adequate surgical anesthesia. Signs of systemic absorption such as tremulousness and shivering are frequently seen. Other problems are also associated with larger doses, such as occasional back pain associated with large quantities of 2-chloroprocaine. There is also a greater risk of unintentional intravascular or subarachnoid injection. Careful test-dosing and observation cannot be sacrificed in the interest of speed. The problem of cardiotoxicity (e.g., arrythmias) is not usually encountered because bupivacaine, the drug most commonly associated with this complication, is rarely used in the ambulatory setting. Similarly, the specific neurotoxicity of the previous bisulfite-containing commercial preparation, Nesacaine (Astra Pharmaceutical Products, Inc., Westboro, MA), is less of a concern since the bisulfite-free preparation appeared on the market in October 1987.[29] Nevertheless, the patient must be protected against the undesirable effects of systemic toxicity or total spinal anesthesia by careful observation with these large dose requirements.

The techniques of lumbar epidural anesthesia are the same as those used for the inpatient. Procedures appropriate for peridural blockade are essentially the same as those for which spinal anesthesia can be applied, as indicated in Table 14-2. This basically includes procedures on the lower extremities, perineum, groin, or lower abdomen. Vaginal procedures often present a challenge, since caudal anesthesia may not provide sufficient blockade of the T10–12 dermatomes to block the sensation of cervical dilatation, but lumbar epidural anesthesia may not provide sufficient perineal anesthesia to avoid the discomfort of vaginal examination. With either technique, a longer time period may be required for onset of sufficient anesthesia. The caudal approach to the peridural space is more appropriate for foot or perianal procedures. Knee arthroscopy, hernia repair, and laparoscopy are all suitable procedures for lumbar epidural blockade.

A frequent concern is the appropriateness of lumbar epidural anesthesia for pelvic laparoscopy. There is inevitably some infringement on the excursion of the diaphragm when the abdominal cavity is insufflated with gas. Thin, young healthy patients will tolerate this without developing hypoxemia,[9] but this technique may not be appropriate in obese patients who have poor ventilatory reserve, nor will it be well-tolerated in extremely anxious patients who may become agitated by their perception of difficulty in breathing. This situation commonly occurs with the young patient undergoing laparoscopy as part of a fertility evaluation. The advantages of the patient's participation in the diagnostic procedure must be weighed against the potential of extreme anxiety which may require doses of sedation that would negate the advantages of the regional technique.

One of the better examples of the appropriate use of epidural anesthesia for abdominal surgery is the application of this technique to inguinal hernia repair. An epidural anesthetic performed with a short-acting local anesthetic agent is combined with generous infiltration of the wound with 0.25 percent bupivacaine. The rapid recovery from the epidural anesthesia and the 6 to 8 hours of postoperative analgesia provided by bupivacaine facilitate early discharge from the outpatient unit.[5] The use of local anesthesia infiltration in combination with other regional techniques needs to be further encouraged.

The major decision to be made in peridural anesthesia is whether an indwelling catheter should be used. The placement of the catheter adds a small degree of increased complexity to the procedure and appears to increase the potential risk for vascular puncture from approximately 3 percent to 8 percent.[30] Nevertheless, the use of a catheter adds considerable flexibility in adjusting the duration of the peridural blockade to match the duration of the procedure. Basically, for procedures of reliably predictable duration, such as laparoscopic tubal ligation, a single injection technique may be appropriate. For procedures associated with less predictable duration, such as arthroscopy of the knee, the continuous technique may be more appropriate.

The choice of drugs is primarily a function of anticipated duration of the surgical procedure (Table 14-1). 2-Chloroprocaine is probably the ideal drug for most surgical procedures lasting 30 to 45 minutes, which may include the majority of laparoscopy, arthroscopy, and herniorrhaphy procedures in most institutions. Lidocaine is a more appropriate choice for an extended arthroscopic procedure, particularly when the potential for significant surgical intervention is present. Mepivacaine may be suitable for longer surgical procedures. It can produce up to 2 hours of surgical anesthesia, but its duration of total blockade may be greater than 4 hours in lithotripsy patients, and a total time to discharge may approach 6 hours from beginning of anesthesia. Longer-acting agents, such as bupivacaine, ropivacaine, and etidocaine, probably have no use in the outpatient setting. For the short-acting drugs, lower concentrations (2 percent chloroprocaine, 1.5 percent lidocaine) will produce adequate sensory anesthesia, but higher concentrations are needed to produce motor blockade. Lidocaine possesses a frequency-dependent component of blockade that clinically produces sensory anesthesia significantly outlasting motor blockade.[31] A 3 percent chloroprocaine anesthetic will actually provide a longer motor blockade than an equal dose of 1.5 percent lidocaine.

Peripheral Nerve Blocks

Arm

Regional anesthesia of the upper extremity epitomizes the advantages of regional anesthesia for the outpatient. Blockade of the entire extremity is relatively easily attained because of the close proximity of all the nerves of the brachial plexus as they exit the spinal column and traverse the first rib and the axilla. Sensory anesthesia can be used for the operative site on the arm without interfering with ambulation. The residual analgesia following the block allows a patient to go home with minimal discomfort and without the side effects of oral analgesics. If sedation is kept to a minimum, there is no interference with postoperative eating or rapid return to normal function. The ideal arm block will allow a patient to leave the recovery unit within 30 minutes of the procedure's completion.

There are some drawbacks to this otherwise ideal technique. More time is usually required to perform a block of the brachial plexus, and there is greater delay in the onset of full surgical anesthesia than is the case in spinal or intravenous regional anesthesia. The functional loss of one arm for some period of time requires the patient to protect that anesthetized extremity from further trauma following the procedure. Nevertheless, regional blockade of the brachial plexus is an ideal technique for outpatients undergoing operations on the upper extremity.

The choice of specific approach to the brachial plexus is a matter of debate. The simplest approach to anesthesia of the upper extremity is the use of an intravenous regional technique, as discussed in Chapter 13. This block has the advantages of rapid onset, simplicity of performance, and high reliability, although many hand surgeons express concern about operating in the "weeping" edematous fields produced by this form of anesthesia. Another problem with the intravenous regional technique is the lack of postoperative analgesia.

The other approaches to the brachial plexus blockade are the axillary, the supraclavicular, and the interscalene. Two factors influence the choice of specific technique. First, each of these blockades produces a different distribution of anesthesia in the forearm.[32] The interscalene block is most suited for operations of the shoulder and upper arm, but has a 15 to 20 percent probability of inadequate blockade of the ulnar distribution of the forearm. Supraclavicular technique is the most likely to anesthetize all four major branches of the forearm. The axillary approach usually gives excellent anesthesia below the wrist, but frequently misses the musculocutaneous branch, which departs the neurovascular bundle high in the axillary sheath (Figs. 14-3 and 14-4). The second consideration is possible side effects. Although the supraclavicular is potentially the most effective blockade, it is also associated with the highest incidence of pneumothorax. In experienced hands, this complication is rare but it is one that potentially requires hospitalization. This may be a major deterrent to the performance of this block in the outpatient setting. The interscalene has a lower risk of pneumothorax when properly performed, but, in many settings, the axillary approach is the technique of choice for the outpatient.

The choice of drug is a matter of preference. Lidocaine will produce adequate anesthesia of the upper arm for 3 to 4 hours if a 1 percent solution with epinephrine is used. Bupivacaine will produce a significantly longer anesthesia, perhaps as long as 10 to 24 hours following surgery. Some patients are disturbed by the duration of this blockade and express concern over how long after their discharge it will take for normal function to return. The use of mepivacaine in a 1 percent concentration will give a blockade of intermediate duration; this may be most appropriate to provide a period of anesthesia sufficient to allow the patient to go home as he or she is beginning to experience the return of function. As in all peripheral nerve blocks, the higher concentrations of local anesthetics should be avoided. Adequate sensory anesthesia can be obtained by using moderate volumes of a more dilute local anesthetic preparation.

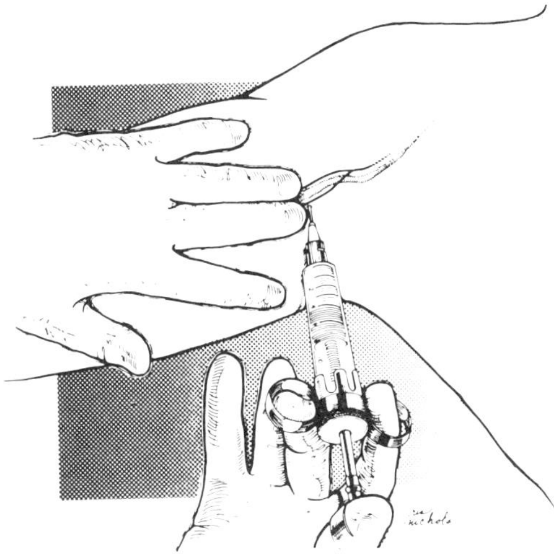

Fig. 14-3. Position for injection of axillary block. The arm is held at 90 degrees abduction, with the elbow flexed at 90 degrees also. The brachial artery is marked as high in the axilla as practical and the area prepared aseptically. Two fingers of equal length straddle the artery while the needle is introduced parallel to the axis of the vessel with the central angulation. The palpating fingers serve not only to identify the vessel but also to compress the perivascular sheath and encourage the spread of anesthetic solution centrally. (From Mulroy,[33] with permission.)

There is also a potential for the surgeon to perform local infiltration of the peripheral nerves of the forearm, either at the elbow or at the wrist, at the time of surgery. The onset of anesthesia in this procedure will take slightly longer than in a properly performed brachial plexus blockade, particularly if that blockade cannot be performed by an anesthesiologist in a separate induction area prior to surgery, and must occur

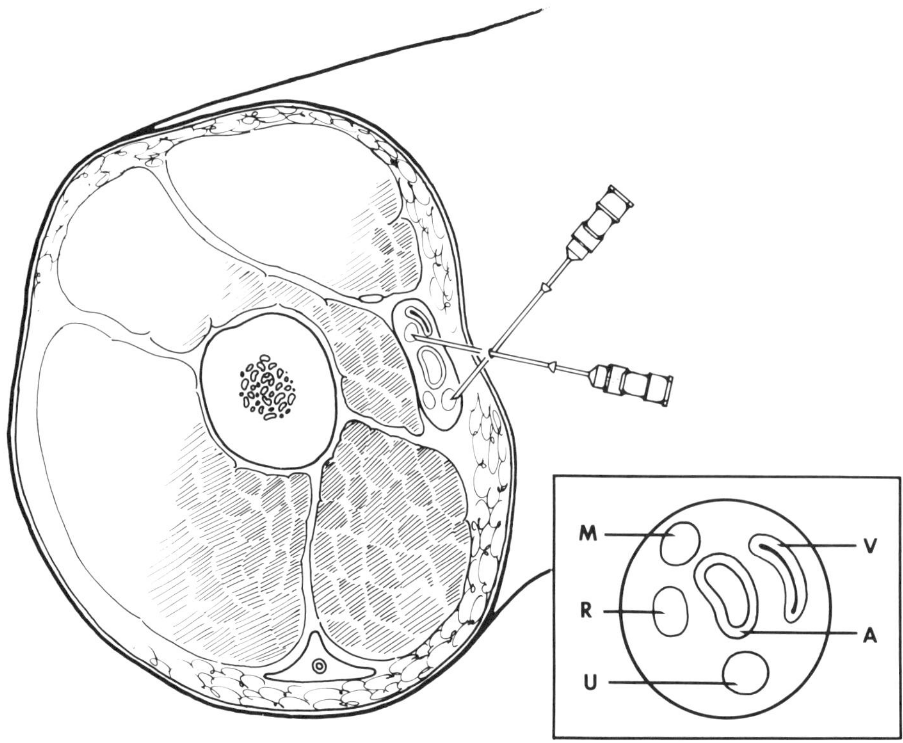

Fig. 14-4. Technique of axillary blockade. The median (M) and musculocutaneous nerves lie on the superior side of the artery (A), although the latter may have already departed the axillary sheath at the level of injection. The ulnar (U) lies inferior, and the radial (R) is inferior and posterior. The vein (V) lies in a variable position superior to the artery. These positions vary with individual patients, and the two positions demonstrated are the most common patterns. The most common technique of blockade involves paresthesias of at least two of the nerves, usually starting with the branch innervating the proposed surgical site. A total of 20 to 40 cc of solution are required to reach all of the branches; a separate injection may be needed for the musculocutaneous nerve if anesthesia of this branch is required for surgery. (Adapted from Partridge et al.[34] as appears in Mulroy,[33] with permission.)

during the positioning and preparation of the operative site.

Leg

Anesthesia of the lower leg can be induced by peripheral nerve blockade of the sciatic and femoral plexus, but the nerves in this location are not as conveniently "bundled" as in the upper extremity. Blockade is more time-consuming and less reliable than spinal or epidural blockade of the same area. Paresthesias are usually required, and their elicitation may be uncomfortable to the unsedated outpatient. Overcoming this discomfort by the use of generous intravenous sedation and nerve stimulator may negate the major advantages of regional techniques. Nevertheless, plexus anesthesia may be useful when surgery is performed on only one extremity, or when a patient refuses axial blockade. Generally, it is less applicable in outpatient surgery, but in several centers peripheral nerve block of the lower extremity is used for operations of the knee or foot.

The two common approaches to the lumbar plexus are the multiple nerve injection (sciatic/femoral/lateral-femoral-cutaneous injections) or the "three-in-one" plexus block described by Winnie et al.[35] Both have been used in the outpatient setting. Patel and colleagues have described the use of the Winnie blockade for knee surgery.[10] They found that this technique was satisfactory for knee arthroscopy, although the success rate was improved if local infiltration of the lateral femoral cutaneous nerve was added to the femoral nerve block. Although recovery time in the regional anesthesia group was at least 30 minutes shorter than that for general anesthesia, the difference in induction times was not given. In overall time there may be no clear advantage between the two methods. In addition, the technique of Patel et al. may not be suitable for operations involving major surgery of the knee. Specifically, the posterior compartment might require additional local anesthesia at the sciatic nerve branches on the back of the leg. If sciatic nerve block is included, this may double the amount of time required for the production of regional anesthesia in the lower extremity.

For operative procedures below the knee, regional anesthesia can be obtained with a single injection of the sciatic nerve in the popliteal fossa at the bifurcation of the two main branches.[36] This technique requires the patient to lie in the prone position and again relies on elicitation of paresthesias (Fig. 14-5). The Mayo Clinic group reports an 85 percent success rate in the application of this technique, which takes less than 15 minutes to perform in experienced hands. Again, adequate time is required for the onset of anesthesia. The block may require supplemental injection to anesthetize the femoral nerve as it crosses the medial head of the tibia if anesthesia of the dorsum of the foot or the big toe is required. Since it does not produce any anesthesia of the quadriceps muscle group, which might interfere with the patient's ability to ambulate, this technique is useful for foot sur-

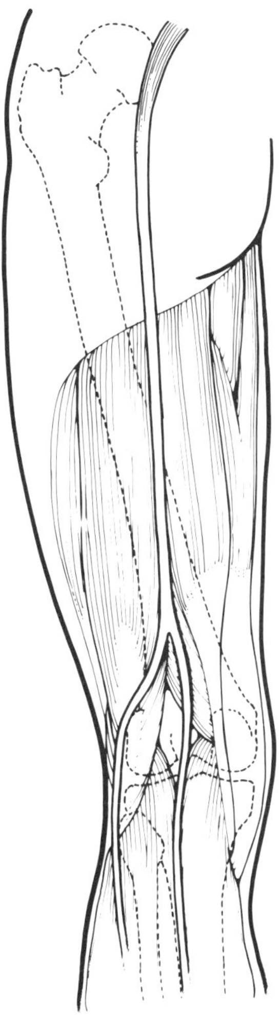

Fig. 14-5. Sciatic nerve block at the popliteal fossa. The two major trunks of the sciatic nerve bifurcate in the popliteal fossa 7 to 10 cm above the knee. To find the trunks near the bifurcation, a triangle is drawn using the heads of the biceps femoris and the semitendinosus muscles and the skin crease of the knee. A line is drawn from the skin crease that bisects this triangle; a long needle is inserted 1 cm lateral to a point 5 cm cephalad from the crease on this line. The needle is directed at a 45-degree angle to explore for the nerve, and 35 cc of solution is injected when a paresthesia to the foot is obtained. (Adapted from Rorie et al.[36] as appears in Mulroy,[33] with permission.)

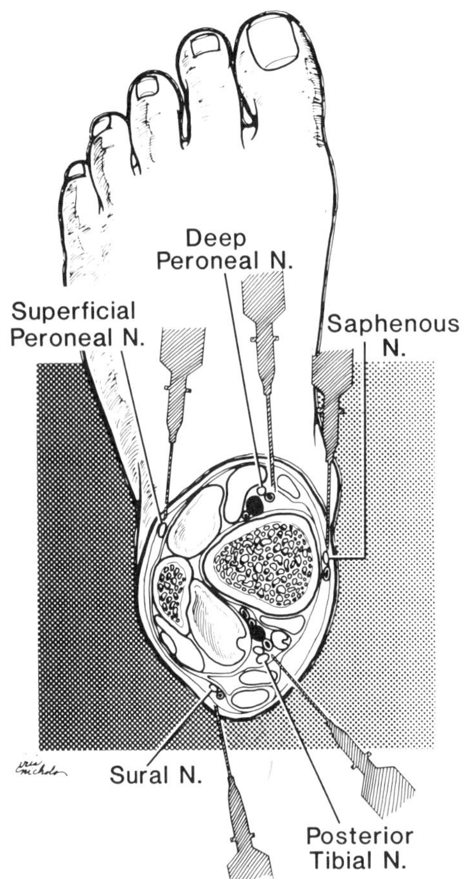

Fig. 14-6. Ankle block. Injections are made at five separate nerve locations. The superficial peroneal nerve, the sural nerve, and the saphenous are usually blocked simply by subcutaneous infiltration, since they may have already generated many superficial branches as they cross the ankle joint. Paresthesias can be sought in the posterior tibial nerve or the deep peroneal, but the bony landmarks will usually suffice to provide adequate localization for the deeper injections. The block can be performed by making the anterior injections while the patient is supine; the posterior injections are then given in the prone position. Alternatively, the patient can flex the knee and rest the sole of the foot on the table so that both sides can be reached in one position. (From Mulroy,[33] with permission.)

gery. One drawback is that it does not provide anesthesia for the discomfort associated with a tourniquet placed on the thigh.

An alternative for anesthesia of the foot is the ankle block (Fig. 14-6).[37] This technique produces the least disruption of ambulatory function and can provide residual postoperative analgesia, particularly if a long-acting local anesthetic is used. However, it is time consuming: as many as five separate injections of local anesthetic may be required, and the patient may have to assume two separate positions for the block to be performed. The number of separate nerves to be anesthetized increases the possibility of inadequate anesthesia in any one area. The multiple injections may also increase administration time, although this technique can be performed with considerable speed if paresthesias are not sought. As always with peripheral nerve blocks, a sufficient delay must be allowed for the onset of anesthesia. Peripheral blockade at the ankle will not provide adequate anesthesia for the ischemic discomfort from a tourniquet placed on the calf. In this situation, a more proximal block or a distal tourniquet is needed.

DISCHARGE CONSIDERATIONS

Patients receiving regional techniques require the same postoperative care as any other outpatient. This includes reasonable resolution of any sedative effects of medication, appropriate adult escort home and observation for the rest of the day, and precautions against any activity requiring normal concentration or coordination. There is no need to delay discharge until all analgesia in an extremity has resolved. In fact, this would negate one of the salient advantages of regional techniques. Those patients who have residual analgesia of an extremity must be specifically cautioned to protect that extremity from any trauma, since the normal warning sensations and reflexes are absent. A sling is all that is needed for a numb arm, but a numb foot should receive a bulky dressing to serve as additional protection against injury. Crutches must be supplied to all patients with knee or foot surgery, and instructions concerning their use and supervision of the patient's first efforts to ambulate should be provided. In patients with impaired mobility, the assistance of an adult escort is critical. All discharge instructions should be in written form and included in the patient's take-home package, both for clarity and for the medicolegal protection of the institution.

Although residual local anesthetic may provide temporary analgesia for the trip home, patients nonetheless will require an oral analgesic. They must be instructed not to be alarmed at the onset of pain as the neural blockade resolves, and they must be counselled concerning the detection of compression or ischemic pain if a cast has been applied. Patients should also be instructed about the possible side effects of oral analgesics, particularly the potential for nausea. The necessity of elevating the extremity after surgery must be stressed, especially in the young patient who frequently attempts to resume normal activity while the local anesthetic is effective. These patients must be warned that excessive activity will not only increase swelling and pain but may also jeopardize the surgical repair.

Discharge following axial blockade is more complicated. Full return of sensory, motor, and autonomic function is required before the patient attempts to ambulate, since premature ambulation can result in hypotension. These patients should be allowed to sit up only after all sensation has returned (particularly in the perianal region) and, after sitting for a while without evidence of postural hypotension, they may be allowed to walk with assistance. The main drawback of axial blockade, as discussed in the spinal anesthesia section, is the potential problem of bladder dysfunction. Urination is generally a mandatory requirement for discharge after procedures involving spinal or epidural blockade. Inability to void usually indicates the need for catheterization of the bladder. Although some patients may simply be catheterized once and discharged, common practice is to admit the patient and leave an indwelling catheter in place overnight.

All patients receiving regional blockade should be contacted the next day to ensure full return of neurologic function. Any residual hypesthesia or pain should be evaluated if it persists more than 48 hours. Patients receiving spinal anesthesia must be evaluated at least once (at 24 hours), and advised that postspinal headaches may occur 2 to 3 days following the procedure. Patients should be given a phone number that will provide 24-hour contact with an anesthesiologist to allow early diagnosis and appropriate management of postoperative complications.

SUMMARY

Regional anesthesia has several distinct advantages over general anesthesia in the patient scheduled for ambulatory surgery. Particular advantages are the presence of residual analgesia and the lower incidence of postoperative nausea and vomiting. With appropriate choice of regional technique and local anesthetic, earlier ambulation and discharge are often possible. These advantages, however, may be negated by the use of excessive sedation. Careful patient selection is also required. Because regional anesthesia requires more time to administer than general anesthesia, it may not be readily accepted by surgeons in a busy outpatient unit. Selected application of regional techniques will help convince surgeons, anesthesiologists, and nurses of the advantages of regional blockade and may ultimately lead to greater patient and surgeon satisfaction.

REFERENCES

1. Bridenbaugh LD: Regional anaesthesia for outpatient surgery—a summary of 12 years' experience. Can Anaesth Soc J 30:548, 1983
2. Beskin JL, Baxter DE: Regional anesthesia for ambulatory foot and ankle surgery. Orthopedics 10:109, 1987
3. Meridy HW: Criteria for selection of ambulatory surgical patients and guidelines for anesthetic management. Anesth Analg 61:921, 1982
4. Fahy A, Marshall M: Postanaesthetic morbidity in out-patients. Br J Anaesth 41:433, 1969
5. Ryan JA, Adye BA, Jolly PC, Mulroy MF: Outpatient inguinal herniorrhaphy with both regional and local anesthesia. Am J Surg 148:313, 1984
6. Hinkle AJ: Percutaneous inguinal block for the out-patient management of post-herniorrhaphy pain in children. Anesthesiology 67:411, 1987
7. Hannallah RS, Broadman LM, Belman AB, et al: Comparison of caudal and ilioinguinal/iliohypogastric nerve blocks for control of post-orchiopexy pain in pediatric ambulatory surgery. Anesthesiology 66:832, 1987
8. Burke RK: Spinal anesthesia for laparoscopy, a review of 1,063 cases. J Reprod Med 21:59, 1975
9. Bridenbaugh LD, Soderstrom RM: Lumbar epidural block anesthesia for outpatient laparoscopy. J Reprod Med 23:85, 1979
10. Patel NJ, Flashburg MH, Paskin S, Grossman R: Regional anesthetic technique compared to general anesthesia for outpatient knee arthroscopy. Anesth Analg 65:185, 1986
11. Moore DC, Chadwick HS, Ready LB: Epinephrine prolongs lidocaine spinal: pain in the operative site most accurate method of determining local anesthetic duration. Anesthesiology 67:416, 1987
12. Chambers WA, Littlewood DG, Logan MR, Scott DB: Effect of added epinephrine on spinal anesthesia with lidocaine. Anesth Analg 60:417, 1981
13. Smith HS, Carpenter RL, Bridenbaugh LD: Epinephrine increases the effectiveness of tetracaine spinal anesthesia. Anesthesiology 71:33, 1989
14. Caplan RA, Ward RJ, Posner K, Cheney FW: Unexpected cardiac arrest during spinal anesthesia: a closed claims analysis of predisposing factors. Anesthesiology 68:5, 1988
15. Pflug AE, Aasheim GM, Foster C: Sequence of return of neurological function and criteria for safe ambulation following subarachnoid block (spinal anaesthetic). Can Anaesth Soc J 25:133, 1978
16. Axelsson K, Mollefors K, Olsson JO, et al: Bladder function and spinal anaesthesia. Acta Anaesthesiol Scand 29:315, 1985
17. Bridenbaugh LD: Catheterization after long- and short-acting local anesthetics for continuous caudal block for vaginal delivery. Anesthesiology 46:357, 1977
18. Vandam LD, Dripps RD: Long-term follow-up of patients who received 10,098 spinal anesthetics: syndrome of decreased intracranial pressure (headache and ocular and auditory difficulties). JAMA 161:586, 1956
19. Flaaten H, Raeder J: Spinal anaesthesia for outpatient surgery. Anaesthesia 40:1108, 1985
20. Atkinson RS, Lee JA: Spinal anaesthesia and day case surgery? Anaesthesia 40:1059, 1985
21. Jones RJ: Role of recumbency in prevention and treatment of post-spinal headache. Anesth Analg 53:788, 1974
22. Carbaat PAT, van Crevel H: Lumbar puncture headache: controlled study on the preventive effect of 24 hours bed rest. Lancet 2:1133, 1981
23. Thornberry EA, Thomas TA: Posture and post-spinal headache. Br J Anaesth 60:195, 1988
24. Perz RR, Johnson DL, Shinozaki T: Spinal anesthesia for outpatient surgery. Anesth Analg 67:S168, 1988
25. Mulroy MS, Neal JM, Bridenbaugh LD, Palmen B: Is post-spinal headache more frequent in outpatients? Reg Anesth 14(2S):2, 1989
26. Mihic DN: Postspinal headache and relationship of needle bevel to longitudinal dural fibers. Reg Anesth 10:76, 1985

27. Mulroy MF: Spinal headaches: management and avoidance. p. 602. In Brown DL (ed): Problems in Anesthesia. Regional Anesthesia at the Virginia Mason Medical Center: A Critical Perspective. Vol. 1, No. 4. JB Lippincott, Philadelphia, 1987
28. Bromage PR: Epidural Analgesia. Ch. 9. WB Saunders, Philadelphia, 1978
29. Gissen AJ, Datta S, Lambert D: The chloroprocaine controversy II: is chloroprocaine neurotoxic? Reg Anesth 9:135, 1984
30. Verniquet AJW: Vessel puncture with epidural catheters. Anaesthesia 35:660, 1980
31. Scurlock JE, Meymaris E, Gregus J: The clinical character of local anesthetics: a function of frequency-dependent conduction block. Acta Anaesth Scand 22:601, 1978
32. Lanz E, Theiss D, Jankovic D: The extent of blockade following various techniques of brachial plexus block. Anesth Analg 62:55, 1983
33. Mulroy MF: Regional Anesthesia: An Illustrated Procedural Guide. Little, Brown, Boston, 1989
34. Partridge BL, Katz J, Benirschke K: Functional anatomy of the brachial plexus sheath: implications for anesthesia. Anesthesiology 66:743, 1987
35. Winnie AP, Ramamurthy S, Durrani Z: The inguinal paravascular technique of lumbar plexus anesthesia. "The 3-in-1 block." Anesth Analg 52:989, 1973
36. Rorie DK, Nelson DO, Sittipong R, Johnson KA: Assessment of block of the sciatic nerve in the popliteal fossa. Anesth Analg 59:37, 1980
37. McCutcheon R: Regional anesthesia of the foot. Can Anaesth Soc J 12:465, 1965
38. Kopacz D, Mulroy MS: Chloroprocaine and lidocaine decrease hospital stay and admission rate after outpatient epidural anesthesia. Reg Anesth 15:30, 1990

15

General Anesthesia

Robert J. Fragen

The basic components of general anesthesia are hypnosis, amnesia, analgesia, and, when necessary, muscle relaxation. A single inhaled anesthetic agent such as halothane, enflurane, or isoflurane can provide all these components, or each can derive from a separate intravenously administered drug. Alternatively, a local or regional anesthetic can provide analgesia and muscle relaxation with a sedative-hypnotic drug added to cause sedation or sleep. This chapter contains a discussion of the drugs and agents that can produce the components of general anesthesia, emphasizing those most appropriate for adult outpatients.

Early philosophy concerning outpatient surgery restricted it to healthy, American Society of Anesthesiologists status I or II patients having operations of a maximum 1 hour's duration. That policy has changed. Today, sicker patients undergo longer surgery on an outpatient basis; thus, drugs of longer duration may be appropriate.

Drugs used in outpatient anesthesia must meet certain performance criteria. Induction should be pleasant, rapid (one arm-brain circulation time), and should cause no untoward effects or reactions. Depth of anesthesia should be easily adjustable and recovery from anesthesia should be rapid without nausea, vomiting, or other side effects. The faster the drug leaves the body, the less the residual anesthetic effect; thus, high-clearance drugs are desirable. An examination of currently available drugs and those still under investigation shows that newer drugs seem to differ from their predecessors by having shorter durations of action at equipotent doses and/or shorter elimination halflives.

It is important to monitor the effects of general anesthesia during outpatient surgery using the same standards applicable to inpatient procedures. In addition to the effects of drugs on the patient, the functioning of the anesthesia delivery system (anesthesia machine or infusion system) should be monitored. Minimal patient monitoring includes measurement of blood pressure, heart rate, heart sounds, cardioscope tracing, body temperature, oxygenation, and expired carbon dioxide (see Ch. 11). Following surgery, patients should be taken to a specialized recovery area supervised by trained personnel where patients can recover from the effects of general anesthesia until they meet the discharge criteria established for the unit.

Sedative, hypnotic, and opioid drugs given prior to induction of anesthesia may prolong recovery from general anesthesia, depending on the drug, dose, and time of administration (see Ch. 17). Perhaps the most important job of the anesthesiologist is to properly evaluate a patient preoperatively and to choose the anesthetic drugs and techniques that are most appropriate for the patient and the scheduled surgical procedure.

The anesthesiologist usually injects a

drug or drug combination intravenously to induce anesthesia. To maintain the anesthetic state, an inhalation anesthetic agent is used, generally a potent volatile anesthetic and nitrous oxide. However, administration of volatile agents alone or with opioids is another option, as is the use of opioids, hypnotics, or both combined with nitrous oxide; the latter is often called "balanced anesthesia." Another alternative, likely to become more common in the future, is total intravenous anesthesia, in which, as the name implies, all the anesthetic components are injected intravenously. Muscle relaxants facilitate tracheal intubation and may be indicated for a few outpatient surgical procedures.

INTRAVENOUS ANESTHETIC AGENTS

The anesthetic induction agents suitable for outpatient anesthesia include the three barbiturates (thiopental, thiamylal, and methohexital), ketamine, etomidate, and propofol. The benzodiazepines, diazepam and midazolam, are suitable as intravenous sedatives when given in small doses, but they are inappropriate for outpatient anesthetic induction. Recovery from these benzodiazepines is slower than after other agents, and antegrade amnesia can last beyond the initial recovery period.[1] Figure 15-1 shows the structural formulae for the agents used for induction of general anesthesia.[3] The opioids, fentanyl, sufentanil, and alfentanil can induce anesthesia, but in doses high enough to produce unconsciousness, they are associated with chest wall rigidity, delayed recovery, postoperative respiratory depression, and nausea. Alfentanil also causes hypotension. The opioids are most useful as adjunctive drugs for outpatient anesthesia, not as induction agents.

The injected dose of a sedative-hypnotic or opioid drug mixes into the central volume of distribution, which presumably includes the blood and the highly perfused organs, such as the brain and heart. After rapidly achieving a drug concentration at central nervous system (CNS) receptors, the drug redistributes to the muscle mass where much of it is deposited.[3] Subsequently, it distributes to less well-perfused tissue, mainly fat (Fig. 15-2). As the drug passes from the central volume of distribution to the total body volume of distribution, the CNS concentration and drug effect decrease until recovery occurs, unless a large dose, multiple injections, or a continuous infusion of the drug keep the CNS concentration within the therapeutic range. Elimination clearance also influences the termination of clinical effects of drugs given in very high doses or by continuous infusion. Therefore, high-clearance drugs are best suited for administration by continuous infusion, as they leave fewer residual effects after administration of the drug ceases. The pharmacokinetics of the sedative-hypnotic drugs are presented in Table

Table 15-1. The Pharmacokinetics of Intravenous Anesthetic Agents (Mean Values)

Drug	Vd_{ss} (L/kg)	Cl_E (ml/kg/min)	T½ β (hr)	Protein binding (%)
Thiopental	2.3	3.4	12.0	83.4
Methohexital	2.2	10.9	3.9	73.0
Etomidate	2.5	17.9	2.9	77.0
Ketamine	3.1	19.1	3.1	12.0
Propofol	2.8	59.4[a]	0.9	97.0
Midazolam	1.1	7.5	2.7	94.0
Diazepam	1.1	0.4	46.6	98.0

[a] Whole blood clearance versus plasma clearance for the other drugs.
(Modified from Fragen and Avram,[2] with permission.)

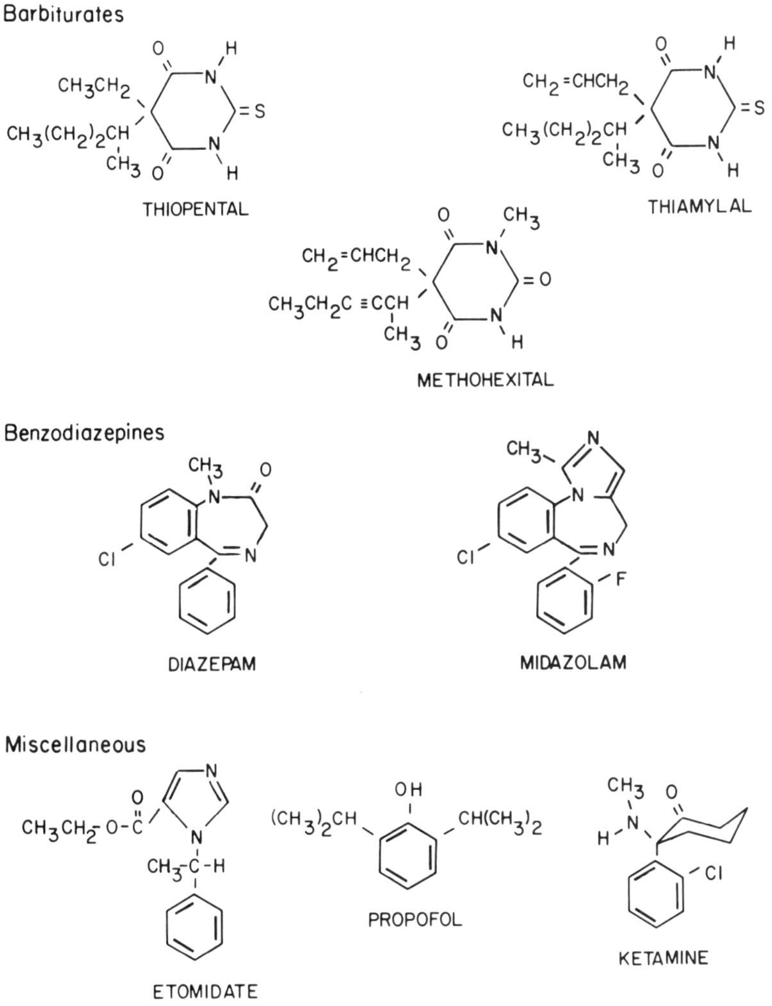

Barbiturates

THIOPENTAL

THIAMYLAL

METHOHEXITAL

Benzodiazepines

DIAZEPAM

MIDAZOLAM

Miscellaneous

ETOMIDATE

PROPOFOL

KETAMINE

Fig. 15-1. The structural formulae of the agents used for the induction of general anesthesia. (From Fragen and Avram,[2] with permission.)

15-1. Although any of these drugs can be given by continuous intravenous infusion to maintain unconsciousness, those most suitable for outpatient anesthesia are the highly cleared drugs (e.g., methohexital, etomidate, ketamine, and propofol).

Pharmacokinetics and pharmacodynamics can be influenced by a number of factors. Volatile anesthetic agents decrease hepatic blood flow and possibly hepatic metabolism; although they may decrease the elimination clearance of other drugs with high hepatic extraction ratios, they do not affect thiopental.[2] With increasing age, people have a larger total volume of distribution and slower elimination clearance[2]; consequently, a given drug dose can have a longer-lasting effect. Furthermore, the elderly are reported to be more sensitive to all intravenous anesthetic agents, making it necessary to reduce doses. To avoid overdosing the obese, it is best to administer doses initially on the basis of lean body mass and add more drug if necessary.

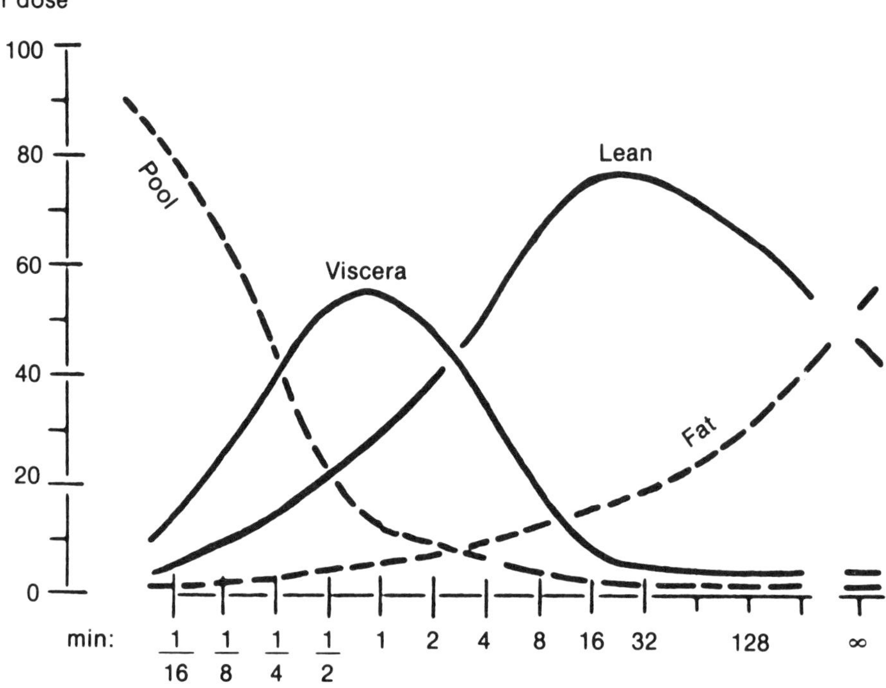

Fig. 15-2. The calculated distribution of drug in various tissues after a single injection of thiopental. (From Price et al.,[3] with permission.)

Thiopental

Thiopental, introduced for medical use in 1934 by Waters at the University of Wisconsin[4] and by Lundy at the Mayo Clinic,[5] has been the "gold standard" of intravenous induction agents for at least 50 years, despite its disadvantages and its misuse in World War II.[6] Investigators have attempted to find a substitute for thiopental, seeking an agent that would cause less local toxicity, less cardiovascular and respiratory depression, and more rapid recovery of mental function. Nevertheless, thiopental remains the most widely used drug in anesthesia.

Thiopental must be reconstituted for clinical use, using sterile water or 0.9 percent sodium chloride to provide a 2.5 percent solution; it contains 6 percent anhydrous sodium carbonate to buffer atmospheric CO_2. The alkaline pH (10 to 11) of this solution causes occasional pain when it is injected into small veins in the hand; tissue irritation and possible slough result if there is extravasation into tissue. Arterial spasm can occur with possible loss of blood supply to the hand following intra-arterial injection.[7] The alkaline pH also causes a precipitate to form when thiopental is mixed in the same syringe or in an intravenous administration set with almost any other drug used in anesthesia practice.

The usual adult induction dose of 3 to 5 mg/kg of thiopental injected intravenously acts rapidly within the CNS to produce unconsciousness. Although there are a number of theories regarding anesthetic action in the CNS,[8] the most widely accepted suggests that thiopental, the other barbiturates,[9,10] etomidate,[11] the benzodiazepines,[12] and probably propofol, act by enhancing γ-amino-butyric acid neurotransmission, thereby interfering with transmembrane electrical activity.

The side effects of thiopental during induction include a low incidence of fine muscle tremors, mild pain on injection into hand or wrist veins, and skin flush. There is also a low incidence of respiratory upset which may consist of cough, hiccough, laryngospasm, or bronchospasm, although the latter two are probably due to the insertion of an artificial airway or the effect of secretions in a lightly anesthetized patient.

Thiopental reduces intraocular pressure which may be important for certain ophthalmologic conditions. The degree of intraocular pressure reduction is similar for all the intravenous sedative-hypnotics with the exception of ketamine, for which pressure change is minimal[13–16] (Table 15-2).

Thiopental causes a dose-related decrease in the rate and depth of breathing and may cause a brief period of apnea when normal induction doses are administered.[17] Respiratory depression is usually greater when the drug is injected rapidly or when it is preceded by an opioid premedicant.[18]

Thiopental directly depresses the myocardium, reducing stroke volume and cardiac output.[19] It dilates capacitance vessels and, to a lesser extent, may decrease systemic vascular resistance (SVR). Sympathetic output from the CNS decreases, but reflex baroreceptor-mediated sympathetic stimulation of heart rate occurs.[20] Thus, hypotension and tachycardia may occur. Hypotension would be greater in the presence of hypovolemia, increased resting sympathetic tone as occurs in nervous, unpremedicated outpatients, β-adrenergic blockade, or a blunted baroreflex. After tracheal intubation or surgical stimulation, blood pressure returns toward (or even exceeds) pre-induction baseline values. Thiopental is not dysrhythmogenic.

Thiopental has no adverse clinical effects on any other organ system of the body. Initial recovery after induction doses of thiopental is fairly rapid, but patients experience a "hangover" for several hours, even after induction for short-lasting anesthetics. Recovery time from thiopental anesthesia depends on the induction dose, whether it is used during maintenance, what other anesthetic agents are given, and the duration of anesthesia. Recovery is usually described as "smooth" and is without excitement, bad dreams, prolonged amnesia, or venous sequelae such as thrombosis or phlebitis.

Table 15-2. Intraocular Pressure Changes With Intravenous Anesthetic Agents

Drug	Change from preoperative control values (%)
Thiopental	31
Etomidate	32
Propofol	30
Midazolam	41
Diazepam	34
Ketamine	8

(Data from Fragen and Hauch[13] and Mirakhur et al.[15])

Thiamylal

Thiamylal is usually constituted in a 2 percent solution. Respiratory depression appears slightly less intense after thiamylal than after thiopental; thiamylal affects tidal volume more than respiratory rate, and there is less tendency for airway complications.[21] Otherwise, the 3 to 5 mg/kg induction dose as well as the other points mentioned in the thiopental discussion are also applicable to thiamylal.

Methohexital

Methohexital, a methylated oxybarbiturate, is produced in a 1 percent solution. Because of its high clearance rate and shorter elimination halflife, methohexital is theoretically a "shorter-acting" drug than thiopental and thus more suitable for outpatient anesthesia. The recommended dose of 1.5 mg/kg lasts about the same time as 4 mg/kg of thiopental, but may have less "hangover" effect. Reports comparing patients' speed of recovery after receiving either methohexital or thiopental are equivocal. Studies generally show a more rapid initial recovery after methohexital[22–24]; however, fine motor skills may take as long to recover as after thiopental injection,[25] irrespective of whether these drugs are given by single injection or continuous infusion. Methohexital is less irritating than the other barbiturates if extravasated into tissues; however, methohexital induction has a higher incidence of pain on injection, excitement phenomena, and respiratory upset such as cough and hiccough than thiopental induction. These side effects can be minimized by using a slow injection time and by intravenous administration of an opioid[26] such as fentanyl, sufentanil, or alfentanil prior to administration of methohexital. Reflex tachycardia may also be greater after methohexital than after the other barbiturates.[26] Thus, for a slightly faster recovery time, the anesthesiologist must contend with a greater number of side effects.

Ketamine

Ketamine, formulated in a 1 to 10 percent solution which is moderately acidic, contains a preservative and is stable. A dose of 2 mg/kg given slowly over 1 minute produces unconsciousness which lasts approximately 10 to 15 minutes. Ketamine probably interacts with brain muscarinic acetylcholine and opiate receptors.[27] It is the only induction agent to have analgesic properties; for surgery that causes only somatic pain, it can be used without additional anesthetic agents. Ketamine infusions have been used in outpatients.[28,29] Its high clearance rate makes it a good infusion drug, and it has the beneficial properties of causing bronchodilation and respiratory stimulation, while producing no cardiovascular depression and virtually no induction side effects. Ketamine also can be antiarrhythmic against epinephrine and digitalis-induced dysrhythmias.[30] However, centrally mediated sympathetic nervous system stimulation caused by ketamine leads to increased heart rate, blood pressure, SVR, pulmonary artery pressure, and myocardial oxygen consumption. In addition, ketamine increases both intracranial and intraocular pressure. Although laryngeal reflexes remain intact after ketamine induction, protective reflexes are not necessarily intact as originally thought.[31] Ketamine also stimulates secretions, so an antisialagogue should be given before ketamine induction. Major disadvantages of ketamine in outpatients are prolonged drowsiness and psychotomimetic effects consisting of hallucinations and bad dreams, which may occur for up to 24 hours in the postoperative period. Barbiturates and benzodiazepines given with ketamine can blunt the cardiovascular stimulation and psychotomimetic effects, but they prolong sleep time. There is no particular advantage of ketamine in the adult outpatient.

Etomidate

Etomidate is dissolved in 35 percent propylene glycol at a concentration of 2 mg/ml in a 10 ml ampule. It remains stable in solution at room temperature for over 2 years. The recommended induction dose of 0.2 to 0.3 mg/kg should be injected slowly into a rapidly running intravenous infusion, preferably in a large vein; it should be preceded by a small intravenous dose of an opioid to minimize the prominent induction side effects of pain on injection and myoclonic movements.[32] Unconsciousness occurs rapidly and the duration of effect of an induction dose is about the same as that after the administration of barbiturate induction agents. When used for short surgical procedures, etomidate is associated with a higher incidence of nausea and vomiting than other induction agents.[33] After larger doses of etomidate, emergence excitement may occur from the time of initial arousal until complete awakening.[34]

Etomidate's advantages over thiopental are that it causes less respiratory depression and essentially no cardiovascular depression. Compared with other intravenous anesthetics, etomidate produces the best balance between myocardial oxygen demand and supply. It also has a mild nitroglycerin-like effect on the coronary circulation.[35]

An infusion scheme for etomidate can lead to recovery approximately 10 minutes after infusion stops.[34] A short-term infusion of etomidate used during outpatient anesthesia is safe, but long-term infusions may be dangerous because it can suppress the postoperative adrenocortical response to stress.[36,37]

Because outpatients are relatively healthy, etomidate seems to offer little or no advantage over thiopental, but it could be advantageous for outpatients with coronary artery disease (e.g., angina) or cerebrovascular insufficiency because of its ability to maintain hemodynamic stability during induction of anesthesia.

Benzodiazepines

Induction of general anesthesia can be accomplished with either diazepam or midazolam. Midazolam is water soluble in acidic solution as supplied by the manufacturer, while diazepam requires an organic solvent, propylene glycol. Midazolam is preferable to diazepam for induction because it causes less pain on injection and less postoperative thrombophlebitis, and in equipotent doses has a shorter duration of effect and a greater amnestic effect. The onset of effect after midazolam is quicker than that of diazepam because of its higher lipid solubility at physiologic pH. Likewise, midazolam's residual effects are of shorter duration than those of diazepam because midazolam has a shorter elimination halflife and less active metabolites. Compared with other induction agents, these benzodiazepines have a slower onset of effect and slower recovery after short surgical procedures.[38–40] Amnesia for 2 hours or longer after injection of midazolam can present a problem: patients may not remember instructions given them in the recovery area and the elderly may not remember any event that takes place on the day of surgery. These disadvantages outweigh the advantages of less respiratory depression and less cardiovascular depression than occur after thiopental.

A specific benzodiazepine antagonist, flumazenil (Fig. 15-3), can reverse almost all the CNS effects of the benzodiazepines, but may not completely reverse the depressed response to hypoxia or the depressed CO_2 response curve.[41] The duration of effect of flumazenil is limited. It has an elimination halflife of approximately 1 hour[42] compared with midazolam's elimination halflife of 2.5 to 4 hours. Therefore, the recommended method of titrating flumazenil by 0.1 to 0.2 mg increments until awakening occurs may allow the effect of the antagonist to wear off and the effect of the agonist, midazolam, to recur.[43] This resedation over time may be similar to the renarcosis that follows naloxone reversal of

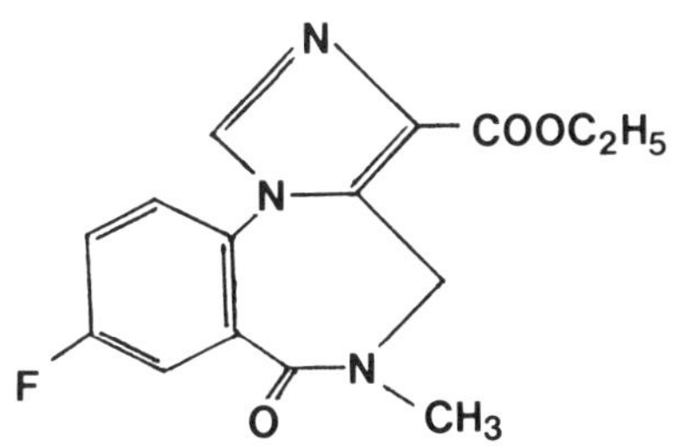

N
$COOC_2H_5$
N
F
N
O
CH_3

Fig. 15-3. The structural formula of flumazenil, a specific benzodiazepine antagonist.

opioids. Further doses of flumazenil by either intravenous, intramuscular, or oral routes can maintain the reversal. At this time, however, there is no evidence that this would safely reduce the postoperative patient observation time. Therefore, it could be hazardous to expand the use of midazolam for anesthetic induction in outpatient surgery when this benzodiazepine antagonist is approved for clinical use in the United States.

This discussion of the injectable benzodiazepines and their antagonist should not be misinterpreted. Midazolam is an excellent drug for sedation for outpatients undergoing diagnostic procedures or receiving local anesthesia or regional anesthesia (see Chs. 12 and 13); a lower dose is required for these indications than for anesthetic induction, and the effects are, therefore, of shorter duration. Midazolam should be titrated in 0.5 to 1.0 mg bolus doses until the patient is calm. This careful titration is especially important when opioids are given with midazolam, because marked respiratory depression can occur, especially in the elderly. Midazolam must be used cautiously by fully trained personnel in outpatient settings.

Propofol

Propofol is a hydrophobic liquid at room temperature and requires an organic solvent. Formulated as 1 percent egg lecithin emulsion, consisting of 10 percent soya bean oil, 2.2 percent glycerol, and 1.2 percent egg phosphatide,[44] it is stable at room temperature. Instructions on the propofol ampule say to store below 25°C, avoid freezing, and shake before use. Propofol has the highest clearance of any of the intravenous hypnotics (Table 15-1) and may be the best intravenous induction agent and maintenance hypnotic for outpatient anesthesia. However, only time can tell if it will ultimately replace thiopental as the most frequently used outpatient anesthetic induction agent.

The solvent is an intralipid-type substance that causes neither pulmonary diffusion problems nor allergic reactions, even in patients with allergy to egg albumin. It is a milky white substance, clearly different from other drugs used in the operating room. The usual induction dose of 1.5 to 2.5 mg/kg acts in one arm-brain circulation time and lasts 3 to 5 minutes.[45,46] The dose should be reduced for the elderly, from 2.25 mg/kg to 1.75 mg/kg according to one study (Table 15-3).[47] Propofol causes pain on injection, especially when injected into small hand or wrist veins,[48] and occasional erythema of the arm or trunk, but no thrombophlebitis or allergic reactions. It may cause fine muscle tremors similar to those occurring after thiopental.[49] Intraocular pressure is significantly decreased after propofol and vecuronium than after propofol and succinylcholine.[50] Respiratory depression is similar to that produced by thiopental.[51]

The main side effect of propofol is cardiovascular depression. It is a direct myocardial depressant,[52] a potent venodilator, and, in some studies, an arteriolar dilator.[53] Its effect on SVR may depend on the sympathetic tone while at rest; the greater the tone, the greater the decrease in both blood pressure and SVR. The baroreflex is reset so that there is a lower heart rate for a given blood pressure.[54] It also may have a central vagotonic effect. In various studies, heart rate decreased, increased slightly, or had no change.

Table 15-3. Frequency (%) of Adequate Induction of Anesthesia With Single Bolus Doses of Propofol in Two Age Groups

Dose (mg/kg)	Under age 60 (yr)	Over age 60 (yr)
1.25	—	[a]100 (30
1.50	53 (13)	97 (3)
1.75	83 (17)	100 (0)
2.00	87 (10)	97 (0)
2.25	97 (0)	[a]100 (0)
2.50	100 (0)	—

Figures in brackets indicate rapid lightening of anesthesia. (N = 30; [a] indicates N = 20.)

(Modified from Dundee et al.,[47] with permission.)

In healthy patients, blood pressure decreases 0 to 25 percent but returns toward control values with tracheal intubation or surgical incision.[55] However, in older patients or in those with poor ventricular function, blood pressure may decrease 40 percent or more; the same result may occur when propofol is combined with narcotic.[56,57] When an opioid such as fentanyl is given with propofol, cardiovascular depression is greater because of vasodilation, decreased stroke volume, and decreased heart rate.[55,58] The degree of depression will depend on the dose of each drug administered. If propofol induction is followed by succinylcholine, severe bradycardia can result unless patients are premedicated with atropine.[59] In healthy patients undergoing outpatient anesthesia, the short-term hypotensive effect is not a problem.

Propofol does not suppress the adrenocortical response to stress,[60] it is safe to use in porphyric patients,[61] and it has no adverse effects on other organ systems. Its effect in patients susceptible to malignant hypothermia is unknown.

The great advantage of propofol is the ease with which patients recover from its effects; patients recover faster from propofol than from other induction agents, regardless of whether the drugs are given by single injection,[62] intermittent injection,[63,64] or continuous infusion during anesthetic maintenance.[65,66] Patients reach a clearheaded state sooner and have a lower incidence of nausea and vomiting[67]; both factors contribute to an earlier discharge from the surgical facility. Some studies suggest that after a propofol-nitrous oxide anesthetic, patients may be eligible for discharge approximately one-half hour sooner than those receiving a thiopental-isoflurane-nitrous oxide anesthetic.[68] Propofol is superior to etomidate as an intravenous hypnotic for microlaryngeal surgery because it provides more stable anesthesia and a faster recovery.[69] Potentially, propofol is the induction and maintenance agent of choice for outpatient anesthesia because of its smooth induction and rapid, smooth recovery. If earlier discharge is possible, the cost savings could more than offset the higher price of propofol compared with thiopental.

Propofol may also be used for sedation during local or regional anesthesia.[70,71] After an initial dose of 1 to 2 mg/kg, a continuous infusion of 3 to 4 mg/kg/hr can keep patients lightly asleep but easy to arouse. If a surgical procedure happens to outlast the regional anesthetic, the infusion rate can be increased to 10 mg/kg/hr and nitrous oxide added to convert to a general anesthetic from which awakening will be rapid.[70] Propofol may be inappropriate for patients receiving outpatient electroconvulsive therapy because it decreases seizure duration.[72]

INHALED ANESTHETICS

An inhaled anesthetic should have the following properties: it should be stable in solution, nonflammable, resistant to biodegradation, rapid in action, nonarrhythmogenic, and, possibly, a good muscle relaxant. It should neither increase cerebral blood flow nor cause cardiovascular side effects. The approved volatile anesthetics, halothane, enflurane, and isoflurane, can be inhaled without the addition of intravenous agents or nitrous oxide, so that both anesthetic induction and maintenance can be provided with one agent. Abolishing the response to surgical stimulation usually requires 1.25 times the minimal alveolar concentration (MAC) value (Table 15-4);

Table 15-4. Comparative Potencies of Volatile Anesthetics

Agent	Minimal alveolar concentration[a]
Halothane	0.74
Isoflurane	1.15
Enflurane	1.68
Sevoflurane	1.70
Desflurane (I-653)	5.09[b]

[a] Thirty to 55 years old, 37°C, 760 mmHg.
[b] Estimated on the basis of animal data.[73]

however, MAC decreases as patients' ages increase. Using one anesthetic agent may sound advantageous, but when one component of anesthesia, usually analgesia, must be increased, all the effects of the single agent, including the side effects, are also increased. That is why most anesthesiologists today use nitrous oxide, hypnotics, analgesics, and muscle relaxants in addition to volatile anesthetics. Because of their low margin of safety, all volatile anesthetics require precision vaporizers that can control concentrations to a fraction of a percent. Mass spectrometry or infrared detectors can be used to identify a specific agent. Analyzing inspired and expired concentrations of these drugs provides for safer administration of volatile agents. Figure 15-4 shows the structural formulae of the available volatile agents. Following an intravenous induction, any of the three approved volatile agents (halothane, enflurane, and isoflurane) can provide outpatients a smooth anesthetic with fairly rapid recovery.

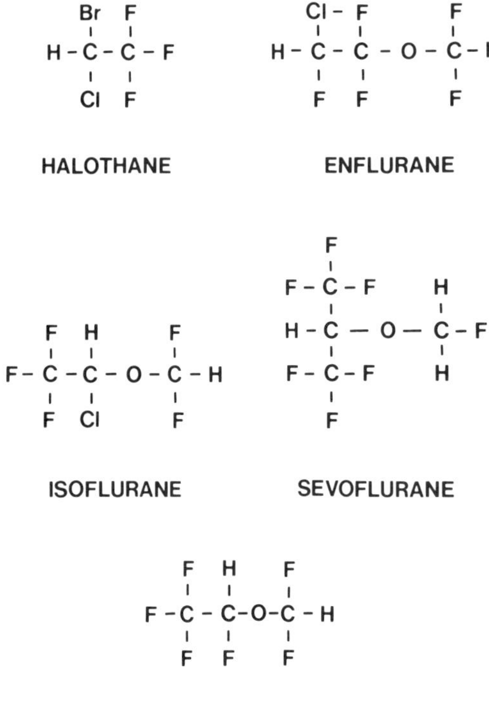

Fig. 15-4. The structural formulae of the volatile anesthetics.

Nitrous Oxide

Discovered by Sir Humphrey Davey in 1800,[74] nitrous oxide (N_2O) provides the basis for many anesthetic techniques. By itself, nitrous oxide cannot be used as an anesthetic because it has an MAC of over 100 percent; anesthesia machine safety devices require administration of at least 30 percent oxygen to prevent inhalation of hypoxic mixtures. However, N_2O reduces the MAC of the volatile anesthetics by 1 percent for each percent of nitrous oxide administered and adds to both the analgesic and hypnotic components of a "balanced" anesthetic technique. Thus, lower concentrations of volatile anesthetics are necessary.[75] Induction is accelerated because nitrous oxide can increase the uptake of volatile anesthetics by the "second gas effect" and "concentration effect."[76] Emergence is more rapid because nitrous oxide is the least soluble of all the inhaled anesthetics and is readily eliminated.

Nitrous oxide has a pleasant odor and is easy to inhale. It is not a respiratory depressant and, for the majority of outpatients, there are no important cardiovascular depressant effects.[77] Sympathetic stimulation offsets the mild cardiovascular depressant effect of nitrous oxide. When combined with volatile agents at a given total MAC, there is less cardiovascular depression than when the same MAC is achieved with halothane,[78] enflurane,[79] or isoflurane[80] alone. Nitrous oxide has some disadvantages. Because it is less soluble than nitrogen, it diffuses into air-containing spaces, increasing the pressure within these spaces; the pressure increase is time-related. The bowel dilates, air containing cysts dilate, and nitrous oxide in the middle ear makes tympanoplasty difficult. There is contradictory evidence about the tendency of N_2O to increase postoperative nausea and vomiting.[81–83] When the anesthetic is discontinued, movement of N_2O from the blood to the alveoli dilutes both alveolar oxygen and carbon dioxide leading to "diffusion hypoxemia" and reduced respiratory drive[84]; this can be avoided by administering oxygen-enriched air or 100 percent oxygen for the first 5 to 10 minutes after N_2O is discontinued. A few anesthesiologists advocate avoiding nitrous oxide because it interferes with vitamin B_{12} metabolism, methionine synthetase activity, and DNA formation.[85] Because there is no clinical evidence that this is detrimental in relatively healthy patients, N_2O continues to be used widely.

Halothane

In 1951, Suckling synthesized halothane, and Raventos and Johnston studied it prior to its approval in 1956.[74] Its introduction was monumental because halothane, when given in clinically useful concentrations, represented the first potent nonflammable, nonexplosive inhaled anesthetic.

Halothane is the easiest of the three currently approved volatile agents to inhale because it is the least irritating to the airways and has a fruity, nonirritating odor. It is a clear liquid with the preservative thymol added. Thymol remains in the vaporizer after the vaporization of halothane and can cause malfunction of vaporizers over time if they are not occasionally drained and cleaned.

Halothane, like the intravenous hypnotics, reduces intraocular pressure (IOP).[86] It causes an increased respiratory rate, a decreased tidal volume, and bronchodilation.

Halothane is a myocardial depressant, but has fewer peripheral vascular effects than enflurane or isoflurane. It may decrease heart rate.[87] Halothane sensitizes the heart to both exogenous and endogenous catecholamines,[88] which means tachyarrhythmias are more likely to occur with surgical stimulation under "light" anesthesia following atropine administration and with hypercarbia. Approximately 20 percent of inspired halothane undergoes metabolic degradation in the body. Oxidation, reduction, and dehalogenation of halothane may form metabolites; the reductive metabolites are implicated as the cause of potentially fatal massive hepatic necrosis in approximately 1 in 10,000 patients.[89,90] Although there is no proven cause and effect relationship, this potentially fatal complication has caused most anesthesiologists to abandon the use of halothane for adult outpatients.

Enflurane

Enflurane was synthesized by Ross Terrell in 1963 and approved for general use in 1972.[74] It is a clear liquid with a pungent, ethereal odor that can be tolerated by awake adults if the concentration is increased gradually. It has a moderately low blood-gas partition coefficient of 2.0 and, with its high potency, allows rapid induction. Of the three volatile agents, it has the lowest tissue-blood solubility, which leads to rapid recovery.[91] In comparative studies, recovery after enflurane is more rapid than after halothane[92,93] or isoflurane,[94] but the differences are not clinically important.[95]

Enflurane, in concentrations above 4 percent, can cause seizure-like activity both clinically and on the electroencephalogram, especially when $PaCO_2$ is less than 30 mmHg. It has intracranial and intraocular effects similar to those of halothane. Enflurane causes depression of both tidal volume and respiratory rate; it produces bronchodilation in a dose-related manner. It also causes a dose-related cardiovascular depression, depressing the myocardium directly and decreasing SVR. The peripheral effects predominate. It causes little or no change in heart rate, does not sensitize the heart to catecholamines, and does not cause dysrhythmias.[95] Organ toxicity is unlikely because only 3 to 5 percent of inhaled enflurane is metabolized, but a rare report suggests that enflurane might cause hepatic toxicity.[96]

Isoflurane

In 1965, Ross Terrell also synthesized isoflurane, an isomer of enflurane, but it was not released for general use until 1981.[74] It is the most biologically stable of the volatile anesthetics with biotransformation of <1 percent.[97] This clear liquid with a pungent, ethereal odor has the lowest blood:gas partition coefficient (1.4), making the onset of its effect rapid when it is used following an intravenous induction agent.[98] Its pungency, however, impedes its use as an inhalation induction agent.[99]

Isoflurane causes cerebral effects similar to those of the other volatile agents, but to a lesser degree,[100] and it also reduces IOP. A bronchodilator, it depresses both the rate and depth of breathing. When given too rapidly or to a patient who is too lightly anesthetized, it can provoke coughing and breathholding. Isoflurane causes less direct myocardial depressant effects than enflurane, but both agents reduce systemic vascular tone. Isoflurane does not sensitize the heart to catecholamines, but it causes tachycardia in some patients.[98] In patients with coronary artery disease, it has the ability to cause maldistribution of coronary blood flow and myocardial ischemia,[101] an unlikely effect of halothane.

Isoflurane has no adverse effects on other organ systems. It is currently the most widely used volatile anesthetic agent because of its low potential for toxicity. An inhalation anesthetic that might improve on isoflurane for outpatient anesthesia would have the same low toxicity but be less soluble, which would allow faster induction and recovery. Two such agents are under investigation, seroflurane and I-653.

Sevoflurane

Sevoflurane (Fig. 15-3) is a potent volatile anesthetic with a low blood:gas partition coefficient of 0.686.[102] The low solubility of sevoflurane should lead to rapid induction and emergence, making it a potentially good outpatient induction and maintenance agent. The MAC of this nonpungent drug is 1.7 percent.[103] In anesthetic concentrations, sevoflurane, like enflurane and isoflurane, causes both dose-dependent cardiovascular and respiratory depression,[104] and it fails to sensitize the myocardium to catecholamines.[105]

Despite these beneficial properties for outpatient anesthesia, sevoflurane is unlikely to be approved for anesthetic use in the United States because it undergoes degradation to formaldehyde, hydrofluoric acid, methanol, and olefin at elevated temperature in the presence of soda lime.[105–107] It is not clear whether these potentially toxic products would be retained in soda lime, inhaled by patients, or metabolized to nontoxic products. Also, serum inorganic fluoride concentration increases with 1.2 to 1.8 MAC hours of sevoflurane use, although this concentration is not near that necessary to cause renal toxicity.[107]

Desflurane

Desflurane (I-653) should be an improvement over today's most popular inhaled agent, isoflurane, having both less pungency and lower solubility (Fig. 15-4). Chemically, I-653 differs from isoflurane by the substitution of fluorine for the chlorine atom. Its blood:gas partition coefficient is 0.42 and its oil:gas partition coefficient is 18.7 at 37°C; both coefficients are lower than those of isoflurane.[108] It also has lower tissue:gas and tissue:blood partition coefficients in human tissue.[109] Clinical investigation of I-653 in humans is just starting at the time of this writing, and tests in rats and pigs make investigators optimistic about its usefulness for humans; it undergoes minimal biodegradation,[110] is nontoxic,[111,112] and is very stable in soda lime.[113] Minimal alveolar concentration is 5.7 percent inspired in rats,[114] which awaken five times faster from I-653 than from isoflurane at equivalent MAC concentrations.[115] The projected MAC in humans is 5.09.[73] Dose-related cardiovascular effects of equal MAC concentrations of I-653 or isoflurane were similar in swine.[116] Because I-653 has the same cardiovascular profile as isoflurane, it might possibly cause coronary artery vasoconstriction, coronary artery steal, and regional myocardial dysfunction.

Available data from animal studies imply that I-653 is a potentially desirable volatile anesthetic agent for use in outpatient anesthesia, mainly because its lower blood:gas and tissue solubilities are likely to lead to faster patient recovery.

ANALGESICS

Of all the drug effects mentioned in this chapter, only analgesia should persist in the postoperative period. It would be a significant breakthrough if analgesia could be provided without drowsiness, dizziness, nausea, vomiting, and, most importantly, respiratory depression; the analgesics used intraoperatively are opioids that have these negative side effects. Before the mid1960s, only long-acting analgesics were available for intraoperative use. Now, shorter-acting, more potent drugs are available. The intensity and duration of their effects are dose-related. For outpatient anesthesia, opioids are used in doses recommended as adjuncts, not in the high doses recommended for cardiac surgery or neurosurgery. Opioids are not recommended for use as anesthetic induction agents nor as sole anesthetic agents for outpatients, because the doses necessary would last too long, have too many side effects, and would not guarantee unconsciousness or amnesia for the surgical procedure. Because both "traditional opioids," morphine and meperidine, have a relatively long duration of action, fentanyl, sufentanil, and alfentanil are more appropriate for outpatient use (Fig. 15-5); these are μ agonists that produce dependence, euphoria, miosis, nausea and vomiting, respiratory depression, and supraspinal analgesia. They are included in balanced anesthetic techniques because they minimize fluctuation in cardiovascular hemodynamics, reduce the volatile agent requirement, and provide greater postoperative analgesia.

If there is an inadvertent opioid overdose, titrated 0.1 mg doses of naloxone can be administered to reverse CNS and respiratory depression. Occasionally, excitement and hypertension occur after naloxone administration. Depending on the opioid and its dose, renarcotization can occur when naloxone's duration of action and elimination halflife are shorter than those of the opioid. When the anesthesiologist allows spontaneous recovery from large doses of fentanyl or its derivatives, renarcotization can occur within the first hour postoperatively.[117]

Fentanyl

Fentanyl, a synthetic opioid related to the phenylperidines, has been the anesthesiologist's intraoperative analgesic of choice for many years. It is 75 to 125 times more potent than morphine. It has a rapid onset of action and a shorter duration of effect than morphine due to its high lipid solubility. For outpatient anesthesia, doses of 2 to 10 μg/kg are often satisfactory as part of a balanced anesthetic technique with nitrous oxide and a hypnotic drug. These doses rarely cause changes in blood pressure, even in patients with decreased ventricular function, because plasma histamine levels remain normal.[118] Bradycardia may occur from central vagal stimulation and can be treated with a belladonna alkaloid, such as

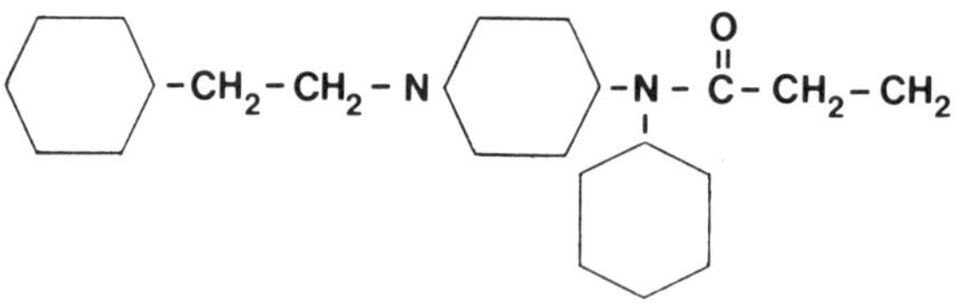

FENTANYL

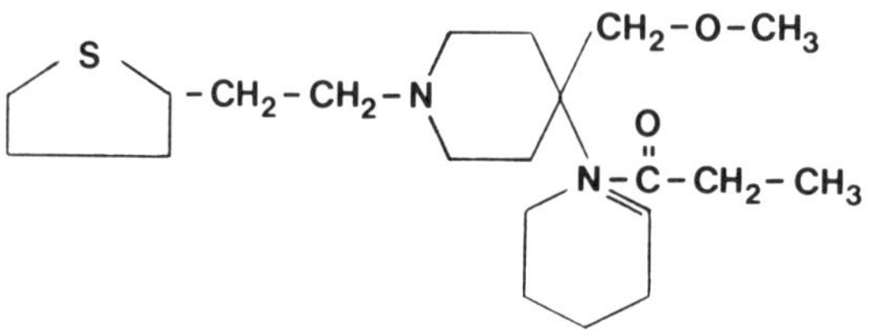

SUFENTANIL

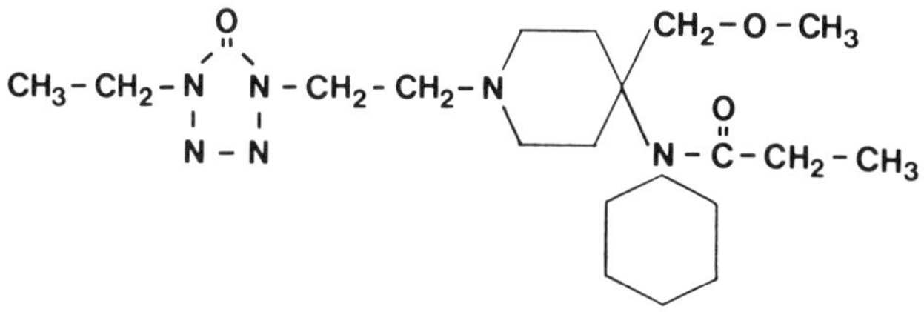

ALFENTANIL

Fig. 15-5. The structural formulae of the opioids appropriate for outpatient anesthesia.

atropine, if necessary. Peak dose-related respiratory depression occurs 5 to 10 minutes after injection and some respiratory depression, including a depressed slope of the CO_2 response curve[119] and a depressed hypoxic ventilatory curve, may persist for hours, even after small doses,[120] especially in the elderly.

Sufentanil

Sufentanil and fentanyl used in small, equivalent doses are comparable in their onset of action, duration of effect, and side effect profile. Although sufentanil is approximately ten times more potent than fentanyl, each is commerically available as a citrate salt in the same concentration, 50 μg/ml. For safety reasons, each ml of sufentanil should be diluted with saline to 10 ml (0.5 μg/ml). In rats, the therapeutic index of sufentanil is approximately 100 times that of fentanyl. The differences between sufentanil and fentanyl are mainly pharmacodynamic. Sufentanil binds to the μ receptor with ten times the affinity of fentanyl, and it is twice as soluble in fat.[121] The volume of distribution is between that of alfentanil and fentanyl, and it has a very high hepatic extraction ratio.[122] In doses likely to be the upper limit for "balanced" anesthesia in outpatients, both sufentanil, 0.7 μg/kg, and fentanyl, 7 μg/kg, cause minimal cardiovascular effects—a slight decrease in heart rate, mean arterial pressure, and cardiac index—and no change in SVR.[123]

Alfentanil

Alfentanil, produced in an aqueous solution of 0.5 mg/ml in 5-, 10-, or 20-ml ampules, is the opioid most suited pharmacologically to outpatient anesthesia. Compared with other opioids, it is distributed less extensively and has a slower clearance rate and a shorter elimination halflife. It is highly protein-bound, but much less ionized at physiologic pH.[124] Alfentanil can readily cross biologic membranes including the blood-brain barrier to act rapidly on the CNS, where its peak effect occurs only 1 to 2 minutes after intravenous injection compared with 3 to 5 minutes for fentanyl.[124] It has a brief duration of action because it redistributes rapidly to other tissues.[125] Doses of 0.5 to 1 mg IV will act for only a few minutes. The pharmacokinetics of alfentanil are compared with other opioids in Table 15-5.

When used as a component of balanced anesthesia on a double-blind basis for gynecologic laparoscopy, a total mean dose of 2.06 mg of alfentanil or 0.21 mg of fentanyl given by intermittent injection produced similar times to extubation, response to verbal command, and orientation to time and place. Normal respiration resumed after reversal of muscle relaxation, but the incidence of nausea was high after both drugs.[126] Intravenous infusion can be used as an alternative to frequent intermittent injections of alfentanil.[127] A convenient infusion pump is commercially available for administration of either bolus doses or continuous infusion of alfentanil based on body weight.[128] A dose of 15 μg/kg will usually depress respiration for less than 20 minutes.[129] For clinical use, approximately 6.5 μg of alfentanil can provide equivalent analgesia to 1 μg of fentanyl with a faster return to normal ventilation.

Alfentanil is supposedly one-third as potent as fentanyl and has one-third the duration of action. To suppress the hemodynamic response to laryngoscopy and tracheal intubation at the time of barbiturate induction, 10 μg/kg of alfentanil is sufficient in the elderly,[130] but younger patients require up to 30 μg/kg.[131] The recovery period is not greatly prolonged by supplemental doses of alfentanil given to control sympathetic responses during anesthetic maintenance. Age has little effect on the plasma concentration-effect relationship,[132] but dose requirements are lower in older patients than in younger patients.[133] Also, muscle rigidity occurs more often in the older patients.

Alfentanil produces the typical opioid effects of respiratory depression, chest wall rigidity, bradycardia, hypotension, and nausea and vomiting. Although the incidence and severity of these symptoms are

Table 15-5. Pharmacokinetics of the Opioids Fentanyl, Sufentanil, and Alfentanil Compared With Morphine

	Morphine	Fentanyl	Sufentanil	Alfentanil
pKa	7.9	8.4	8.0	6.5
% Unionized at pH 7.4	23.0	8.5	19.7	89.0
Lipid solubility (octonal-water partition coefficient)	6.0	826.0	1757.0	129.0
Protein binding (%)	63	84	93	92
Vd_{ss} (L/kg)	3.4	4.0	1.7	0.7
Cl (ml/kg/min)	2.3	12.6	12.7	5.1
t½ β (hr)	1.7	3.6	2.7	1.6

(Data from Dundee and Wyant.[26])

dose-related, they can occur even with low doses. Rigidity can be accompanied by hypertonus of pharyngeal or laryngeal muscles and can lead to partial airway obstruction.[134] This can be prevented with a small dose of a muscle relaxant. Although highly controversial, there is some evidence that the incidence of nausea is higher after alfentanil than after fentanyl.

Less alfentanil is required for a continuous infusion than for an intermittent bolus technique.[127] When alfentanil is administered with a computer-assisted infusion, anesthesia is smoother and there is less postoperative respiratory depression.[135] Each anesthesiologist must determine the dose that will obliterate the response to surgery for an individual patient by varying the infusion rate, much as one varies the concentration of a volatile anesthetic. The interindividual dose requirement or blood level required to obliterate responses to surgery varies widely when alfentanil is administered with nitrous oxide.[136]

Alfentanil can have a prolonged effect if given to patients taking erythromycin,[137] because erythromycin apparently interferes with the metabolism of alfentanil. No other important drug interactions have been reported.

MUSCLE RELAXANTS

The goals for muscle relaxants in outpatient anesthesia are rapid onset of action, short duration of action matching the need for muscle relaxation during surgery, a rapid recovery index, no interaction with other anesthetic drugs, no side effects, and easy pharmacologic reversal. Because medical conditions such as hypokalemia or undiagnosed myasthenia gravis can occur in outpatients, a careful history is required to avoid administering muscle relaxants to patients with diseases or conditions that make them more sensitive to these drugs. Muscle relaxants may be needed only to facilitate tracheal intubation, or they may be necessary for surgical procedures including bronchoscopy, esophagoscopy, laryngoscopy, gynecologic laparoscopy, or lithotripsy. Electively, they may be used as part of a balanced anesthetic technique.

Investigators are still trying to develop more appropriate drugs for short surgical procedures. A new classification of muscle relaxants based on their time course is illustrated in Fig. 15-6.[138] Currently, the only ultrashort-acting muscle relaxant available is succinylcholine, a depolarizing muscle relaxant. Clinical trials will begin soon with nondepolarizing relaxants in this category, but it is unknown when they or others will be approved for clinical use. When approved, they could become the muscle relaxants of choice for outpatient anesthesia. The short-acting class now includes only mivacurium, a drug currently undergoing extensive clinical trials in the United States.

Until more rapid and shorter-acting drugs become available for clinical use, the most appropriate muscle relaxants for outpatient anesthesia will remain the intermediate-acting relaxants, atracurium and vecuronium. Following an ED_{95} dose of atracurium or vecuronium, maximum block occurs in 5 minutes; following twice the ED_{95} dose, 2.5 to 3 min are required to achieve maximal blockade. To hasten the onset of block for earlier tracheal intubation, either the priming principle[139] or higher initial doses[140] of these two muscle relaxants must be used. However, these dose manipulations seem unnecessary for elective outpatient anesthesia. For patients having a greater risk of aspiration, such as those who are obese or who have a hiatal hernia or other condition that delays gastric emptying, succinylcholine remains the choice to facilitate tracheal intubation. Older patients usually require the same initial dose of the nondepolarizing muscle relaxants as younger patients, but a given dose will last longer.[141]

The long-acting relaxants currently available are gallamine, metocurine, d-tubocurarine, and pancuronium, all of which are excessively long-acting for the needs of most outpatient procedures. Two new drugs in this long-acting category, doxacurium and pipecuronium, are under clinical investigation. Unlike the currently available long-acting relaxants, they have no cardiovascular effects. Instead of a long-acting muscle relaxant, atracurium, vecuronium, mivacurium, or succinylcholine can be given by repeated injections of half the ED_{95} for each, or by continuous infusion when it is necessary to prolong their effects. Cumulation is not a clinical issue when these relaxants are given in this way. Spontaneous recovery is faster, and their effects are easier to reverse pharmacologically than those of the longer-acting relaxants.

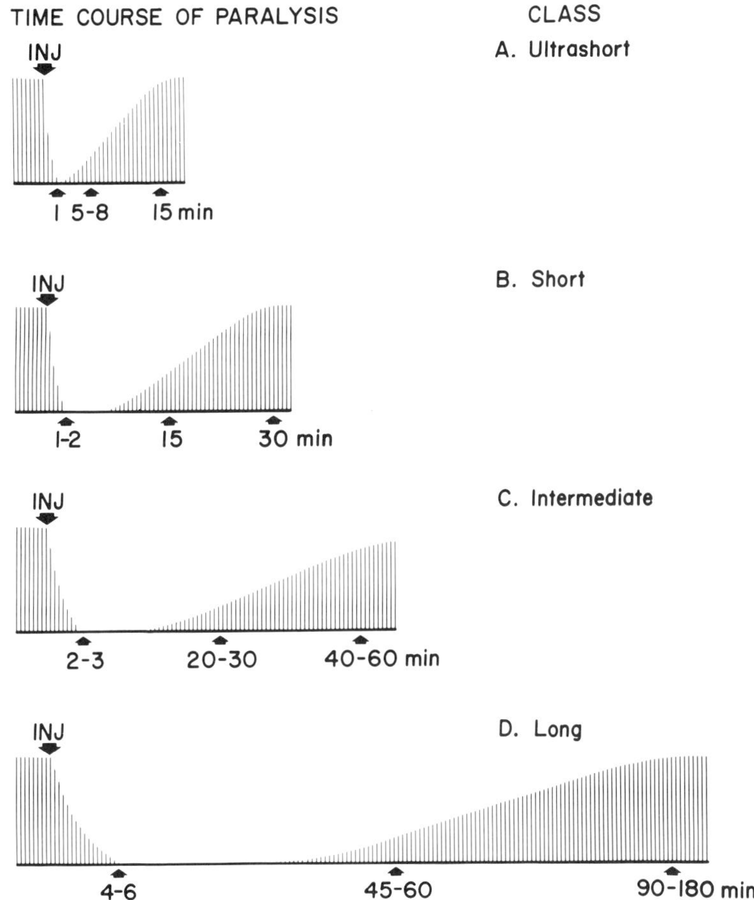

Fig. 15-6. A classification of muscle relaxants based on the time course of paralysis. Three measurements of this time course differentiate each class of relaxant: ultrashort, short, intermediate, and long. The first measurement is the onset of effect, the time from injection to maximum blockade, represented by the arrow on the left of each time line. The second measurement is the duration of surgical relaxation or the time from injection to 25 percent recovery of twitch height, represented by the middle arrow on each time line. The third measurement is the time from injection to clinical recovery or 95 percent of twitch height and is represented by the arrow on the right of each time line. (From Fragen and Shanks,[138] with permission.)

Succinylcholine

Succinylcholine is widely used to facilitate tracheal intubation and to provide profound relaxation for up to 10 minutes. After injection, it is rapidly hydrolyzed to succinylmonocholine and, subsequently, to the inactive succinic acid and choline. The depolarizing action at the myoneural junction and other nicotinic receptors results in a long list of potential side effects. It is likely to cause a higher incidence of myalgia in outpatients who ambulate soon after surgery,[142] as well as muscular patients[143] or females.[144] Fasciculations after succinylcholine are unnecessary for the occurrence of myalgia.[145] A nondepolarizing muscle relaxant with significant prejunctional effects, such as 0.05 mg/kg of d-tubocurarine given approximately 3 to 5 minutes before succinylcholine, can reduce the incidence and severity of postsuccinylcholine myalgia,[146] but pretreatment may result in signs of muscle weakness,[147] such as diplopia, difficulty in swallowing, or dyspnea. After pretreatment with a nondepolarizing relaxant, the dose of succinylcholine should be increased to 1.5 to 2 mg/kg. Aspirin, 600 mg PO, given 1 hour before anesthesia, is as effective as d-tubocurarine in reducing the incidence of myalgia, and the normal 1 mg/kg dose of succinylcholine could be used.[148]

Prolonged apnea occurs if succinylcholine is given to patients who have abnormal or low levels of pseudocholinesterase, the enzyme responsible for the breakdown of succinylcholine. The enzyme can be congenitally low or reduced by drugs patients are taking, such as lithium or magnesium, echothiophate iodide eye drops, monoamine oxidase inhibitors, or cyclophosphamide. A careful history should be taken to elicit these possibilities. Succinylcholine given by continuous infusion can cause tachyphylaxis and a phase II block which is not reversible with an anticholinesterase drug.

Potential Side Effects of Succinylcholine

- Cardiac dysrhythmias
- Hyperkalemia
- Increased intracranial pressure
- Increased intragastric pressure
- Increased intraocular pressure
- Phase II block
- Postanesthesia myalgias
- Prolonged apnea with abnormal pseudocholinesterase
- Tachyphylaxis with continuous infusion
- Triggering agent for malignant hyperpyrexia

Atracurium

Atracurium, a benzylisoquiniline (Fig. 15-7), was deliberately developed to break down spontaneously in the body.[149] The acidified solution of 1 mg/ml can be left at room temperature for up to 2 weeks, but generally should be refrigerated to prevent loss of potency. Atracurium is inactivated by Hofmann elimination, nonspecific ester hydrolysis, and organ elimination.[150] The metabolites have no clinical neuromuscular activity, and the metabolite laudanosine does not reach a concentration high enough to cause CNS excitation. The pharmacokinetics of atracurium, vecuronium, and mivacurium in normal patients are compared in Table 15-6.[151,152] The clinical effects of atracurium are similar over a wide age range.

In normal or lower induction doses, the clinical duration of atracurium and vecuronium are similar, but the elimination half-life of atracurium is shorter. Intubation may be easily accomplished 2 to 3 minutes

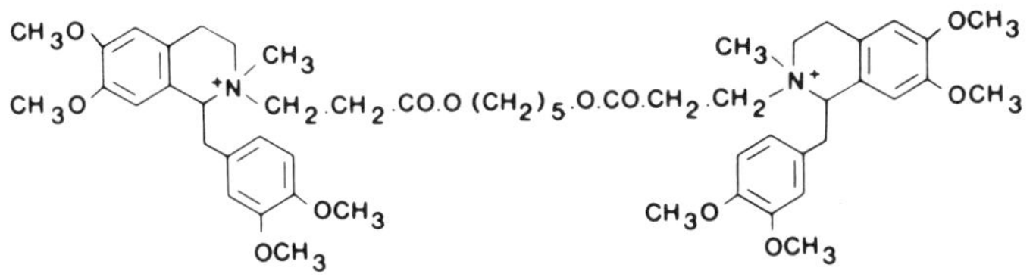

Atracurium

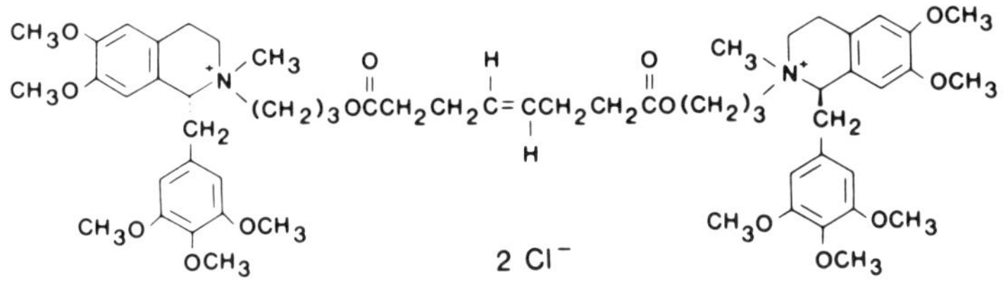

Mivacurium

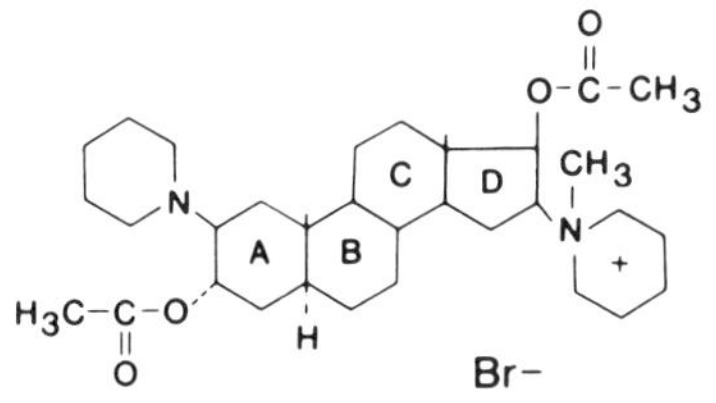

Vecuronium Bromide

Fig. 15-7. The structural formulae of the nondepolarizing muscle relaxants appropriate for outpatient anesthesia. Mivacurium and atracurium, two benzylisoquinolines, differ from each other by the number of methoxy groups, the interonium distance, and the structural configuration between the two nitrogen atoms. Vecuronium is a steroid structure that differs from the longer-acting pancuronium only by the absence of a methyl group on the A-ring.

after the normal intubating dose of 0.5 mg/kg. The time from the onset of effect of this dose to 95 percent recovery is 1 hour. An ED_{95} of 0.2 mg/kg requires 5 minutes before intubation, but has a duration of effect of 20 to 25 minutes. The ED_{95} causes essentially no cardiovascular effects, but the normal intubating dose should be injected slowly over 1 minute to prevent hypotension and skin flush of brief duration. Cutaneous reactions occur after approximately 12.5 percent of atracurium injections without serious accompanying reactions, even in asthmatics or in those with an allergic history.[153] For a longer duration of neuromuscular blockade, a continuous infusion of atracurium 6 μg/kg/min[154] may be used after an initial ED_{95} dose; thereafter, the dose can be adjusted to maintain the response level at either one twitch of the train-of-four stimulation pattern or at 90 percent neuromuscular blockade if a more precise monitor is used. Recovery after infusion or bolus dosing is similar.

Table 15-6. Pharmacokinetics of Atracurium, Vecuronium and Mivacurium in Normal Patients (± SD)

Drug	t½ β (min)	Clearance (ml/kg/min)	V_D (L/kg)
Atracurium	17 ± 2	5.8 ± 2	0.14 ± 0.04
Vecuronium	80 ± 14	3.0 ± 0.3	0.19 ± 0.4
Mivacurium[a]	35 ± 28	18.7 ± 8	0.30 ± 0.2

[a] Basta SJ, personal communication, Boston, MA.
(Data from de Bros et al.[151] and Fahey et al.[152])

Vecuronium

Both vecuronium and pancuronium have a steroid nucleus, but vecuronium has a tertiary nitrogen in the A-ring rather than a quaternary nitrogen (Fig. 15-7). A quaternary nitrogen confers neuromuscular blocking properties and antinicotinic effects in the D-ring, causing atropine-like symptoms or antimuscarinic effects in the A-ring. Vecuronium, therefore, has no side effects in doses up to six times the ED_{95}.[155] It metabolizes to weakly active metabolites that are excreted mainly in the bile and to a lesser degree (about 15 percent) in the urine.

Because vecuronium is unstable in solution, it comes as a freeze-dried powder that must be dissolved in water. Its pharmacokinetics are different from atracurium (Table 15-6), although clinically useful doses have similar durations of effect. When the ED_{95} dose of 0.05 mg/kg of vecuronium is given to outpatients, it has a slightly shorter onset time, duration of effect, and recovery index than an ED_{95} of atracurium. When two to three times the ED_{95} is given, both drugs have similar effects.[156] Thus, vecuronium may be preferable to atracurium in ED_{95} doses for short outpatient procedures.

Unlike a nitrous oxide-narcotic anesthetic, isoflurane and enflurane prolong the action of vecuronium, even when small doses are used for gynecologic laparoscopy.[157] The normal intubating dose of 0.1 mg/kg requires 2 to 3 minutes for maximum neuromuscular block, provides 20 to 40 minutes of surgical relaxation, and allows for recovery of 95 percent control in about 1 hour. The recovery index of this dose, the time from 25 to 75 percent recovery of neuromuscular block, is 11 to 12 minutes.[158] The ED_{95} of 0.05 mg/kg requires 5 minutes for maximum block, and surgical relaxation lasts 10 to 15 minutes.[157]

Vecuronium can also be administered by continuous infusion in a way similar to that described for atracurium. After an ED_{95} dose, the vecuronium infusion should be started at a rate of 1 μg/kg/min.

Mivacurium

Mivacurium (Fig. 15-7), a benzylisoquinoline, differs from atracurium in that it is hydrolyzed by plasma cholinesterase at approximately 88 percent of the rate of succinylcholine; in addition, there may be some hepatorenal elimination.[159] The metabolites of mivacurium are probably inactive at the neuromuscular junction.

When the 2 mg/ml aqueous solution of mivacurium is given in increasing doses, it produces dose-related pharmacologic effects (Table 15-7)[159] and cardiovascular depression.[159] When the recommended intubating dose of 0.2 to 0.25 mg/kg is given (instead of the ED_{95} of 0.1 mg/kg), the time required to reach maximum blockade is shortened from 4 to 2.5 minutes and recovery to 95 percent is lengthened by 5 minutes, namely, 30 minutes instead of 25 minutes. The recovery index over this dose

Table 15-7. Neuromuscular Blocking Properties of Mivacurium Chloride in Humans Receiving "Balanced" Anesthesia (Mean ± SEM)

Dose	Blockade (%)	Onset[a] (min)	25% Recovery (min)	95% Recovery (min)	Recovery Index (min)
0.05	43.7 ± 2.1	5.3 ± 0.8	—	14.4 ± 2	—
0.10	95.7 ± 2.8	3.8 ± 0.5	14.2 ± 1.5	24.5 ± 1.6	7.0 ± 0.5
0.15	100	3.3 ± 0.2	16.8 ± 1.1	26.9 ± 1.6	6.6 ± 0.6
0.20	100	2.5 ± 0.3	19.7 ± 1.8	30.6 ± 2.4	6.9 ± 0.4
0.25	100	2.3 ± 0.3	20.3 ± 1.5	30.4 ± 2.2	6.6 ± 0.5

[a] Measured from end of injection.
(Data from Savarese et al.[159])

range is remarkably stable at 6.6 to 7 minutes. The dose-response curve of mivacurium is shifted to the left and the recovery index is slightly prolonged by isoflurane compared with a nitrous oxide-opioid anesthesia.[160] Thus, intubating doses of mivacurium last half as long as atracurium and twice as long as succinylcholine. When mivacurium is given by the priming principle, the intubating time may be even shorter, approaching 1 minute.[161] In 1- to 2-hour infusions, mivacurium provides at least as fast a recovery time as succinylcholine,[162] making it a good alternative to longer-acting drugs or succinylcholine infusion for maintaining neuromuscular blockade. It can produce the same degree of neuromuscular blockade as a vecuronium infusion, but the time to 25 and 90 percent recovery of twitch height and the recovery index are about half that of vecuronium.[163] The recovery index after single doses of mivacurium is similar to that produced by infusions lasting 30 to 180 minutes.[164] Until a nondepolarizing muscle relaxant in the ultrashort-acting category is available, mivacurium will likely be the best drug to use for intubation and for intermittent injection or continuous infusion during outpatient anesthesia.

A weak histamine-releasing action can cause a temporary decrease in blood pressure and cutaneous flush. The incidence and severity of these side effects can be reduced by slowing the injection time to 1 minute, keeping the dose below 0.2 mg/kg, or using continuous infusion.[165] Hypotension may be more severe in β-blocked patients or those on diuretic therapy. Mivacurium is pharmacologically reversible with an anticholinesterase drug.

Neuromuscular Monitoring

It is important to monitor neuromuscular blockade using either train-of-four[166] or double-burst stimulation.[167] Along with clinical signs, these can indicate the need for further muscle relaxation during surgery or can help determine the adequacy of recovery from neuromuscular blockade at the end of the operation. By itself, visual or tactile assessment of train-of-four is very inaccurate,[168] and little experience has yet been gained with double-burst stimulation, although it is potentially more accurate.[167] Therefore, instead of relying solely on the neuromuscular monitor, the clinical signs of good grip strength, sustained head lift for at least 5 seconds, negative inspiratory force of at least 20 cm H_2O, and the ability to cough provide indications of adequate recovery from neuromuscular blockade.

Pharmacologic Antagonism of Neuromuscular Block

If there is residual neuromuscular block, the block should be antagonized with an anticholinesterase. Antagonism of neuromuscular block depends on the degree of paralysis at the time of antagonism, the pharmacokinetics and pharmacodynamics of the muscle relaxant, the specific antagonist, and the dose of the antagonist. If the second twitch of the train-of-four is visible, edrophonium 0.5 mg/kg with atropine 10 μg/kg, or neostigmine 0.05 mg/kg with glycopyrolate 0.10 μg/kg are equally effective for reversing the block.[169,170] To reverse a deeper block, either the same dose of neostigmine or edrophonium 1 mg/kg can be given.[170] Although both atropine and glycopyrolate can block the muscarinic effects of neostigmine, the time course of glycopyrolate is a better match with neostigmine. There is a lower incidence of nausea and vomiting associated with spontaneous recovery than is present when neostigmine and atropine are used to antagonize neuromuscular block.[171] Therefore, shorter-acting relaxants producing faster spontaneous recovery are preferable for outpatients.

If there is doubt about the recovery of neuromuscular function after the administration of neuromuscular blocking drugs, they should be antagonized pharmacologically. Muscle weakness is not only dangerous in itself, but the ensuing inadequate ventilation can lead to nausea and vomiting; all of these conditions can prolong the recovery period.

SUMMARY

All the general anesthetic agents and adjuncts that are described in this chapter are suitable for use in outpatient surgery. Each has specific advantages and drawbacks that the anesthesiologist must consider when choosing the specific agent or agents most appropriate for a particular patient and surgical procedure. There are no great differences between equivalent doses of the several approved volatile agents, nor between the three opioids. Improvements in the volatile agents, intravenous hypnotics, and muscle relaxants may come in the form of drugs recently under investigation (I-653, propofol, and mivacurium, respectively) or those still being tested.

ACKNOWLEDGMENT

I deeply appreciate the efforts of Michael J. Avram, Ph.D., and Joan A. Fragen for their help in editing this chapter, and to Connie A. Mora for typing it.

REFERENCES

1. Reves JG, Fragen RJ, Vinik HR, Greenblatt DJ: Midazolam—pharmacology and uses. Anesthesiology 62:310, 1985
2. Fragen RJ, Avram MJ: Comparative pharmacology of drugs used for the induction of anesthesia. p. 103. In Stoelting RK, Barash PG, Gallagher TJ (eds): Advances in Anesthesia. Year Book Medical Publishers, Chicago, 1986
3. Price HL, Kovnat PJ, Safer JN, et al: The uptake of thiopental by body tissues and its relation to the duration of narcosis. Clin Pharmacol Ther 1:16, 1960
4. Pratt TW, Tatum AL, Hathaway HR, Waters RM: Sodium ethyl (1-methylbutyl) thiobarbiturate: preliminary experimental and clinical study. Am J Surg 31:464, 1936
5. Lundy JS: Intravenous anesthesia: preliminary report of the use of two new thiobarbiturates. Proc Staff Meetings Mayo Clinic 10:534, 1935
6. Halford FJ: A critique of intravenous anesthesia in war surgery. Anesthesiology 4:67, 1943
7. Davies DD: Local complications of thiopentone. A further report. Br J Anaesth 51:1147, 1979
8. Ueda I, Kamaya H: Molecular mechanisms of anesthesia. Anesth Analg 63:929, 1984
9. Johnston GAR, Willow M: GABA and barbiturate receptors. Trends Pharmacol Sci 3:328, 1982
10. Ho IK, Harris RA: Mechanism of action of barbiturates. Ann Rev Pharmacol Toxicol 21:83, 1981

11. Willow M: A comparison of the actions of pentobarbitone and etomidate on [^{3}H]GABA binding to crude synaptosomal rat brain membranes. Brain Res 220:427, 1981
12. Martin IL: The benzodiazepine receptor: functional complexity. Trends Pharmacol Sci 5:343, 1984
13. Fragen RJ, Hauch T: The effect of midazolam maleate and diazepam on intraocular pressure in adults. p. 245. In Aldrete JA, Stanley TH (eds): Trends in Intravenous Anesthesia. Year Book Medical Publishers, Chicago, 1980
14. Calla S, Gupta A, Sen N, Garg IP: Comparison of the effects of etomidate and thiopentone on intraocular pressure. Br J Anaesth 59:437, 1987
15. Mirakhur RK, Sheppard WFI, Darrah WC: Propofol or thiopentone: effects on intraocular pressure associated with induction of anaesthesia and tracheal intubation (facilitated with suxamethonium). Br J Anaesth 59:431, 1987
16. Corssen G, Hoy JW: A new parenteral anesthetic CI-581: its effect on intraocular pressure. Pediatr Ophthalmol 4:20, 1967
17. Patrick RT, Faulconer AJ: Respiratory studies during anesthesia with ether and with pentothal sodium. Anesthesiology 13:252, 1952
18. Eckenhoff JE, Helrich M: Study of narcotics and sedatives for use in preanesthetic medication. JAMA 167:415, 1958
19. Dwyer EM, Weiner L: Left ventricular function in man following thiopental. Anesth Analg 48:499, 1969
20. Priano LL: Pharmacology of anesthetic drugs and adjuncts. p. 125. In Thomas SJ (ed): Manual of Cardiac Anesthesia. Churchill Livingstone, New York, 1984
21. Helrich M, Papper EM, Rovenstine EA: Surital sodium: a new anesthetic for intravenous use: preliminary clinical evaluation. Anesthesiology 11:33, 1950
22. Carson IW, Graham I, Dundee JW: Clinical studies of induction agents XLII: Recovery from althesin—a comparative study with thiopentone and methohexitone. Br J Anaesth 47:358, 1975
23. Bahar M, Dundee JW, O'Neill MP, et al: Recovery from intravenous anaesthesia: a comparison of disopropofol with thiopentone and methohexitone. Anaesthesia 37:1171, 1982
24. Thornton JA: Methohexitone and its application in dental anaesthesia. Br J Anaesth 42:255, 1970
25. Korttila K, Linnoila M, Ertama P, Hakkinen S: Recovery and simulated driving after intravenous anesthesia with thiopental, methohexital, propanidid or alphadione. Anesthesiology 43:291, 1975
26. Dundee JW, Wyant GM: Intravenous Anaesthesia. 2nd Ed. Churchill Livingstone, Edinburgh, 1988
27. Vincent JP, Corey D, Kameka JM, et al: Interaction of phencylidine with the muscarinic and opiate receptors in the central nervous system. Brain Res 152:176, 1978
28. White PF, Dworsky WA, Horal Y, Trevor AV: Comparison of continuous infusions of fentanyl or ketamine versus thiopental—determining the mean effective serum concentrations for outpatient surgery. Anesthesiology 59:564, 1983
29. White PF: Use of continuous infusion versus intermittent bolus administration of fentanyl or ketamine during outpatient anesthesia. Anesthesiology 59:294, 1983
30. White PF, Way WL, Trevor AJ: Ketamine—its pharmacology and therapeutic use. Anesthesiology 56:119, 1982
31. Taylor PA, Towey RM: Depression of laryngeal reflexes during ketamine anaesthesia. Br Med J 2:688, 1971
32. Korttila K, Tammisto T, Aromaa U: Comparison of etomidate in combination with fentanyl or diazepam with thiopentone as an induction agent for general anaesthesia. Br J Anaesth 51:115, 1981
33. Fragen RJ, Caldwell NJ: Comparison of a new formulation of etomidate with thiopental—side effects and awakening times. Anesthesiology 50:242, 1979
34. Fragen RJ, Avram MJ, Henthorn TK, Caldwell NJ: A pharmacokinetically designed etomidate infusion regimen for hypnosis. Anesth Analg 62:654, 1983
35. Kettler C, Sonntag H, Wolfram-Donath W, et al: Haemodynamics, myocardial function, oxygen requirements and oxygen supply of the human heart after administration of etomidate. p. 81. In Doenicke EA (ed):

Etomidate—An Intravenous Hypnotic Agent. Springer-Verlag, New York, 1977
36. Fragen RJ, Shanks CA, Molteni A, Avram MJ: Effects of etomidate on hormonal response to surgical stress. Anesthesiology 61:652, 1984
37. Wagner RL, White PF: Etomidate inhibits adrenocortical function in surgical patients. Anesthesiology 61:647, 1984
38. Berggren L, Eriksson I: Midazolam for induction of anaesthesia in outpatients. A comparison with thiopentone. Acta Anaesthesiol Scand 25:492, 1981
39. Fragen RJ, Caldwell NJ: Recovery from midazolam used for short operations. Drug Res 31:2261, 1981
40. Verma R, Ramasubramanian R, Sacher RM: Anesthesia for termination of pregnancy: midazolam compared with methohexital. Anesth Analg 64:792, 1985
41. Barakat T, Lechat JP, Laurent P, et al: Ventilatory effects of flumazenil on midazolam-induced sedation. Anesthesiology 69:A817, 1988
42. Klotz U, Ziegler G, Reimann IW: Pharmacokinetics of the selective benzodiazepine antagonist RO 15-1788 in man. Eur J Clin Pharmacol 271:151, 1984
43. Raeder JC, Hole A, Arnulf V, Grynne BH: Total intravenous anaesthesia with midazolam and flumazenil in outpatient clinics. A comparison with isoflurane or thiopentone. Acta Anaesthesiol Scand 31:634, 1987
44. Glen JB, Hunter SC: Pharmacology of an emulsion formulation of ICI 35,868. Br J Anaesth 56:617, 1984
45. Cummings GC, Dixon J, Kay NH, et al: Dose requirements of ICI 35 868 (propofol, Diprivan) in a new formulation for induction of anaesthesia. Anaesthesia 39:1168, 1984
46. Rolly G, Versichelen L: Comparison of propofol and thiopentone for induction of anaesthesia in premedicated patients. Anaesthesia 40:945, 1985
47. Dundee JW, Robinson FP, McCollum JSC, Patterson CC: Sensitivity to propofol in the elderly. Anaesthesia 41:482, 1986
48. Hynynen M, Korttila K, Tammisto T: Pain on I.V. injection of propofol (ICI 35,868) in emulsion formulation: short communication. Acta Anaesthesiol Scand 29:651, 1985
49. Edelist G: A comparison of propofol and thiopentone as induction agents in outpatient surgery. Can J Anaesth 34:110, 1987
50. Mirakhur RK, Shepherd WRI, Elliott P: Intraocular pressure changes during rapid sequence induction of anaesthesia: comparison of propofol and thiopentone in combination with vecuronium. Br J Anaesth 60:379, 1988
51. Grounds RM, Maxwell DL, Taylor MD, et al: Acute ventilatory changes during IV induction of anaesthesia with thiopentone or propofol in man. Br J Anaesth 59:1098, 1987
52. Martin C, Saux P, Albanese J, et al: Right ventricular end-systolic pressure-volume relation during propofol infusion. Anesthesiology 69:A141, 1988
53. Andrew A, Rouby JJ, Leger P, et al: Peripheral vascular effects of propofol. Anesthesiology 69:A567, 1988
54. Cullen PM, Turtle M, Prys-Roberts C, et al: Effect of propofol anesthesia on baroreflex activity in humans. Anesth Analg 66:1115, 1987
55. Van Aken H, Meinshausen E, Prien T, et al: The influence of fentanyl and tracheal intubation on the hemodynamic effects of anesthesia induction with propofol/N_2O in humans. Anesthesiology 68:157, 1988
56. Coates DP, Monk CR, Prys-Roberts C, Turtle MJ: Hemodynamic effects of infusions of the emulsion formulation of propofol during nitrous oxide anesthesia in humans. Anesth Analg 66:64, 1987
57. Monk CR, Coates DP, Prys-Roberts C, et al: Haemodynamic effects of a prolonged infusion of propofol as a supplement to nitrous oxide anaesthesia—studies in association with peripheral vascular surgery. Br J Anaesth 59:954, 1987
58. Lepage JM, Pinaud ML, Helias JH, et al: Left ventricular function during propofol and fentanyl anesthesia in patients with coronary artery disease: assessment with a radionuclide approach. Anesth Analg 67: 949, 1988
59. Baraka A: Severe bradycardia following propofol-suxamethonium sequence. Br J Anaesth 61:482, 1988

60. Fragen RJ, Weiss HW, Molteni A: The effect of propofol on adrenocortical steroidogenesis: a comparative study with etomidate and thiopental. Anesthesiology 66:839, 1987
61. Mitterschiffthaler G, Theiner A, Hetzel H, Fuith LC: Safe use of propofol in a patient with acute intermittent porphyria. Br J Anaesth 60:109, 1988
62. Heath PJ, Kennedy DJ, Ogg TW, et al: Which intravenous induction agent for day surgery? A comparison of propofol, thiopentone, methohexitone and etomidate. Anaesthesia 43:365, 1988
63. Sung Y-F, Freniere S, Tillette T, Powell RW: Comparison of propofol and thiopental anesthesia in outpatient surgery: speed of recovery. Anesthesiology 69: A562, 1988
64. Milligan KR, O'Toole DP, Howe JP, et al: Recovery from outpatient anaesthesia: a comparison of incremental propofol and propofol-isoflurane. Br J Anaesth 59:1111, 1987
65. Doze VA, Wesphal LM, White PF: Comparison of propofol with methohexital for outpatient anesthesia. Anesth Analg 65: 1189, 1986
66. Doze VA, Schafer A, White PF: Propofol-nitrous oxide versus thiopental-isoflurane-nitrous oxide for general anesthesia. Anesthesiology 69:63, 1988
67. McCollum JSC, Milligan KR, Dundee JW: The antiemetic action of propofol. Anaesthesia 43:239, 1988
68. Korttila K, Faure E, Apfelbaum J, et al: Less nausea and vomiting after propofol than after enflurane or isoflurane anesthesia. Anesthesiology 69:A564, 1988
69. DeGrood PMRM, Mitsukuri S, Van Egmond J, et al: Comparison of etomidate and propofol for anaesthesia in microlaryngeal surgery. Anaesthesia 42:366, 1987
70. Mackenzie N, Grant IS: Propofol for intravenous sedation. Anaesthesia 42:3, 1987
71. Jessop E, Grands RM, Morgan M, Lumley J: Comparison of infusions of propofol and methohexitone to provide light general anesthesia during surgery with regional blockade. Br J Anaesth 57:1173, 1985
72. Simpson KH, Halsall PJ, Carr CME, Stewart KG: Propofol reduces seizure duration in patients having anaesthesia for electroconvulsive therapy. Br J Anaesth 61:343, 1988
73. Doorley BM, Waters SJ, Terrell RC, Robinson JL: MAC of I-653 in beagle dogs and New Zealand white rabbits. Anesthesiology 69:89, 1988
74. Fragen RJ: History of inhalation anesthesia. p. 1. In Booij LHDJ (ed): Current Status of Inhalation Anesthetics. Binge Scientific Publishers, Utrecht, 1982
75. Saidman LJ, Eger EI II: Effect of nitrous oxide and of narcotic premedication on the alveolar concentration of halothane required for anesthesia. Anesthesiology 25:302, 1964
76. Epstein RM, Rackow H, Salnitre E, et al: Influence of the concentration effect on the uptake of anesthetic mixtures: the second gas effect. Anesthesiology 25:364, 1964
77. Eger EI II, Gaskey NJ: A review of the present status of nitrous oxide. AANA 54:1, 1986
78. Bahlman SH, Eger EI II, Smith NT, et al: The cardiovascular effects of nitrous oxide-halothane anesthesia in man. Anesthesiology 35:274, 1971
79. Smith NT, Calverley RK, Prys-Roberts C, et al: Impact of nitrous oxide on the circulation during enflurane anesthesia in man. Anesthesiology 48:345, 1978
80. Dolan WM, Stevens WC, Eger EI II, et al: The cardiovascular and respiratory effects of isoflurane-nitrous oxide anesthesia. Can Anaesth Soc J 21:557, 1974
81. Melnick BM, Johnson LS: Effects of eliminating nitrous oxide in outpatient anesthesia. Anesthesiology 67:982, 1987
82. Alexander GD, Skupski JN, Brown EM: The role of nitrous oxide in postoperative nausea and vomiting. Anesth Analg 63:175, 1984
83. Korttila K, Hovorka J, Erkola O: Omission of nitrous oxide does not decrease the incidence or severity of emetic symptoms after isoflurane anesthesia. Anesth Analg 66:S98, 1987
84. Sheffer L, Steffenson JL, Birch AA: Nitrous oxide-induced diffusion hypoxia in patients breathing spontaneously. Anesthesiology 37:436, 1972
85. Eger EI II: Should we not use nitrous

oxide? In Eger EI II (ed): Nitrous Oxide. Elsevier Publishing, New York, 1985
86. Merkel G, Eger EI II: A comparative study of halothane and halopropane anesthesia. Anesthesiology 24:346, 1963
87. Hickey RF, Eger EI II: Circulatory pharmacology of inhaled anesthetics. p. 649. In Miller RD (ed): Anesthesia. 2nd Ed. Churchill Livingstone, New York, 1986
88. Johnston RR, Eger EI II, Wilson C: A comparative interaction of epinephrine with enflurane, isoflurane and halothane in man. Anesth Analg 55:709, 1976
89. Rehder KI, Forbes J, Alter H, et al: Biotransformation in man: a quantitative study. Anesthesiology 31:560, 1967
90. Lindenbaum J, Leifer E: Hepatic necrosis associated with halothane anesthesia. N Engl J Med 268:525, 1963
91. Eger EI II: Anesthetic Uptake and Action. Williams & Wilkins, Baltimore, 1974
92. Stanford BJ, Plantevin OM, Gilbert JR: Morbidity after day care gynaecological surgery. Comparison of enflurane with halothane. Br J Anaesth 51:1143, 1979
93. Padfield A, Mullins SRC: Recovery comparison between enflurane and halothane techniques: a study of outpatients undergoing cystoscopy. Anaesthesia 35:508, 1980
94. Korttila K, Valanne J: Recovery after outpatient isoflurane and enflurane anesthesia. Anesth Analg 64:239, 1985
95. Eger EI II: Enflurane (Ethrane). Anaquest, Madison, 1985
96. Lewis JH, Zimmerman HJ, Ishak KIG, et al: Enflurane hepatoxicity. Ann Intern Med 98:984, 1983
97. Davidkova T, Kikuchi H, Fujii K, et al: Biotransformation of isoflurane: urinary and serum fluoride ion and organic fluorine. Anesthesiology 69:218, 1988
98. Eger EI II: Isoflurane (Forane). Anaquest, Madison, 1985
99. Buffington CW: Clinical evaluation of isoflurane. Reflex actions during isoflurane anesthesia. Can Anaesth Soc J 29:S35, 1982, (suppl)
100. Todd MM, Drummond JC: A comparison of the cerebrovascular and metabolic effect of halothane and isoflurane in the cat. Anesthesiology 60:276, 1984
101. Khambatta HJ, Sonntag H, Larsen R, et al: Global and regional myocardial blood flow and metabolism during equipotent halothane and isoflurane anesthesia in patients with coronary artery disease. Anesth Analg 67:936, 1988
102. Strum DP, Eger EI II: Partition coefficients for sevoflurane in human blood, saline and olive oil. Anesth Analg 66:654, 1987
103. Katoh T, Ikeda K: The MAC of sevoflurane in humans. Anesthesiology 66:301, 1987
104. Doi M, Kazuyuki I: Respiratory effects of sevoflurane. Anesth Analg 66:241, 1987
105. Wallin RF, Regan BM, Napoli MD: Sevoflurane: a new inhalation anesthetic agent. Anesth Analg 64:758, 1975
106. Strum DP, Johnson BH, Eger EI II: Stability of sevoflurane in soda lime. Anesthesiology 67:779, 1987
107. Holaday DA, Smith FR: Clinical characteristics and biotransformation of sevoflurane in health human volunteers. Anesthesiology 54:100, 1981
108. Eger EI II: Partition coefficients of I-653 in human blood, saline, and olive oil. Anesth Analg 66:971, 1987
109. Yasuda N, Targ AG, Eger EI II: Solubility of I-653, sevoflurane, isoflurane and halothane in human tissues. Anesthesiology 69:A615, 1988
110. Koblin DD, Eger EI II, Johnson BH, et al: I-653 resists degradation in rats. Anesth Analg 67:534, 1988
111. Eger EI II, Johnson BH, Ferrell LD: Comparison of the toxicity of I-653 and isoflurane in rats: a test of the effect of repeated anesthesia and use of drug soda lime. Anesth Analg 66:1230, 1987
112. Eger EI II, Johnson BH, Strum DP, Ferrell LD: Studies of the toxicity of I-653, halothane and isoflurane in enzyme-induced hypoxic rats. Anesth Analg 66:1227, 1987
113. Eger EI II: Stability of I-653 in soda lime. Anesth Analg 66:983, 1987
114. Eger EI II, Johnson BM: MAC of I-653 in rats, including a test of the effect of body temperature and anesthetic duration. Anesth Analg 66:974, 1987
115. Eger EI II, Johnson BH: Rates of awakening from anesthesia with I653, halothane,

isoflurane, and sevoflurane: a test of the effect of anesthetic concentration and duration in rats. Anesth Analg 66:977, 1987
116. Weiskopf RB, Holmes MA, Eger EI II, et al: Cardiovascular effects of I-653 in swine. Anesthesiology 69:303, 1988
117. Mahla ME, White SE, Moneta MD: Delayed respiratory depression after alfentanil. Anesthesiology 69:593, 1988
118. Moss J, Rosow CE: Histamine release by narcotics and muscle relaxants in humans. Anesthesiology 59:330, 1983
119. McClain DA, Hug CC: Intravenous fentanyl kinetics. Clin Pharmacol Ther 28:106, 1986
120. Becker LD, Paulson BA, Miller RD, et al: Biphasic respiratory depression after fentanyl-droperidol or fentanyl alone used to supplement nitrous oxide anesthesia. Anesthesiology 44:291, 1976
121. Stahl KD, van Bever W, Janssen P, Simon EJ: Drugs for affinity and pharmacological potency of a series of narcotic analgesics, anti-diarrheal and neuroleptic drugs. Eur J Pharmacol 46:199, 1977
122. Bovill JH, Sebel PS, Blackburn CL, et al: The pharmacokinetics of sufentanil in surgical patients. Anesthesiology 61:502, 1984
123. Borel JD: New narcotics in anesthesia. p. 1. In Brown BR Jr (ed): New Pharmacologic Vistas in Anesthesia. Contemporary Anesthesia Practice. FA Davis, Philadelphia, 1983
124. Scott JC, Poganis KV, Stanski DR: EEG quantitation of narcotic effect: the comparative pharmacodynamics of fentanyl and alfentanil. Anesthesiology 62:234, 1985
125. Hug CC Jr: Lipid solubility, pharmacokinetics and the EEG: are you better off today than you were four years ago? Anesthesiology 62:221, 1985
126. Brown EM: Comparison of alfentanil versus fentanyl for outpatient surgery. p. 98. In Estafanous FG (ed): Opioids in Anesthesia. Butterworth Publishers, Boston, 1985
127. White PF, Coe V, Shafer A, et al: Comparison of alfentanil with fentanyl for outpatient anesthesia. Anesthesiology 64:100, 1986
128. Avram MJ, Henthorn TK: What's new in pharmacokinetics and pharmacodynamics? p. 251. In Fragen RJ (ed): New Anesthetic Drugs, Anesthesiology Clinics of North America. WB Saunders, Philadelphia, 1988
129. Scamman FL, Ghoneim MM, Korttila K: Ventilatory and mental effects of alfentanil and fentanyl. Acta Anaesth Scand 28:63, 1984
130. Kirby IJ, Northwood D, Dodson ME: Modification by alfentanil of the haemodynamic response to tracheal intubation in elderly patients. A dose-response study. Br J Anaesth 60:384, 1988
131. Black TE, Kay B, Healy TEJ: Reducing the haemodynamic response to laryngoscopy and intubation. Anaesthesia 39:883, 1984
132. Lemmens HJM, Bovill JG, Hennis PJ, Burm AGL: Age has no effect on the pharmacodynamics of alfentanil. Anesth Analg 67:956, 1988
133. Scott JC, Stanski DR: Decreased fentanyl and alfentanil dose requirements with increasing age. A simultaneous pharmacokinetic and pharmacodynamic evaluation. J Pharmacol Exp Ther 240:159, 1987
134. Benthuysen JL, Smith NT, Sanford TJ, et al: Physiology of alfentanil-induced rigidity. Anesthesiology 64:440, 1986
135. Ausems ME, Vuyk J, Hug CC Jr, Stanski DR: Comparison of a computer-assisted infusion versus intermittent bolus administration of alfentanil as a supplement to nitrous oxide for lower abdominal surgery. Anesthesiology 68:851, 1988
136. Ausems ME, Hug CC Jr, Stanski DR, et al: Plasma concentrations of alfentanil required to supplement nitrous oxide anesthesia for general surgery. Anesthesiology 65:362, 1986
137. Bartkowski RR, Larijani GE, Goldberg ME, Boerner TF: Erythromycin treatment inhibits alfentanil metabolism. Anesthesiology 69:A590, 1988
138. Fragen RJ, Shanks CA: Is there an ideal outpatient muscle relaxant? p. 69. In Wetchler BV (ed): Problems in Anesthesia, Outpatient Anesthesia. JB Lippincott, Philadelphia, 1988
139. Schwarz S, Illas W, Lackner F, et al: Rapid

tracheal intubation with vecuronium. The priming principle. Anesthesiology 62:388, 1985
140. Cossen WR, Jones RM: Vecuronium-induced muscular blockade: the effect of increasing dose in the speed of onset. Anaesthesia 41:354, 1986
141. O'Hara DA, Fragen RJ, Shanks CA: The effect of age on the dose-response curves for vecuronium in adults. Anesthesiology 63:542, 1986
142. Churchill-Davidson HC: Suxamethonium (succinylcholine) chloride and muscle pains. Br Med J 1:174, 1954
143. Newman PTF, Lauden IM: Muscle pain following administration of suxamethonium: the aetiological role of muscular fitness. Br J Anaesth 38:533, 1966
144. Burtles R, Tunstall ME: Suxamethonium chloride and muscle pains. Br J Anaesth 33:24, 1961
145. Brodsky JB, Ehrenwerth J: Postoperative muscle pain, suxamethonium. Br J Anaesth 52:215, 1980
146. Lichtiger M, Wetchler BV, Philip BK: The adult and geriatric patient. p. 175. In Wetchler BV (ed): Anesthesia for Ambulatory Surgery. JB Lippincott, Philadelphia, 1985
147. Engbaek J, Viby-Mogenson J: Precurarization—a hazard to the patient? Acta Anaesthesiol Scand 28:61, 1984
148. McLaughlin C, Nesbitt GA, Howe JP: Suxamethonium-induced myalgia and the effect of pre-operative administration of oral aspirin. Anaesthesia 43:565, 1988
149. Stenlake JB, Waigh RD, Urwin J, et al: Atracurium: conception and inception. Br J Anaesth 55:3S, 1983
150. Fisher DM, Canfell PC, Fahey MR, et al: Elimination of atracurium in humans: contribution of Hofmann elimination and ester hydrolysis versus organ elimination. Anesthesiology 65:6, 1986
151. de Bros FM, Lai A, Scott R, et al: Pharmacokinetics and pharmacodynamics of atracurium under isoflurane anesthesia in normal and anephric patients. Anesth Analg 64:207, 1985
152. Fahey MR, Morris RB, Miller RD, et al: Pharmacokinetics of ORG NC 45 (Norcuron) in patients with and without renal failure. Br J Anaesth 53:1049, 1981
153. Rowlands DE: Harmless cutaneous reactions associated with the use of atracurium. Br J Anaesth 59:693, 1987
154. Shanks CA: Pharmacokinetics of the nondepolarizing neuromuscular relaxants applied to calculation of bolus and infusion dosage regimens. Anesthesiology 64:72, 1986
155. Morris RD, Cahalan MK, Miller RD, et al: The cardiovascular effects of vecuronium (ORG NC 45) and pancuronium in patients undergoing coronary artery bypass grafting. Anesthesiology 58:438, 1983
156. Robertson FN, Booij LHDJ, Fragen RJ, Crul JF: A comparison of atracurium and vecuronium (ORG-NC-45) in anaesthetized man. Br J Anaesth 55:125, 1983
157. Fragen RJ, Shanks CA: Neuromuscular recovery after laparoscopy. Anesth Analg 63:51, 1984
158. Baird WLM, Savage DS: Vecuronium—the first years. p. 347. In Norman J (ed): Neuromuscular Blockade. Clinics in Anaesthesiology. WB Saunders, London, 1985
159. Savarese JJ, Ali HH, Basta SJ, et al: The clinical neuromuscular pharmacology of mivacurium chloride (BW B1090U). Anesthesiology 68:723, 1988
160. Weber S, Brandom BW, Powers DM, et al: Mivacurium chloride (BW B1090U)-induced neuromuscular blockade during nitrous oxide-isoflurane and nitrous oxide-narcotic anesthesia in adult surgical patients. Anesth Analg 67:495, 1988
161. Savarese JJ, Ali HH, Basta SJ, et al: Sixty-second tracheal intubation with BW B1090U after fentanyl-thiopental induction. Anesthesiology 67:A351, 1987
162. Savarese JJ: The newer muscle relaxants. 1986 ASA Annual Refresher Course Lectures #142
163. Basta SJ, Ali HH, Savarese JJ, et al: Comparative infusions of vecuronium and the new relaxant BW B1090U. Anesth Analg 66:S4, 1987
164. Ali HH, Savarese JJ, Embree PB, et al:

Clinical pharmacology of BW 1090U continous infusion. Anesthesiology 65:A282, 1986
165. Savarese JJ, Basta SJ, Ali HH, et al: Cardiovascular effects of BW B1090U in patients under nitrous oxide-oxygen-thiopental-fentanyl anesthesia. Anesthesiology 63:A319, 1985
166. Lee C: Train-of-four quantitation of competitive neuromuscular block. Anesth Analg 54:649, 1975
167. Ueda N, Viby-Mogensen J, Engbaek J, et al: New stimulation pattern for manual evaluation of neuromuscular transmission "Double" burst stimulation. Jpn J Anesthesiol 37:716, 1988
168. Viby-Mogensen J, Jensen NH, Engbaek J, et al: Tactile and visual evaluation of the response to train-of-four nerve stimulation. Anesthesiology 63:440, 1985
169. Rupp SM, McChristian JW, Miller RD, et al: Neostigmine and edrophonium antagonism of varying intensity neuromuscular blockade induced by atracurium, pancuronium or vecuronium. Anesthesiology 64:711, 1986
170. Yang E, Lee C, Tran B: Optimum dose of edrophonium for reversal of atracurium neuromuscular block. Anesth Analg 63:283, 1984
171. King MJ, Milazkiewicz R, Carli F, Deacock AR: Influence of neostigmine on postoperative vomiting. Br J Anaesth 61:403, 1988

16

Anesthesia for the Geriatric Outpatient

Charles H. McLeskey
David M. Nibel

An absolute definition of a geriatric patient based on age is not possible because arbitrary limits are constantly changing. For example, many studies of surgery in the elderly have been published since the early 1900s, but the definition of "elderly" varies widely throughout. An early report in 1907 described 167 operations performed on patients more than 50 years of age and described this advanced age as a contraindication to surgery.[1] Twenty years later, Ochsner suggested that "an elective operation for inguinal hernia in a patient older than 50 years was not justified."[2] In 1937, Brooks reported a series of 293 operations in patients more than 70 years of age; subsequently, most investigators have considered patients older than the ages of 65 to 70 years as being elderly.[3] For convenience in this chapter, geriatric patients will be considered those 65 years of age or older. However, with the not infrequent recent reports of anesthesia and surgery performed on patients older than the age of 80 years, there is no consensus today as to the definition of "geriatric" in medical practice, and the arbitrary age defining a geriatric patient very likely will be increasing in the near future. For example, Djokovic and Hedley-Whyte have reported the prediction for outcome after surgery in 500 patients older than age 80.[4] Miller et al. have described anesthesia and surgery in 147 patients ranging in age from 90 to 102 years.[5] In 1985, Catlic reported six patients older than the age of 100 who had anesthesia and surgery.[6] Hosking et al. recently reported 795 patients who were over age 90 and who underwent operative procedures at the Mayo Clinic. Of these, 13 patients were over the age of 100.[7] Catlic has perhaps best reflected on today's changed mood of medicine when he stated that "elective surgery should not be deferred nor emergency surgery denied (even for) centenarians on the basis of chronologic age."[6]

Older patients are undergoing surgical procedures more frequently, in part due to medical advances, but also in part due to the aging of the American society. The 1980 census indicated that 11.3 percent of the American population was more than 65 years of age. By the early 21st century, it is predicted that the elderly will comprise 16 percent of the U.S. population (approximately 52 million). Inpatient operations performed on patients older than 65 increased by 43 percent from 1975 to 1980, while the overall increase for all age groups was only 11.5 percent. Patients in this age group accounted for 21 percent of all inpatient operative procedures and 38.4 percent of total hospital days. Surgical rates on patients 90 years of age or older have increased nearly fivefold over the past 10 years.[8] A specific example of the increasing age of the surgical population may be found in a series from the Cleveland Clinic in which, over a 15-year period, more than 5,000 patients over age 65 underwent coronary artery bypass surgery (Fig. 16-1).[9] Thus, the trend is obvious; surgery performed on older patients is becoming more and more widespread. It is estimated that 50 percent of Americans who are presently older than age 65 will have at least one operative procedure before death.

Older patients are also more frequently undergoing surgery in an outpatient setting. In a 1983 Federated Ambulatory Surgery Association survey from 40 ambulatory care centers, 10.4 percent of patients undergoing surgery in the outpatient setting were over age 60. It appears that in the near future, the majority of elective surgical procedures will be performed in an outpatient setting. The Medicare program, as well as other third-party payment systems, are

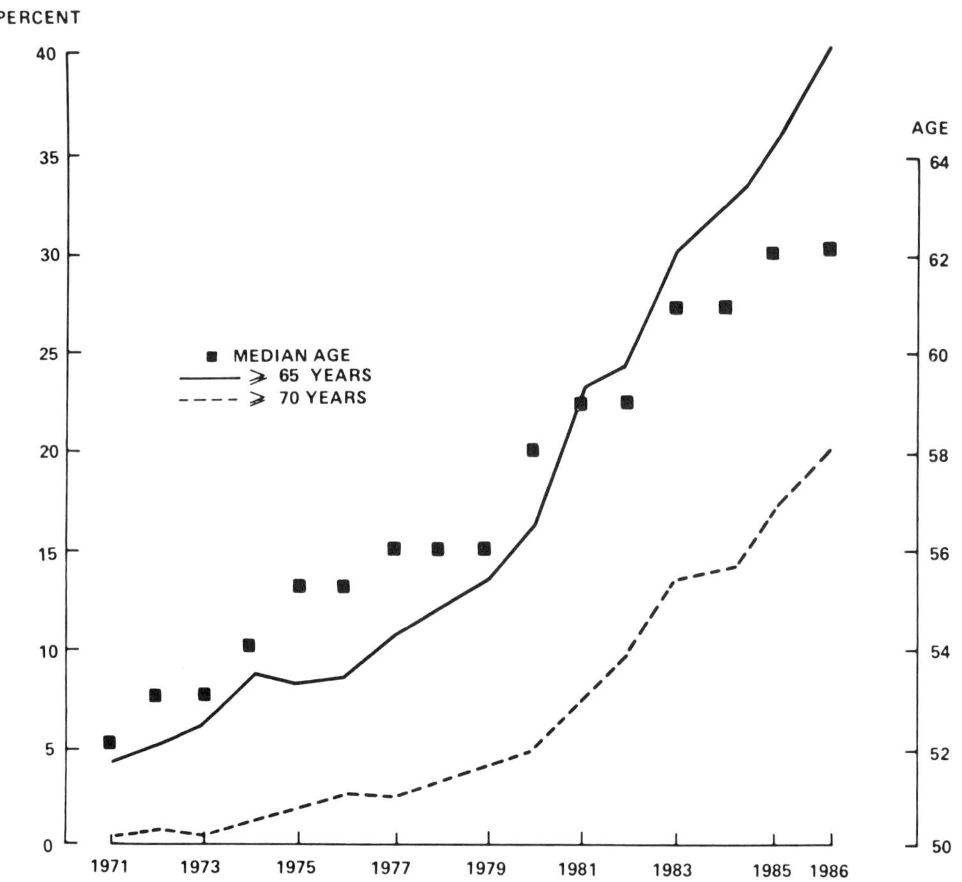

Fig. 16-1. The median age of patients who underwent cardiac bypass surgery at the Cleveland Clinic in 1986 increased to age 62. The percentage of cardiac surgical candidates greater than age 65 exceeded 40 percent of the surgical volume and there has also been an increase in the percentage of the surgical population above age 70, which in 1986 exceeded 20 percent of all surgical bypass patients. (From Loop et al.,[9] with permission.)

more frequently mandating that surgical procedures be performed on geriatric patients on an outpatient basis. The importance to the anesthesiologist is obvious—an increasing number of surgical candidates belong to the geriatric age group and an increasing percentage of their procedures will be performed on an outpatient basis. Thus, the anesthesiologist needs to be aware of the differences in dealing with the geriatric population, especially in an outpatient setting, and of how pharmacologic and physiologic changes associated with increasing age may influence anesthetic and analgesic requirements for outpatient surgical procedures.

Ambulatory surgery should be viewed as a potentially beneficial experience for the geriatric patient. Advantages afforded the geriatric patient when undergoing surgery in this setting include limited separation from their family, friends, and familiar environment, with more rapid return to normal surroundings postoperatively. There is less severe disruption in routine, diet, medication, and sleep. In an outpatient setting, geriatric patients receive fewer medications and the close presence of relatives and friends contributes to a lower incidence of postoperative confusion. Over one-half of hospitalized geriatric patients experience transient confusion postoperatively.[10]

AGE-RELATED PERIOPERATIVE RISK

Because the aging process varies from person to person and from one organ system to another, elderly patients do not present to us as a homogeneous entity. There is little correlation between chronologic age and biologic age. People appear to reach their peak physiologic function in their late 20s or early 30s and from then on it is, in general, a "down-hill course."[11] The amount of physiologic function that remains in people of advanced age varies greatly. For example, one patient may physiologically appear as a relatively young octogenarian compared with another who physiologically appears as a relatively old septuagenarian. It is difficult to predict the physiologic function of an elderly patient simply from chronologic age, which is a primary reason why older citizens present a higher risk when undergoing anesthesia and surgery.

It is widely believed that compared with younger patients, elderly patients (even those free from concomitant disease) having major surgery have a significantly higher incidence of complications or death. In an English survey, approximately 50 percent of intraoperative deaths occurred in geriatric patients, although this group of patients represented only 5 percent of the overall surgical population.[12] As shown in Table 16-1, age, per se, appears to predict increased perioperative morbidity and mortality.[13] A large study from Cardiff of 108,878 anesthetics between the years 1972 and 1977 also supported the concept of a higher mortality for both men and women of older age groups (Table 16-2).[14] As shown in Table 16-3, Santos and Gelperin reviewed operative mortality within 10 days of surgery for a group of patients aged 50 to 90+ years undergoing a total of 2,186 operations.[15] An apparently clear age-related mortality rate

Table 16-1. Mortality Within 7 Days of Anesthesia in Consecutive Surgical Patients

Age (yr)	No. of Patients	No. of Deaths (%)
<1	3,396	56 (1.6)
1–10	3,650	30 (0.8)
11–20	5,608	25 (0.45)
21–30	5,192	41 (0.8)
31–40	3,962	55 (1.4)
41–50	4,129	97 (2.3)
51–60	4,063	126 (3.1)
61–70	2,941	130 (4.4)
71–80	1,162	79 (6.8)
>81	73	6 (8.2)
Total	34,140	645 (1.9)

(Modified from Marx et al.,[13] with permission.)

Table 16-2. Mortality by Age and Sex

	Men			Women		
Age (yr)	Deaths	Total	Mortality (%)	Deaths	Total	Mortality (%)
0–14	105	8,041	1.3	59	4,601	1.3
15–24	46	5,695	0.8	27	9,683	0.3
25–44	121	9,488	1.3	94	22,411	0.4
45–64	428	14,174	3.0	331	15,925	2.1
>65	578	9,749	5.9	612	9,111	6.7

(Modified from Farrow et al.,[14] with permission.)

Table 16-3. Surgical Mortality by Age Group

Age Group (yr)	No. of Procedures	No. of Deaths (%)
Under 50	212	2 (0.9)
50–59	220	7 (3)
60–69	467	15 (3)
70–79	603	21 (3)
80–89	568	33 (5)
90+	116	10 (7)
Total	2,186	88 (3.9)

(Modified from Santos and Gelperin,[15] with permission.)

was observed. In addition, a large French survey conducted between 1978 and 1982 followed 190,389 anesthetic procedures in approximately 500 institutions.[16] In that study, the overall frequency for anesthetic accidents was one death in 2,410 anesthetics or an incidence of 0.04 percent. However, a sharp increase in incidence to approximately two to three deaths per 1,000 anesthetics occurs beyond age 65. As shown in Table 16-4, Gersh et al. demonstrated a mortality rate in patients 75 years of age or older that is approximately twice that of patients aged 65 to 69 and far greater than that of patients who are younger than age 65.[17] Similarly, Acinapura et al. compared 685 patients over age 70 with 3,142 patients under age 70; both age groups were undergoing coronary artery bypass surgery.[18] Hospital mortality was 8 percent for patients over age 75 compared with a mortality rate less than 2 percent for patients under age 70. Pottecher et al. surveyed 198,103 anesthetics in France and determined the overall frequency of cardiac arrest under anesthesia to be one per 1,665 anesthetics or an incidence of 0.06 percent.[19] The greatest number of arrests occurred in patients between the ages of 55 and 74 years. These investigators constructed a comparative risk coefficient (CRC) that was determined to be the incidence of occurrence of cardiac arrest divided by the number of anesthetics for patients of different ages. As shown in Fig. 16-2, the CRC values were age-related and highest in patients over age 85. This age-related mortality also seems to be borne out in the very oldest surgical patients. As Hosking et al. have observed (Table 16-5), the mortality rate of patients within 30 days of surgery was approximately 8 percent in patients in their early 90s, yet almost doubled in patients over age 100.[7]

Table 16-4. Perioperative Mortality in Coronary Artery Bypass Surgery Patients

Age (yr)	No. of Patients	No. of Deaths (%)
<65	7,827	151 (1.9)
65–69	803	37 (4.6)
70–74	241	16 (6.6)
75–84	42	4 (9.5)

(Modified from Gersh et al.,[17] with permission.)

Table 16-5. Surgical Mortality in the Very Old

Age (yr)	No. of Patients	Percent Mortality (within 30 d)
90–94	671	8.1
95–99	111	9.4
100+	13	15.4

(Modified from Hosking et al.,[7] with permission.)

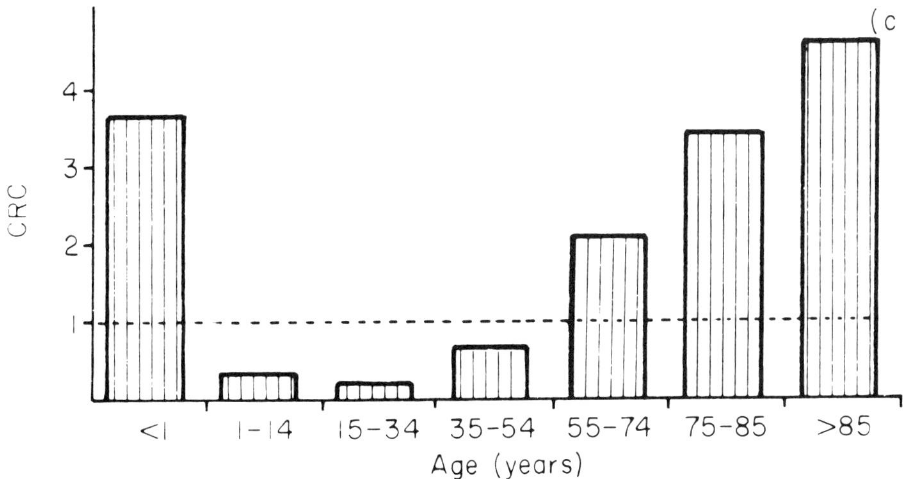

Fig. 16-2. Comparative risk coefficient (CRC) related to age. The CRC is equal to the cardiac arrests (percentage) per anesthetics (percentage) by age distribution. Older patients apparently have the highest risk for intraoperative cardiac arrest and perioperative complication. (From Pottecher et al.,[19] with permission.)

However, not all studies concur with the notion that patients who are older will necessarily have a higher complication rate during the perioperative period. For instance, in a series of 500 patients having anesthesia and surgery, Djokovic and Hedley-Whyte found no consistent increase in the incidence of death as patients' ages increased from 80 to 95 years.[4] In 1983, Filzweiser and List reported a prospective study of 500 consecutive patients older than 70 and did not find a single intraoperative death.[20] Similarly, Hatton et al. reported an actual reduction in deaths resulting from anesthesia in patients older than 80.[21] In view of the controversy, one wonders if there is a factor other than age alone that better predicts potential complications and deaths in geriatric patients undergoing the stress of anesthesia and surgery.

When the role that age plays as a risk factor for geriatric patients having anesthesia and surgery is examined, the distinction between physiologic age and chronologic age becomes important. Compared with younger patients, elderly patients may be at greater risk for perioperative complications and deaths because of two factors: first, a decline in basic organ function (independent of disease) resulting from aging and second, an increased prevalence of age-related concomitant disease. We will examine each of these factors.

PATHOPHYSIOLOGY OF AGING

Should aging influence perioperative morbidity and mortality in elderly patients, it likely does so, in part, as a result of the gradual decline in physiologic reserve in a variety of organ systems. Physiologic function that remains despite the readily apparent progressive decline in function with age is nevertheless sufficient to allow the elderly person to carry out the normal requirements of living. However, their ability to respond to stress and to overcome complications is reduced. Response to cellular injury is impaired, and the ability to summon resources of increased organ function necessary to respond to complications after surgery is so dramatically limited that what would be a minor complication in a younger person may produce a domino-like cascade of progressive complications that may lead to death in the elderly surgical patient.

In this section, we will discuss the pathophysiologic changes of aging that affect major organ systems and that subsequently impact on our choice of anesthetic techniques.

Cardiovascular System

Perhaps the most important age-related physiologic changes that affect the anesthetic management of the elderly patient are those that occur in the cardiovascular system. Many of these physiologic changes once thought to reflect the aging process itself now appear to be manifestations of age-related disease and/or a lifestyle resulting in prolonged deconditioning. Since major lifestyle changes occur and the prevalence of disease increases sharply with advancing age, it is difficult to determine the effects of the process of aging itself on the cardiovascular system.

The cardiovascular changes associated with aging include impaired myocardial pump function and reduced cardiac output. Increasing fibrosis of the endocardial lining of the cardiac chambers and valves leads to progressive endocardial thickening and rigidity. Calcification of valves, especially in the region of the annulus, may produce distortion of valvular leaflets, resulting in progressive valvular incompetence. In addition, loss of elasticity throughout the vascular tree with age produces a progressive loss of arterial distensibility and increased impedance to left ventricular output, resulting in a progressive compensatory hypertrophy of the left ventricle. With age-induced diminished caliber and elasticity of coronary arteries, maximum coronary perfusion decreases. Not surprisingly, many of these factors combine to contribute to an increased incidence of hypertension and ischemic heart disease in elderly patients.

Vascular Elasticity and Blood Pressure

Large artery elasticity is, in general, reduced during the aging process, resulting in stiffening of the arterial vasculature. The histologic and morphologic changes seen in the aging aorta and arterial tree resemble those of younger patients who suffer from essential hypertension.[22] As a consequence, there is an age-related increased impedance to ejection of blood with each contraction of the heart, resulting in an increase in systolic blood pressure. Probably as an adaptive mechanism to maintain normal wall stress, a concentric hypertrophy of the left ventricular wall that approximates 30 percent develops between the ages of 30 and 80 years. Long-term longitudinal studies of patients, such as that reported in the Framingham study, demonstrate an increase in systolic blood pressure of 25 to 35 mmHg.[23] Hypertension in the elderly is frequently inadequately treated, and if diastolic blood pressure is chronically greater than 100 to 110 mmHg, plasma volume depletion is likely.[24] Pre-existent hypovolemia in poorly treated elderly hypertensive patients makes intraoperative blood pressure lability likely and also renders the patient poorly tolerant of sudden changes in posture, intrathoracic pressure, or blood loss.

Heart Rate and Adrenoreceptor Responsiveness

Although the resting heart rate and heart rate response to submaximal exercise loads in the elderly are similar to that of younger patients, the maximum heart rate that can be generated by an elderly patient is considerably less. Regulation of chronotropic and inotropic cardiac function is partly dependent on catecholamine effect. During exercise, an increase in serum catecholamines in elderly subjects in excess of that seen in younger subjects has been observed.[25] Thus, failure to synthesize and release catecholamines during stress cannot explain the apparent diminution in adrenergic response manifested by a reduced maximal heart rate and ejection fraction. Instead, an age-related decrease in target organ responsiveness due to a reduced number of receptors[26] or a reduced receptor sensitivity has been suggested.[27] The number of adrenergic receptors has been documented to decrease in the aging heart. Thus, catecholamine effects that enhance calcium ion transport in the myocardium and improve calcium ion availability are less marked in elderly patients, partly explaining the reduced myocardial myofibril contraction and the reduced maximum heart rate in elderly subjects.

Many studies have also demonstrated a reduced chronotropic response to a variety of exogenously administered drugs and a reduced autonomic response in the elderly. For example, older patients have a reduced tachycardiac response to atropine compared with younger patients.[28] At age 50 or older, the heart rate is increased by only 4 to 5 beats/min following atropine administration, whereas the same dose in younger subjects produces a far more dramatic response. Similarly, a multicenter clinical evaluation demonstrated an increase in heart rate in response to isoflurane administration in younger patients that was of minimal significance in the elderly.

In summary, it is difficult to determine on brief inspection of an elderly individual if cardiac function has been well-maintained during the aging process. To make this decision, a skilled anesthesiologist will attempt to discover if an elderly individual has developed age-related cardiac disease or has allowed a sedentary lifestyle to interfere with the maintenance of long-term cardiovascular fitness. It is reassuring to know that a significant percentage of our elderly patient population may have surprisingly well-maintained cardiac function and will be able to compensate to meet the demands of stressful situations. However, it is unnerving to realize that it is difficult to determine on superficial evaluation what sort of cardiac reserve the average elderly patient may have. More than half of elderly individuals will have significant coronary artery disease whether or not they are symptomatic.

Coronary Artery Disease

Although a high percentage of elderly individuals have coronary stenosis at autopsy, a much lower percentage demonstrates clinical manifestations, such as angina pectoris or myocardial infarction. Thus, coronary artery disease is occult during life in a large number of elderly individuals. An estimate of the prevalence of coronary disease in men aged 51 to 90 will be markedly low and inaccurate if one relies only on resting criteria, such as a history of angina pectoris, previous myocardial infarction, and/or an abnormal ECG.[22] On the other hand, with more intensive evaluation of coronary perfusion, such as using radionuclide imaging of the myocardium, coupled with ECG monitoring during a treadmill stress test, many more individuals with significant coronary artery disease may be identified. In fact, it appears that individuals 70 years of age or older have at least a 50 percent chance of developing significant coronary artery disease whether or not they are symptomatic.

Many studies have contributed to the classically held belief that cardiac output gradually declines approximately 1 percent per year beyond age 30. A typical example is a study by Brandfonbrener et al.[29] in which a 50 percent decline in cardiac index from the ages of 20 to 80 was observed. Unfortunately, the population tested in many of these classic studies was comprised of patients who were housed in hospital wards and were being treated for either acute or chronic disease.

The Baltimore Longitudinal Study on Aging is a program that, on a longitudinal basis, follows volunteer subjects who are carefully screened, viewed to be healthy, and are not affected by disease or deconditioning. These individuals return to Baltimore every other year for a complete physical evaluation. Recently, data from this study group has yielded a divergent view of the change that has classically been thought to occur in resting cardiac output as a result of age. Rodeheffer et al.[30] demonstrated that there is no significant age-associated decline in cardiac output at rest or during exercise in healthy adults between the ages of 25 and 79 years. Therefore, it appears that elderly individuals may have a decline in cardiac output with age if they have maintained a sedentary lifestyle or if they are affected by age-related disease. On the other hand, healthy elderly individuals who have maintained an active lifestyle do not necessarily have a predetermined age-related obligatory decline in cardiac output.

Respiratory System

In general, aging produces reduced maximum ventilatory functions and decreased efficiency of gas exchange. An approximate 10 percent reduction in total lung capacity develops from the ages of 20 to 70 years.[31] This is contributed to by a narrowing of the intervertebral disc spaces, resulting in a shortening of overall body height. The bellows function of the lung is further impaired by rigidity of the thoracic cage due to stiffening of cartilage and replacement of elastic tissue in the costal, intercostal, and intervertebral areas. Progressive kyphosis and/or scoliosis produces upward and anterior rotation of the ribs and sternum, which leads to an increase in the anteroposterior chest diameter, further restricting chest expansion. The gradual loss of skeletal muscle mass with aging results in diaphragm and intercostal muscle wastage, further reducing an elderly individual's ability to ventilate. All of these changes contribute to an age-related reduction in vital capacity, total lung capacity, and maximum breathing capacity.

At 20 years of age, maximum voluntary ventilation is approximately 100 L/min, or 12 to 15 times that needed to meet basal metabolic needs. However, maximum voluntary ventilation reduces to approximately 30 to 40 L/min, representing a ventilatory reserve of approximately sevenfold in the healthy nonagenarian. This is more than adequate to meet ventilatory needs for the average nonstressed healthy elderly individual. However, if other age-related diseases or the damaging effects on ventilation that anesthesia and surgery produce are superimposed on this pattern, ventilatory reserve may, in fact, be quite limited. For instance, if a patient presenting for ambulatory surgery has pre-existent pulmonary disease (e.g., emphysema) maximum voluntary ventilation may be reduced. Furthermore, if a patient undergoes a surgical procedure through an upper abdominal or thoracic incision, postoperative splinting will further reduce the ability to ventilate. Residual effects of anesthetic agents and muscle relaxants may reduce the ventilatory capability still further. On the other side of the equation, the requirement for ventilation may be increased in an elderly patient postoperatively. A patient who is septic or who has an acute infection or other medical illness will have greater ventilatory requirements to meet the needs of an increased basal metabolic rate. Superimposed on this, if the patient arrives in the recovery room hypothermic and shivering, basal needs may be further increased. Thus, it is easy to understand why elderly individuals with reasonably adequate ventilatory reserve under normal preoperative conditions may postoperatively quickly find their pulmonary reserves inadequate. Not surprisingly, therefore, elderly patients will more commonly require ventilatory support postoperatively until their metabolic needs are reduced and their ability to ventilate returns toward preoperative levels.

Age-induced parenchymal changes of the lung mimic those of emphysema.[32] Alveolar septi are lost and alveolar spaces expand, resulting in decreased alveolar surface area and diminished pulmonary capillary bed density. The progressive diminution in functional alveoli with age reduces elastic recoil of the lung, resulting in an increase in the ratio of residual volume to total lung capacity and the ratio of functional residual capacity to total lung capacity. In addition, since alveolar septi produce radial traction or tethering of the terminal bronchioles, a reduction in their quantity during aging makes the support framework for the terminal bronchioles less stable in geriatric patients. Thus, small airways will collapse at larger lung volumes, producing an age-related increase in the "closing volume" of the lung. As closing volume increases with age, greater portions of tidal ventilation occur at lung volumes below closing volume, thus producing air trapping and V/Q mismatch. As a result, resting PaO_2 normally declines with age at a rate described by the following equation:[33–35]

$$PaO_2 = 100 - (0.4 \times \text{age [yr]})\ \text{mmHg}$$

Elderly patients must be observed more closely postoperatively since their protective mechanisms against hypoxia and hypercapnia are less effective than those of younger patients. Higher inspired concentrations of oxygen may be required intraoperatively for elderly individuals because of their lower resting PaO_2 values and reduced efficiency of ventilatory exchange. Supplemental inspired oxygen should be considered until adequate oxygenation resulting from breathing room air resumes.

Central Nervous System

Age-related central nervous system (CNS) disease is not uncommon in the elderly. Dementia may be due to localized areas of microemboli or due to organic brain syndrome (a neuropsychiatric disorder associated with impaired brain tissue function). A common variety of this, Alzheimer's disease, is associated with cerebral atherosclerosis that results in a gradual reduction of cerebral blood flow and CNS activity.

Although an obligatory age-induced decline in cerebral cognitive function remains controversial, it is generally agreed that geriatric patients have a reduced requirement for anesthetic agents. This may not be distinguishable in any given patient, but it is observed in cross-sectional studies comparing elderly to younger individuals and is believed to be due, at least in part, to a reduction in pre-existent CNS activity. Muravchick[36] suggests that we think of anesthetic requirement as resistance to loss of consciousness and that elderly individuals may have a reduced anesthetic requirement due to a decrement in this resistance.

A classic example of age-related reduced anesthetic requirement is the reduced minimum alveolar concentration necessary in elderly patients to produce anesthesia with either cyclopropane, halothane, or isoflurane.[37–39] The requirement for these inhalational agents decreases linearly with patient age. Munson et al. noted that the requirements for all three agents closely parallel each other when age comparisons are made.[39]

The reduced anesthetic requirement for geriatric patients applies not only to inhalational anesthetics but also to local anesthetics, narcotics, barbiturates, benzodiazapines, and other intravenous anesthetic agents. Elderly patients achieve a comparable level of sedation at diazepam plasma concentrations significantly lower than those required by younger adults. Equivalent EEG suppression occurs at lower plasma concentrations of both fentanyl and alfentanil in the aged.[40] Similar to narcotics, the induction dose of barbiturates required in 70-year-old adults is approximately 30 percent less than that required for individuals four to five decades younger. However, for the barbiturates it has been suggested that the increased sensitivity to the same dose of drug in the elderly may relate more to differences in pharmacokinetics than to an increased pharmacodynamic sensitivity. Homer and Stanski,[41] using the "spectral edge" determination of EEG activity as a measure of anesthetic depth, found that the serum concentration of thiopental required to induce anesthesia in elderly patients was no different from that of younger patients. Their explanation of the greater sensitivity of the elderly to the same dose of thiopental was based on the reduced initial volume of distribution in the elderly that resulted in a higher plasma concentration following the same administered dose.

Thus, it appears that elderly individuals may demonstrate greater sensitivity to different drugs on the basis of pharmacokinetic and/or pharmacodynamic differences associated with aging. The CNS and peripheral nervous system undergo progressive anatomic and functional changes during the aging process that may influence the dose-response relationship of elderly individuals to anesthetic agents. Multiple observations have been proposed to explain the enhanced responsiveness of the elderly to anesthetic drugs.

First, there is a continual loss of neuronal substance with advancing age. On average, a daily attrition of perhaps as many as 50,000 neurons from an initial neuron pool of approximately 10 billion occurs during the life span of an individual.

A second and closely related explanation for the greater sensitivity of the elderly to anesthetic agents is a reduced number of receptor sites or reduced affinity in the brain for hormonal and drug actions. For example, the pharmacology of the autonomic nervous system is altered, necessitating increased plasma norepinephrine levels in elderly patients to produce the same effects as lower levels in younger patients.[42] It is thought that this is secondary to a reduced number of receptor sites or a reduced receptor response. β-Receptor density has also been observed to decrease in the cerebrum and cerebellum of both rats and humans. The reduced sensitivity of the elderly to β-adrenergic agents has been suggested to result from a functional alteration in β-receptor affinity or uncoupling of the β-receptor–adenylate cyclase system.[43] These age-related observations in the CNS parallel the reduced number of receptor sites and changes in receptor affinity that has been noted in the cardiovascular system of the elderly.

A third theory proposed for the reduced anesthetic requirements of the elderly involves the rate of synthesis of neurotransmitters. A progressive and significant decrease in the concentration of enzymes that synthesize neurotransmitters is consistently seen in aging neural tissues.[44]

Although the exact explanation for why elderly individuals may be more sensitive to many anesthetic agents remains unclear, the observation of their greater sensitivity to most agents is not questioned. The anatomic and functional changes occurring in the CNS with aging that result in a reduced anesthetic requirement for the elderly may also increase their risk for postoperative deterioration of mental function. This may be an issue of equal or even greater importance, affecting the quality of an elderly patient's perioperative experience. This takes on special importance when considering management of the elderly patient in an outpatient setting.

Body Composition

Important age-related changes in body composition include a loss of skeletal muscle (lean body mass), an increase in percentage of body fat, and intracellular dehydration. There is an approximate 10 percent decline in skeletal muscle mass (lean body mass) with aging. The average loss of muscle mass is estimated to be 6 kg at age 80, and is more dramatically observed in women.

The increase in percentage of body fat that occurs with age results in an increased availability of lipid storage sites and a greater reservoir for deposition of lipid soluble anesthetic drugs. The sequestration of anesthetic agents in the lipid storage tissues of the elderly allows for a more gradual and protracted elution of anesthetic agents from these storage sites, increasing the time period required for elimination, and resulting in greater residual plasma concentrations of drug and prolonged anesthetic effects.

Renal Function

Similar to the deterioration of other organ functions, the number of effective renal glomeruli decreases with age. Glomerular filtration rate is reduced approximately 1 ml/min per year or about 1 to 1.5 percent per year.[45] In addition to reductions in glomerular function (filtration), tubular function (excretion) also shows a parallel decline during aging. As a result, renal clearance of drugs is adversely affected.

The linear decrease in glomerular filtration rate is far more dramatic than the modest age-associated loss of renal tissue mass,[46] suggesting that reduced renal plasma flow may be the primary explanation for loss of renal function with age. The reduced renal plasma flow associated with increased age is due to a reduction in the magnitude of the renal vascular bed produced by a disproportionately large loss of cortical renal tissue mass (glomeruli), and may be contributed to by an overall age-associated decrease in cardiac output.

These renal changes result in a reduced ability of elderly individuals to excrete administered drugs, both in their unchanged form and in their metabolized by-product form. For example, creatinine, a normal metabolic by-product of muscle creatine, is less efficiently excreted in the elderly patient, measured as a decrease in creatine clearance rate.[47] However, healthy geriatric patients will have approximately the same circulating level of serum creatinine as do younger patients because there is less skeletal muscle and, thus, less creatinine production.[48] Measurement of serum creatinine levels in an attempt to determine renal function is therefore inaccurate and, to gain an accurate assessment of renal function, clearance of creatinine or another substance is a more appropriate test. Elevated serum creatinine levels in an elderly patient imply a decrement in renal function even greater than that normally observed with aging. The reduced capacity for renal clearance in elderly individuals also affects their ability to clear anesthetic drugs and contributes to a longer duration of action of these drugs.

Hepatic Function

Although results of standard liver function tests, such as serum bilirubin, albumin, and alkaline phosphatase levels, may be normal in geriatric patients, other tests truly reveal the decrement in hepatic function that parallels age. For example, impaired bromosulfaline excretion with resultant increased retention may be first noted in patients over 50 years of age and may become progressively worse with increasing age.[49]

The most likely explanation for reduced hepatic clearance of a variety of substances in elderly individuals is the marked reduction in hepatic size that occurs with the aging process.[46,50]

The effect of an age-associated reduction of hepatic blood flow and a potential reduction in microsomal enzyme fraction impairs the ability of the liver to metabolize anesthetic drugs. This, combined with the reduced filtration and excretory capability of the aging kidney, results in a more gradual decline in plasma concentration of anesthetic agents in the elderly (a prolonged β-elimination halflife) and contributes to a longer duration of effect from anesthetic drug administration in the elderly.

Basal Metabolic Rate and Thermoregulation

Basal metabolic rate declines approximately 1 percent per year in individuals beyond age 30. Thus, all anesthetic agents may be expected to be metabolized and excreted more slowly in elderly patients. In addition, the age-related incidence of postoperative hypothermia in elderly patients is at least partly explained by the decrease in metabolic rate with aging. Goldberg and Roe, in a study of 101 adult surgical patients, showed that the difficulty in maintaining normothermia during general anesthesia is age-related.[51] Elderly patients showed exaggerated intraoperative decreases in rectal temperature compared with younger patients, even during short and relatively minor surgical procedures. Not surprisingly, the development of intraoperative hypothermia correlated with the length of operation. These investigators attributed a portion of anesthetized young patients' abilities to more easily maintain body temperature intraoperatively to their greater endogenous heat production as a result of a greater basal metabolic rate. In turn, the lesser basal heat production of older patients contributed to a more exaggerated intraoperative heat loss in this patient group.

Thus, as a result of impaired heat production and a reduced ability to thermoregulate, it is not surprising that Vaughn et al. showed that patients more than 60 years of age are both admitted to and discharged from the postanesthesia care unit (PACU) with a lower measured body temperature compared with younger patients.[52] The lower temperatures on discharge from the PACU in elderly patients relate to the fact that there is no difference in the rate of temperature return in older patients compared with younger ones. Older subjects thus demonstrated a longer duration of hypothermia in the PACU than that seen in younger patients. Several adverse effects can result from hypothermia. The first problem is the incidence of shivering. The greater the severity of hypothermia of patients on arrival in the PACU, the greater the incidence of shivering.[52,53] Shivering in the postoperative period may represent a risk to the elderly patient, since shivering results in a marked increase in basal metabolic rate. Oxygen consumption must necessarily increase as much as 400 to 500 percent,[54] which places increased demands on the cardiac and pulmonary systems. Arterial hypoxemia may result in shivering patients. In addition, shivering may cause myocardial ischemia in geriatric patients (who frequently have occult coronary artery disease) due to the increased myocardial oxygen demand resulting from the increased requirements for cardiac output in the presence of peripheral vasoconstriction. Protracted hypothermia in the postoperative period in elderly patients also reduces the elimination rate of residual anesthetic agents.

Close attention to maintenance of body temperature intraoperatively is desirable in all patients, especially in geriatric patients. Methods to reduce temperature loss, such as warming intravenous fluids, administering humidified and warmed inspired gases, reducing radiation losses by providing adequate blankets and drapes, and maintaining a warm room temperature, are of obvious benefit to elderly patients.

EFFECTS OF CONCOMITANT DISEASE

Multiple concomitant diseases are the rule, rather than the exception, in the elderly patient. A current surgical illness is likely to be present in patients in whom old injuries, prior illnesses, past operations, and a variety of chronic disorders, including cataracts, osteoarthritis, anemia, osteoporosis, and diabetes mellitus, may be observed. Malignancy, cerebral vascular accidents, parkinsonism, dementia, and fractures of the femur are observed with increased frequency in this patient group. For instance, pathologic findings were observed on medical examination in 92 percent of patients 81 years of age or older.[55] Of these, cardiovascular abnormalities including atherosclerosis and hypertension were seen in 78 percent of patients, whereas mental dysfunction occurred in 30 percent and pulmonary, endocrine, and neurologic abnormalities were observed in 14 percent, 12 percent, and 10 percent of patients, respectively. Stephen reported the frequency of abnormalities encountered in 1,000 patients older than age 70.[56] Once again, hypertension, atherosclerosis, and renal disease led the list of concomitant disease states in geriatric patients interviewed before operation.

Which of the common pre-existing conditions correlate most closely with an increased risk of perioperative complications and death in elderly patients? Rowe et al. found that ischemic heart disease, dementia, and diabetes seemed to correlate most closely with an increased risk.[48] On the other hand, Farrow et al. found that cardiac failure, impaired renal function, and angina were the preoperative conditions most indicative of a high-risk perioperative death.[14] These conditions were associated with mortality 10 to 30 times greater than the overall 0.5 percent mortality observed in patients without these preoperative medical conditions. Hosking et al.[7] observed that renal disease, CNS disease, or biliary tract disease contributed to poorer long-term survival in patients over age 90. They also noted that postoperative morbidity within 48 hours of surgery was more commonly observed in patients who had prior atrial arrhythmias. This is similar to another study which demonstrated that patients with chronic atrial fibrillation have an increased mortality rate.[57]

Thus, a variety of different preoperative medical conditions have been credited with producing increased risk in elderly patients. The type of preoperative medical condition as well as the number of associated diseases may be important in determining the rate of perioperative complications. As mentioned above, Tiret et al. appeared to demonstrate in a large study that the rate of anesthesia-related complications correlated directly with the patient's age.[16] However, on closer examination (Fig. 16-3), it is clear that the complication rate relates far more closely to the number of associated diseases with which the patient presented rather than the patient's age.

The greater incidence of complications and death in older patients most likely reflects the fact that these patients more commonly present for surgery with a greater number of associated pre-existent diseases. Stephen's analysis of a large number of elderly surgical patients showed that 36 percent developed a nonfatal complication and that 66 percent of these had three or more preoperative functional abnormalities.[56] In addition, while he observed an overall mortality rate of 5.8 percent in elderly patients, 84 percent of those who died had more than three pre-existent medical conditions. Similarly, Denney and Denson reported a mortality rate of 29 percent among patients older than age 90 who had disease in multiple organ systems, compared with a strikingly lower mortality of 4.9 percent in a group of healthy persons of similar age.[58] The study of Goldman et al. of cardiac risk factors also suggests that pre-existent medical conditions may be more important than a patient's age when attempting to predict the risks associated with anesthesia and surgery.[59] "Points" in the Goldman risk index are assigned to patients before operation, with greater point values given to those criteria more likely to result in perioperative complications and death. Age greater than 70 years is assigned a point value, indicating

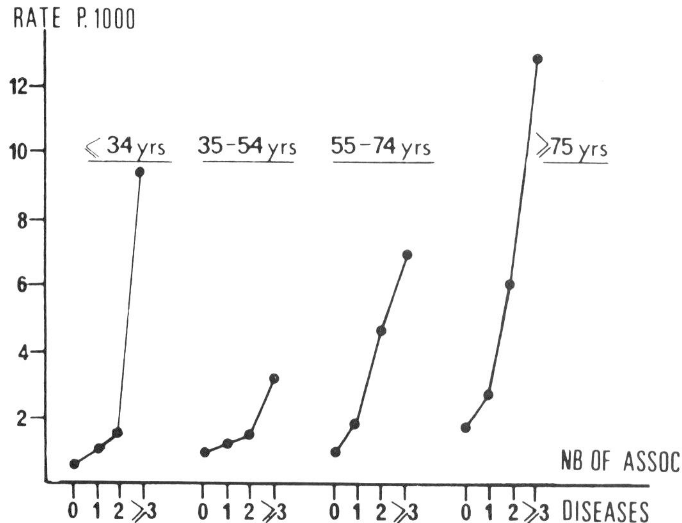

Fig. 16-3. Perioperative death rate per 1,000 anesthetics related to the number of pre-existent diseases in patients of four different age groups. Pre-existent disease (physiologic age) is more important than chronologic age alone in predicting perioperative morbidity and mortality. (From Tiret et al.,[16] with permission.)

that age alone may be a risk. However, age is intermediate in importance and has a point value less than that assigned to certain preoperative medical conditions, such as a recent myocardial infarction or signs of congestive heart failure. Finally, Gersh et al.[60] have also shown that long-term (5-year) survival in patients older than 65 years was affected by the number of concurrent diseases. In patients with no concurrent diseases, there was an 89 percent 5-year survival rate in patients recovering from coronary artery bypass surgery compared with a 71 percent rate in patients presenting to surgery with two or more pre-existent diseases.

VALUE OF PHYSICAL STATUS CLASSIFICATION SYSTEM IN PREDICTING RISK

The American Society of Anesthesiologists (ASA) Physical Status Classification is not affected by patient age, but rather by the number and severity of pre-existent medical conditions.[7] The ASA classification system predicts with reasonable accuracy the risks of elderly patients undergoing anesthesia and surgery. For instance, in a study of 500 patients older than age 80, only one of 187 ASA class II patients died in the perioperative period compared with 14 of 56 (25 percent) ASA class IV patients.[4] Similarly, a prospective study of almost 200,000 anesthetics demonstrated an incidence of complications that related directly to the patient's ASA physical status.[16] Del Guercio and Cohn showed a similar relationship: in patients over age 65, those that were ASA class II had a mortality rate less than 10 percent, whereas ASA class III patients had a mortality rate between 10 and 15 percent and ASA class IV patients had a mortality rate greater than 20 percent.[61] In patients over 90 years of age, Hosking et al. found an increasing incidence of perioperative morbidity, and an increasing mortality rate (both at 48 hours and 30 days postoperatively) in patients of higher ASA classification.[7] Similarly, in a large French study, ASA physical status class I patients had an accident rate of approximately 1 per 1,000 anesthetics, which increased to a rate of 17 per 1,000 anesthetics for ASA class IV and V patients. These investigators found no deaths in ASA class I patients, but a death rate of 8.8 per 1,000 for physical status class IV and V patients.[21]

In 1973, Marx et al. found that increased physical status classification indicated increased perioperative risk far more reliably than did increased age.[13] More recently, Cohen et al. showed the same phenomenon when observing more than 100,000 patients for the first 7 postoperative days. Although their data demonstrated that advanced age is an independent predictor of increased mortality, when viewed in comparison, the relative risk predicted by increased age was far less dramatic than the relative risk predicted by poor physical status.[62] For example, advanced age increased the relative risk of perioperative deaths by approximately 13-fold; however, poor physical status as reflected by an ASA physical status score of III to V was an even more important determinant of relative risk.

From all of the information presented, it appears that the presence of age-related disease, especially as reflected in a higher ASA physical classification score, plays a greater role than does age itself in contributing to perioperative complications and death in elderly patients.

ANESTHETIC MANAGEMENT OF GERIATRIC PATIENTS

Patient Selection

A successful outpatient program for elderly patients depends on careful selection of patients and operations. An understanding of the physiologic changes of aging described above explains why an ASA physical status I geriatric patient is a rarity. Geriatric patients more frequently present with multiple medical problems and therefore deserve a thorough evaluation before being considered as acceptable to undergo surgery on an outpatient basis. Early preanesthesia screening for the geriatric outpatient provides both the anesthesiologist and the patient with information, and enables the decision to be made if additional consultations or laboratory studies are required. Consultation with the patient's physician as well as a responsible family member may aid in the presentation of a properly prepared patient for surgery and anesthesia. If a preoperative interview of the patient and the patient's family is impossible, preoperative telephone contact by the anesthesiologist is essential. Ideally, interviews by the staff as far in advance of surgery as possible are valuable. All instructions to the patient and family must be given in writing and compliance must be checked on arrival. Older patients frequently become confused over requirements regarding NPO status, medication regimens, and arrival times.

In addition to a detailed history, an evaluation of the patient's past medical history, review of systems, and a complete drug history should be taken using past medical records and relatives as necessary. In addition to the routine laboratory evaluations, including a complete blood cell count and urinalysis, geriatric patients should also have preoperative chest x-rays and ECGs, with an attempt to date any pathologic changes noted.

Perhaps the most important preoperative assessment we can make regarding geriatric patients is an assessment of the quality of home care that will be provided postoperatively. We believe that preoperatively interviewing the family member who will be taking care of the patient postoperatively is as important as interviewing the patient. The 88-year-old spouse of an 86-year-old patient may be either mentally or physically incapable of postoperatively managing a patient who is experiencing difficulties. Every outpatient, with the exception of those receiving local anesthesia only, must have a responsible person to take them home and monitor them for the first postoperative day. If a geriatric patient has no responsible person at home, then either one must be found for them from among relatives or health care providers or the procedure must be scheduled on an inpatient basis.

Special Considerations

In general, geriatric patients should be brought into the outpatient center earlier than usual on the morning of surgery. Older patients move slower, comprehend slower, and react slower. With these individuals, everything takes longer to accomplish. It takes longer for them to enter the surgical facility, longer to register, and longer to respond to a questionnaire. They must be scheduled for more time for their preoperative visit, arriving at the hospital, registration, and preparing for surgery. They must be scheduled for longer discharge times and for slower dressing when leaving the hospital.

Geriatric patients are physically more difficult to handle. Wetchler[63] suggests that step stools with handles are helpful in allowing patients to get on or off stretchers more easily. Wheelchairs are also, of course, a necessity. The more fragile physical nature of geriatric patients also makes their positioning both intraoperatively and postoperatively more crucial. Geriatric patients poorly tolerate radical positions designed to facilitate surgical approach. For example, when the neck of an elderly patient is rotated, significant reductions in vertebral artery flow may be produced. When geriatric patients are positioned in a hyperlordotic position (in order to enhance bladder or prostate exposure from an abdominal surgical approach), stretch can be placed on the artery of Adamkiewicz, resulting in reduced perfusion to the spinal cord and potential for producing anterior spinal artery syndrome. A similar position in a younger patient may produce no symptoms whatsoever due to larger and more effective collateral perfusion. Extreme attention must be paid to positioning older patients gently while attempting to accomplish surgery with less radical positioning.

Communication with elderly citizens is more difficult. Because of impaired hearing and comprehension, it is frequently more difficult for instructions necessary for a smooth outpatient experience to be understood and followed. Older patients who wear hearing aids should have them left in place as long as possible and returned to them as soon as possible in the PACU. The older patient adapts less well to new environments and may become disoriented or demonstrate psychological defenses in order to cope with the stress of being placed in a new environment. Active efforts by the staff of the outpatient center to communicate and maintain contact with the patient will reduce the likelihood of agitation or confusion.

Finally, because geriatric patients have a slower basal metabolic rate and a lesser effectiveness of autonomic neuronal function that serves to reduce peripheral perfusion and insulate the patients from a cold environment, elderly patients tend to cool more readily when placed in cool environments. As a result, during the anesthetic procedure, the clinician needs to take more active efforts in maintaining patient warmth, especially by providing a warmer operating room environment. In addition, during the recovery phase, the PACU must be kept adequately warm to minimize metabolic stress during emergence from anesthesia.

Premedication

When visiting with elderly patients before surgery, the anesthesiologist need not alter the normal interview practice. Elderly people generally have emotions under good control and are frequently placid. Having seen many of life's problems over a long period of time, these patients generally are less intimidated by the threat of upcoming surgery than are younger patients. Nevertheless, verbal reassurance is still important for allaying anxiety.

In general, premedicant drugs must be administered with caution to elderly patients, who will manifest a greater sensitivity and a longer duration of drug effect compared with their younger counterparts. Normal adult premedication doses may produce an exaggerated effect in elderly patients and can create unwanted confusion and agitation. If there is doubt, pharmacologic premedication should be omitted.

Belladonna drugs useful in younger patients to dry secretions are generally unnecessary in older patients, in whom a lesser degree of salivation is present. Scopolamine and other belladonna alkaloids may cause hallucinations or disorientation in the geriatric patient population. It is our perference to avoid premedicant sedative/hypnotic/opioid drugs in the elderly outpatient unless specifically indicated.

Monitoring

Monitoring the geriatric outpatient should be identical to monitoring the geriatric inpatient and should not be influenced by the fact that the patient will be going home postoperatively. The intensity of monitoring in this setting should be determined by the patient's physiologic condition and the magnitude of the surgical procedures. Because of limited physiologic reserves and a reduced margin for error in elderly patients, monitoring should be generally more intense for this patient group than for younger patients. However, in deciding on the intensity of monitoring for any given elderly patient, it is important to weigh the fact that complications from invasive monitoring are also more likely to be observed in this group. Thus, every monitoring technique has a cost-benefit relationship that must be assessed individually in view of the patient's age, physical status, and proposed surgical procedure. In general, however, intensity of monitoring should not be altered simply because a geriatric patient is undergoing a surgical procedure as an outpatient.

Selection of Anesthetic Type

To some extent, all anesthetic agents are protein bound to plasma proteins. Not all drugs or classes of drugs are equally bound. For instance, in the narcotic class, fentanyl is 80 percent protein bound, whereas morphine and meperidine are only 30 to 40 percent bound. In contrast, alfentanil and sufentanil are both approximately 90 percent protein bound. The portion of the drug that is bound to protein is unable to cross membranes to produce the desired drug effect. On the other hand, the portion that remains free in plasma is able to equilibrate across membranes, including the blood-brain barrier, and is responsible for drug effect.

Because protein binding of anesthetic drugs is less efficient in elderly individuals, the CSF or brain concentration will more closely approach the plasma concentration at all times for this patient group. Thus, for the very same plasma concentration, one would predict a higher CSF or brain level of an anesthetic drug and a more dramatic anesthetic effect.

Before the selection of anesthetic type and agent is made, consideration must be given to the pharmacokinetic and pharmacodynamic changes of aging that affect different anesthetic agents.

General Anesthesia

Induction

Onset of induction of anesthetic agents in the elderly population is changed in predictable ways. First, since cardiac output and heart rate tend to be somewhat diminished as a patient ages, circulation time can be prolonged. Therefore, onset of effect following administration of intravenous agents will be delayed.[64] Caution must thus be exercised when administering intravenous drugs to ensure that adequate time has elapsed from administration of one dose to the administration of the next. If the drug has not had sufficient time to reach its target organ(s), and another dose is given due to lack of observed effects, the patient may receive an overdose from which he or she may not have the reserves to recover.

Inhalational agents are not as predictable as intravenous agents. Due to decreased circulation, the partial pressure of the agent in the alveoli will tend to be greater, which suggests that inhalational agents will have a faster onset of action.[64] However, because of pulmonary and pharmacokinetic changes with aging, this effect may not be observed.[65] In general, the behavior of inhalational agents in geriatric patients is similar to their behavior in younger adults.

Duration

Along with delayed onset, anesthetic agents also tend to have longer halflives in elderly patients. A number of factors contribute to this. First, decreased cardiac output will also prolong the duration of anesthetic agents by decreasing the rate of redistribution of the drug. Declining renal and hepatic function result in prolongation of the halflives of drugs. The aging kidney with reduced glomerular and tubular function loses its ability to efficiently clear drugs and their metabolites, while the oxidative capacity of the liver's microsomal enzyme system becomes impaired with age and thus slows in its ability to metabolize drugs. Thus, drugs and their metabolites tend to remain in the circulation longer, producing calculated increases in β-elimination halflife and suggesting longer clinical duration of drug effect.

Contributing to the increased halflives of anesthetic agents seen in older patients is the alteration of body composition, in which total body fat increases while total body water decreases.[66] Therefore, in elderly patients the steady-state volume of distribution will be larger and, hence, the bioavailability of lipid-soluble anesthetic agents will be different from that found in younger patients. Therefore, the outpatient anesthesiologist should attempt to use the shortest-acting agent in every drug class in order to speed emergence and reduce the likelihood of an unplanned admission of a geriatric patient.

Response

In general, less agent is required in the elderly patient to produce a given effect. Part of the explanation for this can be deduced from the decreased metabolism and clearance of drugs in the elderly, which results in higher serum concentrations than would be found in a younger patient. In addition, the decreased binding capacity of serum proteins in geriatric patients allows more free, unbound, and, hence, active drug to be present; this is interpreted clinically as increased sensitivity. Additionally, the number of CNS receptors and neurotransmitters decline with age, producing a pharmacodynamic-enhanced sensitivity to drugs of many classes. On the gross level, brain weight decreases with age, as does cerebral blood flow and oxygen consumption. All of these features culminate in a decrease in CNS function and an increase in anesthetic sensitivity. Thus, when titrating a drug to effect, or when considering giving a standard dose, it should be remembered that the elderly population will respond more intensely than younger patients, and drugs are likely to produce side effects (e.g., drowsiness, hypotension) out of proportion to the dose.[65]

In summary, the elderly patient is best managed by administering a smaller dose of drug than that required by the typical younger surgical patient. Due to age-related changes in pharmacokinetics, the drugs used will be present for longer periods of time, so that maintenance doses will also be smaller than usual. For the outpatient anesthesiologist, this is vital to bear in mind, as use of long-acting drugs will prolong recovery time and potentially lead to greater complications, requiring an unplanned admission.

Regional Anesthesia

To date, it has not been possible to demonstrate the superiority of a specific anesthetic technique for the elderly outpatient.[67] However, regional anesthesia (depending on the adjuvantive narcotic or sedative hypnotic agents given) may be associated with less deterioration of cerebral function postoperatively when compared with general anesthesia.[68] In addition, in geriatric patients undergoing major hip surgery, regional anesthesia appears to be associated with a reduced incidence of deep vein thrombosis, reduced intraoperative blood loss, less postoperative hypoxemia, and a lower death rate within 4 weeks of surgery.[69] In the past, for less invasive surgical procedures, there has been little hard data to recommend one anesthetic technique over another. However, there now appears to be a swell of enthusiasm among surgeons and anesthesiologists who recommend local or regional anesthesia whenever possible in geriatric patients. New studies support the concept that surgical procedures in geriatric outpatients accomplished under local anesthesia or regional anesthesia with mild sedation are associated with a lower complication rate and a lower requirement for hospital admission. For example, in a series of 5,636 patients older than age 60 at the Methodist Ambulatory SurgiCare Center, Wetchler observed that of those patients undergoing surgery with local anesthesia without sedation, an unanticipated admission rate of 0.4 percent occurred. Patients undergoing surgery via regional anesthesia had a 0.8 percent admission rate and patients who received local anesthesia with sedation had a 2.8 percent admission rate. All of these rates compared favorably with an unanticipated admission rate of 4.1 percent in elderly patients undergoing general (inhalational) anesthesia. The overall 1.1 percent admission rate in this series for geriatric patients was slightly higher than the unanticipated admission rate of 0.8 percent for all outpatients.[63] Among patients requiring admission, the reasons for admission, in order of decreasing frequency, were for further observation and evaluation, surgery more extensive than planned, postoperative bleeding, syncope or abnormal blood pressure, and, finally, because no responsible person was available to care for the patient at home after surgery.

Local anesthesia and regional anesthesia may have several other specific advantages that recommend their use for geriatric outpatient surgery. Recovery time is significantly shorter and there is a reduction in side effects following general anesthesia, such as sore throat, muscle pains, airway trauma, dizziness, nausea, and vomiting. When administered by an anesthesiologist adept at regional techniques, spinal anesthesia and epidural anesthesia are perfectly acceptable and, at times, desirable for use in elderly outpatients.

Outpatients receiving regional anesthesia must be as carefully evaluated and prepared as those who receive general anesthesia. The outpatient may be on chronic medications, such as anticoagulants, that are contraindications to a major regional anesthesia (spinal, epidural). There is still some controversy concerning the safety of performing regional anesthesia for patients on "minidose" heparin anticoagulation.

Cataract procedures may be easily performed in an outpatient setting under local anesthesia with or without supplemental sedation. Occasionally, a patient will become agitated and a change to general anesthesia will be required. However, if properly counseled preoperatively, the vast majority of patients will undergo this procedure successfully via local anesthesia.[70]

Lower abdominal procedures, such as inguinal herniorrhaphy, penile prothesis implantation, and surgery on the prostate or bladder, are particularly amenable to regional anesthesia performed in an outpatient setting. Inguinal hernia repair in the elderly patient has become a predominantly outpatient procedure. Under these circumstances, local infiltration of the operative site with dilute solutions of local anesthetics is probably the simplest and safest technique. Local anesthesia alone is associated with the most rapid recovery, the fewest postoperative side effects, and the lowest incidence of unexpected admissions after ambulatory surgical procedures. Although a certain percentage of patients will require intravenously administered sedative or analgesic drugs, most patients will tolerate local anesthetic infiltration or field block without intravenous supplementation. The elderly outpatient undergoing a hernia procedure via local anesthesia will more likely be successful in early voiding and ambulation and will have reduced exposure to anesthetic and analgesic medication. These patients have been found to have fewer wound hematomas and other surgical complications while being satisfied with their ability to go home on the same surgical day.[71]

In addition, local anesthesia has been suggested for outpatient implantation of penile prostheses.[72] For patients undergoing a bit more invasive perineal surgery or prostate surgery, a spinal or epidural anesthesia may be particularly advantageous. Mental function of patients following spinal anesthesia tends to be superior to that of patients receiving general anesthesia.[73] Patients receiving spinal anesthesia for transurethral resection of the prostate have less postoperative mental confusion than do patients who receive general anesthesia.[74] The incidence of postlumbar puncture headache is less than 1 percent when subarachnoid block is performed on an older outpatient. However, residual sympathetic blockade and an inability to void may delay discharge. For brief surgical procedures limited to a single extremity, an intravenous regional block, a regional block of the brachial plexus, or sciatic-femoral-obturator nerve block may be useful.

Good communication between the anesthesiologist, the surgeon, and the patient is essential to ensure selection of the proper anesthetic technique (including regional block) for the surgical procedure contemplated. Because morbidity and mortality associated with surgery and general anesthesia increase with time of surgery, it has been advised that outpatient procedures be restricted to those of less than 2 hours' duration. However, a peripheral somatic nerve block with a long-acting local anesthetic drug may alleviate some of this concern. It should be remembered that duration of nerve blocks is a function of the selected local anesthetic drug rather than the technique. Selection of a regional anesthetic technique in the geriatric outpatient should be determined, in part, on the basis of physiologic response to the block and the risk of complications. Clearly, a pure somatic nerve block without any degree of sympathetic trespass will have fewer effects on pulse, blood pressure, early ambulation, and so forth, than would a spinal or epidural anesthetic. Second, although some complications will manifest in the operative or immediate postoperative period, others have a latent onset. It is probably inadvisable to select nerve block techniques that may have complications that will not become apparent until after the patient is discharged. This would include nerve block techniques that might produce pneumothorax or hematoma formation (e.g., intercostal nerve blocks). In the properly informed and instructed patient, the risk of postlumbar puncture headache is not felt to be a contraindication to spinal and epidural blockade for outpatient surgery in the geriatric patient population.

In choosing the appropriate local anesthetic for outpatient nerve blocks, duration of action is the primary criterion. Although 2-chloroprocaine is the shortest acting of the local anesthetic agents and would be ideal for very brief outpatient procedures, its use is not recommended for intravenous regional anesthesia, nor is it favored by some for use in epidural anesthesia because of its ability to produce backaches. Lidocaine and mepivacaine are probably the agents of choice for most of the regional anesthetic techniques in outpatients. These drugs will still permit patients a predictable discharge from the recovery unit and provide additional operative time as well. For these intermediate-acting local anesthetic agents, the use of adrenaline in a concentration of 1:200,000 will not only provide additional duration, but will significantly reduce the peak plasma concentration of local anesthetic produced. Caution should be used when selecting a long-acting local anesthetic agent, such as bupivacaine, for outpatient procedures. However, it may have application when used in a purely somatic block of the body trunk or when infiltrated along the margins of the incision for postoperative analgesia. Following extremity block, one must caution patients regarding the need for postoperative protection of the denervated extremity, as well as the need for elevation to prevent vascular engorgement during the period of sympathetic blockade.

Again, there is no single type of anesthetic that is best for all situations. The selection should be based on agreement between the patient, the surgeon, and the anesthesiologist. However, due to the considerations discussed above, the outpatient anesthesiologist should select an anesthetic technique that produces the least postoperative central nervous system depression. Not only will this serve to reduce complications and expedite recovery (and thus discharge), but it also has the advantage of allowing the patient to remain awake and able to verbally report significant events, such as angina and clouding of thought.

This is not to say that general anesthesia should never be used in the geriatric outpatient, nor does it imply that local and regional techniques are without risk in this population. As with general anesthesia, decreased blood flow will prolong the effects of local and regional anesthesia. In the case of spinal or epidural administration, residual sympathetic blockade and inability to void may result in a delay in discharging the elderly outpatient. Hypotension observed with spinal and epidural anesthesia is poorly tolerated in older patients, especially considering their decreased reserves and diminished capacity for activation of compensatory reflexes. However, since regional anesthesia may be associated with fewer perioperative and postoperative complications, shorter recovery times, and decreased postoperative mental confusion, these methods should be considered in an outpatient setting before choosing general anesthesia.

Recovery from Anesthesia and Discharge Criteria

Due to their reduced pulmonary reserves and increased V/Q mismatch, geriatric patients tend to have a lower arterial PO_2 at rest and greater deterioration in arterial PO_2 postoperatively compared with younger adults. This predisposes the elderly patient group to arterial oxygen desaturation, both during movement of the patient to the PACU and also for a period of time prior to discharge. Several recent articles underscore the importance of supplementing oxygen for patients during transport from the operating room to the PACU.[75] After the stimulus of operation has ended, it is not unusual for the patient to have some degree of respiratory depression and/or upper airway obstruction. Resultant hypoxemia may lead to myocardial ischemia or infarction. Restlessness and delirium in the aged may often be due to hypoxia rather than pain. We believe that all geriatric patients should have oxygen delivered by nasal cannula following emergence from anesthesia, during transport of the patient to the PACU, and for a period of time afterward, depending on their measured arterial oxygen saturation.

Outpatient discharge criteria for geriatric patients should not differ from those for the general surgical population. While no standardized discharge criteria have been established especially for geriatric patients, it is generally agreed that the patient should be awake, with a mental status comparable to that of the preoperative evaluation. Postoperative confusion and agitation, while common in geriatric inpatients, is rare in the outpatient setting, probably due to less disruption in the patient's routine. However, Chung et al.[76] showed that even as outpatients, elderly patients do, in fact, have a higher incidence of cognitive impairment than younger adults. Interestingly, in geriatric patients undergoing cataract operation under local anesthesia with sedation, these investigators found that the likelihood of postoperative cognitive impairment was related not only to patient age but also to baseline preoperative mental function as determined by a mini-mental state examination. Postoperative mental confusion must be resolved prior to discharge. Vital signs must be at or near preoperative levels and stable for at least 30 to 60 minutes. Full recovery to preoperative levels of motor, sensory, and urinary function, particularly following spinal and epidural anesthesia, must be attained to assure that no residual depression exists.

Finally, the geriatric patient must be discharged to a responsible party who can ensure that adequate care will be provided at home, and that all postoperative medications will be taken and instructions followed. The nursing staff or physician should assess the adult who is to take the patient home in order to determine whether this individual is a responsible person and is someone who is not only mentally but also physically capable of taking care of the patient at home. The patient needs detailed instructions, preferably written, of what to do and not do after arriving home. Telephone numbers of the medical facility should be given so the patient will know who to contact should problems develop. It may be wise to have both the patient and the responsible adult sign the medical record, signifying that both have received and understood the verbal and written discharge instructions.

SUMMARY

The average age of our outpatient population is increasing daily. Older patients are undergoing surgical procedures. With cost-containment efforts and the efforts of third-party payers, more surgical procedures are now being undertaken in an outpatient setting. As a result, the anesthesia community will be asked to take care of increasingly older patients undergoing more invasive procedures on an outpatient basis. Factors we need to consider regarding the acceptability of a geriatric outpatient are the patient's physiologic age and physical status, the surgical procedure that the patient is to undergo, the appropriate anesthetic techniques, and, perhaps most importantly, the quality and reliability of home care for the first 24 hours postoperatively. With an improved understanding of the physiologic differences of the elderly individual compared with younger adults, and with modifications in our anesthetic techniques and perianesthetic management in order to provide individualized care for elderly patients, the risk that these patients face when undergoing an operative procedure may be reduced to a level approaching that of a younger patient population. As Meridy has stated regarding the geriatric outpatient, "arbitrary limits placed on the type of surgery, age of the patient, [and] the duration of the procedure . . . appear to be unwarranted."[77]

REFERENCES

1. Smith OC: Advanced age as a contraindication to operation. Med Rec (NY) 72:642, 1907
2. Ochsner A: Is risk of operation too great in the elderly? Geriatrics 22:121, 1927
3. Brooks B: Surgery in patients of advanced age. Ann Surg 105:481, 1937
4. Djokovic JL, Hedley-Whyte J: Prediction of outcome of surgery and anesthesia in patients over age 80. JAMA 242:2301, 1979
5. Miller R, Marlar K, Silvay G: Anesthesia for patients aged over 90 years. NY State J Med 77:1421, 1977
6. Catlic MR: Surgery in centenarians. JAMA 253:3139, 1985
7. Hosking MP, Warner MA, Lobdell CM, et al: Outcomes of surgery in patients 90 years of age and older. JAMA 261:1909, 1989
8. Warner MA, Hosking MP, Lobdell CM: Utilization of surgery among those ≥ 90 years of age: a population-based study in Olmsted County, Minnesota, 1975–85. Ann Surg 207:26, 1988
9. Loop FD, Lytle BW, Cosgrove DM, et al: Coronary artery bypass graft surgery in the elderly. Indications and outcome. Cleve Clin J Med 55:23, 1988
10. Kelly MJ, Reich P: Psychiatric preparation of the surgical patient. p. 218. In Vandam LD (ed): To Make the Patient Ready for Anesthesia: Medical Care of the Surgical Patient. 2nd Ed. Addison-Wesley Publishing, Reading, MA, 1983
11. McLeskey CH: Anesthesia for the geriatric patient. p. 31. In Stoelting RK, Barash PG, Gallagher TJ (eds): Advances in Anesthesia. Year Book Medical Publishers, Chicago, 1985
12. Davenport HT: Anesthesia for the geriatric patient. Can Anaesth Soc J 30:S51, 1983
13. Marx GF, Mateo CV, Orkin LR: Computer analysis of post-anesthetic deaths. Anesthesiology 39:54, 1973
14. Farrow SC, Fowkes FGR, Lunn JN, et al: Epidemiology in anaesthesia. II: factors affecting mortality in hospital. Br J Anaesth 54:811, 1982
15. Santos AL, Gelperin A: Surgical mortality in the elderly. J Am Geriatr Soc 23:42, 1975
16. Tiret L, Desmonts JM, Hatton F, et al: Complications associated with anaesthesia—a prospective survey in France. Can Anaesth Soc J 33:336, 1986
17. Gersh BJ, Phil D, Kronmal RA, et al: Coronary arteriography and coronary artery bypass surgery: morbidity and mortality in patients ages 65 years or older. Circulation 67:483, 1983a
18. Acinapura AJ, Rose DM, Cunningham JN, et al: Coronary artery bypass in septuagenarians. Circulation 78:suppl. I, I-179, 1988
19. Pottecher T, Tiret L, Desmonts JM, et al: Cardiac arrest related to anesthesia: a prospective survey in France (1978–1982). Eur J Anaesthesiol I:305, 1984
20. Filzweiser G, List WF: Morbidity and mortality in elective geriatric surgery. p. 75. In Vickers MD, Lunn JN (eds): Mortality and Anesthesia. Springer-Verlag, Berlin, 1983
21. Hatton F, Tiret L, Vourc'h G: Morbidity and mortality associated with anesthesia—French survey: preliminary results. p. 25. In Vickers MD, Lunn JN (eds): Mortality and Anesthesia. Springer-Verlag, Berlin, 1983
22. Lakatta EG, Fleg JL: Aging of the adult cardiovascular system. p. 1. In Stephen CR, Assaf RAE (eds): Geriatric Anesthesia: Principals and Practices. Butterworth, Boston, 1986
23. Kannel WB, Gordon T: Evaluation of cardiovascular risk in the elderly: the Framingham study. Bull NY Acad Med 54:573, 1978
24. Tarazi RC, Frohlich ED, Dustan HP: Plasma volume in men with essential hypertension. N Engl J Med 278:762, 1968
25. Tuzankoff ST, Fleg JL, Norris AH, Lakatta EG: Age-related increase in serum catecholamine levels during exercise and healthy adult men. Physiologist 23:50, 1980
26. Shocken DD, Roth GS: Reduced beta-adrenergic receptor concentrations in aging man. Nature 267:856, 1977
27. Dillon N, Chung S, Kelly J, O'Malley K: Age and beta adrenoceptor mediated function. Clin Pharmacol Ther 27:769, 1980

28. Grollman A, Grollman EF: Anticholinergic drugs acting on effector organs innervated by postganglionic parasympathetic nerve. p. 338. In Grollman A, Grollman EF: Pharmacology and Therapeutics. 7th Ed. Lea & Febiger, Philadelphia, 1970
29. Brandfonbrener M, Landowne M, Shock NW: Changes in cardiac output with age. Circulation 69:557, 1955
30. Rodeheffer RJ, Gerstenblith G, Becker LC, et al: Exercise cardiac output is maintained with advancing age in healthy human subjects: cardiac dilatation and increased stroke volume compensate for a diminished heart rate. Circulation 69:203, 1984
31. Goldman HL, Becklake MR: Respiratory function tests: normal values at median altitudes and the prediction of normal results. Am Rev Tuberculosis 79:457, 1959
32. Pontoppidan H, Geffins B, Lowenstein A: Acute respiratory failure in the adult. N Engl J Med 287:690, 1972
33. Raine JM, Bishop JM: A difference in O_2 tension and physiological dead space in normal man. J Appl Physiol 18:284, 1963
34. Kitamura H, Sawa T, Ikezono E: Postoperative hypoxemia: the contribution of age to the maldistribution of ventilation. Anesthesiology 36:244, 1972
35. Wahba W: Body build and preoperative arterial oxygen tension. Can Anaesth Soc J 22:653, 1972
36. Muravchick S: Current concepts: anesthetic pharmacology in geriatric patients. Prog Anesthesiol 1:2, 1987
37. Gregory GA, Eger EI II, Munson ES: The relationship between age and halothane requirement in man. Anesthesiology 30:488, 1969
38. Stevens WC, Dolan WM, Gibbons RT, et al: Minimum alveolar concentrations (MAC) of isoflurane with and without nitrous oxide in patients of various ages. Anesthesiology 42:197, 1975
39. Munson ES, Hoffman JC, Eger EI: Use of cyclopropane to test generality of anesthetic requirement in the elderly. Anesth Analg 63:998, 1984
40. Kaiko RF, Wallenstein SL, Rogers AG, et al: Narcotics in the elderly. Med Clin North Am 66:1079, 1982
41. Homer TD, Stanski DR: The effect of increasing age on thiopental disposition and anesthetic requirement. Anesthesiology 62:714, 1985
42. Lake CR, Ziegler MG, Coleman MD, Kopin IJ: Age-adjusted plasma nor-epinephrine levels are similar in normotensive and hypertensive subjects. N Engl J Med 296:208, 1977
43. Feldman RD, Limbird LE, Nadeau J, et al: Alterations in leukocyte-receptor affinity with aging: a potential explanation for altered-adrenergic sensitivity in the elderly. N Engl J Med 310:815, 1984
44. McGeer EG, McGeer PL: Age changes in the human for enzymes associated with metabolism of catecholamine, GABA, and acetylcholine. Adv Behav Biol 16:287, 1975
45. Hollenberg NK, Adams DF, Solomon HS, et al: Senescence and the renal vasculature in normal man. Circ Res 34:309, 1974
46. Muravchick S: The aging patient and age related disease. ASA Annual Refresher Course Lectures 151:1, 1987
47. Hicks R, Dysken MW, Davis JM, et al: The pharmacokinetics of psychotropic medication in the elderly: a review. J Clin Psychiatry 42:374, 1981
48. Rowe JW, Adres R, Tobin JD, et al: The effect of age on creatinine clearance in man: a cross-sectional and longitudinal study. J Gerontol 31:155, 1976
49. Thompson EN, Williams R: Effect of age on liver function with particular reference to bromosulphalein excretion. Gut 6:266, 1965
50. Vestal RE: Drug use in the elderly: a review of problems and special consideration. Drugs 16:382, 1978
51. Goldberg MJ, Roe F: Temperature changes during anesthesia and operations. Arch Surg 93:365, 1966
52. Vaughn MS, Vaughn RW, Cork RC: Postoperative hypothermia in adults: relationship of age, anesthesia and shivering to rewarming. Anesth Analg 60:746, 1981
53. Jones HB, McLaren CAB: Postoperative shivering and hypoxaemia after halothane, nitrous oxide, and oxygen anaesthesia. Br J Anaesth 37:35, 1965
54. Roe CG, Goldberg MJ, Blair CS, et al: In-

fluence on early post-operative oxygen consumption. Surgery 60:85, 1966
55. Haljamae T, Stefannsson T, Wickstrom I: Preanesthetic evaluation of the female geriatric patient with hip fracture. Acta Anaesthesiol Scand 26:393, 1982
56. Stephen CR: The risk of anesthesia and surgery in the geriatric patient. p. 231. In Krechel SE (ed): Anesthesia and the Geriatric Patient. Grune & Stratton, Orlando, FL, 1984
57. Gajewski J, Singer RB: Mortality in an insured population with atrial fibrillation. JAMA 245:1540, 1981
58. Denney JH, Denson JS: Risk of surgery in patients over 90. Geriatrics 27:115, 1972
59. Goldman L, Caldera DL, Nussbaum SR, et al: Multifactorial index of cardiac risks in non-cardiac surgical procedures. N Engl J Med 297:845, 1977
60. Gersh BJ, Phil D, Kronmal RA, et al: Long-term (5 year) results of coronary bypass surgery in patients 65 years old or older: a report from the coronary artery surgery study. Circulation 68:suppl. II, II-190, 1983b
61. Del Guercio LRN, Cohn JD: Monitoring operative risk in the elderly. JAMA 243:1350, 1980
62. Cohen MM, Duncan PG, Tate RB: Does anesthesia contribute to operative mortality? JAMA 260:2859, 1988
63. Wetchler BV: The geriatric outpatient. p. 128. In Wetchler BV (ed): Problems in Anesthesia. Vol 2. JB Lippincott, Philadelphia, 1988
64. McLeskey CH: Anatomical and physiological changes of aging. Can J Anaesth 34:156, 1987
65. Brown LL: Anesthesia in the geriatric patient. Clin Plast Surg 12:51, 1985
66. Mitenko PA: Changes in drug disposition. Can J Anaesth 34:159, 1987
67. Wickstrom I, Holmberg I, Stefansson T: Survival of female geriatric patients after hip fracture surgery. A comparison of 5 anesthetic methods. Acta Anaesth Scand 26:607, 1982
68. Hole A, Terjesen T, Breivik H: Epidural versus general anesthesia for total hip arthroplasty in elderly patients. Acta Anaesth Scand 24:279, 1980
69. Davis FM, Laurenson VG: Spinal anaesthesia or general anaesthesia for emergency hip surgery in elderly patients. Anaesth Intensive Care 9:352, 1981
70. Vindhya PK, Sheets JH, Tolia NH, Tomlinson LJ: Retrobulbar block using pentothal as a sedative for ambulatory cataract surgery. J Cataract Refract Surg 13:321, 1987
71. Ryan JA, Adye BA, Jolly PC, Mulroy MF: Outpatient inguinal herniorrhaphy with both regional and local anesthesia. Am J Surg 148:313, 1984
72. Scott FB: Outpatient implantation of penile protheses under local anesthesia. Urol Clin North Am 14:177, 1987
73. Chung F, Meier HMR, Lautenschlaeger E: Reduced confusion: spinal or general anaesthesia in the elderly. Anesth Analg 66: S30, 1987
74. Chung F, Meier R: General or spinal anaesthesia: which is better for the elderly? Can Anaesth Soc J 33:S118, 1986
75. Tyler IL, Tantisira B, Winter PM, Montoyama EK: Continuous monitoring of arterial oxygen saturation with pulse oximetry during transfer to the recovery room. Anesth Analg 64:1108, 1985
76. Chung F, Lavell PA, McDonald S, et al: A screening test for elderly outpatients. Anesthesiology 69:A900, 1988
77. Meridy HW: Criteria for selection of ambulatory surgical patients and guidelines for anesthetic management: a retrospective study of 1553 cases. Anesth Analg 61:921, 1982

17

Recovery Period and Discharge

Kari Korttila

Since more extensive operations requiring longer duration of anesthesia are being performed on an outpatient basis, the assessment of recovery from anesthesia is increasingly significant.[1] We must determine how to judge when patients can be sent home safely after outpatient anesthesia and how to anesthetize patients to provide rapid recovery with as little postanesthetic cognitive and psychomotor impairment as possible. Excessive fatigue, nausea, vomiting, or pain can delay discharge from the outpatient facility. Patients with psychomotor impairment also may be prone to accidents during transportation or after arrival home. This chapter focuses on assessing recovery and psychomotor function after anesthesia and presents studies on effects of anesthetics and analgesics on awakening, arousal, and mobilization times. The importance of assessing "home readiness" as distinct from "street fitness" and complete recovery; common side effects and treatment modalities after general, regional, and local anesthesia; and sedation technique in ambulatory surgery settings are also discussed.

STAGES OF RECOVERY

The time course of recovery includes early recovery, intermediate recovery, and late recovery. Early recovery refers to emergence from general and local anesthetic and sedative drugs. Intermediate recovery refers to "home readiness" and discharge from the surgical facility. Patients continue recovery at home until they have resumed normal daily activities, such as driving and returning to work.

Before patients can be considered fully recovered (e.g., fit to drive), their psychomotor performance must return to the preanesthetic level. Most important is to determine if the recovery room patient is at risk if left unattended, if the patient can be safely discharged from the hospital after anesthesia, and when it is safe to allow the patient to drive. Table 17-1 illustrates different stages of recovery after anesthesia.

ASSESSMENT OF "HOME READINESS"

The success of ambulatory surgery depends on appropriate and timely discharge of patients who have had anesthesia. Premature release of patients who later experience postoperative complications requiring unanticipated admission to the hospital or emergency care should rarely (if ever) occur. The major hospital accreditation body in the United States (the Joint Commission of Accreditation of Health Care) requires that policies and procedures be implemented for safe recovery after anesthesia, including examination of the patient and the requirement that the patient have an escort home.[2] It is also required that each patient receive written postoperative instructions which include advice to contact an appropriate physician if problems develop. How can these safety measures be implemented?

For patients who will stay in the hospital after surgery, scoring systems have been developed to guide the transfer from recovery room to ward. The most commonly used method, described by Aldrete and Kroulik in 1970,[3] assigns a numeric score of 0, 1, or 2 for activity, respiration, circulation, consciousness, and skin color; a score of 10 indicates that the patient is in the best possible condition for discharge from the recovery room. This score, however, does not help us in assessing "home readiness" after ambulatory surgery.

Ideally, patients recovering from anesthesia after ambulatory surgery should be evaluated in two separate recovery rooms,[4] the phase I recovery room for recumbent patients and the phase II recovery room (step-down recovery room) for patients who are able to sit and walk. When patients are fully awake and oriented, their ability to stand and walk should be tested. Once they are ambulatory, they should be moved to the phase II recovery room. There they should be offered liquids to take by mouth, and when they have tolerated oral fluids, they should walk to the bathroom and attempt to void. When patients have tolerated oral fluids and voided, have no excessive

Table 17-1. Stages of Recovery and Some Tests for Their Assessment

Stage of Recovery	Test of Recovery
Awakening and recovery of vital reflexes	Patient can open eyes and answer questions. Patient can maintain and guard his or her own airway.
Immediate clinical recovery	Patient can stand unaided.
Home readiness	Patient can walk in a straight line. Paper and pencil tests. Maddox wing test. Simple coordination and reaction time test.
Street fitness	Flicker fusion test. Psychomotor test batteries.
Full recovery (complete psychomotor recovery)	Carefully selected psychomotor test batteries. Real driving tests.
Psychologic recovery	Psychologic tests.

Guidelines for Safe Discharge after Ambulatory Surgery

Patient's vital signs must have been stable for at least 1 hour.

Patient must have no evidence of respiratory depression.

Patient must be

- Oriented to person, place, time
- Able to maintain orally administered fluids[a]
- Able to void[a]
- Able to dress himself or herself
- Able to walk without assistance

Patient must not have

- More than minimal nausea or vomiting
- Excessive pain
- Bleeding

Patient must be discharged by both the person who administered anesthesia and the person who performed surgery, or by their designees. Written instructions for the postoperative period at home, including a contact place and person, need to be reinforced.

Patients must have responsible "vested" adult escort them home and stay with them at home.

[a] The role of these variables as criteria for discharge remains to be established.

pain or vomiting, and are able to walk by themselves, they can be discharged with an escort.[5] At discharge, the patient should be given three phone numbers: that of the surgeon, that of the ambulatory center, and that of the emergency room backup. The minimal criteria for safe discharge are summarized on the previous page.

ASSESSMENT OF RECOVERY USING COGNITIVE AND PSYCHOMOTOR TESTS

Unfortunately, we do not have cognitive or psychomotor tests that could be recommended as standard criteria for discharging patients after anesthesia for outpatient surgery. Table 17-1 presents some tests that have been used in assessing different stages of recovery.

Paper and Pencil Tests

Newman et al.[6] have described a commonly applied test that uses paper and pencil. In this test, called the Trieger test (see Fig. 1-11), patients are asked to connect a series of dots. One method of scoring the results is to add the number of dots not touched by the connecting pencil line to the time it takes to complete the drawing.

More sensitive than the Trieger test is a perceptual speed test in which the patient is instructed to circle the number shown at the beginning of the row (Fig. 17-1), with the score being the number of correct answers completed in 2 minutes.[7] A test similar to the perceptual speed test, called the "p"-deletion test, which requires the patient to cross out the letter "p" from a sheet of paper with 58 closely spaced letters in 3 minutes, has been described by Dixon and Thornton.[8]

One of the most sensitive writing tests for the detection of residual anesthetic effects is the digit symbol substitution test.[9] Patients are shown a code at the top of the form in which the numbers 1 through 9 are matched with simple symbols (Fig. 17-2). The patients are told to place the appropriate symbol below each number in the evaluation form; the score is the number of correct responses completed in, for example, 90 seconds. Current paper and pencil tests are inadequate indicators of a patient's ability to react safely when discharged after receiving anesthesia or sedation;[10] nor can such tests be recommended as guidelines for discharge without outcome studies.

Other Tests

In the tapping board test (Fig. 17-3), the patient is asked to use a stylus to tap metal target areas at alternate ends of a 55-cm board as rapidly as possible.[11,12] This test has the same problems as the paper and pencil tests in terms of the ability to measure "home readiness" or late recovery.

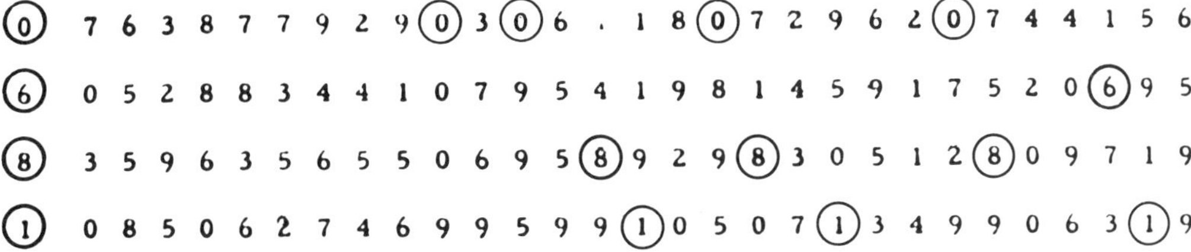

Fig. 17-1. Perceptual speed test. The subject's task is to circle the number indicated at the beginning of the row. The score is the number of correct answers completed in 2 minutes. In order to eliminate the training effect, slightly different but equivalent sheets are used when the test is repeated.

DIGIT SYMBOL SUBSTITUTION TEST	TIME	DATE			ACTUAL TIME
		MO.	DAY	YR.	A.M. P.M.

										SCORE
DIGIT	1	2	3	4	5	6	7	8	9	
SYMBOL	O	⊐	=	L	⊥	Λ	⊔	X	—	

SAMPLES

6	7	6	9	4	2	5	4	1	2	6	9	6	9	3	7	5	8	3	2	8	3	9	4	5

2	7	4	3	5	8	7	1	6	5	9	6	2	3	8	7	9	6	4	3	7	9	1	6	9

4	7	4	1	5	4	3	7	3	9	3	8	1	3	1	6	3	4	2	6	2	6	8	6	8

Fig. 17-2. Digit symbol substitution test. The subject's task is to place the appropriate symbol below each number. The score is the number of correct responses completed in, for example, 90 seconds. In order to eliminate the training effect, different symbols are used when the test is repeated.

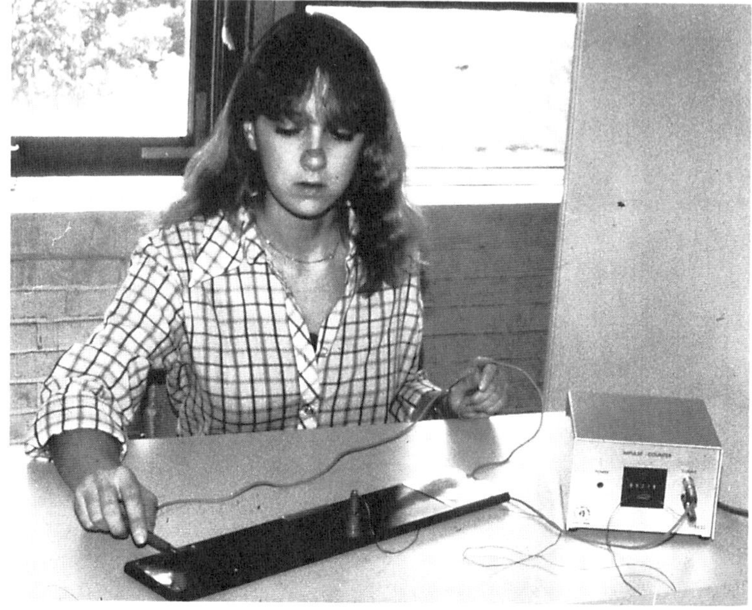

Fig. 17-3. Tapping board test. The subject is asked to use a metal stylus to tap metal target areas at alternate ends of a 55-cm board as rapidly as possible.

In the postbox test, patients are asked to pass as many of 18 shapes as possible (three each of six different shapes) in 20 seconds through the lid of a child's toy postbox.[13] This test measures both attention and eye-hand coordination.

The Maddox wing test[14] measures imbalance of extraocular muscles of the eye (Fig. 17-4). Drugs such as anesthetics decrease muscle tone and can cause the eyes to diverge. This test is relatively sensitive to the effects of benzodiazepines, but it

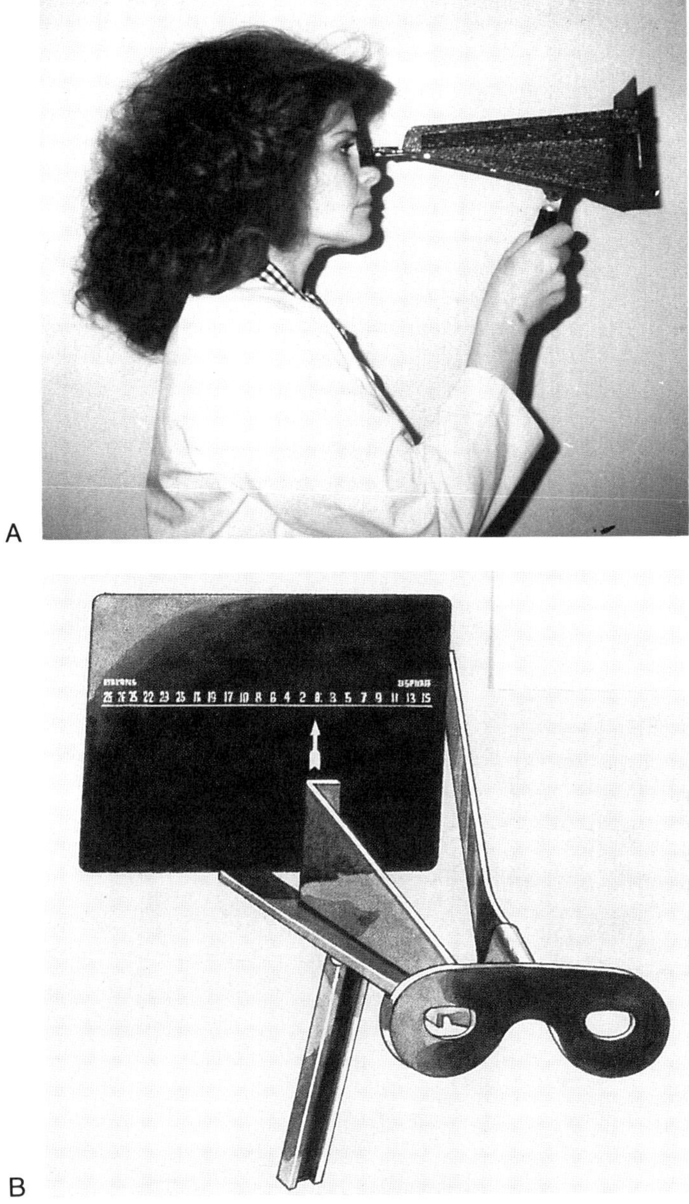

Fig. 17-4. **(A)** Maddox wing test. **(B)** The subject's right eye sees an arrow and the left eye sees a number. The subject states the number the arrow is pointing at as a measure of disconjugation of the eyes in diopters (esophoria or exophoria).

more adequately assesses relaxation of extraocular muscles than overall recovery of cognitive or psychomotor function.[15]

The flicker fusion test, which assesses a patient's ability to discriminate the fusion of flickering light, has been used to test central integral activity in many studies of drugs, including sedatives,[16] analgesics,[17] and anesthetics.[18] However, the test is difficult to perform in clinical practice and has not proved to be very helpful in assessing "home readiness" after outpatient anesthesia.

A test that records postural sway on a force platform may be useful in objectively assessing how long a patient must stay after anesthesia; however, the device is expensive, and more clinical experience with it is necessary.[12]

Although psychomotor and cognitive tests provide useful objective data on residual drug effects, their validity in assessing a patient's suitability for discharge after ambulatory surgery should be more fully documented.[19] The main problems associated with the clinical use of these tests are twofold: test results improve when tests are repeated (training effect), and the effect of individual test results vary greatly. Nevertheless, the primary purpose of these tests is to assess "home readiness" regardless of the variability in patient responses to anesthetic and analgesic drugs.

Assessment of Late Recovery

Assessment of complete recovery (e.g., when a patient is ready to drive a car or resume normal daily activities) requires sophisticated laboratory tests that cannot be used in routine clinical practice (Fig. 17-5).[20] Because it is impractical to test a patient on this level of recovery, clinicians must know which drugs have a long duration of action and prolonged residual ef-

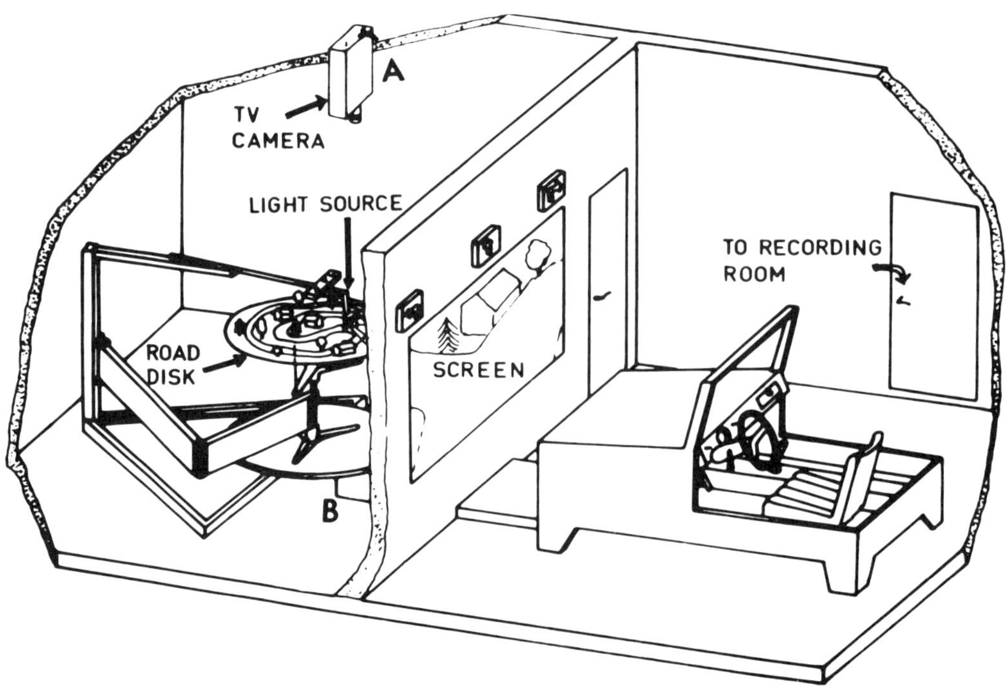

Fig. 17-5. Driving simulator test. The subject looks at a view with a road and "drives" the car on a movie screen. Safe driving skills that can be measured with this test include the ability to follow the road, obey instructions, and brake in good time.

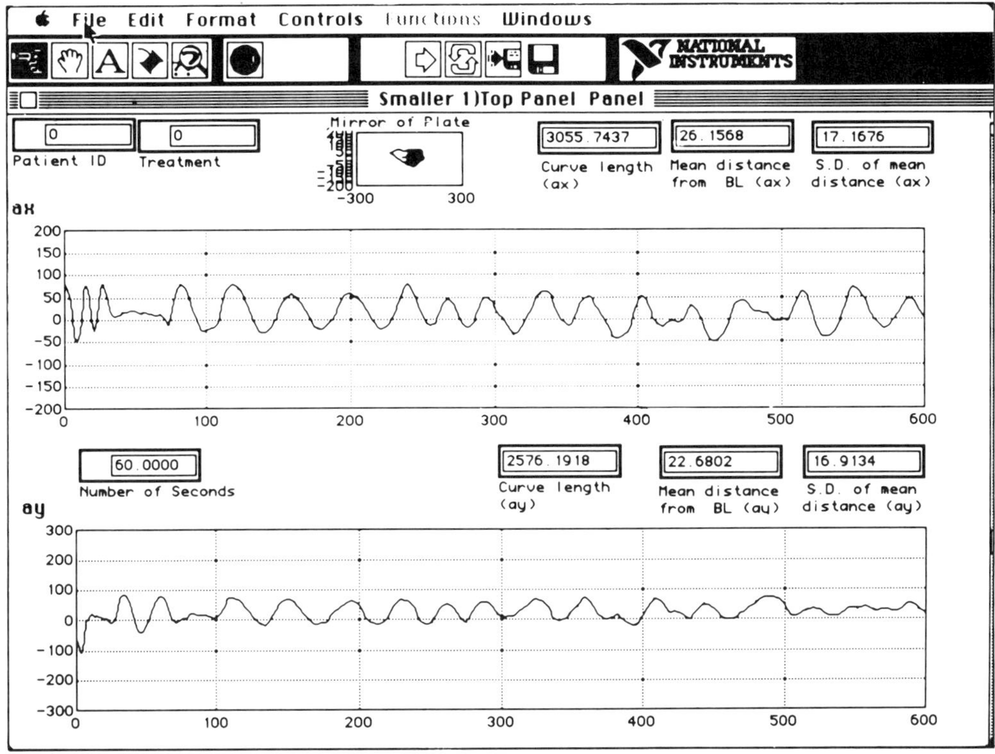

Fig. 17-6. A sample recording of body sway using a force plate and a microcomputer in which the subject tested for 60 seconds is illustrated. In this procedure, the subject stands on a force platform and his or her ability to maintain equilibrium is immediately recorded (analogue converted signals) on a computer screen. ax, sway curve in lateral direction; ay, sway curve in anteroposterior direction; mirror of plate, overall sway pattern. The computer also immediately displays curve length as well as mean and standard deviation, with the ax and ay curves representing zero.

fects.[19] Driving skills have been tested after brief anesthesia and sedation in volunteers,[17,21,22] but studies in patients undergoing anesthesia for ambulatory surgery need to be performed. Computer-assisted testing of recovery from anesthesia can be used to assess all levels of recovery (Figs. 17-6 to 17-8).

COMMON SIDE EFFECTS AND TREATMENT MODALITIES

Nausea and Vomiting

Prolonged drowsiness and fatigue are not the only reasons which delay "home readiness." Patients' discharge from the hospital may also be postponed because of nausea and vomiting or postoperative pain.[23] Although emesis may prolong the hospital stay, it rarely causes a patient to be admitted to the hospital or to return to the hospital after discharge.[19] Some clinicians believe that droperidol decreases nausea and vomiting in outpatients, and consequently they will give a dose of 0.01 mg/kg IV either prophylactically or in the recovery room; this dose can be repeated if necessary without producing extensive sedation.[24] Millar and Hall[25] suggest that 0.25 to 0.5 mg of intravenous droperidol significantly reduces postoperative nausea and vomiting without any delay in immediate recovery or discharge in patients undergoing termination of pregnancy. The total dose of dro-

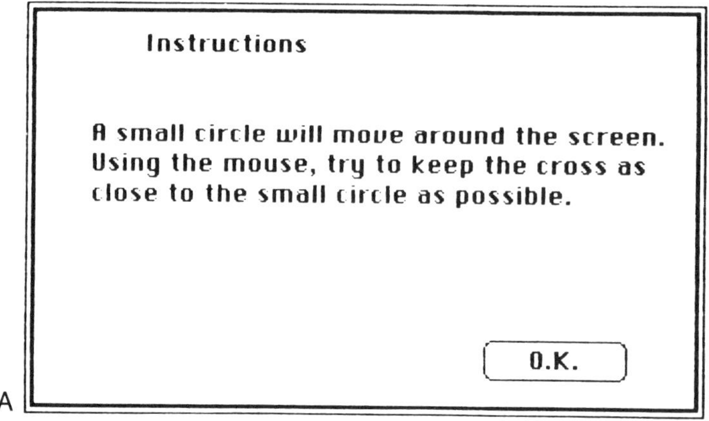

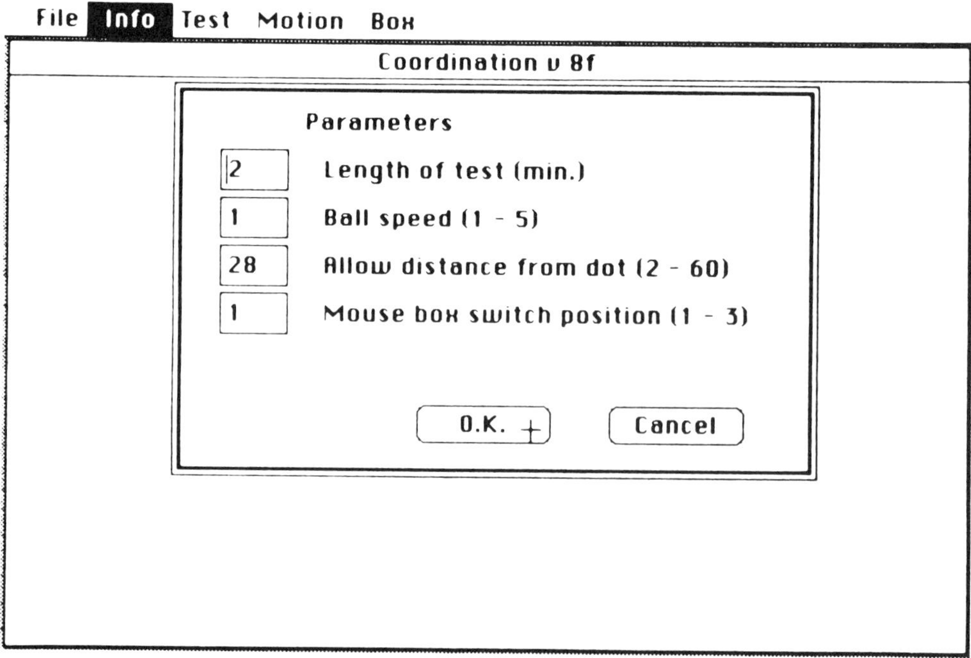

Fig. 17-7. A microcomputer, keyboard, and mouse can be used to test recovery from anesthesia. (**A**) An example of instructions for hand-eye coordination test. (**B**) The difficulty of the test (length, speed, required accuracy, etc.) can be modified to test all levels of recovery. (*Figure continues.*)

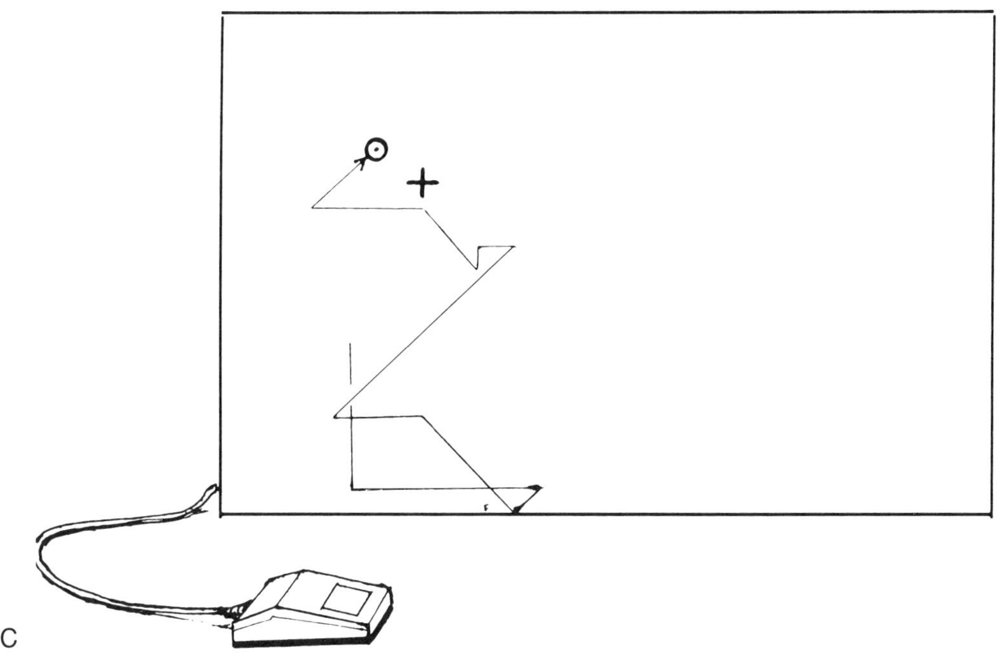

C

File Info Test Motion Box

Coordination v 8f

STATISTICS

Patient id 007-Rx

Mouse box switch position 1

Seconds outside circle 3 3

Length of test (in seconds) 120 016

Cumulative distance from center 1977 476

Mean distance from center 9 646 +/- 9 553

Mistakes 11

Press space bar to clear screen

D

Fig. 17-7 (*Continued*). **(C)** An imaginary path of the target (circle) is displayed on the screen. **(D)** Results are displayed on the screen.

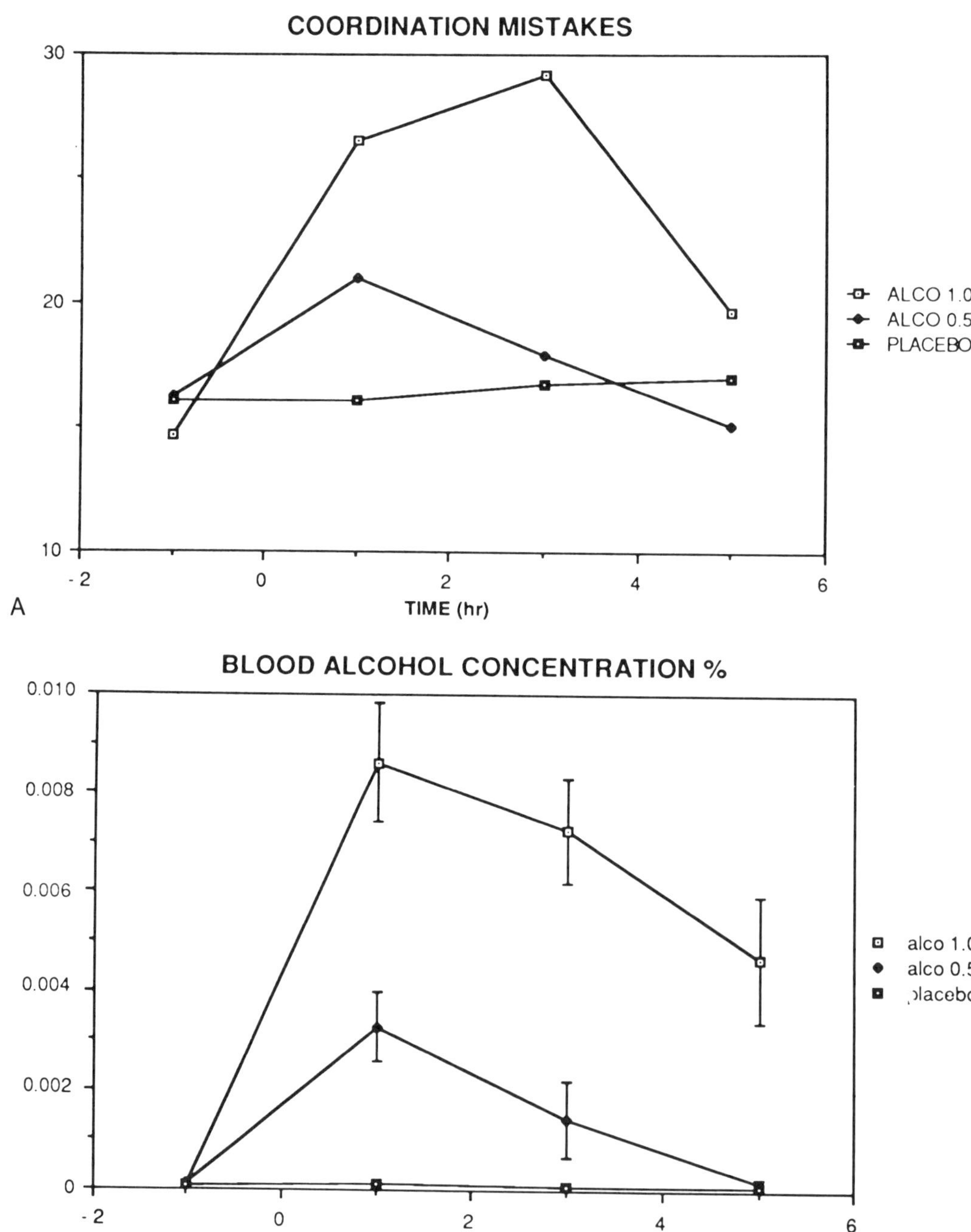

Fig. 17-8. **(A)** An example of hand-eye coordination during alcohol-induced inebriation. Mean results of 10 healthy volunteers before and after ingestion of alcohol (0.5 and 1.0 mg/kg) or placebo. **(B)** Corresponding alcohol blood levels in the same volunteers. Note that impaired hand-eye coordination is consistent with blood alcohol levels and residual effects of anesthetics can be compared with alcohol-induced inebriation when tests are applied during recovery from anesthesia.

peridol should not exceed 1.25 mg, because larger doses are likely to cause excessive drowsiness and disorientation and may jeopardize safe discharge.[26,27]

Postoperative Pain

Excessive pain after an outpatient operation may cause a patient to be admitted to the hospital unexpectedly. Postoperative pain should be controllable either with oral analgesics (e.g., acetaminophen alone or in combination with codeine, or nonsteroidal anti-inflammatory analgesics) or with one or two doses of 0.05 mg IV fentanyl. If larger doses or long-acting opioid agonists are needed for pain, it may be necessary to admit the patient to the hospital. In the same context, if the ambulatory surgical procedure is associated with postoperative pain, it may not be ideal to use anesthetics that provide ultrafast recovery because more analgesics would be needed after anesthesia than with longer-acting anesthetics.[28]

Unanticipated Hospital Admissions

The incidence of hospitalization after ambulatory surgery varies from 0.68 percent to 4.1 percent.[29] The reasons for hospital admission are usually surgical or medical rather than anesthesia related. Table 17-2 lists some reasons for unanticipated hospital admission.

CHOICES OF ANESTHESIA AND THE SPEED OF RECOVERY

Proper choice of anesthetic technique influences the time needed for patients to meet the criteria for discharge after undergoing anesthesia.

Regional Versus General Anesthesia

Studies comparing the complications with general versus regional anesthesia are difficult to design and often yield inconclusive results. However, one study suggests that the use of regional anesthesia decreases recovery times and is associated with few side effects when compared with an inhalational technique.[30] Intravenous regional anesthesia is suited for outpatient hand surgery and is associated with earlier discharge. Although patients can be discharged quickly after regional anesthetic techniques, the long-acting local anesthetics may impair psychomotor performance for at least 2 hours.[31]

Premedication

If rapid recovery is desired, it is best to avoid premedication. Meridy[32] retrospectively studied 1,553 ambulatory surgical patients and reported that patients who received either meperidine or morphine premedication were discharged 30 minutes

Table 17-2. Reasons for Unanticipated Hospital Admission

Reason for Admission	Details
Surgical	More extensive surgery, positive biopsy results. Problems (bleeding, uterine perforation, bowel burn, bladder puncture).
Medical	Pre-existing disease (poorly controlled diabetes). Perioperative complications (chest pain, dysrhythmias).
Anesthesia	Prolonged nausea and vomiting, intractable pain, slow recovery and prolonged somnolence, aspiration.
Social	Patient's request, surgeon's request, no escort.

later than patients who received no premedication. Discharge criteria were not presented in that study. In a prospective study, however, Clark and Hurtig[33] found no difference in home readiness in patients premedicated with meperidine and atropine for outpatient surgery compared with patients who received no premedication. When meperidine (versus saline) premedication was used, less diazepam was needed to provide proper sedation in patients undergoing hand surgery under intravenous regional anesthesia,[34] which may in part explain why meperidine does not necessarily prolong recovery.

In one study, scopolamine was found less appropriate for outpatients than atropine because of its comparatively prolonged residual effects on cognitive performance.[35] However, discharge criteria were not presented in that study. In another study, patients who had been given glycopyrrolate showed no significant cognitive changes after surgery, whereas those who received atropine (1.6 mg) showed short-term postoperative memory deficit.[36]

Although premedication with diazepam[32] or meperidine[33] may not delay discharge, both drugs have a long duration of action and may impair cognitive and psychomotor performance after patients are discharged from the hospital.[17] Lorazepam premedication is not recommended for day surgery because it may cause prolonged fatigue and has lingering residual effects on psychomotor skills.[37] In contrast, intramuscular midazolam 5 mg (versus saline) does not delay recovery after short outpatient procedures under general anesthesia.[38] Lichtor et al.[39] studied the effect of intravenous midazolam premedication on recovery in patients undergoing ambulatory laparoscopic tubal ligation and found that time to discharge home was not affected by intravenous midazolam when compared with a control group receiving saline.

Choice of Local Anesthetic Agents

Effects of local anesthetics can contribute to delayed recovery and impaired psychomotor skills after day surgery. On the other hand, the surgical procedure itself may be associated with impaired cognitive skills. Kjaergård et al.[40] showed that patients' postural stability after hand surgery was impaired for up to 40 minutes after perivascular axillary block using mepivacaine with epinephrine. Delayed reaction times seen after local dental anesthesia are believed to result from the stress of the procedure regardless of the local anesthetic used.[41,42] However, adjunctive use of sedative-hypnotic drugs for sedation may have contributed to the postural instability.

Studies in healthy volunteers indicate that in high doses some local anesthetics may impair psychomotor skills. Psychomotor performance was impaired for 1 to 1.5 hours after 200 mg of plain lidocaine, whereas 500 mg of lidocaine with epinephrine or 3 mg/kg plain mepivacaine or 3 mg/kg prilocaine did not impair psychomotor skills.[43,44] Similar studies with long-acting local anesthetics suggest that bupivacaine (1.3 mg/kg) and etidocaine (2.6 mg/kg) may impair psychomotor performance for at least 2 hours.[45] Cognitive or psychomotor skills have not been assessed after 2-chloroprocaine, which is commonly used in the United States, but it is likely to have no or only minimal residual effects owing to its rapid breakdown in plasma, presumably by circulating esterase.[46]

In clinical practice it is unlikely that fatigue caused by systemic effects of local anesthetics delays safe discharge of patients, but one should not have a false sense of security that local anesthetics (e.g., large doses of bupivacaine for peripheral nerve blocks) do not affect complete recovery.

Choice of Inhaled Agents

Because of its rapid recovery time, nitrous oxide offers an ideal supplementation for outpatient anesthesia.[12,47,48] For example, supplementation of intravenous anesthesia with nitrous oxide enables the use of lower dosages of intravenous anesthetics, which consequently results in more rapid recovery and in fewer residual effects.[49]

Low concentrations of nitrous oxide are used with oxygen in dentistry. Recovery from such low concentrations is fast but not instantaneous.[11] In healthy volunteers, a distinct impairment in hand-eye coordination 12 minutes after cessation of the administration of 30 percent nitrous oxide (Fig. 17-9) suggests that even young and healthy outpatients need supervision for at least 20 to 30 minutes after nitrous oxide sedation and analgesia.

Carter et al.[13] compared the use of halothane, enflurane, and isoflurane to supplement methohexitone–nitrous-oxide–oxygen anesthesia in patients undergoing dilatation and curettage. They found no major differences in the three groups in terms of recovery when they assessed patients with the p-deletion and postbox tests. Patients undergoing outpatient oral surgery were able to ambulate better after isoflurane than after enflurane anesthesia (Fig. 17-10).[50]

Theoretically, the duration of administration should affect rapidity of recovery after inhalational anesthesia because the pharmacokinetics of inhaled anesthetics depend on the length of time they are administered.[51] Carpenter et al. studied healthy

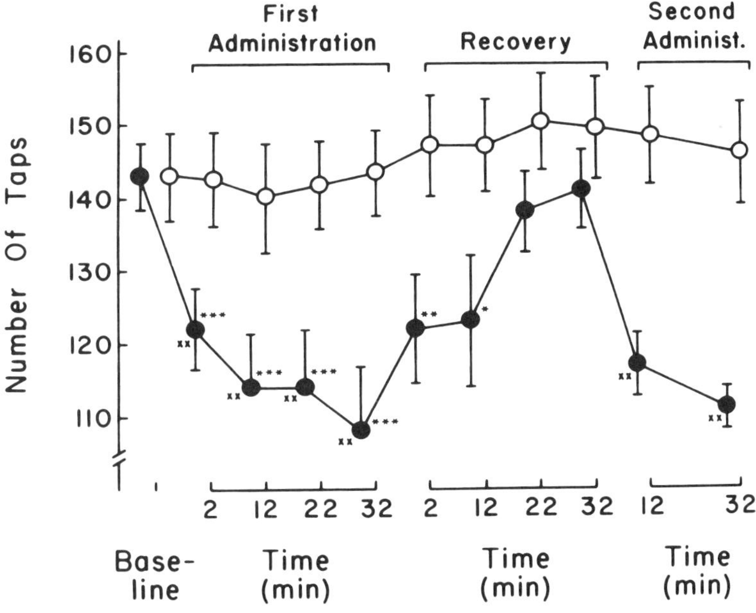

Fig. 17-9. Recovery time from nitrous oxide as indicated by the results of the tapping board test. The graph shows the mean number of taps recorded through the first and second administrations of 30 percent nitrous oxide (●) or oxygen (○). Note that during recovery it takes 22 to 32 minutes after discontinuation of nitrous oxide for hand coordination to return to baseline. (From Korttila et al.,[11] with permission.)

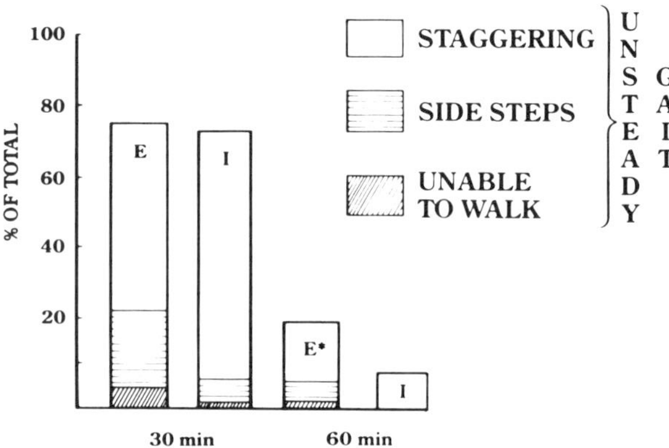

Fig. 17-10. Chart showing percentage of patients with unsteady gait 30 to 60 minutes after anesthesia with enflurane (E) or isoflurane (I) for outpatient restorative dentistry and/or oral surgery. An asterisk indicates a significance of $P < .05$ for unsteady gait after enflurane compared with isoflurane. After 60 minutes, patients who had received isoflurane were ambulating better than those who had received enflurane. (From Valanne and Korttila,[50] with permission).

volunteers and found that the alveolar washout was more rapid after a 30-minute administration of halothane or isoflurane compared with a 120-minute administration (Fig. 17-11). Clinically, the rapidity of recovery with enflurane was influenced more by the duration of anesthesia than was the case with isoflurane.[50] Prolonged enflurane anesthesia (more than 90 minutes) was associated with slower recovery than enflurane anesthesia administered over brief periods (less than 40 minutes). Equally prolonged isoflurane anesthesia did not appear to be associated with delayed recovery.[51]

Sevoflurane is less soluble in blood than isoflurane and might prove useful for outpatients in allowing a faster recovery. However, sevoflurane is not stable in soda lime, and additional toxicologic studies are required to evaluate its products of degradation.[52] The other new inhaled anesthetic, I-653, is even less soluble to blood than sevoflurane,[53] and studies in rats[54] suggest that recovery from I-653 is likely to be very rapid in humans.

Choice of Intravenous Agents

Before the introduction of propofol, intravenous anesthetics were used more often for induction than for maintenance of anesthesia.

Although waking and clinical recovery are more rapid with methohexital than with thiopental, complete recovery (e.g., normalization of driving skills) takes the same length of time when both agents are administered for brief periods.[21,55,56] Because metabolites of methohexital do not contribute to its prolonged action on the central nervous system,[57] it is likely that the parent compound itself is responsible for these effects, although it disappears faster from blood than thiopental.[58] If repeated injections or infusions of barbiturates are used to maintain anesthesia, the shorter elimination halflife of methohexital, compared with that of thiopental, is likely to be associated with faster overall and complete recovery. Because methohexital causes more pain on injection, as well as more hiccough and movement, most anesthesiolo-

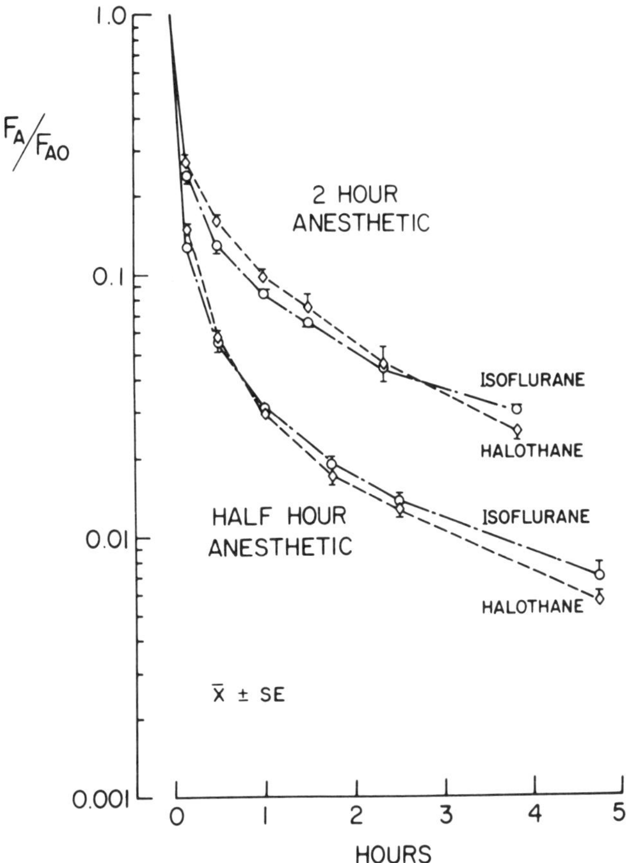

Fig. 17-11. Rate of elimination of inhaled agents after short and long periods of anesthesia. The decline in the alveolar concentration is expressed as a ratio of the alveolar concentration at a given time (F_A) to the alveolar concentration immediately before discontinuation of anesthetic (F_{AO}) and is plotted against time for both the 30-minute (n = 7) and 2-hour (n = 9) anesthetic administrations. Note that the F_A/F_{AO} ratio decreases more rapidly after the shorter anesthetic administration with both halothane and isoflurane. (From Carpenter et al.,[51] with permission.)

gists prefer to use thiopental rather than methohexital for anesthesia induction in outpatients.

Large doses of ketamine (> 2 mg/kg IV in adults or > 8 mg/kg IM in children) should be avoided (if possible) in ambulatory practice because ketamine has greater residual effects on performance than thiopental.[59]

Because of the relatively high incidence of pain on injection and of involuntary muscle movements, etomidate must be combined with other agents to produce satisfactory anesthesia without side effects.[60] Recovery from such combinations may not be faster than that from thiopental alone, which tends to restrict the use of etomidate in ambulatory practice.

Propofol has a short elimination halflife, and recovery from propofol may be faster than from thiopental or methohexital anesthesia.[61,62] However, such a quick recovery

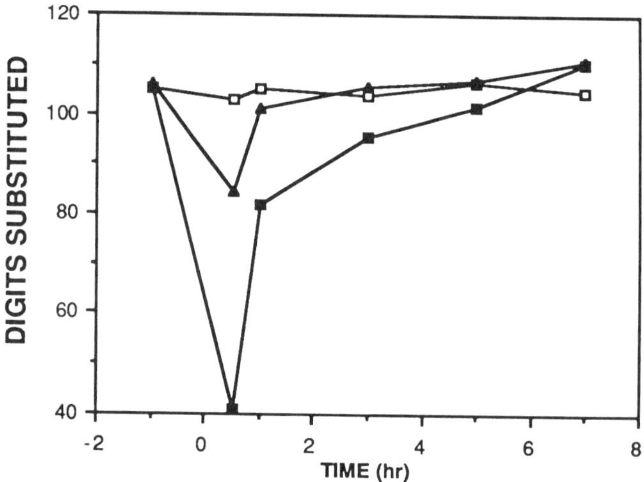

Fig. 17-12. Recovery of cognitive and psychomotor performance after intravenous anesthesia. Plotting represents the number of digits substituted in the digit symbol substitution test (see text) before administration of and at intervals of 30 minutes and 1, 3, 5, and 7 hours after injection of either saline (control) (□), propofol (▲, 2.5 plus 1.0 mg/kg), or thiopental (■, 5.0 plus 2.0 mg/kg). Note that performance returns near baseline and near control 1 hour after propofol anesthesia, whereas it takes as long as 5 hours to reach baseline and control after thiopental anesthesia. (From Korttila et al.,[65] with permission.)

has not been reported by all investigators.[63,64] Logan et al.[64] compared propofol (3 mg/kg) with methohexital (2 mg/kg) as a single-shot intravenous anesthetic in patients undergoing outpatient dental surgery and did not find any difference in several parameters of recovery 40 minutes after propofol or methohexital anesthesia. However, recent studies in healthy volunteers[65] indicate that recovery (ambulation as well as cognitive and psychomotor performance) from propofol is definitely faster than from thiopental (Figs. 17-12 and 17-13) and may be faster than from methohexital. Agreeing with the volunteer study,[65] Millar and Jewkes[66] recently confirmed that day surgery patients are fit for discharge faster if propofol or propofol with alfentanil is used for brief urologic or gynecologic procedures instead of thiopental with enflurane. If the induction of propofol anesthesia is followed by maintenance of anesthesia with inhaled anesthetics (e.g., enflurane), there is no difference between methohexital and propofol in rapidity of recovery or time to discharge.[67] However, if anesthesia is induced and maintained with intravenous agents, propofol allows the patient to recover and walk sooner than with methohexital anesthesia.[68] Similarly, when propofol was used for induction and maintenance of anesthesia in patients undergoing ambulatory surgery, patients receiving propofol infusions (6 to 9 mg/kg/hr) had less nausea and vomiting and were ready for discharge approximately 1 hour sooner than patients receiving thiopental for induction and isoflurane for maintenance of anesthesia during similar procedures (Table 17-3).[69] Doze et al.[70] reported significantly less psychomotor impairment after propofol-nitrous oxide versus thiopental–isoflurane–nitrous-oxide general anesthesia, and concluded that the rapid recovery profile for propofol following its use during short nonmajor procedures makes it a useful alternative for ambulatory surgery.

Many outpatients will not undergo re-

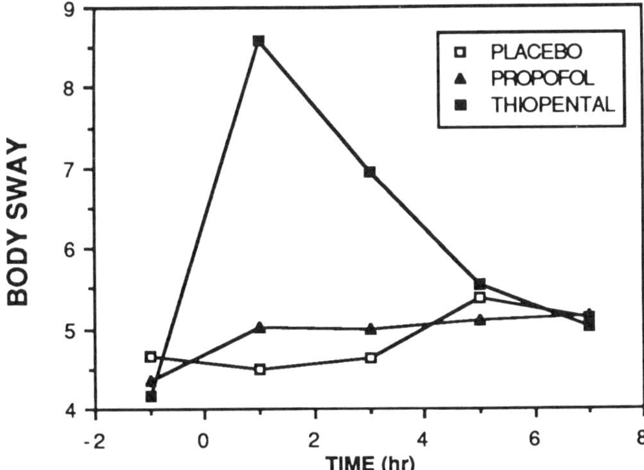

Fig. 17-13. Ability to stand after intravenous anesthesia and sedation. Plotting indicates body sway (mean sway units of 12 volunteers) when standing on a force platform before and 1, 3, 5, and 7 hours after saline (control), propofol (2.5 plus 1.0 mg/kg), or thiopental (5.0 plus 2.0 mg/kg) anesthesia. Note that body sway (i.e., ability to maintain equilibrium) is not affected 1 hour or later after propofol anesthesia, whereas it takes as long as 5 hours after thiopental anesthesia until body sway returns to baseline and control. (From Korttila et al.,[65] with permission.)

gional anesthetic techniques without sedation.[71] So far, diazepam has been the intravenous sedative chosen most often for such purposes. Midazolam has recently gained popularity as an intravenous sedative because of its shorter halflife in blood and the rare incidence of venous irritation and phlebitis after its administration.[71]

Clinicians should be aware that the rapid disappearance of midazolam from blood is not related to a more rapid recovery after intravenous sedation.[72,73] With patients

Table 17-3. Recovery from Propofol Infusions Versus Thiopental-Isoflurane in Patients Undergoing Outpatient Anesthesia

	Propofol	Thiopental-Isoflurane
Patients		
No.	19	30
Age (yr)	34 ± 2.9	35 ± 1.7
Weight (kg)	70 ± 3.0	63 ± 2.4
Duration of anesthesia	85 ± 12[a]	57 ± 5.2
Recovery[b]		
Response to command	3.5 ± 0.6[a]	6.1 ± 0.6
Eyes open	4.0 ± 0.7[a]	6.3 ± 0.6
Able to sit	59 ± 5.3	73 ± 6.5
Able to stand	68 ± 6.0	87 ± 8.0
Able to walk	70 ± 7.2	96 ± 9.6
Tolerates oral fluids	61 ± 4.5[a]	130 ± 17
Able to void	102 ± 15[a]	173 ± 16
Ready for discharge	138 ± 18[a]	206 ± 16

[a] $P < .05$ versus thiopental-isoflurane.
[b] Minutes after cessation of nitrous oxide administration.
(From Korttila et al.,[69] with permission.)

Table 17-4. Ambulation After Intravenous Sedation for Bronchoscopy

	Diazepam (0.2 mg/kg)	Midazolam (0.05 mg/kg)	Midazolam (0.1 mg/kg)
No. of patients	27	25	24
Unable to stand steadily (%)			
After 30 min	56	32	67[a]
After 60 min	7	17	17
After 120 min	0	0	8
Unable to walk along a straight line (%)			
After 30 min	63	56	83
After 60 min	22	20	58[b]
After 120 min	0	4	17[c]

[a] $P < .05$ versus midazolam 0.05 mg/kg.
[b] $P < .05$ versus diazepam and midazolam 0.05 mg/kg.
[c] $P < .05$ versus diazepam.
(From Korttila and Tarkkanen,[72] with permission.)

who had bronchoscopic examinations, immediate clinical recovery, which entailed standing and walking in a straight line, after midazolam sedation was similar or prolonged compared with patients receiving equivalent doses of diazepam (Table 17-4).[72] In another study in which recovery was evaluated thoroughly with six psychomotor tests repeated over 5 hours, there was no evidence that the midazolam-treated group recovered more quickly than the diazepam-treated groups.[73] Animal studies indicate that both diazepam and midazolam occupy receptors rapidly and disappear from receptors at the same rate (Fig. 17-14),[74] paralleling the onset and duration of the sedative and amnesic properties of these drugs after acute administration to humans.[31,71] It is possible that the "hangover" effect of diazepam results in part from its long acting principal metabolite. Clinical sedation can also recur as a result of increased diazepam blood levels after food intake (Fig. 17-15) when diazepam is used for intravenous sedation,[75] a phenomenon that may not occur with midazolam.

Muscle Relaxants and Recovery

In the past, succinylcholine was the only muscle relaxant applicable for outpatient anesthesia. Pancuronium or other long-acting, nondepolarizing muscle relaxants should be avoided in ambulatory practice because it is not clear to what extent and for how long possible residual relaxation[76,77] may impair psychomotor skills in some patients. Today it appears that both atracurium and vecuronium are suitable for ambulatory surgery[78,79] and are unlikely to cause residual relaxation, which might impair psychomotor skills.[80] Ali et al.[81] have shown that spontaneous recovery after mivacurium chloride, a new short-acting, nondepolarizing muscle relaxant, is twice as fast as that of comparable doses of atracurium or vecuronium. Mivacurium may be useful in day surgery.[81,82]

Inhaled Versus Intravenous Agents

Simpson et al.[83] compared recovery of mental efficiency (performance in three different paper and pencil tests) after either thiopental–fentanyl–pancuronium–nitrous-oxide or thiopental–halothane–nitrous-oxide anesthesia in patients undergoing hernia repair. At first there was an advantage for the fentanyl group in that they awoke earlier, but after 6 hours the halothane patients were equal to them in per-

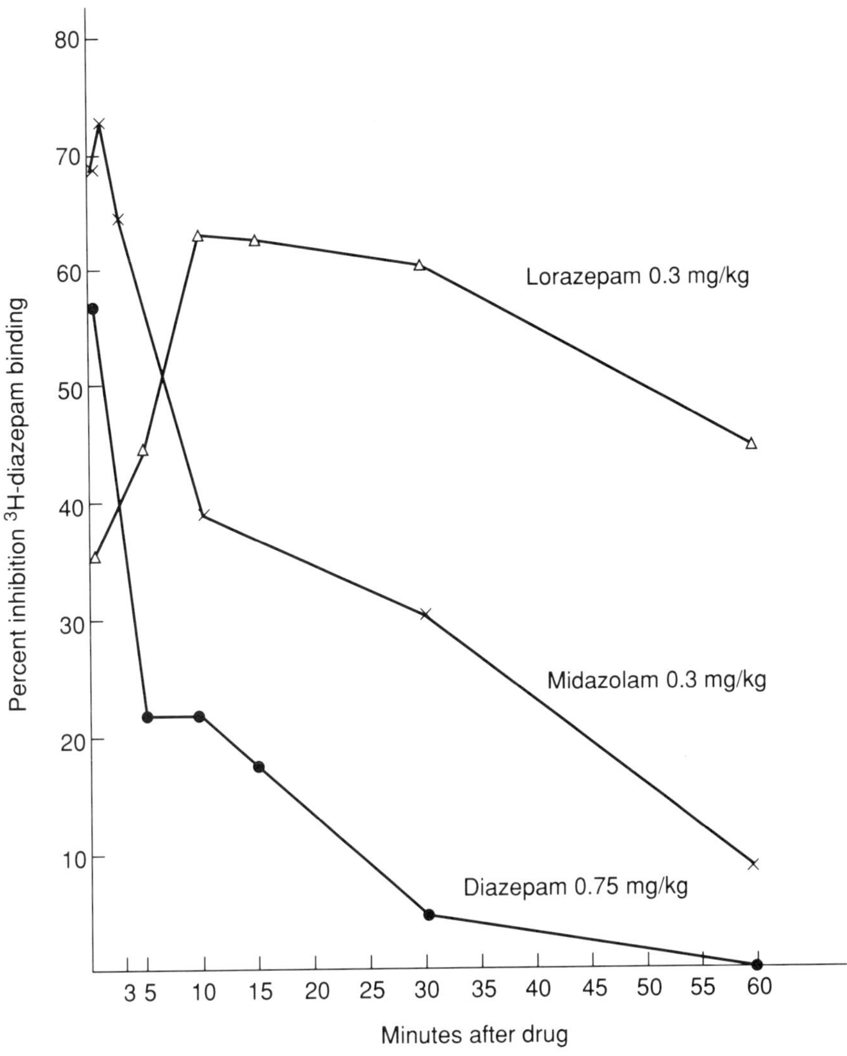

Fig. 17-14. Ex vivo receptor binding profile after intravenous administration of three benzodiazepines. The percent inhibition of ^{3}H-diazepam binding in rat cortex is shown as a function of time following intravenous administration of diazepam, midazolam, and lorazepam to 150-g male rats. Note that both diazepam and midazolam occupy receptors rapidly and disappear from them relatively quickly, whereas lorazepam both occupies and disappears slowly from benzodiazepine receptors. (From Jack et al.,[74] with permission.)

formance and from that point improved more rapidly than the fentanyl group.

Metter et al.[23] also found no difference in times of discharge in outpatients after isoflurane or fentanyl–nitrous-oxide–oxygen anesthesia for laparoscopic examination. When Moss et al.[84] used alfentanil and Zuurmond and Leeuwen[85] used sufentanil to maintain anesthesia, they reported that emergence (awakening) was more rapid when the newer narcotics were used as part of a "balanced" anesthetic compared with inhalational techniques with halothane or isoflurane; however, no differences were

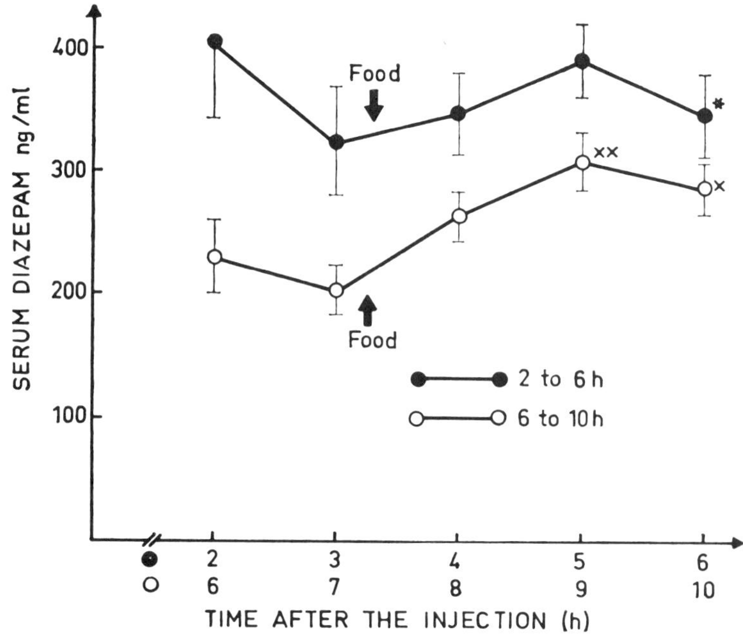

Fig. 17-15. Serum diazepam concentrations (means ± SEM) of seven subjects at 2, 3, 4, 5, and 6 hours (●) and 6, 7, 8, 9, and 10 hours (○) after intravenous injection with diazepam 0.3 mg/kg. Arrows indicate food intake. Note that food intake 3 or 7 hours after sedation increases diazepam blood levels. (From Korttila et al.,[75] with permission.)

noted with respect to "home readiness." As mentioned earlier, propofol infusions have been compared with thiopental-isoflurane anesthesia in patients having ambulatory surgery,[69,70] and the results indicate that propofol anesthesia provides faster recovery than isoflurane anesthesia. When the criteria for home readiness were followed (see guidelines on page 370), patients were discharged approximately 1 hour earlier after propofol than after isoflurane.[69]

Discharge After Regional Anesthesia

Patients recovering from regional anesthesia must meet the same discharge criteria as do patients who are discharged after general anesthesia (see guidelines on page 370). Extremity or major peripheral nerve block is seldom associated with delayed recovery or problems meeting the discharge criteria. Although the use of peripheral nerve block techniques are well-accepted, many ambulatory surgery centers try to avoid using spinal or epidural anesthesia because urinary retention and postspinal headache may occur later, when the patient is at home. However, some investigators think that spinal anesthesia is extremely well-suited to the outpatient setting.[86]

If spinal or epidural anesthesia has been used for outpatient surgery, it is important to determine when the patient can safely walk. Hypotension and syncope may occur if the sympathetic nervous system is still blocked when the patient stands up. Obviously, a patient must recover proprioception and motor function for standing, walking, and use of the toilet. Actually, a patient's ability to walk to the bathroom and urinate may be the best recovery test after epidural or spinal anesthesia, because these abilities reflect the recovery of motor and sympathetic function.

Obviously, no motor block should be present when a patient tries to stand or walk. The ability to move the legs and feet freely is indication that the motor block is no longer functioning. To test this, one can ask the patient to touch both the right and left heel to the opposite big toe and to run each heel up and down the opposite leg to the knee.[87] After spinal anesthesia, it is of utmost importance that young outpatients be warned about the possibility of spinal headache; a follow-up telephone call the day after surgery is helpful in documenting the absence of headache.

In one study, patients who had outpatient laparoscopic examination were discharged home earlier after chloroprocaine epidural anesthesia than those given general anesthesia.[30] As discussed earlier in this chapter, one must remember that the central nervous system effects of local anesthetics may prolong complete recovery after regional anesthetics.

ANTAGONISTS

If anesthetic and analgesic drugs are properly titrated, antagonist drugs are of limited clinical value. Although they effectively reverse the residual effects of intravenously administered sedatives or general anesthetics, the postoperative benefits are unproven.

The duration of action of naloxone is too short to warrant its routine use in outpatient anesthesia, and a rebound effect may occur in narcotic action as the action of naloxone wears off. Nalmefene, an experimental narcotic antagonist, is longer acting than naloxone and may prove useful in the outpatient setting.[83] It has been studied in volunteers,[88,89] and it should be studied in outpatients to ascertain its effectiveness for ambulatory surgery.

Aminophylline may partially reverse oversedation caused by benzodiazepines,[90,91] but is does not seem to hasten the recovery of outpatients. Similarly, aminophylline has been suggested to reduce the depth and duration of sedation with barbiturates in patients undergoing termination of pregnancy,[92] but further studies are needed to assess if this drug has any clinical implications in outpatient surgery.

The recently synthesized selective benzodiazepine receptor antagonists are effective in reversing residual benzodiazepine-induced sedation and amnesia. Preliminary clinical studies have tested flumazenil's (RO-1788) ability to reverse benzodiazepine sedation, and some have also assessed its use in day surgery.[93–95] In patients having urologic surgery who received midazolam for sedation, flumazenil produced immediate reversal of residual sedation and improved the ability to respond to verbal commands.[95] However, these antagonists must be studied in more detail before one can estimate their applicability in ambulatory practice. The brevity of flumazenil's action may be a drawback for use with outpatients because its duration may not be long enough to guarantee permanent reversal of benzodiazepine sedation.[96] Pharmacokinetic studies indicate that the elimination halflife of flumazenil is approximately 1 hour,[97] which may explain signs of "rebound" sedation when benzodiazepine sedation is reversed with this antagonist. Raeder et al.[98] gave total intravenous anesthesia using midazolam and alfentanil in patients undergoing outpatient dilatation and curettage. With flumazenil reversal, patients woke up faster, cooperated better, and were less tranquil 15 to 30 minutes after anesthesia (Fig. 17-16). However, no difference in recovery parameters was noted 7 hours after operation. Although flumazenil reversed sedation and tranquillity, it did not reverse impaired performance on cognitive and psychomotor tests, suggesting that flumazenil may not reverse all benzodiazepine effects. Additional studies must be per-

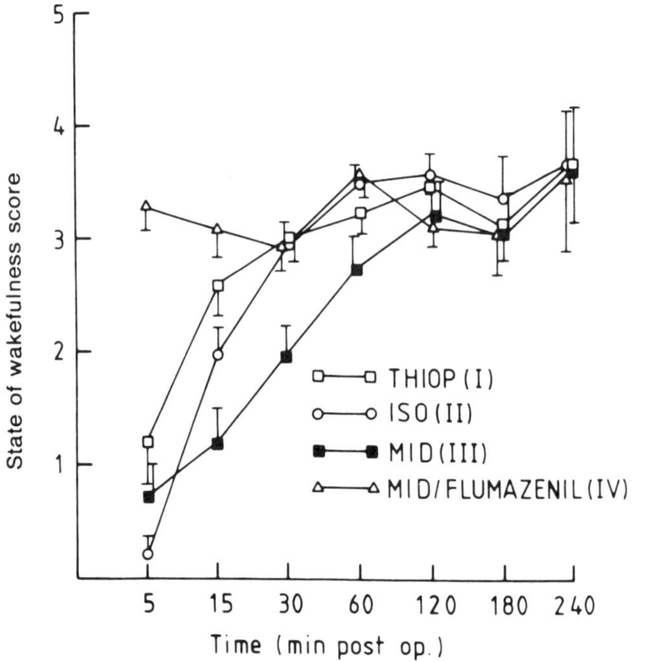

Fig. 17-16. The influence of flumazenil on awakening. The graph shows the state of wakefulness (0, not arousable; 1, arousable after tactile stimulus; 2, arousable after verbal stimulus; 3, sleepy or drowsy; 4, awake, normal; and 5, awake, agitated) after four different anesthetic techniques in patients undergoing outpatient dilatation and curettage. I, alfentanil plus thiopental; II, alfentanil, midazolam plus isoflurane; III, alfentanil plus midazolam and saline for reversal; and IV, alfentanil plus midazolam and flumazenil (0.5 mg) for reversal. Note that with flumazenil, reversal patients woke up faster and were less sedated 15 to 30 minutes after anesthesia compared with other groups, but no difference was noted 2 hours after anesthesia. (From Raeder et al.,[98] with permission.)

formed with flumazenil in volunteers and day surgery patients.

DRIVING AFTER ANESTHESIA

To assess the effects of anesthesia on driving, several studies have been performed to measure psychomotor skills in healthy volunteers after they were exposed to different analgesics, sedatives, and anesthetics.[20,31] Many drugs impaired psychomotor and cognitive skills for as long as 10 to 12 hours after administration. When a sensitive choice–reaction-time test was used in patients who had hernia repair during halothane anesthesia, it was reported that reaction times were impaired for as long as 1 or 2 days after surgery.[99] However, from these results it cannot be concluded whether such impaired reaction times resulted from surgery and anesthesia or from bedrest, because bedrest alone has been shown to be associated with substantial impairment of cognitive and psychomotor function.[100]

In recent years, it has been recommended that patients not drive after anesthesia and sedation for periods ranging between 24 and 48 hours. A convenient guideline is the following: if the duration of anesthesia is less than 30 minutes, patients should refrain from driving for 24 hours; if the duration of anesthesia is 2 hours or more, it is safer to advise patients not to drive for at least 48 hours.

LEGAL CONSIDERATIONS

Timely discharge is important in outpatient anesthesia (Table 17-2). An interesting study in Scotland in 1972 reported that 31 percent of 100 ambulatory surgical patients who had halothane anesthesia went home unescorted. Of 41 car owners, 9 percent drove themselves home and 73 percent drove within 24 hours.[101]

Recently, a case of premature discharge resulted in litigation when a patient had dental extraction with methohexital–nitrous-oxide–oxygen anesthesia. The patient was discharged unaccompanied, fell, and had a knee fracture. A $40,000 settlement was reached in 1982.[102] Thus, it is important that all safety measures are implemented and that they are documented in the patient's medical record. To protect against a possible challenge of inappropriate discharge, a physician (or the recovery room nurse) must have evidence that he or she carefully assessed the patient for home readiness.

SUMMARY

In the near future, it is likely that almost 50 percent of all surgery will be performed as day surgery. To provide safe discharge after longer and more extensive operations performed in ambulatory surgical facilities, the clinician must carefully evaluate patients for home readiness and instruct them in such a way that they receive and understand all relevant information. Minimal criteria for discharge home should be established by every surgical facility. Today, we do not have cognitive or psychomotor tests that could be recommended as standard criteria for discharging patients after anesthesia for ambulatory surgery; we have to rely on clinical criteria in assessment of home readiness. When patients have tolerated oral fluids and voided, have no excessive pain or vomiting, and are able to walk out by themselves, they can be discharged with an escort. If a patient does not have an escort home, the procedure should be canceled or the patient should be admitted to the hospital. Recommendations not to drive after anesthesia or sedation vary between 24 and 48 hours, depending on the duration of anesthesia. As the complexity of cases and scheduled surgical procedures increases, patient safety and satisfaction probably will depend to an even greater degree on anesthesiologists' medical skills and administrative abilities.

REFERENCES

1. Wetchler BV (ed): Preface. Anesthesia for Ambulatory Surgery. JB Lippincott, Philadelphia, 1985
2. Joint Commission of Accreditation of Hospitals: Ambulatory Health Care Standards Manual, Standards No. 9: Surgical and Anesthesia Services, Chicago, 1986
3. Aldrete JA, Kroulik D: A postoperative recovery score. Anesth Analg 49:924, 1970
4. Korttila K: The outpatient facility. p. 339. In Brown B, Nunn J, Utting J (eds): General Anaesthesia. 5th Ed. Butterworths, 1988
5. Korttila K: Practical discharge criteria. Probl Anesth 2:144, 1988
6. Newman MG, Trieger N, Miller JC: Measuring recovery from anesthesia—a simple test. Anesth Analg 48:136, 1969
7. Gelfman SS, Gracely RH, Driscoll EJ, et al: Comparison of recovery test after intravenous sedation with diazepam-methohexital and diazepam-methohexital and fentanyl. J Oral Surg 37:391, 1979
8. Dixon RA, Thornton JA: Tests of recovery from anaesthesia and sedation: intravenous diazepam in dentistry. Br J Anaesth 45:207, 1973
9. Wechsler Adult Intelligence Scale Revised Record Form. Psychological Corporation, New York, 1981

10. Korttila K: Recovery after intravenous sedation: a comparison of clinical and paper and pencil tests used in assessing late effects of diazepam. Anaesthesia 21:31, 1976
11. Korttila K, Ghoneim MM, Jacobs L, et al: Time course of mental and psychomotor effects of 30 percent nitrous oxide during inhalation and recovery. Anesthesiology 54:220, 1981
12. Korttila K, Ghoneim MM, Jacobs L, Lakes RS: Evaluation of instrumented force platform as a test to measure residual effects of anesthetics. Anesthesiology 55:625, 1981
13. Carter JA, Dye AM, Cooper M: Recovery from day-case anaesthesia. The effect of different inhalational agents. Anaesthesia 40:545, 1985
14. Hannington-Kiff JG: Measurement of recovery from outpatient general anaesthesia with a simple ocular test. Br Med J 3:132, 1970
15. Hannington-Kiff JG: Residual postoperative paralysis. Proc R Soc Med 63:73, 1970
16. Korttila K, Linnoila M: Psychomotor skills related to driving after intravenous sedation: dose-response relationship with diazepam. Br J Anaesth 47:457, 1975
17. Korttila K, Linnoila M: Psychomotor skills related to driving after intramuscular administration of diazepam and meperidine. Anesthesiology 42:685, 1975
18. Grove-White IG, Kelman KR: Critical flicker frequency after small doses of methohexitone, diazepam and sodium-4-hydroxybutyrate. Br J Anaesth 43:110, 1971
19. Korttila K: How to assess recovery from anesthesia. p. 1. In Barash P (ed): American Society of Anesthesiologists Refresher Course Lectures. Vol 16. JB Lippincott, Philadelphia 1988
20. Korttila K: Recovery and driving after brief anaesthesia. Anaesthesist 30:377, 1982
21. Korttila K, Linnoila M, Ertama P, Häkkinen S: Recovery and simulated driving after intravenous anesthesia with thiopental, methohexital, propanidid or alphadione. Anesthesiology 43:291, 1975
22. Korttila K, Tammisto T, Ertama P, et al: Recovery, psychomotor skills, and simulated driving after brief inhalational anesthesia with halothane or enflurane in combination with nitrous oxide and oxygen. Anesthesiology 46:20, 1977
23. Metter SE, Kitz DS, Young ML, et al: Nausea and vomiting after outpatient laparoscopy: incidence, impact on recovery room stay and cost. Anesth Analg 66:S116, 1987
24. Valanne J, Korttila K: Effect of a small dose of droperidol on nausea, vomiting and recovery after outpatient enflurane anesthesia. Acta Anaesthesiol Scand 29:359, 1985
25. Millar JM, Hall PJ: Nausea and vomiting after prostaglandins in day case termination of pregnancy. The efficacy of low dose droperidol. Anaesthesia 42:613, 1987
26. Korttila K, Linnoila M: Skills related to driving after intravenous diazepam, flunitrazepam or droperidol. Br J Anaesth 46: 961, 1974
27. Cohen SE, Woods WA, Wyner J: Antiemetic efficacy of droperidol and metoclopradime. Anesthesiology 60:67, 1984
28. Editorial: New awakening in anaesthesia—at a price. Lancet 2:1469, 1987
29. Natof H: Complications. p. 321. In BV Wetchler (ed): Anesthesia for Ambulatory Surgery. JB Lippincott, Philadelphia, 1985
30. Bridenbaugh LH: Anesthesia and outpatient surgery. Reg Anesth 21:157, 1982
31. Korttila K: Postanesthetic cognitive and psychomotor impairment. Int Anesthesiol Clin 24:59, 1986
32. Meridy HW: Criteria for selection of ambulatory surgical patients and guidelines for anesthetic management: a retrospective study of 1553 cases. Anesth Analg 61:921, 1982
33. Clark AJ, Hurtig HB: Premedication with meperidine and atropine does not prolong recovery to street fitness after outpatient surgery. Can Anaesth Soc J 28:390, 1981
34. Korttila K, Tarkkanen L, Aittomäki J, et al: The influence of intramuscularly administered pethidine on the amnesic effects of intravenous diazepam during intravenous regional anesthesia. Acta Anaesthesiol Scand 25:323, 1981
35. Anderson S, McGuire R, McKeown D: Comparison of the cognitive effects of premedication with hyoscine and atropine. Br J Anaesth 57:169, 1985

36. Simpson KH, Smith RJ, Davies LF: Comparison of the effects of atropine and glycopyrrolate on cognitive function following general anaesthesia. Br J Anaesth 59:966, 1987
37. Seppälä T, Korttila K, Häkkinen S, Linnoila M: Residual effects and skills related to driving after single oral administration of diazepam, medazepam and lorazepam. Br J Clin Pharmacol 3:831, 1976
38. Shafer A, Urquhart ML, Doze VA, White PF: Outpatient premedication with intramuscular midazolam. Anesthesiology 67: A419, 1987
39. Lichtor LJ, Korttila K, Lane BS, et al: The effect of preoperative anxiety and premedication with midazolam on recovery from ambulatory surgery. Anesth Analg 68:S163, 1989
40. Kjaergård H, Larsen TK, Rasmussen PS, Brondum L: Impairment of postural stability following perivascular axillary block with mepivacaine. Acta Anaesthesiol Scand 28:508, 1984
41. Tetsch P: Reaktionzeitmessungen by zahnärtzlichchirurgischen Eingriffen in Analgosedierung. Dtsch Zahnartzl Z 28:618, 1973
42. Tetsch P, Machtens E, Voss M: Reaktionzeitmessungen by operativen Eingriffen in örtlicher Schmerzausschaltung. Schweiz Monatsschr Zahnheilkd 83:229, 1972
43. Korttila K: Psychomotor skills related to driving after intramuscular lidocaine. Acta Anaesthesiol Scand 18:290, 1974
44. Korttila K: Lack of impairment in skills related to driving after intramuscular administration of prilocaine or mepivacaine. Acta Anaesthesiol Scand 21:31, 1976
45. Korttila K, Häkkinen S, Linnoila M: Side effects and skills related to driving after intramuscular administration of bupivacaine and etidocaine. Acta Anaesthesiol Scand 19:384, 1975
46. Ritchie JM, Greene NM: Local anesthetics: fate of local anesthetics. p. 308. In Gilman AG, Goodman LS, Rall TW, et al (eds): The Pharmacological Basis of Therapeutics. 7th Ed. Macmillan, New York, 1985
47. Fuchs E, Karpinski HP: Lachgas-Analgesie und Verkehrstüchtigkeit. Zahnartl Welt 61:170, 1960
48. Trieger N, Loskota WJ, Jacobs AW, Newman MG: Nitrous oxide—a study of physiological and psychomotor effects. J Am Dent Assoc 82:142, 1971
49. Driscoll EJ, Christenson GR, White CL: General anesthesia for ambulatory dental patients. J Oral Surg 23:431, 1965
50. Valanne J, Korttila K: Recovery following general anesthesia with isoflurane or enflurane for outpatient dentistry and oral surgery. Anesth Prog 35:48, 1988
51. Carpenter RL, Eger EI, Johnson BH, et al: Does the duration of anesthetic administration affect the pharmacokinetics or metabolism of inhaled anesthetics in humans? Anesth Analg 66:1, 1987
52. Strum DP, Johnson BH, Eger EI: Stability of sevoflurane in soda lime. Anesthesiology 67:779, 1987
53. Eger EI: Partition coefficients of I-653 in human blood, saline and olive oil. Anesth Analg 66:971, 1987
54. Eger EI, Johnson BH: Rates of awakening from anesthesia with I-653, halothane, isoflurane, and sevoflurane: a test of the effect of anesthetic concentration and duration in rats. Anesth Analg 66:977, 1987
55. Doenicke A, Kugler J, Laub M: Evaluation of recovery and "street fitness" by e.e.g. and psychodiagnostic tests after anaesthesia. Can Anaesth Soc J 14:567, 1967
56. Dubois M, Scott DF, Savege TM: Assessment of recovery from short anaesthesia using the cerebral function monitor. Br J Anaesth 50:825, 1978
57. Korttila K, Ghoneim MM, Chiang C, et al: Metabolites of methohexital do not contribute to its prolonged action on the central nervous system. Anesthesiology 69: A426, 1988
58. Korttila K: Pharmacokinetics of intravenous non-narcotic anesthetics. p. 13. In Aldrete JA, Stanley TH (eds): Trends in Intravenous Anesthesia. Yearbook Medical Publishers, Chicago, 1980
59. Thompson GE, Remington JM, Millman BS: Experiences with outpatient dental anesthesia. Anesth Analg 52:881, 1974
60. Korttila K, Tammisto T, Aromaa U: Comparison of etomidate in combination with fentanyl or diazepam, with thiopentone as an induction agent for general anaesthesia. Br J Anaesth 51:1151, 1979

61. O'Toole DP, Milligan KR, Howe JP, et al: A comparison of propofol and methohexitone as induction agents for day case isoflurane anesthesia. Anaesthesia 42:373, 1987
62. Johnston R, Noseworthy T, Anderson B, et al: Propofol versus thiopental for outpatient anesthesia. Anesthesiology 67:532, 1987
63. Zuurmond WWA, Leeuwen L, Helmers JH: Recovery from propofol infusion as the main agent for outpatient arthroscopy. A comparison with isoflurane. Anaesthesia 42:356, 1987
64. Logan MR, Duggan JE, Levack ID, Spence AA: Comparison of 2, 6 di-isopropyl phenol and methohexitone. Br J Anaesth 59:179, 1987
65. Korttila K, Nuotto E, Lichtor L, et al: Recovery and psychomotor effects after brief anesthesia with propofol and thiopental. Anesth Analg 68:S150, 1989
66. Millar JM, Jewkes CF: Recovery and morbidity after daycase anaesthesia. A comparison of propofol with thiopentone enflurane with and without alfentanil. Anaesthesia 43:738, 1988
67. Valanne J, Korttila K: Comparison of methohexitone and propofol (Diprivan) for induction of enflurane anaesthesia in outpatients. Postgrad Med J 61:138, 1985
68. Doze VA, Westphal LM, White P: Comparison of propofol with methohexital for outpatient anesthesia. Anesth Analg 65: 1189, 1986
69. Korttila K, Faure E, Apfelbaum J, et al: Recovery from propofol versus thiopental-isoflurane in patients undergoing outpatient anesthesia. Anesthesiology 69:A564, 1988
70. Doze VA, Shafer A, White PW: Propofol-nitrous oxide versus thiopental-isoflurane-nitrous oxide for general anesthesia. Anesthesiology 69:63, 1988
71. Korttila K: Clinical effectiveness and untoward effects of new agents and techniques used in intravenous sedation. J Dent Res 63:848, 1984
72. Korttila K, Tarkkanen J: Comparison of diazepam and midazolam for sedation during local anaesthesia for bronchoscopy. Br J Anaesth 57:581, 1985
73. Skelly AM, Boscoe MJ, Dawling S, Adams AP: A comparison of diazepam and midazolam as sedatives for minor oral surgery. Eur J Anaesthesiol 1:253, 1984
74. Jack ML, Colburn WA, Spirt NM, et al: A pharmacokinetic/pharmacodynamic/receptor binding model to predict the onset and duration of pharmacological activity of the benzodiazepines. Prog Neuropsychopharmacol Biol Psychiatry 7:629, 1983
75. Korttila K, Mattila MJ, Linnoila M: Prolonged recovery after diazepam sedation: the influence of food, charcoal ingestion and injection rate on the effect of intravenous diazepam. Br J Anaesth 48:333, 1976
76. Henegan C, McAuliffe R, Thomas D, Radford P: Morbidity after outpatient anaesthesia. Anaesthesia 36:4, 1981
77. Kurer FL, Welch DB: Gynaecological laparoscopy: clinical experiences of two anaesthetic techniques. Br J Anaesth 56:1207, 1984
78. Fragen RJ, Shanks CA: Neuromuscular recovery after laparoscopy. Anesth Analg 63: 51, 1984
79. Sengupta P, Skacel M, Plantevin OM: Post-operative morbidity associated with the use of atracurium and vecuronium in day-case laparoscopy. Eur J Anaesthesiol 4:93, 1987
80. Sosis M, Goldberg ME, Marr AT, et al: Atracurium and vecuronium do not affect extraocular muscle function after outpatient surgery. Anesthesiology 68:465
81. Ali HH, Savarese JJ, Embree PB, et al: Clinical pharmacology of mivacurium chloride (BW1090U) infusion: comparison with vecuronium and atracurium. Br J Anaesth 61:541, 1988
82. Scott RFP, Norman J: Editorial: do we need more muscle relaxants? Br J Anaesth 61:528, 1988
83. Simpson JEP, Glynn CJ, Cox AG, Folkard S: Comparative study of short-term recovery of mental efficiency after anaesthesia. Br Med J 1:1560, 1976
84. Moss E, Hindmarch I, Pain AJ, Edmonson RS: Comparison of recovery after halothane or alfentanil for minor surgery. Br J Anaesth 59:970, 1987
85. Zuurmond WWA, Leeuwen L: Recovery

from sufentanil anaesthesia for outpatient arthroscopy: a comparison with isoflurane. Acta Anesthesiol Scand 31:154, 1987

86. Ramsey D, Thompson GE: The case for regional anesthesia for adult outpatient surgery. Anesthesiol Clin North Am 5:97, 1987
87. Farhie SE: Postoperative care after regional anesthesia. Int Anesthesiol Clin 21: 157, 1982
88. Konieczko KM, Barrowcliffe MP, Jordan C, Jones JG: Antagonism of morphine-induced respiratory depression: comparison of nalmefene with naloxone. Br J Anaesth 58:1333P, 1986
89. Gal TJ, DiFazio CA, Dixon R: Prolonged blockade of opioid effects with oral nalmefene. Anesthesiology 65:A343, 1986
90. Arvidsson S, Niemand D, Martinell S, et al: Aminophylline reversal of diazepam sedation. Anaesthesia 39:806, 1984
91. Gürel A, Elevli M, Hamulu A: Aminophylline reversal of flunitrazepam sedation. Anesth Analg 66:333, 1987
92. Krintel JJ, Wegmann F: Aminophylline reduces the depth and duration of sedation with barbiturates. Acta Anaesthesiol Scand 31:352, 1987
93. Alon E, Baitella L, Hossli G: Double-blind study of the reversal of midazolam-supplemented general anaesthesia with RO-1788. Br J Anaesth 59:455, 1987
94. Kirkegaard L, Knudsen L, Jensen S, Kruse A: Benzodiazepine antagonist Ro 15-1788. Antagonism of diazepam sedation in outpatients undergoing gastroscopy. Anaesthesia 41:1184, 1986
95. Sage DJ, Close A, Boas RA: Reversal of midazolam sedation with anexate. Br J Anaesth 59:459, 1987
96. Doenicke A, Suttman H, Kapp W, et al: On the action of the benzodiazepine-antagonist Ro 15-1788. Anaesthesist 33:343, 1984
97. Roncari G, Ziegler WH, Guentert TW: Pharmacokinetics of the new benzodiazepine antagonist Ro 15-1788 in man following intravenous and oral administration. Br J Clin Pharmacol 22:421, 1986
98. Raeder JC, Hole A, Arnulf V, Grynne BH: Total intravenous anaesthesia with midazolam and flumazenil in outpatient clinics. A comparison with isoflurane or thiopentone. Acta Anaesthesiol Scand 31:634, 1987
99. Herbert M, Healy TEJ, Bourke JB, et al: Profile of recovery after general anaesthesia. Br Med J 286:1539, 1983
100. Edwards H, Rose EA, Schorow M, King TC: Postoperative deterioration in psychomotor function. JAMA 245:1342, 1981
101. Ogg TW: An assessment of postoperative outpatient cases. Br Med J 4:573, 1972
102. Montedonico J, Tarraza PM: Legal considerations of outpatient anesthesia. Anesthesiol Clin North Am 5:227, 1987

18

Postoperative Complications

Surinder K. Kallar
Gareth W. Jones

In 1981, the Federated Ambulatory Surgery Association (FASA) defined a complication as an untoward response or abnormal condition resulting from treatment and care associated with ambulatory surgery. Natof[1] expanded this to define a major complication as "an untoward response or abnormal condition having the potential for serious harm" and a minor complication as "an untoward response with minimal or no potential for serious harm." Major complications include hemorrhage, infection, serious anesthetic complications, (e.g., arrhythmias, bronchospasm), persistent nausea and vomiting, and any medical problem that requires hospitalization. Minor complications include transient nausea and vomiting, weakness, headache, myalgia, sore throat, and dizziness.

Natof[1] has also postulated three concepts for complications in ambulatory surgery: (1) many major complications are related to the type of surgery and will be independent of the surgical setting; (2) other complications may have a decreased incidence as a result of the surgery being performed in an ambulatory care institution (e.g., infection or patient identification errors); and (3) owing to the large throughput of patients, all types of complications will eventually occur.

Complications can occur in the operating room, in the postanesthesia care unit (PACU), or after discharge. The etiology may be related to surgery, anesthesia, preexisting disease, or some other factor. Natof,[2] in a review of 40 centers, has demonstrated that 86 percent of complications occur after surgery has been completed, which emphasizes the need for vigilance and a high level of nursing care in the PACU. The type of anesthesia may influence the complication rate. In Natof's study,[2] the incidence of complications following local infiltration and sedative technique was one in 106; general anesthesia produced a rate of one in 120, and patients receiving regional anesthesia had the lowest complication rate.

In this chapter, we will discuss the etiology and treatment of complications that occur in the PACU.

NAUSEA AND VOMITING

Nausea and vomiting following surgery in the ambulatory care facility is a significant problem, as it is distressing to the patient and prolongs the time to ambulation and subsequent discharge from the unit. It has also been shown to be a significant cause of unexpected hospital admission from the PACU.[3] With newer anesthetic agents, the time to full recovery of consciousness is decreasing and, consequently, postoperative nausea and vomiting become more obvious and objectionable to the patient.

Many of our patients have previous experience of postoperative nausea and vomiting and this is often their major concern regarding the conduct of the anesthesia. It is important, therefore, for the anesthesiologist to undertake all possible measures to reduce the incidence of this difficult problem.

A wide variety of stimuli can influence the vomiting center, either directly or indirectly via the chemoreceptor trigger zone, autonomic input from the GI tract, and the eighth nerve connect with the vomiting center. Input from the chemoreceptor trigger zone is stimulated by both analgesics and anesthetics (Fig. 18-1).[4]

The incidence of postoperative nausea and vomiting is affected by a number of different factors (Table 18-1).[93] Predisposing medical conditions include obesity, diabetes mellitus, and pregnancy. Postoperative nausea and vomiting is particularly common in children and tends to decrease with age. The incidence is equal between the sexes until puberty, when it becomes more common in females[5,6]; this may be related to gonadotrophin levels. Motion sickness and a previous experience of postoperative nausea and vomiting increase the likelihood of developing postoperative emetic symptoms.

The choice of anesthetic agents can influence the incidence of nausea and vomiting following outpatient anesthesia. Morphine and meperidine have long been recognized for their emetic side effects, and their halflives ensure that the effect will persist into the postoperative period. If premedication is desirable, these agents should be avoided and hypnotics used as a substitute. Narcotics used intraoperatively also effect the postoperative recovery; the incidence of nausea and vomiting is higher when a "balanced" technique using a nar-

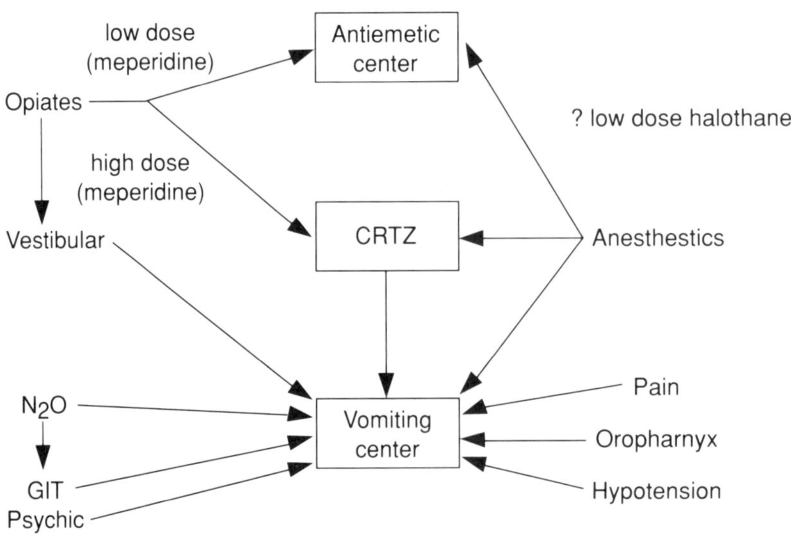

Fig. 18-1. Schematic representation of anesthesia-related stimuli which can influence activity at the vomiting center, including input from the chemoreceptor trigger zone (CRTZ) and the gastrointestinal tract (GIT). (From Palazzo and Strunin,[4] with permission.)

Table 18-1. Common Etiologies of Nausea and Vomiting in Outpatients

Predisposing factors
Age
Female gender
Motion sickness
Morbid obesity
Early pregnancy
Increased gastric volume
Excessive anxiety
Noncompliance
Premedicants
Narcotic analgesics (e.g., fentanyl)
Anesthetic agents
Inhaled drugs (e.g., isoflurane, N_2O)
Intravenous drugs (e.g., etomidate)
Surgical procedures
Laparoscopy
Strabismus correction
Insertion of PE tubes in ears
Orchiopexy
Postoperative factors
Hypotension
Pain

(From White and Shafer,[93] with permission.)

cotic is compared with a relaxant-volatile agent-nitrous oxide technique,[7] although the supplementation of fentanyl does reduce recovery time.[8] Pollard[9] has shown that the incidence of nausea and vomiting after a "balanced" technique, to which droperidol is added, is comparable to isoflurane anesthesia.

Nitrous oxide has been implicated as a cause of postoperative nausea and vomiting,[3,10,11] but recent studies by Muir et al.[12] and Korttila et al.[13] found no association between nausea and the use of nitrous oxide. Of the induction agents, methohexital is less likely to cause postoperative nausea than either thiopental or etomidate. Propofol has been shown to have a low incidence of nausea and vomiting.[14]

Surgical procedures and the conduct of the anesthesia may affect postoperative nausea and vomiting. Patients undergoing laparoscopy, dilatation and curettage, strabismus correction, and orchiopexy frequently develop nausea and vomiting. The longer the surgery and anesthesia, the greater the incidence of emetic symptoms. Assisted mask ventilation also causes nausea and vomiting which may be related to inflation of the stomach, as the incidence decreases in correlation with the experience of the anesthesiologist.[15] Pitocin and ergometrine are potent emetics and their effects will last into the postoperative period.

Postoperative factors include pain and early ambulation. Comroe and Dripps[16] demonstrated that nausea and vomiting increased following narcotic injections in ambulatory patient compared with those lying down. Anderson and Krohg[17] investigated the relationship between pain and postoperative nausea; in their study, nausea was relieved by effective analgesia. It should also be noted that hypotension can precipitate nausea and vomiting.

General measures that help reduce nausea and vomiting include reassurance and adequate preoperative explanation of the procedure to allay anxiety. In the PACU, the patient should be rewarmed and caution taken in moving the patient on the stretcher; nasopharyngeal suction should not be so excessive that it stimulates the gag reflex.

Promethazine, cyclizine, benzquinamide, prochlorperazine, and hydroxyzine have been used to control postanesthetic nausea and vomiting, but with limited success.[18,19] In addition, promethazine and hydroxyzine are associated with significant discomfort if given intramuscularly.

At present, low-dose droperidol seems to be the most effective antiemetic. Wetchler et al.[20] found droperidol, 0.625 to 1.25 mg IV, immediately following intubation for laparoscopic tubal sterilization, to be effective. In addition, as a result of the decreased nausea and vomiting, the patients receiving droperidol had a shorter stay in the PACU than the control group. More recently, Pandit et al.[21] compared the effect of droperidol 20 μg/kg with droperidol 10 μg/kg and a placebo group, and found that 20 percent of the patients in the high-dose group, 25 per-

Table 18-2. Incidence of Nausea Only or Nausea and Vomiting in the Recovery Room

Group	None (%)	Nausea only (%)	Nausea and vomiting (%)
Metoclopramide 5 mg + placebo	45	35	25
Metoclopramide 10 mg + placebo	55	25	20
Placebo + droperidol 5 μg/kg	60	20	20
Placebo + droperidol 10 μg/kg[a]	75	20	5
Placebo + droperidol 20 μg/kg[a]	80	10	10
Placebo + placebo	35	25	40
Metoclopramide 10 mg + droperidol 10 μg/kg[a]	75	20	5

[a] χ^2 test, $P < .05$. Placebo + placebo significantly different from placebo + droperidol 10 μg/kg, placebo + droperidol 20 μg/kg, and metoclopramide 10 mg + droperidol 10 μg/kg.
(From Pandit et al.,[21] with permission.)

cent in the low-dose group, and 65 percent in the placebo group suffered nausea and vomiting. In addition, they found that the high-dose group did not require any further antiemetic after discharge (Table 18-2).

A combination of metoclopramide 10 to 20 mg IV and droperidol 0.5 to 1.25 mg IV has been shown to be more effective than metoclopramide alone.[22–24] For pediatric patients, strabismus surgery and orchiopexy have a high incidence of nausea and vomiting. Droperidol has been used in doses of up to 75 μg/kg.[25–27] If given 30 minutes before the end of surgery, the incidence of emetic symptoms is reduced (Table 18-3). Lerman et al.[28] demonstrated that a further reduction could be obtained if droperidol (75 μg/kg) was given during induction of anesthesia.

The combination of ephedrine 25 mg IV and hydroxyzine 25 mg IM given on admission to the PACU has been studied in patients with a history of motion sickness and previous postanesthetic nausea and vomiting.[29] The regimen was shown to be effective in reducing symptoms.

Transdermal scopolamine 0.5 mg effectively reduces nausea and vomiting when given as a premedicant commencing 72 hours before surgery, but it is associated with a high incidence of anticholinergic side effects.[30] Acupuncture has also been shown to effectively reduce nausea and vomiting when compared with cyclizine and metoclopramide,[31] but further evaluation will be required before it becomes part of routine practice.

PAIN

Prompt and effective treatment of pain reduces analgesic requirements and prevents the complications of nausea and vomiting which result from untreated severe pain. It is customary to administer intra-

Table 18-3. Antiemetic Action of Droperidol 75 μg/kg: Effects on Recovery After Outpatient Pediatric Strabismus Surgery

	Control recovery time[a] (%)	Droperidol recovery time[a] (%)
Vomiting		
Severe[b]	369 ± 15 (39)	—
Mild	354 ± 23 (46)	348 ± 21 (43)
No vomiting	211 ± 18 (15)	284 ± 23 (57)
Overall	338 ± 16	309 ± 17

[a] Mean time (± SEM) required to achieve an Aldrete score of 10 (minutes).
[b] Vomiting requiring antiemetic therapy.
(Modified from Abramowitz et al.,[25] with permission.)

muscular narcotic analgesics in the PACU,[32] but the intravenous route can be used for a faster onset; however, smaller incremental doses are advised.

Postoperative pain control should commence intraoperatively by supplementing the anesthetic technique with a short-acting narcotic analgesic or a regional block.

In their study, Epstein et al. divided patients undergoing voluntary interruption of pregnancy or dilatation and curettage procedures into two groups.[8] The control group received thiopental and nitrous oxide in oxygen; the study group received thiopental, nitrous oxide in oxygen, and supplemental fentanyl. These investigators found a significantly higher incidence of pain and a slightly higher incidence of excitement during recovery in those patients who did not receive fentanyl. Analgesics were required in five of 25 patients in the control group and in only one of 14 in the fentanyl group. Although there was a higher incidence of nausea and vomiting in the fentanyl group, these patients recovered significantly faster than those in the control group, as defined by the time taken to walk unaided and demonstrate a negative Romberg test. Therefore, the total time spent in the PACU was decreased. At 24 hours, the fentanyl group had lower pain scores than the control group. Hunt and colleagues[33] administered a single dose of fentanyl (75 to 125 μg) intravenously at induction of anesthesia to a group of patients undergoing dilatation and curettage. When assessed both in the PACU and during the first evening at home, it was found that the addition of fentanyl significantly reduced incidence of abdominal pain.

Local anesthetic agents can be used as an effective method of providing postoperative analgesia. The techniques available are local infiltration of the incision site, intra-articular injection, and nerve or regional blockade; this is more fully discussed in Chapter 14 concerning regional techniques.

Fentanyl is the drug of choice for postoperative pain relief. Intravenous fentanyl is given in small incremental doses of 12.5 μg at 5-minute intervals, up to a total dose of 100 μg. The patient should be re-evaluated if this dose needs to be exceeded.

When the patient has resumed intake of oral fluids, oral analgesics can be administered to make the journey home more comfortable (see Ch. 19).

ASPIRATION PNEUMONITIS

There is a constant danger of this serious complication in the ambulatory surgical patient. Patients "at risk" for developing acid aspiration syndrome have been defined as those with gastric pH below 2.5 and a gastric fluid volume above 25 ml.[34,35] Morbidity and mortality associated with aspiration vary, depending on the volume and the chemical nature of the aspirate.

The clinical picture produced by aspiration of gastric contents depends on the nature, acidity, and volume of the aspirate. Signs and symptoms may be delayed and the patient may appear quite well for a few minutes after aspiration. Generalized wheezing, rales, and expiratory rhonchi may be present in the chest and may be likened to an asthmatic attack.[36]

Tachycardia, dyspnea, cyanosis, pulmonary edema, and hypotension may develop rapidly. The patient is hypoxic, mildly hypercapnic, and shows a metabolic acidosis. The chest x-ray may be normal for some time after the injury, and the full extent of pneumonitis may not be radiologically evident for several hours. The early diagnosis is based on arterial blood gases, and the only reliable sign is hypoxemia. If the PaO_2 is greater than 60 mmHg, there is no respiratory distress, and the vital signs are stable, then therapy should include oxygen and vigorous chest physical therapy. When significant aspiration occurs with severe hypoxemia, treatment must include endotracheal intubation, suctioning, and mechanical ventilation with positive end-expiratory pressure and a high F_{IO_2}. Pulmonary lavage has not been shown to be beneficial. Lavage with saline solution decreases compliance and increases the intrapulmonary shunt. Prophylactic use of antibiotics does not alter the course of aspiration pneumonitis and should only be used if indicated.[37] The use of corticosteroids to alter the outcome is no longer indicated and may be harmful.[38,39] Some degree of pulmonary edema occurs after every episode of aspiration. Once the airway is cleared of aspirated material, further suctioning to remove pulmonary edema fluid accomplishes little and only delays proper oxygenation of the patient.

Aspiration pneumonitis is not restricted to patients who have general anesthesia but may occur with regional techniques or in any patient whose level of consciousness is impaired by disease or sedation. Patients at increased risk include those with hiatal hernia, obesity, pregnancy, peptic ulceration, extreme nervousness, old age, and upper abdominal surgery. Habitual smokers do not have an increased risk of aspiration.[40] The common factors which precipitate vomiting during anesthesia are partial respiratory obstruction, and "light" anesthesia; other factors include insertion of an oropharyngeal airway, strong autonomic stimulation (peritoneal traction, traction of the ocular muscles), narcotic premedication, and glycopyrrolate.[41]

Regurgitation may be encouraged by the Trendelenberg position, the prone position, and palpation of the abdomen. Aspiration occurs at the end of the operation with nearly the same frequency as it does during induction.[42]

The incidence of regurgitation has been reported as 7 to 8 percent[43]; 8.6 percent of these patients inhaled gastric contents. A survey of 181 institutions performing ambulatory surgery during the calendar year 1985 revealed an annual incidence of regurgitation of 1.7 episodes per 10,000 procedures (Kallar SK, Keenan RL, personal communication). The same institutions reported their 10-year experience (1976 to 1985); there were 81 definite cases of aspiration and 185 cases of suspected aspiration. Of all of these cases, 47.5 percent were intubated for the procedure. Aspiration was most likely to occur during induction. Hospitalization was necessary in just over half of the patients, but no death or permanent disability occurred (Table 18-4).[94]

Anesthetic deaths due to aspiration are extremely rare. Harrison[44] reported two deaths from aspiration in a survey of 240,483 anesthetics, and Natof[1] reported only one suspected aspiration and no deaths in a survey of 32,001 outpatient procedures. A study from Sweden reported an incidence of aspiration of 4.7 per 10,000 anesthetics with a mortality of 0.2 per 10,000 anesthetics,[95] which contrasts with an earlier reported mortality of 40 percent following confirmed aspiration.[45]

Table 18-4. Aspirations in 10 Years (1976 to 1985)

	No. of aspirations (%)
Total reported	266 (100.0)
Suspected	185 (69.5)
Definite	81 (80.5)
Intubated	126 (47.5)
Not intubated	140 (52.5)
Time of aspiration	
Induction	166 (62.5)
Maintenance	28 (10.6)
Emergence	72 (26.9)
Not hospitalized	122 (45.9)
Hospitalized	144 (54.1)
Length of hospitalization	
1 d	71 (49.3)
2–3 d	54 (37.5)
4 or more d	19 (13.2)
Deaths/disability	0

(From Kallar,[94] with permission.)

Ong et al.[46] demonstrated that ambulatory patients may be at increased risk of aspiration due to their high residual gastric fluid volumes. Eighty-six percent of outpatients had volumes greater than 25 ml. Coté et al.[47] demonstrated that 76 percent of pediatric patients had a pH of less than 2.5 and a gastric volume in excess of 0.4 ml/kg.

Various drug therapies have been suggested to either increase the pH or decrease the volume of gastric juice. Martin et al.[48] demonstrated that intramuscular cimetidine reduced the number of breast biopsy patients "at risk" to zero. Metoclopramide is a dopamine antagonist which augments lower esophageal sphincter tone and stimulates gastric motility. A 10-mg dose has been shown to be effective in decreasing gastric volume.[49] Rao and co-workers[50] showed that administering a combination of 300 mg cimetidine and 10 mg metoclopramide by mouth more than 2 hours before induction significantly decreased gastric volume and increased gastric pH in all patients compared with either cimetidine or metoclopramide alone.

Other effective regimens include a preoperative oral dose of 300 mg cimetidine at bedtime and another on the morning of surgery, or a combination of oral and intramuscular dose.[51,52]

In pediatric outpatients, 7.5 mg/kg cimetidine syrup orally 1 hour before surgery has been shown to decrease gastric acid volume and increase gastric pH.[53]

Ranitidine 150 mg by mouth at bedtime and again on the morning of surgery has been shown to effectively reduce gastric acid volumes and raise pH.[54] Intravenous ranitidine 50 mg 1 hour before induction decreases gastric pH but does not reduce gastric acid volume. Although adverse reactions have been reported with both ranitidine and cimetidine, ranitidine is considered superior because of its longer duration of action.

Due to the limitation of control in the preoperative period, one would suspect aspiration to be a recurring problem in ambulatory patients. The incidence of aspiration is in fact low (1.7 per 10,000) with a very low mortality; this favorable finding may be due to the special emphasis placed on preoperative instructions and the thorough questioning of patients about ingestion of food and liquids upon arrival at the ambulatory surgery center, as well as competent and experienced personnel administering anesthesia in ambulatory units.

Whether every ambulatory patient should receive prophylaxis against acid aspiration remains a topic for debate. Individual ambulatory surgery centers must make their own decisions according to their past experiences with patients and estimates of cost-effectiveness. It seems reasonable that high-risk patients (i.e., hiatal hernia, obesity, pediatric, old age, late midtrimester pregnancy) should receive prophylaxis against acid aspiration.

POSTOPERATIVE HYPERTENSION

In a study of 1,800 inpatient admissions to the PACU, Gal and Cooperman[55] found that 3.25 percent of patients developed systolic blood pressures over 190 mmHg, with diastolic pressures in excess of 100 mmHg. The onset of hypertension occurred within 30 minutes of the end of surgery.

The most common cause of postoperative hypertension is a pre-existing hypertensive state. This accounts for more than 50 percent of cases seen in the PACU.[55] The hypertension is more pronounced if antihypertensive medication has been withdrawn preoperatively[56]; therefore, patients should continue to take their medication up to and including the day of surgery. Other factors that may contribute to postoperative hypertension are pain, hypoxia, hypercarbia, the presence of an endotracheal tube, emergence excitement, fluid overload, and a distended bladder.

The morbidity and mortality of postoperative hypertension is related to the magnitude and duration of the hypertension and to the underlying pathology. Severe hypertension increases myocardial demand for oxygen which may precipitate left ventricular failure, dysrhythmia, or myocardial infarction. In addition, the patient is at risk of a cerebral hemorrhage.

The successful management of postoperative hypertension depends on accurately diagnosing the etiology. Pain is a frequent cause, mediated through an increased sympathoadrenal outflow, and should be treated with intravenous narcotic analgesics. Careful attention to maintaining normothermia, postoperative ventilatory function, and the timely extubation of the patient should decrease the incidence of postoperative hypertension. If hypertension occurs despite these measures, specific antihypertensive therapy is indicated. Vasodilators are the drugs of first choice and hydralazine is commonly used in doses of 2.5 to 5.0 mg by slow intravenous injection to a total dose of 20 mg. The maximum effect is seen within 15 to 20 minutes. Its major side effect is a reflex tachycardia.

β-Blockade with propranolol in a dose of 0.5 to 1.0 mg IV may be useful but is contraindicated in the presence of bronchospastic disease. Esmolol is a cardioselective β-blocker with a halflife of approximately 9 minutes. It is gaining increasing popularity as an infusion to treat tachycardia. Labetolol, the mixed α and β receptor antagonist, can be used effectively in incremental doses of 5 to 10 mg IV.

Clonidine, the α-2 receptor agonist, is an oral agent that can be used to treat postoperative hypertension. More importantly, sudden withdrawal can cause acute rebound hypertension; therefore, all patients receiving clonidine therapy should be maintained on that therapy throughout the perioperative period.

HYPOTENSION AND SYNCOPE

Syncope is defined as hypotension accompanied by dizziness, drowsiness, and weakness. The common causes are hypovolemia, position changes, pain, a full bladder, and the administration of narcotics or antiemetics. Pulmonary embolus and myocardial infarction are rare events in ambulatory surgery, but should be excluded as a cause of hypotension. In the PACU, patients will not experience syncope until they are moved to phase II of their recovery period.

To prevent hypoperfusion of vital organs and subsequent ischemic damage, prompt diagnosis and treatment are important. Immediate therapy should include elevation of the legs and administration of intravenous fluids. Hypotension in association with bradycardia is usually the result of vagal stimulation and will respond to atropine 0.5 to 1.0 mg IV.

Hypotension and syncope may occur frequently after termination of pregnancy. Blood loss in combination with a long period of NPO produces hypovolemia in these patients. At the Medical College of Virginia, the incidence of syncope post-termination of pregnancy has been significantly reduced by the routine infusion of 2.0 L of crystalloid solution to all such patients.

If hypotension persists after fluid resuscitation, ephedrine in 5- to 10-mg increments should be given intravenously.

DYSRHYTHMIAS

Dysrhythmias are most commonly seen in patients who have pre-existing heart disease, but may also occur in healthy patients in the postoperative period. Predisposing factors include hypoxia, hypercarbia, hypokalemia, and pain. The common dysrhythmias are sinus tachycardia, sinus bradycardia, and ventricular and atrial premature beats. First-line treatment is to eliminate any predisposing factor, and it is uncommon for further antiarrhythmic medication to be required.

DISSEMINATED INTRAVASCULAR COAGULATION

Disseminated intravascular coagulation has been reported in ambulatory surgical units following midtrimester abortions.[57] At the Medical College of Virginia, there have been 12 laboratory-proven cases in the past 8 years. It commonly presents as excessive vaginal bleeding, which may occur immediately after surgery or during the first postoperative hour. The differential diagnosis includes incomplete curettage, and these patients often have the procedure repeated before the correct diagnosis is made.

In obstetric practice, disseminated intravascular coagulation is associated with abruptio placenta,[58] amniotic fluid embolism,[59] severe pre-eclampsia/eclampsia, the dead fetus syndrome, and saline-induced abortions. In ambulatory surgery, however, it occurs following abortions in which the fetal gestational age is greater than 20 weeks which are associated with a difficult placental and/or fetal extraction.

The clotting and fibrinolytic cascades are probably activated by placental thromboplastin or amniotic fluid which enters the maternal circulation during curettage. This is more likely to occur in midtrimester abortions due to the difficulty sometimes experienced in extracting the large placenta which results in damage to the venous sinuses.

The diagnosis is based on a high index of suspicion and laboratory investigation. The coagulation abnormalities include a prolonged prothrombin time and partial thromboplastin time, a decreased platelet count, and serum fibronigen levels with elevation of the fibrin split products. A whole blood clotting time can be performed at the bedside while awaiting the laboratory results; clot formation may be delayed or alternatively early clot lysis may occur.

Initial treatment is aimed at restoring the intravascular volume; if the coagulations studies are abnormal, prompt administration of the appropriate procoagulant is indicated. Bleeding should be controlled by the administration of platelets and fresh frozen plasma.

In all patients undergoing second trimester abortions, a blood sample should be sent to the blood bank preoperatively for type and crossmatch.

MALIGNANT HYPERTHERMIA

Malignant hyperthermia is a serious and catastrophic complication. If not recognized and treated early, it has a high mortality rate.[60–62] The availability of dantrolene sodium[63] to counteract this hypermetabolic condition has dramatically decreased the morbidity and mortality associated with this syndrome. The incidence of malignant hyperthermia in outpatients is unclear. In his extensive review of complications, Natof[1] found no cases of malignant hyperthermia up to 1982; in 1983 (with 60 centers reporting), he identified three episodes of malignant hyperthermia occurring in the ambulatory setting; two were suspected cases and one was confirmed. Three additional episodes were identified in 1984 (from 40 centers); two were confirmed cases and one was suspected.

Surgery on pediatric patients in ambulatory centers has gained popularity. Halothane and succinylcholine are commonly used in pediatric anesthesia and both can trigger an attack of malignant hyperthermia.[64,65] It is important, therefore, to be aware of the syndrome and to take steps to prevent or treat it should it develop.

Prevention includes thorough evaluation and screening of at-risk patients. It is important to obtain a full history of past anesthetic experience in both the patient and the patient's family. Increased risk factors include a history of strabismus and muscle cramps unrelated to exercise. Suspicious signs in the past anesthetic history include tachycardia during anesthesia, masseter spasm after the administration of succinylcholine, unexplained fever, and unstable blood pressure. Screening and diagnostic tests include serum creatinine phosphokinase level and muscle biopsy.

The patient with a history of malignant hyperthermia is not a candidate for ambulatory surgery, but malignant hyperthermia may develop unexpectedly; therefore, every ambulatory surgery center should develop a plan to treat this catastrophic emergency. A recent study from Texas revealed that 48 percent of the 73 ambulatory surgery centers surveyed were considered incapable of dealing with a malignant hyperthermia case due to inadequate supplies of dantrolene.[66] It is imperative that a malignant hyperthermia cart be stocked and labeled, and since dantrolene is the drug of choice, it is vital to have adequate supplies of the drug available.

Malignant hyperthermia-susceptible patients have been anesthetized in ambulatory facilities. These patients must be observed for a minimum of 6 hours postoperatively and some centers advocate overnight observation.

POSTOPERATIVE HEMORRHAGE

Hemorrhage complicating surgery may manifest itself during the postoperative recovery period. Surgical procedures associated with a relatively high incidence of postoperative hemorrhage include tonsillectomy, adenoidectomy, augmentation mammoplasty, late second trimester abortions, and rhinoplasty. The incidence for hemorrhage after tonsillectomy and adenoidectomy has been recorded as 1.5 to 1.7 percent.[1,67] The management of hemorrhage involves resuscitation and further surgical intervention.

POSTANESTHETIC EXCITEMENT/ DELIRIUM

Postoperative excitement, characterized by restlessness, disorientation, irrational talking, or crying represents a stage between surgical anesthesia and complete orientation. In its extreme form, it is referred to as emergence delirium. These patients can be in a violent, agitated state, often requiring manual restraint to prevent them from doing harm to themselves or the recovery room personnel. It is most common in children and healthy young adults who are apprehensive about their surgery or fear pain. The incidence decreases with age. Although the most common stimulus for this response is pain, several other important factors may be involved, including anxiety, a distended urinary bladder, hypoxia, and hypercarbia. The use of phenothiazines, barbiturates, or scopolamine as premedicants in the absence of a narcotic analgesic increases the incidence of postoperative excitement.[68] It may also be seen in children during emergence from inhalation anesthesia.

Management of these cases includes the exclusion of simple causes and often, a change in the patient's bed position is all that is required. Pain should be relieved with small intravenous doses of narcotics. Physostigmine (1 to 3 mg IV)[69–71] can be used to reverse delirium caused by anticholinergics or benzodiazepines. Awakening and orientation is seen within 2 to 5 minutes, but delirium may recur and requires a repeat dosage. Physostigmine also appears to reverse drowsiness after halothane and disorientation after neuroleptic (droperidol-fentanyl) anesthesia.[72]

The side effects of physostigmine are bradycardia, nausea, increased bronchial secretions, ventricular arrhythmia, and abdominal cramping. Atropine will counteract these muscarinic effects.

POSTINTUBATION CROUP

Ambulatory care units are particularly suitable for the management of pediatric patients. A serious postoperative complication in pediatric practice is postintubation croup, which presents as hoarseness, cough, and stridor, and if untreated may progress to severe airway obstruction. A large number of cases have undoubtedly been the result of poor intubation technique and it is gratifying to see that the incidence of croup, in reported studies, is declining. A survey from Boston reports the incidence as 1 percent.[73] Factors which contribute to croup are age (less than 4 years), trauma on intubation, size of the endotracheal tube, coughing with the endotracheal tube in place, and movements of the patient's head while intubated. In addition, the site and duration of the procedure may also affect the incidence of croup. It should also be noted that faultless technique does not totally eliminate postintubation croup as a complication.

Symptoms manifest themselves at any time from immediately after extubation up to 3 hours after surgery, but symptoms that will require treatment will be present within the first hour in the PACU.

Treatment with cool mist inhalations and dexamethasone 4 to 8 mg IV has been shown to be effective.[74] Postintubation croup will also respond to nebulized epinephrine inhalations: 2.25 percent racemic epinephrine 0.5 ml diluted in 3 ml sterile saline delivered by nebulizer.[67] Following intervention, the patient should be observed for a minimum of 2 hours before a decision on discharge is taken. Factors which influence the decision will include age, severity, and the home circumstances.

AWARENESS DURING ANESTHESIA

Awareness with or without pain during the operation and its later recall are obviously the result of inadequate anesthesia. This may be caused by unintentional anesthetic errors, such as leaks within the breathing system, unnoticed changes in gas flows, or malfunctioning vaporizers, or it may be the result of inadequate dosage of intravenous drugs. Tolerance to central nervous system depressants develops in patients who are heavy drinkers, narcotic, or tranquilizer abusers; these patients may, therefore, be at greater risk of awareness during anesthesia. Awareness occurs mostly with "balanced" or nitrous oxide-narcotic-relaxant techniques, as it is difficult to assess the depth of anesthesia in a patient who is paralyzed. However, there have been reports of awareness with inhalational agents.

Patients appear to have better recall for events perceived by them to be life-threatening. The chances of recall are also increased at the beginning of the operation (between induction of anesthesia and start of the operation) and at the end, when level of anesthesia is light. The sense of hearing is the last to disappear and the first to reappear after general anesthesia. Unfortunately, the noise level in the operating room also increases at the end of the operation and the semiconscious patient may believe that this noise was heard during the intraoperative period.[75,76] Operating room personnel should always be mindful that an unconscious patient may hear off-hand remarks; and, therefore, conversation should be quiet and disciplined.

During the procedure, signs of light anesthesia should not be ignored. These include somatic signs such as wrinkling of the forehead, eyelid movement, and movements of the upper limbs, and autonomic signs such as tearing, sweating, tachycardia, and an increase in blood pressure.[77] In the unpremedicated ambulatory surgery patient, the recall under general anesthesia has been as high as 9 percent. A study by Epstein[78] demonstrated that intravenous diazepam, up to a total dose of 5 mg given 2 to 3 minutes before induction, significantly decreased awareness. In the absence of diazepam, there was a 4.9 percent recall of conversation, a 2.1 percent recall of extubation, and a 0.7 percent recall of pain.

Midazolam and diazepam have been used as premedicants for their amnesic actions. The amnesic effect of midazolam is more intense but shorter lasting than diazepam. Nitrous oxide is also a powerful amnesic; if it is to be discontinued for any reason (e.g., at high altitudes) during balanced anesthesia, substitution with an intravenous agent with known amnestic properties is indicated. Narcotics are notoriously poor amnesics.

In some patients, recall presents little problem, but in others it may lead to a traumatic neurotic syndrome with symptoms of anxiety, irritability, and a preoccupation with death.[79] Although these patients are reluctant to discuss it or even believe that what they remember really happened, it is important that the cause of such symptoms be explored with them. A direct and honest explanation often provides for a dramatic cure.

MINOR COMPLICATIONS

In a study by Fahy and Marshall,[80] 45 percent of the patients developed symptoms related to the anesthesia, but most of these minor complications resolved within 24 hours. The complications included drowsiness, headache, myalgia, nausea and vomiting, malaise, sore throat, hoarseness, and dizziness. They also demonstrated that the following factors increased postoperative morbidity: female sex, first anesthetic experience, endotracheal intubation, and duration of surgery. Ogg[81] studied 100 outpatients and found the following incidence of postoperative symptoms: headache, 27 percent; drowsiness, 26 percent; nausea, 22 percent; and dizziness, 11 percent. Dhamee et al.[82] compared the postoperative morbidity of patients undergoing laparoscopic procedures with halothane, enflurane, or fentanyl-based techniques. The incidence of headache was increased with the volatile agents but nausea and vomiting was more common after the narcotic technique; most of these symptoms had resolved after 48 hours (Table 18-5).

Sore throat is commonly experienced after endotracheal intubation, but it can also be caused by the use of an oropharyngeal airway or the inhalation of dry gases. Myalgias may be caused by the use of succinylcholine; they usually appear within 12 to 24 hours and may last for 1 to 2 days. The muscle pains are described as being similar to those experienced after taking vigorous exercise and commonly involve the proxi-

Table 18-5. Comparative Morbidity After Three Different Outpatient Anesthetic Techniques for Laparoscopy

Time of incidence	Primary anesthetics	Drowsy	Dizzy	Headache	Weak	Nausea	Pain	Myalgias
Incidence at discharge (%)	Halothane/N_2O	68	45	20	70	28	20	—
	Enflurane/N_2O	50	39	6	64	22	6	—
	Fentanyl/N_2O	57	43	14	64	43	14	—
Incidence at 24 hr (%)	Halothane/N_2O	83	50	40	83	10	40	80
	Enflurane/N_2O	75	44	25	83	11	25	75
	Fentanyl/N_2O	64	36	7	71	29	7	57
Incidence at 48 hr (%)	Halothane/N_2O	33	23	30	55	13	30	70
	Enflurane/N_2O	33	28	25	61	3	25	83
	Fentanyl/N_2O	21	14	14	43	0	14	42

(Modified from Dhamee et al.,[82] with permission.)

Table 18-6. Minor Complications Reported (Medical College of Virginia 1985 to 1988)[a]

Contact completed	No. of patients contacted (%)
No problems	5,570 (86.7)
Nausea alone	128 (2.0)
Nausea and vomiting	253 (3.9)
Sore throat	106 (1.6)
Hoarseness	8 (1.6)
Headache	47 (0.7)
Myalgias	55 (0.9)
Fever	56 (0.9)
Bleeding	61 (1.0)
Dizziness	37 (0.6)
Intravenous site problem	3 (0.1)
Peripheral nerve injury	4 (0.1)
Injury to skin, eyes, or lips	9 (0.1)
Prolonged regional block	4 (0.1)
Other	250 (3.9)
Referred to surgeon	218 (3.4)

[a] Computerized prospective study. Total of 6,427 patients contacted.

mal musculature (the neck, back, thorax, and abdomen), but may occasionally affect the jaw and limbs. The use of nondepolarizing agent before the administration of succinylcholine may prevent this complication. Many ambulatory surgery centers, however, have completely eliminated the use of succinylcholine in order to avoid this complication.

In the healthy patient, these minor complications can be disturbing. Preoperative and postoperative instruction is therefore mandatory, and should be extensive and explicit in order to provide the patient with a sense of security and knowledge of what to expect.

At the the Medical College of Virginia, a prospective computerized system has been used in an attempt to follow-up 11,377 patients over a 4-year period (1985 to 1988) by telephone 24 hours after anesthesia in order to obtain information regarding postoperative complications. To avoid leading questions, the patients are asked to volunteer information rather than answer a questionnaire. Contact was attempted in 10,029 cases (no postoperative contact was attempted in the 601 cardiac biopsy patients or the 747 patients without a telephone) and was completed in 6,427 cases (64.1 percent). The reported symptoms are documented in Table 18-6. Three hundred eighty-two patients complained of more than one symptom.

MORTALITY

According to different studies, the incidence of anesthetic deaths is 0.7 to 3.7 per 10,000 inpatients receiving anesthetics.[83] In the ambulatory setting, there is a much lower incidence of anesthetic deaths compared with hospitals. This is summarized in Table 18-7.

In 369,528 procedure results collected by Bruns for FASA, only one death was recorded (0.027 per 10,000), an incidence one-fortieth that of hospitals.[84] Similar low incidences have been reported with properly administered dental anesthetics in the United States[85,86] and the United Kingdom[87]; however, a weakness in all of these studies is that they relied on voluntary retrospective reporting from different centers. Recently, the FASA data was updated to include over 1.1 million carefully collected ambulatory anesthetic cases, there were 17 deaths, for an incidence of 0.15 per 10,000 cases.[1,88] While this is greater than

Table 18-7. Studies of Ambulatory Anesthetic Mortality

Source	Anesthetics	Deaths	Deaths/10,000
Driscoll[85] (1974)	2,445,570	7	0.029
Lyte & Yoon[86] (1980)	2,580,000	3	0.012
Bruns[84] (1982)	369,528	1	0.027
Green & Taylor[87] (1984)	598,000	1	0.016
Natof[1] (1985)	1,100,000	17	0.15

(RL Keenan, personal communication.)

in previous reports, it remains much lower than the rate of mortality for hospital inpatients.

UNANTICIPATED HOSPITAL ADMISSIONS

By definition, the aim of ambulatory care is to discharge all patients home; however, if postoperative complications are severe, they may lead to hospital admission. The incidence of admission from the ambulatory facility to hospital ranges from 0.68 to 4.1 percent.[89] Hospital-affiliated centers have a higher admission rate than freestanding centers, which may be related to the ease with which transfer can be achieved and possibly to differences in the case load. Teaching hospitals may have a higher rate also due to the presence of residents in training.

Table 18-8 shows the reasons for hospital admission from the Methodist Ambulatory Surgery Center (private institution, Peoria, IL).

At the Medical College of Virginia's Ambulatory Surgery Center (hospital affiliated/teaching hospital), 21,140 procedures were performed between 1981 and 1988. The unanticipated admission rate over this period was 1.0 percent; the reasons for admission are shown in Table 18-9. From this sample, there was one case of allergic reaction to methohexital, one case of nitrous oxide embolus during laparoscopy, and one case of muscle stiffness in a child receiving succinylcholine (Table 18-10).

Most freestanding ambulatory care facilities have an admission rate of less than 1 percent.[90] Whether this rate is affected by the age and physical status profile of the patients remains unclear. The Phoenix Surgicenter found that their admission rates increased from 0.2 percent overall to 0.6 percent for patients over the age of 64 years,[90] whereas, Meridy[91] retrospectively reported that extremes of age did not affect either duration of recovery or the incidence of complications.

Table 18-11 shows the relationship between anesthesia technique and the incidence of unexpected admission in elderly

Table 18-8. Reasons for Hospital Admission From Methodist Ambulatory Surgery Center[a]

Reasons	No. of patients
Patient (6%)	
Refused to go home	13
No responsible person	9
Procedure (57%)	
More extensive surgery	124
Positive biopsy	47
Problems	45
Bleeding	
Uterine perforation	
Bladder puncture	
Bowel burn	
Pneumothorax	
Intravenous pyelogram dye reaction	5
Postspinal headache	1
Postanesthesia complications (37%)	
Bleeding	35
Syncope	27
Drowsiness	
Dizziness	
Decreased blood pressure	
Pain	35
Pulmonary	16
Asthma	
Aspiration	
Croup	
Nausea and vomiting	17
Arrhythmias	11
Hypertension	2
Possible myocardial infarction	1

[a] September 15, 1977 through September 14, 1985: 52,449 patients.

(Data from Bernard Wetchler, personal communication, and Levy.[89])

Table 18-9. Reasons for Unanticipated Hospital Admissions (Medical College of Virginia, 1981 to 1988)

Reasons	No. of patients (%)
Surgical	127 (57.5)
Anesthesia	31 (14.0)
Medical	38 (17.2)
Social	25 (11.3)
Total	21,140 (100)

Table 18-10. Anesthetic Reasons for Unanticipated Admission (Medical College of Virginia, 1981 to 1988)

Reasons	No. of patients (%)
Intractable vomiting	4 (13.0)
Aspiration	5 (16.1)
Delayed awakening	2 (6.4)
Hypertension	4 (13.0)
Arrhythmia	4 (13.0)
Syncope/hypotension	3 (9.7)
Drug reaction	2 (6.4)
Transfusion reaction	1 (3.2)
Congestive heart failure/ pulmonary edema	1 (3.2)
Myocardial ischemia	1 (3.2)
Atypical pseudocholinesterase	1 (3.2)
Postoperative croup	1 (3.2)
Muscle stiffness	1 (3.2)
N_2O embolus	1 (3.2)

Total no. of patients, 21,140; total no. of admissions, 221; total no. of admissions for anesthetic reasons, 31.

patients at the Methodist Ambulatory Surgery Center.

The pediatric caseload produces a different spectrum of complications which may lead to admission. Patel and Hannallah[92] studied 10,000 patients and reported an incidence of admission of 0.9 percent. One-third of these admissions were for protracted vomiting (Table 18-12).

Those centers that undertake an increasing number of American Society of Anesthesiologists physical status III patients for ambulatory surgery will have a higher admission rate. In Phoenix, the rate is 1.4 percent for these patients.

Premedication, anesthetic technique, and skill/experience of the anesthetist also influence the admission rate of a unit.[91]

Table 18-11. Anesthetic Technique and Incidence of Unexpected Admissions in the Elderly (Methodist Ambulatory Surgery Center, 1981 to 1985)

Type of anesthesia	No. of patients admitted (%)
Local	4,143(0.4)
MAC	395 (2.8)
Regional	471 (0.8)
General (volatile)	627 (4.1)
Overall	5,636 (1.1)

(B Wetchler, personal communication.)

Table 18-12. Reasons for Admission of Pediatric Patients to the Hospital from Short Stay Recovery Unit[a]

Reasons	No. of patients (%)
Protracted vomiting	30 (33)
Complicated surgery	15 (17)
Croup	8 (9)
Parental request	6 (7)
Fever	6 (7)
Bleeding	3 (3)
Sleepiness	2 (2)
Others	20 (22)
Total	90 (100)

[a] Overnight hospital admission rate is 90/10,000 patients (0.9 percent).

(From Patel and Hannallah,[92] with permission.)

SUMMARY

The etiology and management of postoperative complications have been discussed. Specific complications of regional anesthetic techniques are discussed in Chapter 14.

The postoperative recovery period remains the responsibility of the anesthesiologist and it is important, therefore, that he or she is knowledgeable concerning diagnosis and management of these complications. The practice of modern surgery often dictates that the anesthesiologist is the only physician available during the postoperative recovery period; therefore, a knowledge of surgical complications is also necessary (see Ch. 5). It will be the anesthesiologist who must make the decision (with consultation) to discharge or transfer patients from the PACU.

Minor complications of ambulatory care may persist or occur for the first time after discharge. All patients should be informed of this possibility and reassured; in addition, patients should be provided with the telephone numbers of their physicians, the ambulatory facility, and the emergency room as a precaution against any unusual incident.

The overall incidence of major complications resulting in unexpected admissions to a hospital is low; there is, however, no room for complacency. Our practice of ambulatory surgery can only be improved by implementing an effective quality assurance program for every facility. The information gained can then be judged against nationally accepted published data, and the necessary action taken.

ACKNOWLEDGMENT

The authors would like to thank Annette H. Jackson for her assistance in typing this manuscript.

REFERENCES

1. Natof HE: Complications. p. 321. In Wetchler BV (ed): Anesthesia for Ambulatory Surgery. JB Lippincott, Philadelphia, 1985
2. Natof HE: FASA Special Study I. Freestanding Ambulatory Surgery Association, Alexandria, VA, 1985
3. Alexander GD, Skupski JN, Brown EM: The role of nitrous oxide in postoperative nausea and vomiting. Anesth Analg 63:175, 1984
4. Palazzo MGA, Strunin L: Anesthesia and emesis in etiology. Can Anaesth Soc J 31:178, 1984
5. Smessaert A, Schehr C, Artusio JF: Nausea and vomiting in the immediate postanesthetic period. JAMA 170:2072, 1959
6. Purkis IE: Factors that influence postoperative vomiting. Can Anaesth Soc J 2:335 July 1964
7. Janhunen L, Tammisto T: Postoperative vomiting after different modes of general anaesthesia. Ann Chir Gynaecol 61:152, 1972
8. Epstein BS, Levy ML, Thein MH, Coakley CS: Evaluation of fentanyl as an adjunct to thiopental-nitrous oxide-oxygen anesthesia for short surgical procedures. Anesthesiol Rev 2:24, 1975
9. Pollard J: Clinical evaluation of intravenous vs. inhalation anesthesia in the ambulatory surgical unit: a multicenter study. Curr Ther Res 36:617, 1984
10. Eger EL II: Should we not use nitrous oxide? p. 339. In Eger EL II (ed): Nitrous Oxide. Elsevier, New York, 1985
11. Lonie DS, Harper NJN: Nitrous oxide anaesthesia and vomiting. The effect of nitrous oxide anaesthesia on the incidence of vomiting following gynaecological laparoscopy. Anaesthesia 41;703, 1986
12. Muir JJ, Warner MA, Offord Kp, et al: Role of nitrous oxide and other factors in postoperative nausea and vomiting: a randomized and blinded prospective study. Anesthesiology 66:513, 1987
13. Korttila K, Hovorka J, Erkola O: Nitrous oxide does not increase the incidence of nausea and vomiting after isoflurane anesthesia. Anesth Analg 66:761, 1987
14. Doze VA, Westphal LM, White PF: Comparison of propofol with methohexital for outpatient anesthesia. Anesth Analg 65:1189, 1986
15. Bellville JW, Bross IDJ, Howland WS: Postoperative nausea and vomiting IV: factors related to postoperative nausea and vomiting. Anesthesiology 21:186, 1960
16. Comroe JH, Dripps RD: Reactions to morphine in ambulatory and bed patients. Surg Gynecol Obstet 87:221, 1948
17. Anderson R, Krohg K: Pain as a major cause of postoperative nausea. Can Anaesth Soc J 23:366, 1976
18. Wheaton NE: Comparison of benzquinamide hydrochloride and droperidol in preventing postoperative nausea and vomiting following general outpatient anesthesia. AANA J 53:322, 1985
19. McKenzie R, Wadhwa RK, Vyn TL, et al: Antiemetic effectiveness of intramuscular hydroxyzine compared with intramuscular droperidol. Anesth Analg 60:783, 1981
20. Wetchler BV, Collins IS, Jacob L: Antiemetics effects of droperidol on the ambulatory surgery. Anesth Rev 9:23, 1982
21. Pandit SK, Kothary SP, Pandit UA: Antiemetic efficacy of oral metoclopramide versus intravenous droperidol for outpatient laparoscopic procedures. Anesthesiology 67:A425, 1987

22. Doze VA, Shafer A, White PF: Nausea and vomiting after outpatient anesthesia: Effectiveness of droperidol alone and in combination with metoclopramide. Anesth Analg 66:541, 1987
23. Cohen SE, Words WA, Wyner J: Antiemetic efficacy of droperidol and metoclopramide. Anesthesiology 60:67, 1984
24. Rao TLK, Madhavareddy S, Chinthagada M, et al: Metoclopramide and cimetidine to reduce gastric fluid pH and volume. Anesth Analg 63:1014, 1984
25. Abramowitz MD, Oh TH, Epstein BS, et al: The antiemetic effect of droperidol following outpatient strabismus surgery in children. Anesthesiology 59:579, 1983
26. Abramowitz MD, Epstein BS, Friendly DX, et al: The effect of droperidol in reducing vomiting in pediatric strabismic outpatient surgery. Anesthesiology 55:A329, 1981
27. Hardy JF, Charest J, Gurouard G, et al: Nausea and vomiting after strabismus surgery in preschool children. Can Anaesth Soc J 33:57, 1986
28. Lerman J, Enstis S, Smith DR: Effect of droperidol pretreatment on postanesthetic vomiting in children undergoing strabismus surgery. Anesthesiology 65:322, 1986
29. Freeman LA: Ephedrine and hydroxyzine as treatment for postoperative nausea and vomiting. A study of 40 problem patients. Society for Ambulatory Anesthesia, 3rd Annual Meeting, 1988 (abstr)
30. Jackson SH, Schmidt MN, McGuire J, et al: Transdermal scopolamine as a preanesthetic drug and postoperative antinauseant and antiemetic. Anesthesiology 57:A330, 1982
31. Dundee JW, Fitzpatrick KTJ, Ghaly RG: Is there a role for acupuncture in the treatment of postoperative nausea and vomiting? Anesthesiology 67:A165, 1987
32. Aldrete JA: Are intramuscular injections obsolete in the recovery room? Curr Rev Recovery Room Nurses 5:147, 1983
33. Hunt TM, Plantevin OM, Gilbert JR: Morbidity in gynecological day-case surgery. A comparison of two anaesthetic techniques. Br J Anaesth 51:785, 1979
34. Teabeaut JR: Aspiration of gastric contents. An experimental study. Am J Pathol 28:51, 1952
35. Roberts RB, Shirley MA: Reducing the risk of acid aspiration during caesarean section. Anesth Analg 53:859, 1974
36. Bynum LJ, Pierce AK: Pulmonary aspiration of gastric contents. Am Rev Respir Dis 114:1125, 1976
37. Stewardson RH, Nyhus LM: Pulmonary aspiration—an update. Arch Surg 112:1192, 1977
38. Chapman RL, Downs JB, Modell JH, et al: The ineffectiveness of steroid therapy in treating aspiration of HCL. Arch Surg 108:858, 1974
39. Wynne JW, DeMarco FJ, Hood CI: Physiology of cortical steroids in foodstuff aspiration. Arch Surg 116:46, 1981
40. Adelhoj B, Petring OU, Frosig F, et al: Influence of cigarette smoking on the risk of acid pulmonary aspiration. Acta Anaesthesiol Scand 31:7, 1987
41. Clark JM, Seager SJ: Gastric emptying following premedication with glycopyrrolate or atropine. Br J Anaesth 55:1195, 1983
42. Arandia HY, Grogono AW: Comparison of the incidence of combined "risk factors" for gastric acid aspiration: influence of two anesthetic techniques. Anesth Analg 59:682, 1980
43. Blitt DC, Gutman HL, Cohen DD, et al: Silent regurgitation and aspiration during general anesthesia. Anesth Analg 49:707, 1970
44. Harrison GG: Deaths attributable to anesthesia. A ten-year survey (1967–1976). Br J Anaesth 50:1041, 1978
45. Morgan JG: Pathophysiology of gastric aspiration. p. 1. In Roberts RB (ed): Pulmonary Aspiration. International Anesthesiology Clinics. Vol. 15. Little, Brown and Company, Boston, 1977
46. Ong BY, Palahniuk RJ, Comming M: Gastric volume in outpatients. Can Anaesth Soc J 25:36, 1978
47. Coté CJ, Goudsouzian NG, Liu LMP, et al: Assessment of risk factors related to the acid aspiration syndrome in pediatric patients—gastric pH and residual volume. Anesthesiology 56:70, 1982
48. Martin C, Kallar SK, Ciresi S: The effect of oral bicitra compared to intramuscular cimetidine on gastric pH and volume in outpatient surgery. AANA J 56:515, 1988
49. Wyner J, Cohen SE: Gastric volume in early

pregnancy: effect of metoclopramide. Anesthesiology 57:209, 1982

50. Rao TLK, Suseeda M, El-Etv AA: Metoclopramide and cimetidine to reduce gastric pH and volume. Anesth Analg 63:264, 1984
51. Hodgkinson R, Glassenberg R, Joyce TH, et al: Comparison of cimetidine (Tagamet) with antacid for safety and effectiveness in reducing gastric acidity before elective cesarean section. Anesthesiology 59:86, 1983
52. Weber L, Hirshman CA: Cimetidine for prophylaxis of aspiration pneumonitis: comparison of intramuscular and oral dosage schedules. Anesth Analg 58:426, 1979
53. Somori GJ, Kallar SK: The effects of cimetidine on gastric pH and volume in pediatric patients in an ambulatory surgical center. Anesthesiology 61:3A, 1984
54. Manchikanti L, Colliver JA, Marrero TC et al: Ranitidine and metoclopramide for prophylaxis of aspiration pneumonitis in elective surgery. Anesth Analg 63:903, 1984
55. Gal TJ, Cooperman LH: Hypertension in the immediate postoperative period. Br J Anaesth 47:70, 1975
56. Katz JD, Cronau LH, Barash PG: Postoperative hypertension: hazards of abrupt cessation of antihypertensive medication in preoperative period. Am Heart J 92:79, 1976
57. White PF, Coe V, Dworsky W, Margotis A: Disseminated intravascular coagulation following midtrimester abortions. Anesthesiology 58:99, 1983
58. Sutton DMC, Hanser R, Kulapongs P, Backman F: Intravascular coagulation in abruptio placentae. Am J Obstet Gynecol 109:604, 1971
59. Phillips LL, Davidson CC: Procoagulant properties of amniotic fluid. Am J Gynecol 113:911, 1972
60. Postgraduate Educational Issue: Symposium on malignant hyperthermia. Br J Anaesth 60:251, 1988
61. Nelson TE, Flewellen EH: The malignant hyperthermia syndrome. N Engl J Med 309:416, 1983
62. Gronert GA: Malignant hyperthermia. Anesthesiology 53:395, 1980
63. Britt BA: Dantrolene. Can Anaesth Soc J 31:61, 1984
64. Rosenberg H, Fletcher JE: Masseter muscle rigidity and malignant hyperthermia susceptibility. Anesth Analg 65:161, 1986
65. Carroll JB: Increased incidence of masseter spasm in children with strabismus anesthetized with halothane and succinylcholine. Anesthesiology 67:559, 1987
66. Hein HAT: Lack of availability of dantrolene in American surgical facilities: an estimate of associated mortality. Anesthesiology 69:726A, 1988
67. Wetchler BV: Problem-solving in the postanesthesia care unit. p. 275. In Wetchler BF (ed): Anesthesia for Ambulatory Surgery. JB Lippincott, Philadelphia, 1985
68. Eckenhoff JE, Kneale DH, Dripps RD: The incidence and etiology of postanesthetic excitement. A clinical survey. Anesthesiology 22:667, 1961
69. Larson GF, Hurlbert BJ, Wingard D: Physostigmine reversal of diazepam-induced depression. Anesth Analg 56:348, 1977
70. Hill GE, Stanley TH, Sentker CR: Physostigmine reversal of postoperative somnolence. Can Anaesth Soc J 24:707, 1977
71. Smiler BG, Bartholomew EG, Sivak BJ, et al: Physostigmine reversal of scopolamine delirium in obstetric patients. Am J Obstet Gynecol 116:326, 1973
72. Bidwai AV, Cornelius LR, Standley TH: Reversal of innovar-induced postanesthetic somnolence and disorientation with physostigmine. Anesthesiology 44:249, 1976
73. Koka BV, Jeon IS, Andre JM, et al: Postintubation croup in children. Anesth Analg 56:501, 1977
74. Jordan WS, Graves CL, Elwin RA: New therapy for postintubation laryngeal edema and tracheitis in children. JAMA 212:585, 1970
75. Dubvsky SL, Trustman R: Absence of recall after general anesthesia: implications for theory and practice. Anesth Analg 55:696, 1976
76. Eiscle V, Weinreich A, Bartle S: Preoperative awareness and recall. Anesth Analg 55:513, 1976
77. Bitner RL: Awareness during anesthesia. p. 349. In Orkin FK, Cooperman LH (eds): Complications in Anesthesiology. JB Lippincott, Philadelphia, 1983
78. Epstein BS: Outpatient anesthesia. In

American Society of Anesthesiologist Refresher Course Lectures. 1982

79. Blacher RS: On awakening paralyzed during surgery: a syndrome of traumatic neurosis. JAMA 234:67, 1975
80. Fahy A, Marshall M: Postanesthetic morbidity in outpatients. Br J Anaesth 41:433, 1969
81. Ogg TW: An assessment of postoperative outpatient cases. Br Med J 4:573, 1972
82. Dhamee MS, Gandhi SK, Kalbfleisch JH, et al: Morbidity after outpatient anesthesia: a comparison of different endotracheal anesthetic techniques for laparoscopy. Anesthesiology 57:A375, 1982
83. Keenan RL: Anesthetic disasters: causes, incidence, preventability. Refresher Course Lectures, American Society of Anesthesiologists 242, JB Lippincott, Philadelphia, 1988
84. Bruns K: Postoperative care and review of complications. Int Anesthesiol Clin 20:27, 1982
85. Driscoll EJ: ASOA anesthesia morbidity and mortality survey. J Oral Surg 32:733, 1974
86. Lytle JJ, Yoon C: Anesthesia morbidity and mortality survey: Southern California Society of Oral and Maxillofacial Surgeons. J Oral Surg 38:814, 1980
87. Green RA, Taylor TH: An analysis of anesthesia medical liability claims in the United Kingdom, 1977–1982. Int Anesthesiol Clin 22:73, 1984
88. Wetchler BV: Outpatient anesthesia: no double standard. Anesthesia Patient Safety Foundation Newsletter 2:8, 1987
89. Levy ML: Complications: prevention and quality assurance. Anesth Clin North Am 5:113, 1987
90. Dawson B, Reed WA: Anesthesia for adult surgical outpatients. Can Anaesth Soc J 27:409, 1980
91. Meridy MW: Criteria for selection of ambulatory surgical patients and guidelines for anesthetic management: a retrospective study of 1,553 cases. Anesth Analg 61:921, 1982
92. Patel RT, Hannallah RS: Anesthetic complications following pediatric ambulatory surgery: a 3-year study. Anesthesiology 69:1009, 1988
93. White PF, Shafer A: Nausea and vomiting: causes and prophylaxis. Sem Anesth 6:300, 1988
94. Kallar SK: Aspiration pneumonitis: fact or fiction? p. 29. In Wetchler BV (ed): Outpatient Anesthesia: Problems in Anesthesia. Vol. 2:No 1 JB Lippincott, Philadelphia, 1988
95. Olsson GL, Hallen B, Hambracus Jonzon K: Aspiration during anaesthesia: a computer aided study of 185, 358 anaesthetics. Acta Anaesth Scand 30:84, 1986

19

Postoperative Pain Management

S. Mark Poler
John Zelcer
Paul F. White

> "Slapping the patient on the face and telling him or her that 'it's all over' is a complete inversion of the truth. As far as the patient is concerned, it is just the beginning."[1]

In 1942, Ferguson discussed local and general anesthetic techniques for outpatients in his textbook entitled *Surgery of the Ambulatory Patient*.[2] However, he offered almost no advice to the practitioner regarding modalities for providing postoperative analgesia. The currently available armamentarium of analgesic medications has expanded vastly since that time, but we have not fully exploited it for the benefit of patients undergoing outpatient operations.[3] Management of acute postoperative pain is one of the primary responsibilities of anesthesiologists; however, it poses some unique problems following ambulatory surgery. The increasing number and complexity of operations being performed on an outpatient basis are presenting the practitioner with new challenges with respect to acute pain management. Outpatients undergoing ambulatory procedures require analgesia that is effective, has minimal side effects, is intrinsically safe, and can be easily managed away from the hospital or surgery center.

The adequacy of postoperative pain control is one of the most important factors in determining when a patient can be discharged from an ambulatory facility.[4–7] Since inadequately treated pain is a major cause of unanticipated hospital admissions after ambulatory surgery[8,9] the ability to provide adequate pain relief by simple methods that are readily available to the ambulatory patient in his or her home environment is one of the major challenges for providers of outpatient surgery and anesthesia.

Unfortunately, there are very few well-controlled studies that have examined the incidence and severity of pain after outpatient surgery, or even the adequacy of its treatment. In the majority of postsurgical inpatients, parenteral opiate analgesics administered for moderate or severe pain fail to achieve adequate pain relief.[10,11] In fact, inadequate analgesia is the most common surgically related cause of unanticipated hospital admission after ambulatory surgery.[8,9] On the other hand, use of opioids during the perioperative period can be associated with an increased incidence of postoperative nausea and vomiting in outpatients,[12–15] which may in turn contribute to a delayed discharge from the ambulatory facility.[14,16,17] However, the use of opioid analgesics (as well as nonopioid analgesics and therapeutic modalities) to achieve optimal postoperative pain relief does not prolong recovery,[6,7] may contribute to the relief of nausea,[18] and can actually decrease recovery (discharge) time after more painful procedures.[5]

Although individual patient needs vary widely, the requirement for analgesia is highly predictable. Nevertheless, recovery room nurses often restrict the amount of pain medication they administer because of concerns about side effects and addiction liability, rather than progressively titrating opioid analgesics to achieve adequate relief of postoperative pain.[10,19–23] "Good" patients will suffer quietly, thinking that pain is the necessary accompaniment to surgery. Conversely, the "demanding" patient may tempt the staff either to be excessively liberal with analgesic medication, resulting in excessive sedation, or to simply ignore the demanding type of patient in favor of the "good" patients. Either extreme reflects the inadequate individualization of analgesic therapy, a major problem in postoperative pain management.[24]

Since the opioid blood concentrations associated with sedation and respiratory depression are usually significantly higher than the analgesic threshold concentrations (i.e., minimum effective analgesic concentrations) for patients in pain, carefully titrated doses of opioid analgesics administered to treat acute pain are extremely safe.[25] In addition, there is virtually no risk of addiction when acute postoperative pain is being treated with opioid analgesics for brief, predictable periods of time.[25–27] Teske et al. reported a poor correlation between the observations of nurses regarding whether their patients were experiencing pain and the reports of pain experienced by the patients themselves.[28] Unfortunately, these misconceptions of the medical and nursing staff regarding pain and addiction liability caused them to limit the availability of prescribed analgesic drugs. As a result of the above attitudes and practices, many patients are actually receiving less than 25 percent of the analgesic medication needed to control their postoperative pain.[29] Between 60 percent[29] and 90 percent[21,22] of the inpatients surveyed reported unacceptable pain relief.

The availability of newer opioid and nonopioid analgesics, as well as adaptations of currently available techniques for analgesic administration (e.g., patient-controlled analgesia [PCA], opioid infusions), offer increasing choices in the selection of treatment modalities for the outpatient undergoing an elective ambulatory procedure. Simple adjunctive techniques involving the use of local anesthetic-containing topical creams and aerosols, as well as infiltration and wound perfusion at the surgical site, can decrease the required doses of both oral and parenteral analgesics, while other less invasive techniques (e.g., transcutaneous patches, nasal or buccal sprays) hold promise for the future.

Bonica identified three major factors that contribute to the inadequate provisions for providing optimal patient comfort in the immediate postoperative period: deficiencies in our knowledge of pain and its mechanisms, inadequate application of available knowledge regarding pain and its relief, and poor communication of basic science research results to clinical practitioners.[30] Detailed discussions of pain and its mechanisms, psychological and pathophysiologic consequences, and interventions are available in many review articles and monographs.[3,4,25,31–43]

Before discussing the past, present, and future status of acute pain management in the outpatient setting, we will review the important role of pharmacokinetic and dynamic variability in determining the individual patient's response to a given dose of pain-relieving medication. Both opioid and nonopioid analgesics, which are the mainstays of analgesic therapy after ambulatory surgery, will be discussed (Table 19-1),[24] including the efficacious (but often underutilized) nonsteroidal anti-inflammatory drugs. Uses of parenteral analgesics and local anesthetics will also be discussed in the context of those special situations in which they are appropriate for ambulatory surgery patients. The last section of this chapter will consider evolving methods for providing acute postoperative pain relief. Because of their dependence on trained personnel, sophisticated technology, and/or expensive devices, however, the usefulness of these newer techniques in the practice of outpatient analgesia is presently limited. Acupuncture, electrical nerve stimulation, and hypnosis may eventually find a niche for providing postoperative analgesia to some surgical outpatients.

PHARMACODYNAMIC AND PHARMACOKINETIC VARIABILITY

For individual patients in the early postoperative period, there is wide variability in the relationship between the administered dose of analgesic medication and the pain response.[44,45] Following standard doses of analgesic medication, both the time needed to achieve a peak drug level and the

Table 19-1. Classification of Commonly Used Opioid and Nonopioid Analgesics and Their Antagonists

Drug (trade names)
Opioid agonists
Alfentanil (Alfenta)
Alphaprodine (Nisentil)[a]
Codeine
Dextromethorphan (Tussafed)
Diacetylmorphine (heroin)
Fentanyl (Sublimaze)
Hydrocodone (Synalogos, dihydrocodeinone)
Hydromorphone (Dilaudid, dihydromorphinone)
Levorphanol (Levo-Dromoran)
Meperidine (Demerol, pethidine)
Methadone (Dolophine)
Morphine (MS-Contin, Morphine IR, Roxanol, Roxane)
Oxycodone (Percodan)
Oxymorphone (Numorphan)
Phenoperidine (Lealgin,[b] Operidine[c])
Propoxyphene (Darvon)
Sufentanil (Sufenta)
Opioid partial agonists
Buprenorphine (Buprenex)
Opioid agonist-antagonists
Bremazocine
Butorphanol (Stadol)
Dezocine
Nalbuphine (Nubain)
Nalorphine
Pentazocine (Talwin NX; with naloxone, 0.5 mg)
Opioid antagonists
Naloxazone
Naloxone (Narcan)
Naltrexone (Trexan)
Nonsteroidal anti-inflammatory drugs
Diclofenac (Voltaren)
Diflusinal (Dolobid)
Fenoprofen (Nalfon)
Flurbiprofen (Ansaid)
Ibuprofen (Motrin, Medipren, Midol, Nuprin, Advil, Rufen, Aches-N-Pain)
Indomethin (Indocin)
Ketoprofen (Orudis)
Meclofenamate (Meclomen)
Mefanamic acid (Ponstel)
Naproxen (Naprosyn, Anaprox)
Phenylbutazone (Butazolidin)
Piroxicam (Feldene)
Sulindac (Clinoril)
Suprofen (Suprol)
Tolmetin (Tolectin)
Representative salicylic acid derivatives
Acetaminophen with hydrocodone (Vicodin, many others)
Acetylsalicylic acid (aspirin, Ecotin, Ascriptin, Bufferin)
Choline magnesium salicylate (Trilisate)
Sodium salicylate (Disalcid)
Potassium salicylate/aminobenzoate (Pabalate)
Common combinations
Acetaminophen with codeine (Tylenol #3, etc.)
Aspirin with codeine (Empirin #3, etc.)
Acetaminophen with hydrocodeine (Vicodin)
Acetaminophen with oxycodone (Tylox, Percocet)
Acetaminophen with propoxyphene and caffeine (Darvocet-N, Darvon Compound)
Acetaminophen or aspirin with pentazocine (Talacen or Talwin Compound)

Trade names appear in parenthesis.
[a] Withdrawn from U.S. market; [b] available in Sweden; [c] available in Great Britain.

actual peak level achieved also vary widely (i.e., pharmacokinetic variability). Similarly, individual patients vary pharmacodynamically in their responses to given plasma drug concentrations (Fig. 19-1).[44–47] With standard analgesic dosing regimens, drug levels following intermittent intramuscular injections may be above therapeutic (analgesic) levels for only 35 percent of each 4-hour dosing interval.[44] Maximum cerebrospinal fluid (CSF) opioid concentrations also vary widely after parenteral drug administration.[48,49] Despite the high degree of interpatient variability in opioid blood level and analgesic requirements, the drug concentration required for adequate analgesia in the individual patient is much more consistent (Fig. 19-2).[44,45,50]

A low tolerance for pain has been associated with high scores on anxiety and neuroticism personality scales.[44,51] Pain and anxiety are clearly interrelated. Increasing anxiety will make pain less tolerable and, conversely, increasing pain intensifies anxiety.[52] In a study by Scott et al., the level of preoperative anxiety was shown to be a linear predictor of postoperative pain.[53] Coping styles also appear to be important in determining individual patient differences in their analgesic requirement. For

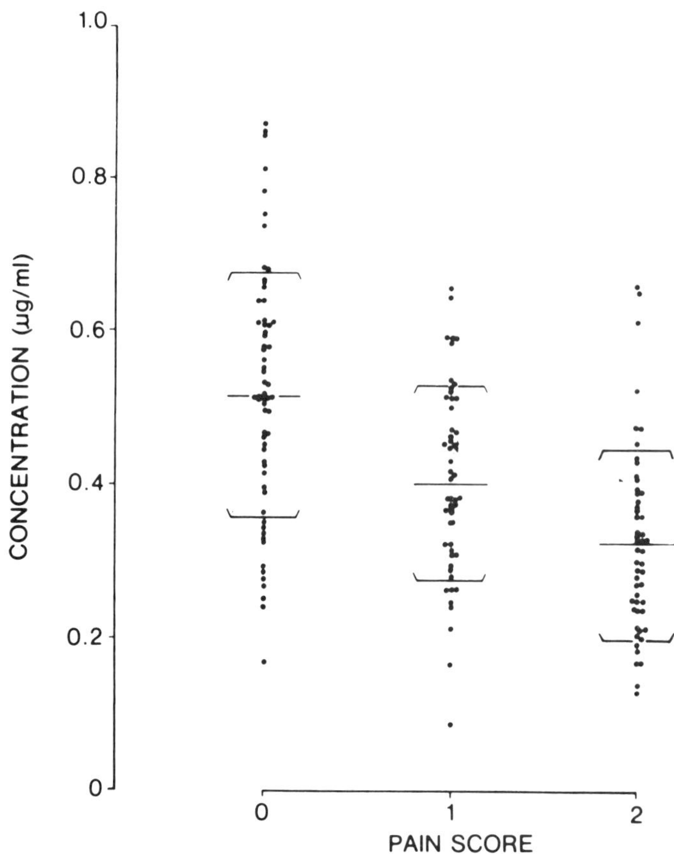

Fig. 19-1. Plasma meperidine levels associated with arbitrary pain scale ratings. There is a wide range of variability in concentrations associated with an analgesic response among individuals. There is also a large overlap of the concentration ranges associated with no analgesia (2), or complete analgesia (0) by different persons. (From Austin et al.,[46] with permission.)

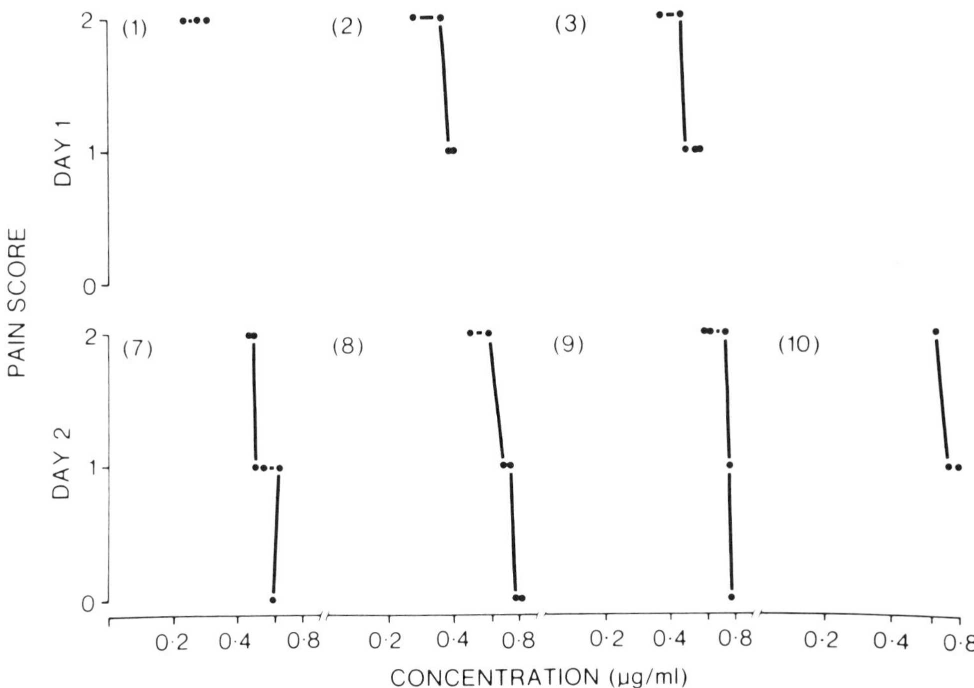

Fig. 19-2. Relationship between blood meperidine concentrations and postoperative pain scores (evaluated as none [0], moderate [1], or severe [2]) in an individual patient after a series of ten intramuscular injections. The numbers in parenthesis on the figure are the sequential injection numbers. Injections (4)-(6) occurred overnight and were not evaluated. The remarkable reproducibility and narrowness of the analgesic concentration range after each injection are noteworthy. (From Austin et al.,[44] with permission).

example, highly aggressive patients consume more medication than patients whose coping styles are more passive. Stoic attitudes on the part of patients and inadequate efforts by the medical and nursing staff to inform patients that effective analgesic medication is available also contributes to the undertreatment of acute postoperative pain.[52,54,55]

Investigations of the influence of age on opioid analgesic requirements have suggested that older patients have an increased sensitivity to opioid analgesics during the perioperative period.[56,57] Alterations in pharmacokinetic factors with increasing age may also result in decreases in the opioid analgesic requirement of geriatric outpatients.[58–61] However, when patients were allowed to titrate their own medication using an "on demand" analgesia delivery system (e.g., PCA), Tamsen et al. reported no age-related differences in the plasma opioid concentrations.[45] Other investigators have reported that a given blood concentration of an opioid analgesic produces greater depression of central nervous system (CNS) activity in the elderly.[60] Although brain receptors may change with increasing age, the effects of aging on the number and affinity of CNS opiate receptors have not been carefully studied. There appears to be wide variability at all ages in patient responses to fixed opioid dosages.[47,62] While analgesic medication is frequently administered on a milligram per kilogram basis, there is little evidence for a direct link between body weight and analgesic requirement.

Investigators have attempted to predict individual analgesic requirements by using physical measurements, pharmacokinetic variables, and personality scores as elements of a database for solving multivariate equations.[63] However, at present, there are no simple or reliable predictors of a given patient's analgesic requirement. All prescriptions for postoperative analgesics should take into consideration the patient's concurrent medications, as well as preexisting medical conditions that might alter their response to these drugs.

ORAL ANALGESICS

Opioid Analgesics

The term *opioids* (narcotics) refers to analgesic drugs that are derived from either natural or synthetic sources. Although opioid analgesics are most often administered parenterally, they can also provide effective pain relief following oral administration. To achieve comparable analgesia, larger doses of opioid medication are required because of the extensive hepatic metabolism after oral absorption (i.e., "first pass" effect) (Table 19-2). Although the onset of analgesia is slower following oral administration, the duration of pain relief is significantly longer after equianalgesic dosages (Fig. 19-3).[64] The term *narcotic* is derived from the Greek word, narkosis, meaning stupor. Historically, the term *opiate* has been used to refer to morphine and other structurally related derivatives of opium. Opioid is currently the preferred nomenclature when referring to morphine-like analgesics. This more general term encompasses natural and synthetic, endogenous

Table 19-2. Equivalent Doses of Opioid Analgesics by Parenteral, Oral, or Rectal Administration for Treatment of Acute Postoperative Pain

Generic name	Dosing interval (h)	Parenteral dose (mg)	Alternate route of delivery	Alternate route dose (mg)
Propoxyphene HCl/Napsylate	3–4	NA	Oral	65/100
Meperidine	2–4	50	Oral	150
Pentazocine	2–4	30	Oral	50–100
Codeine	4–6	30	Oral	30–60
Alphaprodine	2–3	20	NA	NA
Nalbuphine	3–6	10	NA	NA
Oxycodone	4–6	5	Oral	5–10
Morphine sulphate	3–4	5	Oral	10–30
			Rectal	10–20
MS-Contin[a]	8–12	NA	Oral	15–30
Hydrocodeine	4–6	5	Oral	5–10
Methadone	8–12	5	Oral	10
Oxymorphone	4–6	1.5	Rectal	5
Diacetylmorphine	3–4	2.5	Oral	10
Levorphanol	6–8	2	Oral	2–3
Hydromorphone	3–6	2	Oral	2–3
			Rectal	2–3
Butorphanol	3–4	2	Oral (Nasal[b])	2
Buprenorphine	4–6	0.3–0.6	(Sublingual[b])	(0.6–1.2)
Alfentanil	PRN	0.500	NA	NA
Fentanyl	PRN	0.075	NA	NA
Sufentanil	PRN	0.015	NA	NA

All doses are in approximate milligrams for a 70-kg adult. Doses and intervals need to be adjusted for the individual. PRN signifies titrated treatment as needed (intravenously or intramuscularly). NA signifies that the route or dose is not applicable.

[a] Slow-release morphine preparation. Use the same total daily dose as for immediate-release morphine, in two (every 12 hours) or three (every 8 hours) divided doses.

[b] Not an FDA approved use.

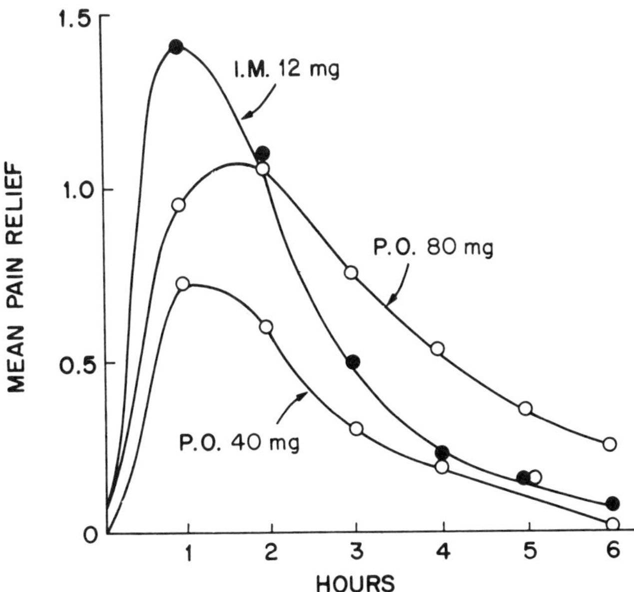

Fig. 19-3. Time-effect curves demonstrating changes on an arbitrary scale after intramuscular and oral morphine doses. The peak effect of the intramuscular dose is earlier and of greater benefit. However, the duration of effect from the oral dose is more prolonged. The effect of first-pass metabolism on analgesic efficacy of two oral doses is also seen. (Modified from Houde et al.[253] as appears in Jaffe and Martin,[64] with permission).

and exogenous substances, including both agonist and antagonist drugs.

These compounds have binding activity at specific opiate receptor subtypes (Table 19-3).[38,65,66] Depending on their interaction with opioid receptors, opioid drugs are classified as either pure agonists, partial agonists, agonist-antagonists, or pure antagonists.[65,67] For opioid agonists, the drug usually has a high affinity for the opioid receptor(s) and activates associated effector mechanisms, while antagonists have specific binding affinity for the opioid receptor(s) but elicit little or no intrinsic activity in the effector processes.

Pure Agonists

Morphine and codeine are both naturally occurring opioid analgesics. Morphine is the prototypic opioid agonist against which all other analgesics must be compared. While the newer opioid compounds may be more potent or have more desirable pharmacologic profiles, there is no better pain-relieving drug than morphine. At equianalgesic doses, opioids that have a reduced affinity for μ-receptors (versus morphine) appear to have an increased incidence of side effects (e.g., constipation, nausea, vomiting, dysphoria). It has been suggested that the more prominent effects are due to interactions with other opioid receptor subtypes.[25] Since morphine is subject to extensive first-pass hepatic metabolism, a dose of about 30 mg PO is required to achieve an analgesic effect which is comparable to 10 mg given parenterally. Because of its side effect profile (e.g., respiratory depression, nausea, vomiting, ileus, sedation), high abuse potential, and low bioavailability, oral morphine is seldom prescribed for acute postoperative analgesia in the outpatient setting.[67]

Table 19-3. Classification of Opioid Receptor Subtypes, Pharmacologic Agonists and Antagonists, and Their Clinical (Pharmacologic) Effects

Subtype	Pharmacologic effects	Prototype agonist	Agonist drugs	Antagonist drugs
μ-1	Supraspinal analgesia	Morphine	β-endorphin morphine and other pure agonist opioids, meptazinol	Naloxone, partial agonists opioids, agonist-antagonist opioids
μ-2	Ventilatory depression, decreased heart rate, constipation, physical dependence, euphoria	Morphine	Pure agonist opioids	Naloxone, agonist-antagonist opioids
δ	Modulation of μ-receptor activity	Vas deferens	Leu-enkephalin	Naloxone, met-enkephalin
ϵ	Analgesia	β-Endorphin	Benzomorphan	(?)
κ	Analgesia, sedation, ventilatory depression, miosis	Ketocyclazine	Dynorphin, MR 2033, partial agonist opioids, agonist-antagonist opioids	Naloxone
σ	Dysphoria, hallucination, hypertension, tachycardia, tachypnea, hypertonia	SKF10047	Ketamine	(?)

Data from Stoelting,[38,66] Neil and Terenius,[65] and other sources.

Codeine is a highly effective analgesic following oral administration because it is less extensively metabolized in the liver than morphine (i.e., it has a higher bioavailability).[68] A drug combination consisting of codeine and acetaminophen or acetylsalicylic acid is the most commonly used oral analgesic following outpatient surgery. A total of 60 mg codeine is equivalent to 600 mg acetaminophen or 650 mg aspirin.[69] When codeine is administered with acetaminophen, the combination is more effective than either analgesic alone.[70] When larger doses (>2 mg/kg) of codeine are administered, its side effect profile becomes similar to morphine, yet with less analgesic benefit. In fact, nausea, vomiting, and constipation are more common with codeine than with morphine because of its reduced affinity for the μ-receptors relative to the other opiate receptor subtypes.

Oxycodone is a codeine derivative that is also orally active. Its analgesic potency is similar to morphine, with a side effect profile similar to codeine. Oxycodone, 5 mg PO, is usually combined with acetaminophen, 325 to 500 mg PO, or acetylsalicylic acid, 325 mg PO, in oral preparations.

Meperidine (50 to 100 mg PO) is a highly effective analgesic which can be used for moderate to severe postoperative pain. Its oral efficacy is limited because of its extensive "first-pass" metabolism. Meperidine is about one sixth to one tenth as potent as morphine parenterally and orally. Since meperidine has a side effect profile and abuse potential similar to morphine, its usefulness as an oral analgesic is limited following outpatient surgery. Accumulation of a metabolite with CNS-stimulating (epileptogenic) properties, normeperidine, can occur with extended use of meperidine in patients with compromised renal function.[71]

Hydromorphone (1 to 2 mg) is a potent

and orally effective derivative of morphine with euphoria as a prominent side effect. Its use for postoperative analgesia in the outpatient setting is limited because of its high abuse potential and relatively short duration of analgesic action (3 to 4 hours).

Methadone (5 to 20 mg) is an orally effective, synthetic opioid that is extremely long-acting (8 to 18 hours) and highly suitable for use in ambulatory surgery (Fig. 19-4).[72,73] However, it can be extremely sedating in analgesic doses.[25] The chemical structure of methadone is different from morphine, allowing for its use in patients who are allergic to morphine or meperidine. However, it has a complex pharmacokinetic profile (i.e., long redistribution and elimination halflives) that makes it difficult to titrate accurately to the outpatient's acute analgesic needs.[25,73–75] Therefore, methadone may be used to provide a basal level of analgesia after the more painful outpatient procedures (e.g., hernia repair, osteotomies, breast augmentation), but it should not be depended on as the primary analgesic. Methadone has minimal associated euphorogenic properties and therefore has little abuse potential.

Propoxyphene is an orally active, synthetic opioid analgesic structurally related to methadone. The commercial products Darvon (propoxyphene HCl, 32 or 65 mg, Eli Lilly and Company, Indianapolis, IN) or Darvon-N (propoxyphene napsylate, 50 or 100 mg, Eli Lilly and Company, Indianapolis, IN) do not contain caffeine. However, Darvon Compound (Eli Lilly and Company, Indianapolis, IN) contains propoxyphene, 32 or 65 mg, as well as aspirin, 325 mg, and caffeine, 32.4 mg. Propoxyphene is at least two thirds as potent as codeine.[67,76] While propoxyphene is not as

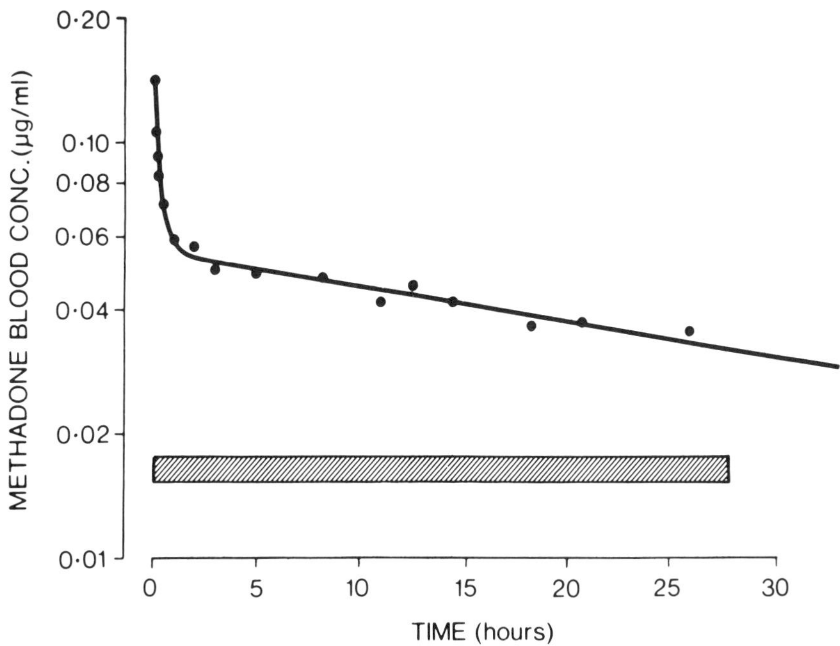

Fig. 19-4. After a single intravenous bolus of 20 mg of methadone, the decreasing plasma concentrations were measured (dots) and fitted to a biexponential decay model (line). The data are plotted on a semilogarithmic scale. The terminal elimination halflife was 36 hours. The period of complete analgesia after repair of a hiatus hernia was 28 hours, denoted by the cross-hatched bar. (From Gourlay et al.,[73] with permission.)

effective as acetaminophen or aspirin alone,[25,77,78] the combination of propoxyphene with a mixture of aspirin (and caffeine) produces greater analgesia than that produced by either propoxyphene or aspirin (and caffeine) administered alone. Therefore, propoxyphene in combination with aspirin may be useful in the management of postoperative pain when aspirin or acetaminophen alone is inadequate.

Partial Agonists

Buprenorphine is a newer, long-acting analgesic that has been described as a partial agonist. Partial agonists interact with the μ-receptors and compete with pure agonists. Like other agonist-antagonists, analgesia is primarily κ-receptor–mediated. However, while antagonism of pure agonists is demonstrable, the unique characteristic distinguishing buprenorphine (and pentazocine to some extent) from other agonist-antagonist opioids is that it produces only a mild withdrawal in opioid-dependent individuals[79]; this is thought to be the result of slow dissociation of the complex it forms with opiate receptors.[80] For this reason, buprenorphine has been used in chemical dependency detoxification programs. It is approximately 30 times more potent than morphine, and has a longer duration of action following an equianalgesic dose. Buprenorphine has a high affinity for the μ-receptor; however, its intrinsic activity is low. These contradictory effects of buprenorphine result in potent analgesic and respiratory depressant activities, with the capability of partially antagonizing pure agonist opioid effects at higher dosages. Because it also possesses some agonist-antagonist type activity at other opioid receptors, the potential for physical dependence is low. It is effective by oral, parenteral (intramuscular), and sublingual[81–83] routes of administration. However, buprenorphine is subject to more than 70 percent first-pass enteric metabolism after oral administration. Even after sublingual administration, only about 50 percent of the administered dose is bioavailable. Side effects include sedation, dizziness, nausea and vomiting, euphoria and hallucinations, as well as occasional cardiovascular changes. Buprenorphine (3 μg/kg) has been successfully used as a premedication alternative to intravenous or intramuscular morphine at the time of surgery, and for analgesia in the first 24 hours following orthopaedic extremity surgery.[84]

Agonist-Antagonists

Agonist-antagonists exert their analgesic effects primarily at the κ-opioid receptors, having limited activity at the μ-opioid receptors. Although they appear to bind to the μ class of opioid receptors, they produce minimal agonist activity after binding. The major advantage of the agonist-antagonist analgesics is related to their "ceiling (plateau) effect" with respect to respiratory depression (Fig. 19-5). However, agonist-antagonists are also characterized by a plateau with respect to analgesia, leading to decreased analgesic efficacy at higher doses.[85,86] Therefore, these compounds are of limited usefulness in the treatment of moderate to severe pain during the early recovery period after outpatient surgery.

Paradoxically, increasing doses of agonist-antagonists reduce their analgesic efficacy because additional blockade of μ-receptors decreases the efficacy of analgesia elicited by binding at κ-receptors.[87,88] The agonist-antagonists are opioids with low abuse potential and limited direct analgesic activity. However, they appear to be suitable for mild to moderate pain in the outpatient setting. Since they are antagonists of μ-receptor binding agonists, their use can also limit the analgesic effectiveness of subsequently administered pure opioid agonists.

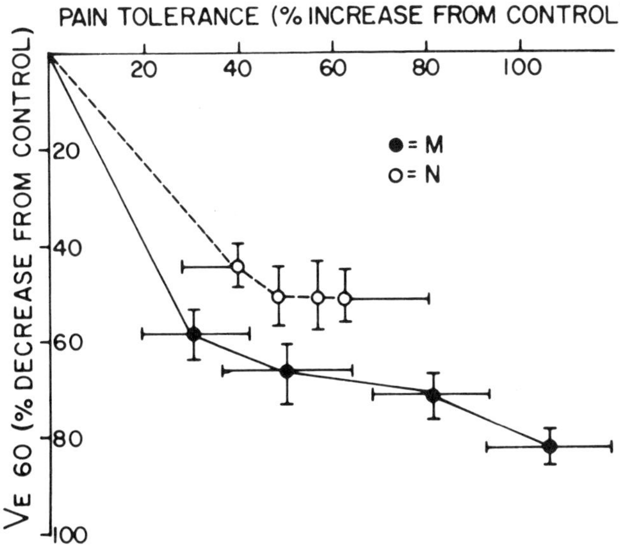

Fig. 19-5. The decrease in the minute volume ($\dot{V}_E$) response provoked by breathing a gas mixture to give an end-tidal carbon dioxide equal to 60 mmHg is plotted against the analgesic response obtained to incremental doses of nalbuphine (N, -○-) or morphine (M, -●-). For every analgesic response, the decrement in breathing response is greater for morphine. However, the blunting of the respiratory response to carbon dioxide challenge, and the maximal analgesia obtained with nalbuphine, are limited at a "ceiling" response, while both responses to increasing morphine doses continue to increase incrementally. (From Gal et al.,[86] with permission.)

Pentazocine was the first agonist-antagonist opioid introduced into clinical practice. It is approximately one third as potent as intramuscular morphine, and almost equipotent to oral codeine. The usual analgesic dose of pentazocine is 50 mg PO every 3 to 4 hours. Its side effects are related to prominent activity at non-μ-opioid receptor subtypes, such as κ (sedation and dizziness) and σ (psychomimetic effects, including anxiety, nightmares, and dysphoria) receptors. At low doses of pentazocine (20 to 25 mg), respiratory depression is disproportionately prominent compared with an equianalgesic dose of morphine; however, its respiratory depressant effects do not continue to increase with higher doses (i.e., plateau effect). Use of pentazocine in opioid-dependent patients can precipitate acute withdrawal symptoms.[67,79] Interestingly, Levine et al. suggested that a low-dose naloxone infusion potentiates the κ-mediated analgesia produced by pentazocine, in contrast to its ability to antagonize μ-mediated analgesics.[89] A commercial oral tablet, Talwin NX (Winthrop Pharmaceuticals, New York, NY), contains 50 mg pentazocine, with 0.5 mg naloxone to minimize the potential for intravenous drug abuse. Perhaps naltrexone, a long-acting opioid antagonist, and pentazocine will also prove to be a useful analgesic combination with minimal abuse potential.

Butorphanol is a more potent agonist-antagonist which is pharmacologically similar to pentazocine; however, its psychomimetic side effect profile is less prominent. An intramuscular dose of butorphanol, 2 to 3 mg, is equivalent to morphine 10 mg intramuscularly with respect to its analgesic and respiratory depressant actions. As expected, increasing doses of butorphanol result in a ceiling effect with respect to its analgesic and respiratory depressant effects. Sedation is a more prominent side effect with butorphanol than with other agonist-antagonist drugs. Like buprenorphine, it can be used to reverse respiratory depression due to pure opioid agonists used intraoperatively, without completely reversing or eliminating opioid-mediated analgesia.

Nalbuphine is another popular agonist-antagonist that acts as a μ-receptor antagonist while producing κ-receptor–mediated analgesia. Unlike buprenorphine, it is a potent opioid antagonist.[79] Nalbuphine is approximately equianalgesic with morphine.[90,91] Thus, it is an effective analgesic for moderate to severe postoperative pain.[90] Its side effect profile includes minimal respiratory[86,92] or cardiovascular depression with doses up to 200 mg/hr.[93] Nalbuphine has minimal psychomimetic effects because of low affinity for σ-receptors. However, it (like pentazocine) can precipitate withdrawal in physically dependent patients.[67,79]

In a comparative clinical trial involving analgesic administration after dental extractions, nalbuphine, 30-60 mg PO, was a more effective analgesic than hydrocodeine, 30 mg PO. Maximal analgesia was achieved in 1.5 hours with nalbuphine compared with 1 hour for hydrocodeine. However, nalbuphine's analgesia persisted throughout the 4-hour observation period compared with only 3 hours for hydrocodeine. Supplemental analgesic medication was required in 33 percent of the patients receiving hydrocodeine compared with 37 percent of the patients receiving nalbuphine, 30 mg PO, and only 12 percent of the patients receiving nalbuphine, 60 mg PO. Side effects typical of opioid analgesics were encountered in all three treatment groups.[94] To provide analgesia in the immediate postoperative period before oral intake recommenced, nalbuphine (0.3 mg/kg IV) was administered at the end of surgery. It was reported to be equivalent to morphine (0.2 mg/kg IV) in providing analgesia after tonsillectomy in children.[95] Both analgesics were superior to placebo, and no adverse effects of nalbuphine were reported.

Nonsteroidal Anti-inflammatory Drugs

A large number of new nonsteroidal anti-inflammatory drugs (NSAIDs) reflecting several different chemical structures have been introduced in the last 20 years (Table 19-1).[66,96] A few of these drugs will be discussed in this section. These compounds are nonopioid analgesics thought to reversibly inhibit prostaglandin synthetase, and appear to produce their analgesic effects by inhibiting the formation of prostaglandin products of arachidonic acid metabolism (principally PGI_2 and PGE_2), thereby limiting tissue inflammation.[96–98,99] However, their mechanism of analgesic action may also include a CNS component. These drugs have proved to be effective adjuvants to opioid analgesics for treating moderate to severe postoperative pain.

The principle advantage of NSAID compounds is the absence of undesirable opioid-related side effects such as sedation, respiratory depression, nausea and vomiting, constipation, ileus, tolerance, and physical dependence. Although some studies suggest that these compounds may be synergistic with respect to analgesia when used in conjunction with opioids, they do not necessarily decrease the incidence of opioid-related side effects.[40] The principle side effects of the NSAIDs include gastrointestinal irritation, occasional deterioration of renal function, and rare hypersensitivity reactions.[98,99] When compared with the opioid analgesics, the NSAIDs produce minimal psychomotor impairment in objective assessments using simulated driving[100] and critical flicker fusion tests.[101–103]

In addition to their analgesic activity, the antiinflammatory and antiplatelet actions of the NSAIDs also vary widely depending on the structural family. Some NSAIDs possess antiinflammatory effects at analgesic doses (e.g., indomethacin, 50 to 100 mg PO), while others do not possess significant antiinflammatory activity at the usual analgesic doses (e.g., naproxen, 500 to 750 mg PO).[104] Intravenous sodium salicylate (a nonacetylated salicylic acid) lacks antiplatelet activity at analgesic doses.[40] Importantly, animal studies suggest that when NSAIDs are used postoperatively, they have the ability to reduce tissue adhesions.[105]

While many studies have demonstrated analgesic efficacy when NSAIDs are used to relieve postoperative pain, others have been unable to demonstrate analgesic actions in the early postoperative period.[106] The inability of NSAIDs to control pain in the early recovery period may result from an inadequate dose of a potentially efficacious NSAID, or inappropriate use of the drug for the treatment of severe acute pain. Although a more prolonged analgesic effect may be achieved with larger doses,[107] some studies suggest that the NSAIDs offer a maximum benefit beyond which higher doses produce no additional analgesia.[77,108] Modification of the chemical structure of currently available NSAIDs may lead to the development of compounds with greater analgesic efficacy in the treatment of postoperative pain. Nevertheless, when the currently available NSAIDs are used alone or in combination for mild to moderate postoperative pain, they appear to be acceptable alternatives to the opioid analgesics.

Acetylsalicylic acid (aspirin) is similar to acetaminophen (Tylenol [McNeil Consumer Products Company, Fort Washington, PA]) with respect to its analgesic potency. These NSAID analgesics are known as analgesic-antipyretics because of their ability to decrease elevated body temperatures in febrile patients. Although it is difficult to make direct comparisons between the opioid analgesics and the nonopioid analgesics, some investigators have suggested that acetylsalicylic acid, 650 mg PO, is equivalent to morphine, 5 to 10 mg IM.

Lysine acetylsalicylate is a water-soluble salt of acetylsalicylic acid administered by intramuscular or intravenous injection. This preparation is metabolized by the liver to the active drug, acetylsalicylate. Korttila et al. found that the onset of analgesia with lysine acetylsalicylate (12.5 to 25 mg/kg) was slower than oxycodone (0.15 mg/kg), but that the quality of analgesia produced by lysine acetylsalicylate was comparable after vein stripping operations.[109] In addition, the antiinflammatory activity of salicylates and other NSAIDs may minimize peripheral components of pain mechanisms, thus reducing the overall postoperative opioid requirement. Aspirin also alters platelet function by irreversibly binding to platelets and inhibiting aggregation, a property unique to the acetylated NSAIDs.[110]

Indomethacin, another widely used NSAID, spared postoperative opioid requirement by about 50 percent when given either by suppository[111] or intravenous infusion.[112,113] In a randomized, double-blind, placebo-controlled clinical trial, the popular NSAID ibuprofen, 500 mg suppositories, given 60 to 90 minutes before surgery and then every 8 hours postoperatively, produced a 20 percent decrease in the morphine PCA requirement.[114] However, pain scores and the incidence of nausea and vomiting were similar in both treatment groups.

Diclofenac is a new, long-acting NSAID available in oral, rectal, and parenteral formulations used primarily for patients with chronic pain due to arthritis.[115] Diclofenac side effects are characteristic of an NSAID compound, principally gastric irritation.[115] In a randomized double-blind study, Nuutinen et al. administered intramuscular diclofenac (75 mg) or oxycodone (10 mg) for postoperative analgesia.[116] The onset of analgesia with diclofenac was slower than oxycodone; however, the pain-relieving effect

1 hour after an intramuscular injection was equivalent in the two drug groups. Furthermore, the interval prior to requesting treatment with a rescue (analgesic) medication was longer in the diclofenac group. In a recent study involving abdominal hysterectomy patients, 70 percent of the patients receiving meperidine, 100 mg IM, required rescue analgesics within 6 hours, yet only 29 percent of the patients treated with diclofenac, 150 mg IM, were rescued within 12 hours.[117] In addition, the number of supplemental analgesic injections required and side effects reported (e.g., nausea, vomiting, and dizziness) were significantly lower in the diclofenac group.[116]

In a double-blind prophylaxis study, Tigerstedt et al. found that an intravenous infusion of diclofenac, 75 mg/h (versus saline), at the completion of intraabdominal or superficial surgery had minimal opioid-sparing effect during the initial 2-hour recovery period.[118] These results were in contrast to the previously reported beneficial effects of lysine acetylsalicylate, dipyridone, or paracetamol in decreasing the postoperative oxycodone requirement.[119,120] In these earlier studies, individual patients were used as their own controls when nonopioid analgesics were administered in response to complaints of pain during the postoperative period. In retrospect, these earlier (positive) results may represent a placebo effect complicating the evaluation of postoperative pain.[121]

The profound opioid-sparing effects of the longer-acting NSAID ketorolac may decrease the likelihood of postoperative ventilatory depression and other opioid-related side effects.[122] Ketorolac, 10-30 mg PO, appears to be equianalgesic to morphine, 3 to 6 mg IM,[122] or acetaminophen, 1 to 2 mg PO.[123] Ketorolac 30–90 mg PO was equivalent to morphine 12 mg IM.[122] While increasing the dose of ketorolac does not improve the quality of the analgesia produced, it does prolong the duration of the analgesic period.[123] Gillies et al. assessed the morphine-sparing effect of ketorolac infusions, 1.5 to 3 mg/hr, using an intravenous PCA titration system.[124] These investigators reported that ketorolac infusions (versus placebo) resulted in lower pain scores and decreased the requirement for supplemental morphine. They also found less ventilatory depression in the ketorolac groups compared with the placebo infusion patients.

Analgesic Combinations

Various combinations of opioid and nonopioid analgesics have been studied to exploit the desired effects of each drug while minimizing their side effects.[125] Other centrally active drugs (e.g., α-2 agonists, respiratory stimulants) have been used in combination with opioid analgesics in an attempt to minimize opioid-related side effects. Recently, investigators reported the use of doxapram to counteract the respiratory depression associated with meperidine administration. However, in the dosages studied (meperidine, 30 mg, with or without doxapram, 45 mg IV), there was no difference in the respiratory rate or the incidence of apnea after cholecystectomy procedures. Furthermore, the use of meperidine did not differ between groups.[126] In fact, the doxapram-treated group complained of greater pain on their visual analog scales.

While opioid analgesics alone or in combination with NSAIDs (and/or local anesthetics) appear to be highly effective in treating surgical pain during the first 24 to 48 hours, NSAIDs can reduce the pain, swelling, and inflammation that develops 24 to 72 hours after surgery. Thus, the use of opioid and nonopioid (NSAID) analgesic combinations is an effective approach to managing acute postoperative pain and may have an additional benefit in decreasing opioid-induced side effects.

Jain et al. compared the NSAID diflusinal and codeine when administered orally alone and in combination. Diflusinal is both analgesic and antiinflammatory, while producing only minimal interference with platelet aggregation. Analgesia was evaluated for 8 hours after lower abdominal procedures and lumbar discectomy operations. Diflusinal, 500 mg PO, alone was superior overall to codeine, 60 mg. However, a combination of the two analgesics was superior to either alone in minimizing opioid-related side effects. The use of the drug combination provided for an earlier onset of analgesia (produced by codeine) and a more prolonged duration of effect (produced by diflusinal). Since there was no statistical evidence of an interaction between the two drugs, it would appear that the degree of analgesia was simply additive.[127] In a similar study, the combination of the investigational NSAID suprofen and codeine was found to be more effective than either drug alone.[128]

The two widely used NSAIDs, ibuprofen[129] and naproxen,[130] also produce additive effects when administered in combination with codeine. Similarly, Or and Bozkurt studied the analgesic effectiveness of a combination of two NSAIDs, aspirin and mefanamic acid.[131] These two drugs were equally effective as analgesics for the pain following third molar extractions; however, the combination was more effective than either drug alone.

Relationship Between Severity of Pain and the Analgesic Drug Regimen

While nonopioid analgesics may be sufficient for treating mild postoperative pain, moderate to severe postoperative pain and acute pain not mediated by inflammatory mechanisms require the analgesic efficacy provided by pure opioid agonists (Table 19-4). To evaluate the severity of pain as a guide to selection of appropriate analgesics and to evaluate the adequacy of the therapy, a pain scale (from 0 to 5) used in the McGill Pain Questionnaire was advocated by Levy.[25] This scale also used verbal descriptors: no pain (0), mild (1, I), moderate/discomforting (2, II), severe/distressing (3, III), very severe/horrible (4, IV), and overwhelming/excruciating (5, V).[132] Based on the severity of the pain, it was possible to devise a treatment regimen involving a number of different analgesic drugs.[25]

The objective assessment of pain is difficult and subjective. For example, patients tend to rate the intensity of pain according to recent experience. Thus, patients who first experience severe pain often evaluate subsequent analgesic therapy as highly effective, while patients who initially experience less intense pain (e.g., after regional conduction block techniques) will later rate their pain as increased and therapy as ineffective.[133] Knos et al. observed this phenomenon in patients having breast biopsies

Table 19-4. Typical Oral Analgesic Regimens[a]

Severity of pain	Non-opioid analgesics	Opioid analgesics
Mild	Aspirin, acetaminophen	Propoxyphene
Moderate	Aspirin, acetaminophen, NSAIDs	Codeine, partial agonists, agonist-antagonists
Severe	NSAIDs	Hydrocodone, oxycodone, methadone, morphine, hydromorphone
	Local anesthetic infiltration or conduction block	

[a] Non-opioid and opioid analgesics may be useful either individually or in combinations. Combinations, either of non-opioids with opioids or of two non-opioids, generally provide additive analgesic effects for increasingly severe pain while minimizing side effects.

under general anesthesia. Patients receiving local anesthetic infiltration (0.5 percent bupivicaine) are often spared intense initial discomfort on awakening from general anesthesia, and will evaluate subsequent pain relative to this initially low intensity pain (compared with untreated control patients who experience their most severe pain initially). However, after 24 hours, the group infiltrated with bupivicaine reported higher pain scores and required more supplemental opioid analgesics.[134] Thus, while an initial assessment may be valuable in initiating a therapeutic regimen, subsequent treatment will need to be adjusted according to the adequacy of the analgesic response. Particular caution is called for with patients having local or regional anesthetic techniques, who should be instructed to begin taking oral analgesics at the first sign of increasing discomfort rather than delaying the first dose until their pain has intensified and becomes more difficult to relieve.

Mild Pain

Mild pain can usually be treated satisfactorily with analgesics such as aspirin or acetaminophen (600 to 1,000 mg). Aspirin should be avoided in patients with a history of gastritis, ulcer, allergic reactions, low platelet counts, or coagulopathy. However, when there is an inflammatory component contributing to the pain, aspirin is a more effective analgesic than acetaminophen. Hepatic compromise is a relative contraindication to acetaminophen-containing compounds because of its associated risk of liver toxicity.

Moderate Pain

Most pain associated with ambulatory surgery is amenable to treatment with oral drugs (e.g., codeine, oxycodone, oxymorphone, and the NSAIDs) that are more potent than those used to treat mild pain (e.g., aspirin, acetaminophen). Tammisto reported good to excellent analgesia for 70 percent to 80 percent of patients treated with oxycodone, 10 to 20 mg IM, after gynecologic and urologic procedures, while 5 percent to 20 percent of the patients surveyed required additional analgesics.[24]

In many cases, the NSAIDs are equal or superior in analgesic effectiveness to the combination of aspirin or acetaminophen with codeine. The time to peak analgesia is typically longer with NSAIDs compared with codeine (and other opioid agonists); however, the overall quality and duration of its analgesia may be greater. As mentioned with respect to the combinations of opioids and acetaminophen or aspirin, the newer NSAIDs produce better analgesia with fewer side effects when administered in combination with the less potent nonopioid analgesics (e.g., acetaminophen and aspirin).[78,125]

Severe Pain

For severe pain to be treated with oral medications requires use of the most efficacious opioid and nonopioid analgesics, often in combination with each other. Combinations of acetaminophen (or aspirin) and oxycodone are the most commonly used treatment regimen for painful ambulatory surgery procedures. Recognizing the wide pharmacologic variability which exists among individual patients, oxycodone (5 to 20 mg PO) will be sufficient for most patients. Since it is difficult to predict which patients may require the higher dosage, preparations containing 325 mg acetaminophen and 5 mg oxycodone (e.g., Percocet [Du Pont Pharmaceuticals, Wilmington, DE]) are usually preferred to those formulations containing larger doses of these drugs alone.

The addition of a NSAID to the potent orally active opioids can be remarkably effective. Unfortunately, their onset of analgesia is slow (compared with parenteral opioid injections), such that anticipation of severe pain is required to rapidly achieve acceptable analgesia with these oral combinations. Therefore, initial control of postoperative pain with incremental doses of potent, rapid-acting intravenous opioid analgesics (e.g., fentanyl 50 to 100 μg IV, sufentanil 5 to 15 μg, hydromorphone 1 to 2 mg, oxymorphone 1.5 to 3 mg, morphine 2 to 4 mg, meperidine 25 to 50 mg, alfentanil 0.5–1 mg) is usually recommended in the recovery room. Alternatively, a long-acting NSAID or opiate premedicant can be used to establish effective analgesia in the immediate postoperative period. Oxymorphone suppositories are also a useful alternative to injected opioids to obtain rapidly effective analgesia until the analgesic effect of the oral opioid is established.

The partial agonists (e.g., buprenorphine) and agonist-antagonists (e.g., nalbuphine) in combination with NSAIDs are also effective analgesics. The combinations can provide long-lasting analgesia with minimal side effects following most outpatient procedures. Nalbuphine with acetaminophen is an effective combination with low abuse potential and less respiratory depression than opioid agonist combinations.[135] To the extent that they antagonize the pure agonists, agonist-antagonists will complicate postoperative pain management if it subsequently becomes necessary to switch to a potent opioid agonist to obtain adequate pain relief.

The most severe postoperative pain can only be satisfactorily treated with potent opioid analgesics alone or in combination with local anesthetic drugs. Morphine, codeine, and their analogs remain the mainstays of treatment for severe pain (as they have been since the 19th century).[136] The opioid-sparing effect of the NSAIDs can potentially minimize the side effects associated with the opioids.

Liquid oral morphine preparations (10 to 100 mg/5 ml) are titratable and well-tolerated by ambulatory cancer patients. In the future, sustained release oral preparations of morphine administered as a premedicant may also prove useful in minimizing postoperative pain in the outpatient setting.[81,137–145] However, the reliability of its absorption and its analgesic effectiveness in postoperative outpatients still needs to be determined.[146–148] Promising sustained-release morphine suppositories have been designed for either initially rapid release or constant release to maintain analgesic plasma levels over 12-hour periods.[149]

Unfortunately, the most effective orally active opioid analgesics (morphine, hydromorphone, and levorphanol) are also the most liable to be abused. Nevertheless, hydromorphone's relatively short duration of action is useful for treating severe pain in the early recovery period. Levorphanol, with a longer dosing interval (6 to 8 hours) would be appropriate for patients with severe pain expected to last for many hours to days (e.g., lumbar laminectomy, knee ligament repairs, shoulder rotator cuff repairs). The use of this analgesic after an outpatient procedure requires a good professional (nursing) support system away from the health care facility, because it is difficult to titrate this potent analgesic to needed analgesia without producing excessive sedation. Currently, most patients requiring these potent opioid analgesics are being admitted to hospitals for overnight "23-hour admission" parenteral analgesic therapy.

Newer Analgesic Drugs and Adjuvants

Newer synthetic opioid analgesics such as dezocine[85,150,151] and pentamorphone (RX 77989)[152] are undergoing extensive laboratory and clinical testing at the present time. More widespread use of the new μ-1 opioid receptor agonist meptazinol has been limited because of its side effect profile.[153] However, meptazinol has been used effectively as a suppository for treating postoperative pain.[154] Picenadol is a mixed agonist-antagonist (a racemic mixture of a D-isomer that is both a μ and a δ agonist, while the L-isomer is an opioid antagonist) that has proven to be a satisfactory analgesic for treating moderate postoperative pain.[155,156]

Although progress in the development of more effective κ and σ opioid receptor agonists has been disappointing (e.g., bremazocine,[157] ketamine[158]), an opioid analgesic that did not produce respiratory depression would be of obvious value. Nefopam is a nonopioid analgesic structurally related to the antihistaminic compound, diphenhydramine, which does not produce respiratory depression; however, its usefulness as a postoperative analgesic is yet to be determined. The side effects of nefopam include moderate tachycardia and diaphoresis.[159]

Even though their main physiologic functions may be unrelated to analgesia per se, many hormonal and synthetic molecules have opioid agonist or antagonist properties. The cholecystokinin antagonist, proglumide, has in vitro activity suggesting that it can bind to δ-opioid receptors.[160] However, a double-blind clinical trial was unable to detect any potentiation of morphine analgesia for postoperative cholecystectomy pain.[161] Another study found that proglumide actually potentiated the antagonistic effect of nalorphine.[162] Hence, proglumide does not appear to be a clinically useful analgesic.

Other more promising drug groups which may prove to be effective in decreasing the postoperative opioid analgesic requirement include the α-2-agonists (e.g., clonidine, dexmedetomidine) and the enkephalinase inhibitors (e.g., SCH 32615 and its structural analogs). Preliminary studies suggest a role for endorphins and enkephalins in the modulation of acute postoperative pain.[50,163] For example, the presence of high CNS levels of endogenous morphine-like substances might be expected to minimize the requirement for exogenous opioid analgesics during the early postoperative period. The concept of providing analgesia by manipulating the CNS's endogenous opioid system has the potential for improved postoperative pain relief while avoiding the peripheral side effects of exogenously administered opioids.

LOCAL ANESTHETICS

Intraoperative infiltration with a local anesthetic solution can obviate the need for any additional analgesics after breast biopsies.[164] Hernia repair with a conduction block and local anesthetic infiltration is highly satisfactory when combined with gentle surgical technique[165,166] and can provide for excellent analgesia in the early postoperative period.[167] Wound instillation of 0.5 percent bupivicaine significantly decreases postoperative pain scores after foot surgery.[168] In a recent report, Moss et al. described the discharge of 40 of 43 cholecystectomy patients. The patients were discharged within 24 hours after their operation if the incision was infiltrated with 0.5 percent bupivicaine and measures to promote gastric motility (e.g., metoclopramide) were undertaken.[169] In contrast, none of the 83 patients receiving conventional parenteral analgesics were discharged in less than 3 days.

Intraarticular bupivicaine is widely held to be effective for pain relief after knee arthroscopic surgery. However, a randomized, double-blind study failed to demonstrate any opioid-sparing effect with respect to the postoperative demand for papaveretum between the control and bupivicaine-treated groups.[170] Interestingly, these investigators did find a statistically significant reduction in the papaveretum requirement and the analog pain scores when patients receiving a femoral nerve block

Table 19-5. Comparative Effects of Parenteral Morphine, Bupivicaine Nerve Block, and Topical Lidocaine for Postoperative Pain Relief After Outpatient Circumcision[a]

	Control (placebo)	Morphine sulfate (0.2 mg/kg)	Nerve block (1.0–1.5 ml)	Lidocaine jelly (0.5–1.0 ml)
Age (yr)	5 ± 2	5 ± 2	4 ± 2	4 ± 2
Pain in postanesthesia care unit (%)	92	27	7[b]	5[b]
Pain-free period (h)	1.1 ± 1.0	4.8 ± 1.7[b]	5.2 ± 1.7[b]	5.3 ± 1.9[b]
Analgesic doses (N)				
0–24 h	1.9 ± 1.0	2.0 ± 0.9	1.5 ± 1.1	1.7 ± 1.1
24–48 h	1.5 ± 1.3	0.7 ± 1.1[b]	1.0 ± 1.1[b]	0.7 ± 1.2[b]

[a] Mean values ± SD.
[b] Significant difference from the control group, $P < .05$.
(Data from Tree-Trakarn and Pirayavaraporn.[176])

were compared with untreated controls and an intraarticular bupivicaine-treated group.[170,254] Continuous[171,172] or intermittent perfusion[167,172–174] of the surgical wound with local anesthetic solutions is also a simple, safe, and effective technique for providing analgesia at the surgical site.

While subcutaneous infiltration of the operative site with local anesthetics remains a popular technique for decreasing the postoperative opioid analgesic requirement in the early recovery period,[164,169] other simplified local anesthetic delivery systems have recently been described. Topical analgesia with lidocaine aerosol has been shown to be highly effective in decreasing pain, as well as the opioid analgesic requirement, after inguinal herniorrhaphy[175] (Fig. 19-6). The simple application of topical lidocaine jelly has also been shown to be as effective as nerve blocks and parenteral opioids in providing pain relief after outpatient circumcision (Table 19-5).[176,177] Intracavitary and wound instillation of local anesthetics is another simple and effective technique for providing pain relief during the early postoperative period.[172]

Regional conduction blocks seem to offer superior analgesia, at least in the initial postoperative period (Table 19-6).[24,178,179] Conduction anesthesia may also have other long-term ramifications for postoperative analgesia due to blockade of the afferent nerve barrage associated with deep tissue injury. Under some circumstances, arrival of a volley of pain impulses carried in C-fibers establishes a field of excessive excitability in the spinal cord, which may become a self-sustaining reflex process. Subsequent nonpainful stimulation from within that sensory field may be interpreted as painful.[33,180]

The combined use of local anesthetics and opioid analgesics may provide additional benefits. While epidural local anesthetic and opioid analgesic combinations are becoming increasingly popular for obstetric analgesia[181,182] as well as for postoperative analgesia,[183,184] dose-response studies are needed to establish optimal con-

Table 19-6. Effect of Anesthetic Technique on the Postoperative Analgesic Requirement

	Time to first request (h)	No analgesic requested (%)	Opioid required in first 2 hours (%)
General anesthesia alone	<2	5	56
With opioid premedication	>5[a]	12	7[b]
Regional anesthesia alone	<8[a]	15	4[b]
With opioid premedication	>9[a]	12	6[b]

[a] $P < .05$.
[b] $P < .01$.
(Adapted from McQuay et al.,[179] with permission.)

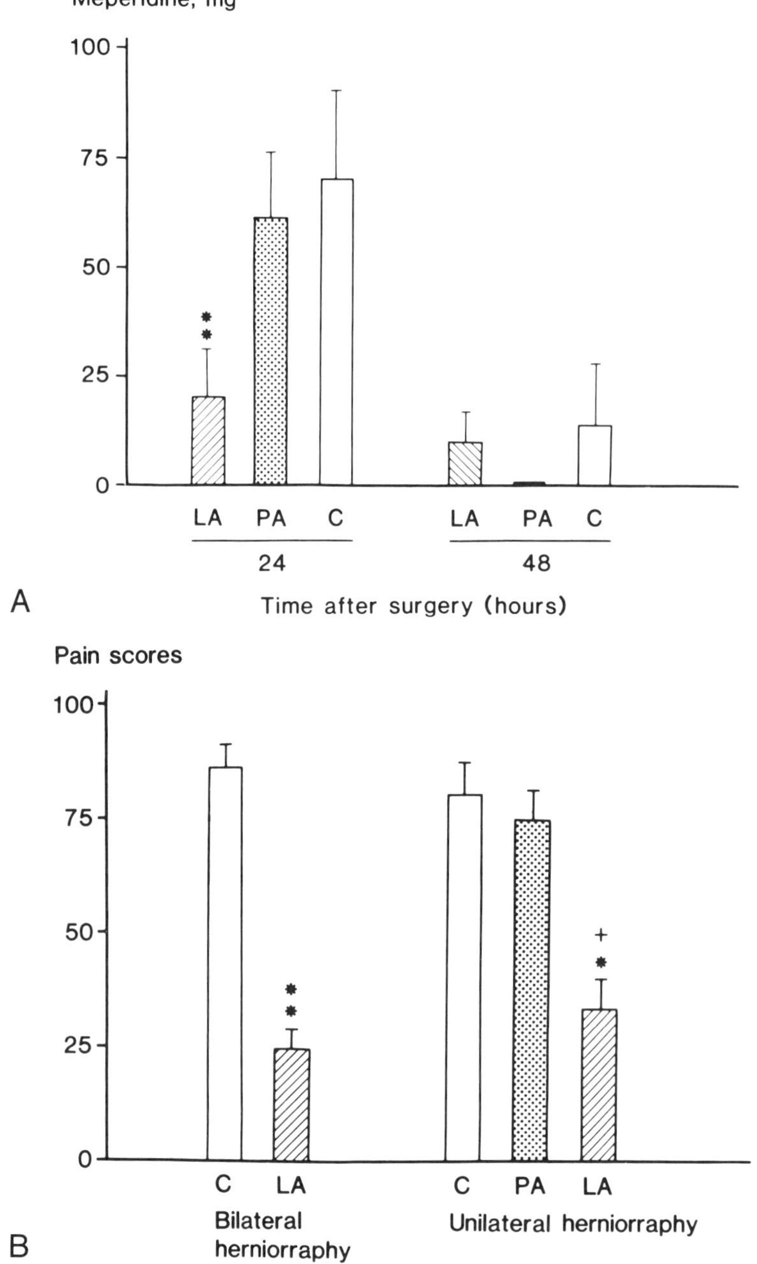

Fig. 19-6. (**A**) Meperidine requirements in the first 24 hours after inguinal hernia repair were significantly reduced for patients treated with lidocaine aerosol (LA) in the surgical wound, compared with patients treated with placebo aerosol (PA) or untreated control patients (C). Bars shows mean requirement, whiskers demarcate SEM.**$P<.01$. (**B**) Twenty-four hours after surgery, pain scores on palpation of the herniorrhaphy wound were significantly less when treated with LA in the wound (left portion of panel). There was a significant reduction of pain scores with LA (**$P<.01$). Seven patients having bilateral hernia repair (right portion of panel) were randomly assigned to treatment on one side with LA or PA, while the other side was left untreated as a paired control. There was a significant response compared with control for LA (*$P<.05$), and for LA versus PA ($^{+}P<.05$). (From Sinclair et al.,[175] with permission.)

centrations (and dosages) of each drug in order to minimize the potential for side effects and untoward drug interactions. In addition, the effects of injected analgesic volume and adjunctive use of vasoconstrictive drugs on the quality and duration of analgesia produced by epidural local anesthetic-opioid combinations needs to be more fully evaluated.

Pediatric Regional Blocks

Use of regional anesthetics for pediatric anesthesia has become one of the most active areas for clinical pain research. The use of regional anesthesia as a supplement to general anesthesia serves two main purposes for ambulatory surgical procedures involving pediatric outpatients.[185] First, it provides excellent analgesia in the immediate postoperative period, facilitating a pleasant emergence and providing better analgesia than oral acetaminophen or indomethacin. Second, use of regional (local) anesthetic techniques minimizes the need for opioid injections.

Caudal blocks were the first to be advocated.[186–188] Subsequently, inguinal[189] or ilioinguinal[190] and hypogastric[191] nerve blocks have been shown to be as effective as caudal anesthesia. More recently, simple wound infiltration[192,193] for hernia and orchiopexy procedures[194–196] and dorsal nerve penile block[197–200] or topical anesthesia for circumcision[176,177,201] have been advocated as highly effective alternatives to the more complicated regional anesthetic techniques. It has been noted that caudal and ilioinguinal nerve blocks require the highest degree of technical skill and are associated with the highest incidence of inadequate analgesia and other unwanted side effects (e.g., weakness and urinary retention).[185]

In pediatric outpatients, simple wound infiltration at the incision site with 0.25 percent to 0.5 percent bupivicaine was as effective as caudal analgesia with bupivicaine, 1 mg/kg, for herniorrhaphy, and had a similar incidence of complications.[192] With local anesthetic infiltration, more satisfactory analgesia was achieved and less supplemental analgesic medication was required than with caudal analgesia.

Effective regional analgesia with a ring block at the base of the penis for circumcision reduced the need for supplemental fentanyl analgesia in the recovery room from about 50 percent to 20 percent.[198] In addition, the time to discharge was decreased by 30 minutes for those patients not requiring fentanyl. While caudal anesthesia provided a pain-free emergence from anesthesia for pediatric patients following circumcision, it also prolonged the time to discharge because of residual motor weakness and sympathetic blockade. Surprisingly, caudal blockade did not necessarily decrease the requirement for hydrocodone following inguinal hernia or orchiopexy procedures.[202]

There are even a few reports describing outpatient pediatric surgical procedures performed with local anesthesia alone. Attwood and Evans reported that they performed corrective surgery of the pinna with local anesthesia[203] on patients more than 9 years of age.

Unpleasant recollections of childhood surgical experiences may persist for many years. Mather and Mackie surveyed postoperative analgesia regimens for 170 hospitalized children in Australia.[204] Remarkably, 25 percent of the children had no postoperative analgesic medication orders, and none were administered in 31 percent of the cases. When both opioid and nonopioid medications were ordered, only the nonopioid was administered in 25 percent of the children. Overall, 75 percent of these children had inadequate pain relief and the pain was rated as "severe" in 20 percent of the children on the day of surgery or the first postoperative day. Unfortunately, there is no similar information available on the incidence and severity of postoperative pain following pediatric outpatient procedures.

In many ambulatory surgery settings, reluctance to prescribe opioid analgesics to pediatric outpatients may result in an even larger fraction of patients receiving inadequate analgesic medication. Simple measures, such as the use of topical local anesthetic preparations (e.g., lidocaine cream/jelly, Eutectic Mixture of Local Anesthetics [EMLA] cream) when performing even minor outpatient procedures (e.g., venipuncture), can minimize the painful stigma associated with surgery.[205,206]

ALTERNATIVE METHODS OF ANALGESIC DELIVERY

Patient-controlled analgesia can provide a partial solution to the inherent pharmacokinetic and pharmacodynamic differences which exist among patients.[207,208] While early studies with intravenous PCA therapy (versus intramuscular injections) suggested that improved analgesia and a more rapid recovery after surgery was possible with less opioid medication,[209–211] more recent studies have not substantiated these opioid-sparing benefits.[212–214] Nevertheless, PCA clearly decreases the need for nursing interventions to provide supplemental analgesic therapy compared with other available therapeutic modalities,[215] while providing analgesia with a high degree of patient acceptance.[216]

Other simplified opioid delivery systems which appear to hold promise for the future include slow-release oral analgesics[217] as well as buccal,[218] sublingual,[81–83,219] transnasal,[220,221] and subcutaneous[222] routes of administration. As mentioned previously (Table 19-2), extensive hepatic metabolism of opioid compounds limits their bioavailability when administered orally (i.e., the so-called "first-pass effect"), thus limiting the usefulness of this route of administration in controlling early postoperative pain.[144]

Although sublingual absorption of morphine is poor, the bioavailability of methadone, fentanyl, and buprenorphine is significantly better using the sublingual route of administration.[223] When opioid compounds are injected into subcutaneous tissue, a larger dose of opioid medication is required.[222] However, subcutaneous PCA with morphine and its analogs (e.g., hydromorphone and oxymorphone) has been shown to be as efficacious as intravenous PCA for managing acute postoperative pain.[222,224] Simplified delivery systems would appear to offer advantages over the more sophisticated drug delivery systems (e.g., epidural opiates and local anesthetics) for patients undergoing less stressful operations (e.g., ambulatory surgery). Studies involving the use of ambulatory PCA following elective outpatient surgery are in progress. These preliminary studies will provide needed insights into the efficacy of ambulatory PCA on an outpatient basis, as well as its technical requirements and safety in that setting.

Current inpatient investigations involving the use of "on demand" epidural opiate and/or local anesthetic administration (epidural PCA) may result in another approach for the future. Concerns about enhanced systemic absorption of the more potent lipophilic narcotic analgesics (e.g., fentanyl, sufentanil) contributing to a higher incidence of drug-induced side effects (e.g., sedation),[225] as well as other technical and safety questions (e.g., catheter migration), are likely to limit the clinical use of this technique in the outpatient setting.

Sublingual Delivery

The sublingual route of administration for opioids is appealing since it is readily accessible, avoids first-pass hepatic drug metabolism, and provides for a rapid onset of analgesia. However, only buprenorphine (a partial agonist) is currently marketed in a sublingual form. In a study designed to determine the fraction of sublingually administered opioid recovered by gastric lavage (i.e., swallowed) after a 10-minute absorption period, the investigators reported that significant amounts of sublingually administered morphine (18 percent), buprenorphine (55 percent), fentanyl (51 percent), and methadone (34 percent) were retrieved. In fact, the estimate of morphine's sublingual absorption may have overestimated its bioavailability. Buffering the oral pH to 8.5 favored the nonionized fraction, and increased methadone's absorption to 75 percent. Absorption of methadone and fentanyl were also time-dependent. Other opioid analgesics (e.g., hydromorphone, oxycodone) were not significantly absorbed sublingually.[223] In one study of patients undergoing knee surgery, sublingual buprenorphine was equivalent to intramuscular morphine or meperidine in all respects except that the morphine group had more frequent shivering in the recovery room.[226] In another report, sublingual buprenorphine provided analgesia comparable to parenteral morphine and meperidine after abdominal surgery, although buprenorphine was associated with more frequent nausea and sedation.[227]

Buccal Transmucosal Administration

Although one report has suggested that morphine administered buccally has greater bioavailability than when administered intramuscularly,[218] possible swallowing of bucally administered morphine was not evaluated in that study. Of greater interest to anesthesiologists is the transmucosal administration of analgesic fentanyl and its analogs.

Oral delivery of fentanyl (as a "lollipop") probably includes both transmucosal and enteric absorption, since onset of analgesia is in part determined by active sucking (versus passive dissolution) and absorption of swallowed drug. Time to increased tolerance for painful stimuli occurred within 20 to 40 minutes and lasted 1 to 2 hours with transmucosal fentanyl, 0.5 to 1.0 mg. Typical opioid-induced side effects (e.g., oxygen desaturation, itching, nausea and vomiting) were reported in the transmucosal fentanyl group. Other opioid-related side effects (e.g., dizziness) were frequently noted on sitting and standing.[228,255] Larger doses (e.g., fentanyl, >15 μg/kg) resulted in longer periods of analgesia; however, its use is associated with an unacceptably high incidence of side effects. Nevertheless, treatment with low-dose transmucosal analgesic delivery systems (e.g., fentanyl, 5 to 15 μg/kg) may be an acceptable low-technology method of administering individualized continuous analgesia in a nonthreatening manner after outpatient procedures resulting in moderate to severe pain. Studies to determine the safety and efficacy of oral transmucosal fentanyl in the treatment of postoperative pain are in progress.

Transdermal Administration

As an alternative to parenteral PCA techniques requiring sophisticated pumps and personnel to monitor postoperative analgesia, a simple and reliable transdermal delivery system for maintaining analgesic plasma opioid concentrations could prove to be extremely valuable. Highly lipophilic opioids (e.g., fentanyl, sufentanil) can be absorbed transdermally after application of skin patches containing an opioid reservoir provided with a diffusional rate-limiting membrane.[229–231] Unfortunately, even with a fentanyl loading bolus, 100 to 200 μg IV (2 hours after patch application), plasma levels of fentanyl increased slowly and required 8 hours to achieve a steady-state "analgesic" blood concentration comparable to those achieved with an intravenous infusion at a fixed rate of 100 μg/h. In addition, plasma clearance is slow (with elimination halflife values of 10 to 25 hours), presumably due to continuing release from a dermal depot. In fact, at 12 hours after patch removal, over two thirds of the patients still had plasma levels >1 ng/ml and, at 24 hours, 10 percent to 20 percent still had fentanyl plasma levels exceeding 1 ng/ml.

Delayed clearance could be considered an advantage for prolonged postoperative analgesia. However, two patients with high plasma fentanyl levels were discontinued from the study protocol when their respiratory rates decreased to less than 8 breaths/min after supplemental morphine analgesia.[232,233] Slow increases in plasma fentanyl levels after application of the patch, and slow decreases after patch removal, increases the potential for adverse drug interactions in the postoperative period, and appears to limit the usefulness of currently available transdermal opioid delivery systems. In addition, fixed doses and rates of drug delivery with opioid patches fail to address the need for titration of analgesic medication to meet the changing needs of individual patients during the early postoperative period.

Rectal Administration

Rectal opioid administration provides for a nonoral, nonparenteral route of administration that also minimizes first-pass hepatic metabolism. The NSAID diclofenac (2 mg/kg) given rectally to children was less sedating and produced less respiratory depression than an opioid mixture (papaveretum) after tonsillectomy.[234] Although complete relief of pain with diclofenac was less frequent than in the opioid group, the requirement for supplemental doses of acetaminophen was decreased in the diclofenac group.[234]

The potent opioid oxymorphone is also available in a rectal suppository form containing 5 mg. Initial onset of analgesia occurs within 10 minutes, and its duration of analgesic action persists for 3 to 6 hours. A cumulative effect equivalent to 25 to 50 mg of parenteral morphine can be achieved with an oxymorphone suppository.

NONPHARMACOLOGIC TECHNIQUES

Transcutaneous electrical nerve stimulation (TENS) has been used as an adjuvant during and after minor outpatient surgical procedures. Given the inherent side effects produced by both opioid and nonopioid analgesics, as well as the local anesthetics, it is not surprising that nonpharmacologic approaches to managing acute postoperative pain have been evaluated in the outpatient setting. Transcutaneous electrical nerve stimulation has been reported to produce a 20 to 50 percent decrease in the halothane anesthetic requirement,[235] as well as the postoperative opioid requirement.[51,236] Pulmonary function was reportedly less depressed in TENS-treated patients than in a sham-treated group.[237] In addition, Jensen et al. reported a more rapid recovery of joint mobility after outpatient arthroscopic surgery (Table 19-7).[238] Nevertheless, other investigative groups have reported no significant decrease in the requirement for opioid analgesic medication or the incidence of postoperative complications when TENS was used for postoperative pain control.[24,239–242] When used after superficial surgical procedures,[243] proper application of the stimulating electrodes and proper patient instruction appear to be important factors if postoperative analgesia is to be achieved with TENS.[244]

Other nonpharmacologic approaches (e.g., cryoanalgesia,[245–247] acupuncture,[248] ultrasound,[249] and hypnosis[250]) have also been evaluated as potentially useful adju-

Table 19-7. Comparative Effects of Transcutaneous Electrical Nerve Stimulation, Sham Stimulation, and Placebo (Control) Treatment After Outpatient Knee Arthroscopy

	Control	Sham	TENS
Number (N)	30	30	30
Pain score			
Day 1	5.8	5.5	4.8
Day 2	5.8	4.5	4.0
Day 3	4.1	3.1	2.9
Total	15.7	13.1	11.7[a]
Analgesic score			
Day 1	3.6	3.3	2.8
Day 2	3.7	2.8	1.8
Day 3	1.9	1.7	1.3
Total	9.2	7.8	5.9[a]
Range of motion			
Week 1	103.2	102.0	111.8
Week 3	119.4	112.4	124.4[a]
Week 7	119.3	119.6	130.0[a]

[a] Significantly different from control group, $P < .05$.
(Data from Jensen et al.[238])

vants to opioid analgesics in the early postoperative period. For most of these modalities, clinical studies have yielded conflicting data.[247]

HOME DELIVERY SYSTEMS FOR ANALGESIC MEDICATION

Until there is more widespread availability of specialized home care nursing services[251] to provide effective long-term outpatient analgesic care with newer treatment modalities (e.g., ambulatory PCA, continuous local and regional anesthetic blocks), it will be difficult to improve currently available postoperative analgesic techniques for outpatients undergoing more extensive surgical procedures. However, the availability of appropriate professional nursing services cannot proceed until the third-party payers agree to reimburse ambulatory (or at-home) nursing and equipment costs as cost-effective alternatives to hospital or convalescent facility admission. As more extensive and painful surgery procedures (e.g., cholecystectomy, laminectomy, knee reconstructions, hysterectomies) are being undertaken on an outpatient basis, health care payers will need to establish suitable reimbursement policies for postoperative pain management. With more sophisticated postoperative analgesic regimens, it should be possible to optimize the benefits of ambulatory surgery for the patient and the health care provider.

It seems likely that in the future there will be an increased reliance on patient-controlled methods for relieving acute postoperative pain in the ambulatory setting. Ambulatory PCA appears to provide excellent analgesia after more extensive outpatient surgery procedures compared with conventional opioid and nonopioid analgesic regimens. However, outcome studies are needed to evaluate the effect of this newer therapeutic approach on postoperative side effects, discharge times, and other important recovery parameters.

Recent studies suggest that factors other than pain per se must be controlled in order to reduce postoperative morbidity.[252] Not surprisingly, the anesthetic technique can influence the analgesic requirement in the early postoperative period (Table 19-6). Although opioid analgesics will continue to play an important role, the adjunctive use of both local anesthetic agents and nonopioid analgesics will likely assume a greater role in the future. Use of drug combinations (e.g., opiates and local anesthetics, opiates and NSAIDs) may provide for improved analgesia with fewer narcotic-induced side effects than opioid analgesics alone. Finally, safer and simpler delivery systems are needed to improve our future ability to provide cost-effective pain relief after ambulatory surgery.

REFERENCES

1. Armitage EN: Postoperative pain—prevention or relief? Br J Anaesth 63:136, 1989
2. Ferguson LK: Surgery of the Ambulatory Patient. JB Lippincott, Philadelphia, 1942

3. Wildsmith JAW (ed): Symposium on aspects of pain. Br J Anaesth 63:135, 1989
4. White PF: Pain management after day-case surgery. Curr Opinion Anaesthesiol 1:70, 1988
5. Wasudev G, Kambam JR, Hazelhurst WM, et al: Comparative study of sufentanil and isoflurane in outpatient surgery. Anesth Analg 66:S186, 1987 (abstr)
6. Pandit SK, Kothary SP: Should we premedicate ambulatory surgical patients? Anesthesiology 65:suppl. 3A, A352, 1986
7. Soni V, Burney R: Anesthetic techniques for laparoscopic tubal ligation. Anesthesiology 55:A145, 1981 (abstr)
8. Meridy HW: Criteria for selection of ambulatory surgical patients and guidelines for anesthetic management: a retrospective study of 1553 cases. Anesth Analg 61:921, 1982
9. Wetchler BV: Problem solving in the postanesthesia care unit. p. 287. In Wetchler BV (ed): Anesthesia for Ambulatory surgery. JB Lippincott, Philadelphia, 1985
10. Cohen FL: Postsurgical pain relief: patients' status and nurses' medication choices. Pain 9:265, 1980
11. Angell M: The quality of mercy. N Engl J Med 306:98, 1982
12. Morrison JD, Hill GB, Dundee JW: Studies of drugs given before anaesthesia. XV. Evaluation of the method of study after 10,000 observations. Br J Anaesth 40:890, 1968
13. Wilton NCT, Burn JMB: Delayed vomiting after paravaretum in paediatric outpatient surgery. Can Anaesth Soc J 33:741, 1986
14. Rising S, Dodgson MS, Steen PA: Isoflurane v. fentanyl for outpatient laparoscopy. Acta Anaesthesiol Scand 29:251, 1985
15. Zuurmond WWA, van Leeuwen L: Alfentanil v. isoflurane for outpatient arthroscopy. Acta Anaesthesiol Scand 30:329, 1986
16. Doze VA, Shafer A, White PF: Nausea and vomiting after outpatient anesthesia—effectiveness of droperidol alone and in combination with metoclopramide. Anesth Analg 66: suppl., S41, 1987
17. Metter SE, Kitz DS, Young ML, et al: Nausea and vomiting after outpatient laparoscopy: incidence, impact on recovery room stay and cost. Anesth Analg 66: suppl., S116, 1987
18. Andersen R, Krohg K: Pain as a major cause of postoperative nausea. Can Anaesth Soc J 23:366, 1976
19. Anonymous: Postoperative pain. Anaesth Intensive Care 4:95, 1976 (editorial)
20. Weis OF, Sriwatanakul K, Alloza JL, et al: Attitudes of patients, housestaff, and nurses toward postoperative analgesic care. Anesth Analg 62:70, 1983
21. Sriwatanakul K, Weis OP, Alloza JL, et al: Analysis of narcotic usage in the treatment of postoperative pain. JAMA 250:926, 1983
22. Marks RM, Sachar EJ: Undertreatment of medical inpatients with narcotic analgesics. Ann Intern Med 78:173, 1973
23. Charap AD: The knowledge, attitudes, and experience of medical personnel treating pain in the terminally ill. Mt Sinai J Med (NY) 45:561, 1978
24. Tammisto T: Analgesics in postoperative pain relief. Acta Anaesthesiol Scand 70:47, 1978
25. Levy MH: Pain management in advanced cancer. Semin Oncol 12:394, 1985
26. Rayport M: Experience in the management of patients medically addicted to narcotics. JAMA 156:684, 1954
27. Porter J, Jick H: Addiction rare in patients treated with narcotics. N Engl J Med 302:123, 1980 (letter)
28. Teske K, Daut R, Cleeland CS: Relationship between nurse's observations and self-report of pain. Pain 16:289, 1983
29. Donovan M, Dillon P, McGuire L: Incidence and characteristics of pain in a sample of medical-surgical inpatients. Pain 30:69, 1987
30. Bonica JJ: Importance of effective pain control. In Benedetti C, Bonica JJ (eds): Recent Advances in Intraspinal Pain Therapy. Acta Anaesthesiol Scand 31: suppl. 85, 1, 1987
31. Benedetti C, Bonica JJ (eds): Recent Advances in Intraspinal Pain Therapy. Acta Anaesthesiol Scand 31:i suppl. 85, 1987
32. Dodson ME: A review of methods for relief of postoperative pain. Ann R Coll Surg Engl 64:324, 1982

33. Fields HL: Pain. McGraw-Hill, New York, 1987
34. Masson AHB: The role of analgesic drugs in the treatment of postoperative pain. Br J Anaesth 39:713, 1967
35. Mitchell RWD, Smith G: The control of acute postoperative pain. Br J Anaesth 63:147, 1989
36. Oden RV (ed): Management of postoperative pain. Anesthesiol Clin N Am 7:1, 1989
37. Raja SN, Meyer RA, Compbell JN: Peripheral mechanisms of somatic pain. Anesthesiology 68:571, 1988
38. Stoelting RK: Current views on the role of opioid receptors and endorphins in anesthesiology. Int Anesthesiol Clin 24:17, 1986
39. Swerdlow M: General analgesics used in pain relief: pharmacology. Br J Anaesth 39:699, 1967
40. Tammisto T, Tigerstedt I: Mild analgesics in postoperative pain. Br J Clin Pharmacol 10:347S, 1980
41. Utting JE, Smith JM: Postoperative analgesia. Anaesthesia 34:320, 1979
42. White PF: Current and future trends in acute pain management. Clin J Pain 5: suppl. 1, S51, 1989
43. Yaksh TL: Spinal opiates: a review of their effect on spinal function with emphasis on pain processing. In Benedetti C, Bonica JJ (eds): Recent Advances in Intraspinal Pain Therapy. Acta Anaesthesiol Scand 31: suppl. 85, 25, 1987
44. Austin KL, Stapleton JV, Mather LE: Relationship between blood meperidine concentrations and analgesic response. Anesthesiology 53:460, 1980
45. Tamsen A, Hartvig P, Fagerlund C, Dahlström B: Patient-controlled analgesic therapy, part II: individual analgesic demand and analgesic plasma concentrations of pethidine in postoperative pain. Clin Pharmacokinet 7:164, 1982
46. Austin KL, Stapleton JV, Mather LE: Multiple intramuscular injections—a major source of variability in analgesic response to meperidine. Pain 8:47, 1980
47. Shafer A, Sung M-L, White PF: Pharmacokinetics and pharmacodynamics of alfentanil infusions during general anesthesia. Anesth Analg 65:1021, 1986
48. Sjöström S, Hartvig P, Persson P, Tamsen A: Pharmacokinetics of epidural morphine and meperidine in humans. Anesthesiology 67:877, 1987
49. Sjöström S, Tamsen A, Persson P, Hartvig P: Pharmacokinetics of intrathecal morphine and meperidine in humans. Anesthesiology 67:889, 1987
50. Tamsen A, Sakurada T, Wahlström A, et al: Postoperative demand for analgesics in relation to individual levels of endorphins and substance P in cerebrospinal fluid. Pain 13:171, 1982
51. Lim AT, Edis G, Kranz H, et al: Postoperative pain control: contribution of psychological factors and transcutaneous electrical stimulation. Pain 17:179, 1983
52. Mindus P: Anxiety, pain and sedation: some psychiatric aspects. Acta Anaesthesiol Scand 32: suppl 88, 7, 1987
53. Scott LE, Clum GA, Peoples JB: Preoperative predictors of postoperative pain. Pain 15:283, 1983
54. Egbert LD, Battit GE, Welch CE, Bartlett MK: Reduction of postoperative pain by encouragement and instruction of patients. A study of doctor-patient rapport. N Engl J Med 270:825, 1964
55. Leigh JM, Walker J, Janaganathan P: Effects of preoperative anaesthetic visit on anxiety. Br Med J 2:987, 1977
56. Bellville JW, Forrest WH, Jr., Miller E, et al: Influence of age on pain relief from analgesics—a study of postoperative patients. JAMA 217:1835, 1971
57. Kaiko RF: Age and morphine analgesia in cancer patients with postoperative pain. Clin Pharmacol Ther 28:823, 1980
58. Koch-Weser J: Drug disposition in old age. N Engl J Med 306:1081, 1982
59. Maitre PO, Vozeh S, Heykants J, et al: Population pharmacokinetics of alfentanil: the average dose-plasma concentration relationship and interindividual variability in patients. Anesthesiology 66:3, 1987
60. Scott JC, Stanski DR: Decreased fentanyl and alfentanil dose requirements with age: a simultaneous pharmacokinetic and pharmacodynamic evaluation. J Pharmacol Exp Ther 240:159, 1987
61. Yate PM, Sebel PS: Abnormal alfentanil pharmacokinetics. Br J Anaesth 59:808, 1987 (letter)

62. O'Connor M, Prys-Roberts C, Sear JW: Alfentanil infusions: relationship between pharmacokinetics and pharmacodynamics in man. Eur J Anaesthesiol 4:187, 1987
63. Mather LE: Pharmacokinetic and pharmacodynamic factors influencing the choice, dose and route of administration of opiates for acute pain. p. 17. In Bullingham RES (ed): Clinics in Anaesthesiology. WB Saunders, London, 1983
64. Jaffe JH, Martin WR: Opioid analgesics and antagonists. p. 506. In Gilman AG, Gilman LS, Gilman A (eds): The Pharmacological Basis of Therapeutics. 6th Ed. MacMillan, New York, 1980
65. Neil A, Terenius L: Receptor mechanisms for nociception. Int Anesthesiol Clin 24:1, 1986
66. Stoelting RK: Opioid Agonists and Antagonists. p. 69. In Stoelting RK: Pharmacology and Physiology in Anesthetic Practice. JB Lippincott, Philadelphia, 1987
67. Wynn RL, Bergman SA: Opioid analgesics. Compendium 8:812, 1987
68. Beaver WT, Wallenstein SL, Rogers A, Houde RW: Analgesic studies of codeine and oxycodone in patients with cancer. I. Comparisons of oral with intramuscular codeine and of oral with intramuscular oxycodone. J Pharmacol Exp Ther 207:92, 1978
69. Cooper SA, Beaver WT: A model to evaluate mild analgesics in oral surgery outpatients. Clin Pharmacol Ther 20:241, 1976
70. Beaver WT: Mild analgesics: a review of their clinical pharmacology. Am J Med Sci 251:576, 1966
71. Szeto HH, Inturrisi CE, Houde RW, et al: Accumulation of normeperidine, an active metabolite of meperidine, in patients with renal failure or cancer. Ann Intern Med 86:738, 1977
72. Gourlay GK, Willis RJ, Wilson PR: Postoperative pain control with methadone: influence of supplementary methadone doses and blood concentration-response relationships. Anesthesiology 61:19, 1984
73. Gourlay GK, Wilson PR, Glynn CJ: Pharmacodynamics and pharmacokinetics of methadone during the perioperative period. Anesthesiology 57:458, 1982
74. Beaver WT, Wallenstein SL, Houde RW, Rogers A: A clinical comparison of the analgesic effects of methadone and morphine administered intramuscularly, and/or orally and parenterally administered methadone. Clin Pharmacol Ther 8:415, 1967
75. Inturrisi CE, Verebely K: The levels of methadone in the plasma in methadone maintenance. Clin Pharmacol Ther 13:633, 1972
76. Jalovaara P, Kiviniemi H, Stahlberg M: Comparison of diflunisal and dextropropoxyphene napsylate in the treatment of post-operative pain. Ann Chir Gynaecol 74:228, 1985
77. Beaver WT: Analgesic efficacy of dextropropoxyphene and dextropropoxyphene-containing combinations: a review. Hum Toxicol 3: suppl, 191S, 1984
78. Beaver WT: Impact of non-narcotic oral analgesics on pain management. Am J Med 84:3, 1988
79. Schmidt WK, Tam SW, Shotzberger GS, et al: Nalbuphine. Drug Alcohol Depend 14:339, 1985
80. Jacob JJ, Michaud GM, Tremblay EC: Mixed agonist-antagonist opiates and physical dependence. Br J Clin Pharmacol 7: suppl 3, 291S, 1979
81. Derbyshire DR, Vater M, Maile CTD, et al: Non-parenteral postoperative analgesia. A comparison of sublingual buprenorphine and morphine sulfate (slow release) tablets. Anaesthesia 39:324, 1984
82. Carl P, Crawford ME, Madsen NB, et al: Pain relief after major abdominal surgery: a double blind controlled comparison of sublingual buprenorphine, intramuscular buprenorphine, and intramuscular meperidine. Anesth Analg 66:142, 1987
83. Edge WG, Cooper GM, Morgan M: Analgesic effects of sublingual buprenorphine. Anaesthesia 34:463, 1979
84. Maunuksela EL, Korpela R, Olkkola KT: Comparison of buprenorphine with morphine in the treatment of postoperative pain in children. Anesth Analg 67:233, 1988
85. Gal TJ, DiFazio CA: Ventilatory and analgesic effects of dezocine in humans. Anesthesiology 61:716, 1984
86. Gal TJ, DiFazio CA, Moscicki JC: Anal-

gesic and respiratory depressant activity of nalbuphine: a comparison with morphine. Anesthesiology 57:367, 1982
87. Sadee W, Rosenbaum JS, Herz A: Buprenorphine: differential interactions with opiate receptor subtypes in vivo. J Pharmacol Exp Ther 223:157, 1962
88. Takemori AE, Ikeda M, Portoghese PS: The mu, kappa, and delta properties of various opioid agonists. Eur J Pharmacol 123:357, 1986
89. Levine JD, Gordon NC, Taiwo YO, Coderre TJ: Potentiation of pentazocine analgesia by low-dose naloxone. J Clin Invest 82:1574, 1988
90. Pinnock CA, Bell A, Smith G: A comparison of nalbuphine and morphine as premedication agents for minor gynaecological surgery. Anaesthesia 40:1078, 1985
91. Beaver WT, Feiser GA: A comparison of the analgesic effect of i.m. nalbuphine with morphine in patients with post-operative pain. J Pharmacol Exp Ther 204:487, 1978
92. Romagnoli A, Keats AS: Ceiling effect for respiratory depression by nalbuphine. Clin Pharmacol Ther 27:478, 1980
93. Kay B, Krishnan A: On-demand nalbuphine for post-operative pain relief. Acta Anaesthesiol Belg 37:33, 1986
94. Kay B, Lindsay RG, Mason CJ, Healy TEJ: Oral nalbuphine for the treatment of pain after dental extractions. Br J Anaesth 61:313, 1988
95. Krishnan A, Tolhurst-Cleaver CL, Kay B: Controlled comparison of nalbuphine and morphine for post-tonsillectomy pain. Anaesthesia 40:1178, 1985
96. Cooper SA: New peripherally acting oral analgesic agents. Annu Rev Pharmacol Toxicol 23:617, 1983
97. Stoelting RK: Nonopioid and nonsteroidal analgesics, antipyretic and antiinflammatory drugs. p. 240. In Stoelting RK: Pharmacology and Physiology in Anesthetic Practice. JB Lippincott, Philadelphia, 1987
98. Kantor TG: Control of pain by nonsteroidal anti-inflammatory drugs. Med Clin N Am 66:1053, 1982
99. Kantor TG: Use of diclofenac in analgesia. Am J Med 80:64, 1986
100. Korttila K, Linnoila M, Ertama P, Häkkinen S: Recovery and simulated driving after intravenous anesthesia with thiopental, methohexital, propanidid or alphadione. Anesthesiology 43:291, 1975
101. Hindmarch I: Information processing, critical flicker fusion threshold and benzodiazepines: results and speculations. Psychopharmacol Ser 6:79, 1988
102. Hindmarch I: A pharmacological profile of fluoxetine and other antidepressants on aspects of skilled performance and car handling ability. Br J Psychiatry 153: suppl 3, 99, 1988
103. Korttila K, Linnoila M: Psychomotor skills related to driving after intramuscular administration of diazepam and meperidine. Anesthesiology 42:685, 1975
104. Aromaa U, Asp K: A comparison of naproxen, indomethacin and acetylsalicylic acid in pain after varicose vein surgery. J Int Med Res 6:152, 1978
105. DeLeon FD, Toledo AA, Sanfilippo JS, Yussman MA: The prevention of adhesion formation by nonsteroidal antiinflammatory drugs: an animal study comparing ibuprofen and indomethacin. Fertil Steril 41:639, 1984
106. Ruedy J, McCullough W: A comparison of the analgesic efficacy of naproxen and propoxyphene in patients with pain after orthopedic surgery. Scand J Rheumatol 2:56 (suppl), 1973
107. Forbes JA, Kolodny AL, Beaver WT, et al: A 12-hour evaluation of the analgesic efficacy of diflusinal, acetaminophen, and acetaminophen-codeine combination, and placebo in postoperative pain. Pharmacotherapy 3:47S, 1983
108. Forbes JA, Yorio CC, Selinger LR, et al: An evaluation of flurbiprofen, aspirin, and placebo in postoperative oral surgery pain. Pharmacotherapy 9:66, 1989
109. Korttila K, Pentti OM, Auvinen J: Comparison of i.m. lysine acetylsalicylate and oxycodone in the treatment of pain after operation. Br J Anaesth 52:613, 1980
110. Anonymous: Drugs for rheumatoid arthritis. Med Lett Drugs Ther 31:61, 1989 (editorial)
111. Thind P, Sigsgaard T: The analgesic effect

of indomethacin in the early post operative period following abdominal surgery. A double-blind controlled study. Acta Chir Scand 154:9, 1988

112. Taivainen T, Hiller A, Rosenberg PH, Neuvonen P: The effect of continuous intravenous indomethacin infusion on bleeding time and postoperative pain in patients undergoing emergency surgery of the lower extremities. Acta Anaesthesiol Scand 33:58, 1989
113. Maunuksela EL, Olkkola KT, Korpela R: Does prophylactic intravenous infusion of indomethacin improve the management of postoperative pain in children? Can J Anaesth 35:123, 1988
114. Owen H, Glavin RJ, Shaw NA: Ibuprofen in the management of postoperative pain. Br J Anaesth 58:1371, 1986
115. Brogden RN, Heel RC, Pakes GE, et al: Diclofenac sodium: a review of its pharmacological properties and therapeutic use in rheumatic diseases and pain of varying origin. Drugs 20:24, 1980
116. Nuutinen LS, Wuolijoki E, Pentikäinen IT: Diclofenac and oxycodone in treatment of postoperative pain: a double-blind trial. Acta Anaesthesiol Scand 30:620, 1986
117. Carlborg L, Lindoff C, Hellman A: Diclofenac versus pethidine in the treatment of pain after hysterectomy. Eur J Anaesthesiol 4:241, 1987
118. Tigerstedt I, Janhunen L, Tammisto T: Efficacy of diclofenac in a single prophylactic dose in postoperative pain. Ann Clin Res 19:18, 1987
119. Tammisto T, Tigerstedt I, Korttila K: Comparison of lysine acetylsalicylate and oxycodone in postoperative pain following upper abdominal surgery. Ann Chir Gynaecol 69:287, 1980
120. Tigerstedt I, Leander P, Tammisto T: Postoperative analgesics for superficial surgery. Comparison of four analgesics. Acta Anaesthesiol Scand 25:543, 1981
121. Swerdlow M, Murray A, Daw RH: A study of postoperative pain. Acta Anaesthesiol Scand 7:1, 1963
122. O'Hara DA, Fragen RJ, Kinzer M, Pemberton D: Ketorolactromethamine as compared with morphine sulfate for treatment of postoperative pain. Clin Pharmacol Ther 41:556, 1987
123. McQuay HJ, Poppleton P, Carroll D, et al: Ketorlac and acetominophen for orthopedic postoperative pain. Clin Pharmacol Ther 39:89, 1986
124. Gillies GWA, Kenny GNC, Bullingham RES, McArdle CS: The morphine sparing effect of ketorlac tromethamine. A study of a new, parenteral nonsteroidal anti-inflammatory agents after abdominal surgery. Anaesthesia 42:727, 1987
125. Beaver WT: Combination analgesics. Am J Med 77:38, 1984
126. Clyburn PA, Rosen M: Patient-controlled analgesia with a mixture of pethidine and doxapram hydrochloride. A comparison of the incidence of respiratory dysrhythmias with pethidine alone. Anaesthesia 43:190, 1988
127. Jain A, McMahon FG, Ryan JR, et al: A double-blind study of diflunisal and codeine compared with codeine or diflunisal alone in postoperative pain. Clin Pharmacol Ther 43:529, 1988
128. Moore PA, Seldin EB, Donoff RB: A clinical trial in oral surgery of the analgesic efficacy of a suprofen/codeine combination. Anesth Prog 34:177, 1987
129. Cooper SA, Engle J, Ladov M, et al: Analgesic efficacy of an ibuprofen-codeine combination. Pharmacotherapy 2:162, 1982
130. Forbes JA, Keller CD, Smith JW, et al: Analgesic effect of naproxen sodium, codeine, a naproxen-codeine combination and aspirin on the postoperative pain of oral surgery. Pharmacotherapy 6:211, 1986
131. Or S, Bozkurt A: Analgesic effect of aspirin, mefenamic acid and their combination in post-operative oral surgery pain. J Int Med Res 16:167, 1988
132. Melzack R: The McGill pain questionnaire: major properties and scoring methods. Pain 1:277, 1975
133. Kay B: Methods of study of post-operative pain. Eur J Anaesthesiol 5:217, 1988 (letter)
134. Knos GB, Sung YF, Powell RW: Effect of local marcaine infiltration on postoperative pain and morbidity. Anesth Analg 68:S149, 1989
135. Forbes JA, Kolodny AL, Chachich BM,

Beaver WT: Nalbuphine, acetaminophen, and their combination in postoperative pain. Clin Pharmacol Ther 35:843, 1984

136. Beaver WT: Analgesic development: a brief history and perspective. J Clin Pharmacol 20:213, 1980
137. Slowey HF, Reynolds AD, Mapleson WW, Vickers MD: Effect of premedication with controlled-release oral morphine on postoperative pain. Anaesthesia 40:438, 1985
138. Coniam SW: Sustained-release morphine for postoperative analgesia. Anaesthesia 40:700, 1985
139. Derbyshire DR, Pinnock CA, Smith G: Sustained release morphine for postoperative analgesia. Anaesthesia 40:1234, 1985 (letter)
140. Simpson KH, Dearden MJ, Ellis FR, Jack TM: Premedication with slow release morphine (MST) and adjuvants. Br J Anaesth 60:825, 1988
141. Brahams D: Death of patient participating in trial of oral morphine for relief of postoperative pain. Lancet 1:1083, 1984
142. Derbyshire DR, Bell A, Parry PA, Smith G: Morphine sulphate slow release. Comparison with i.m. morphine for postoperative analgesia. Br J Anaesth 57(9):858, 1985
143. Pinnock CA, Derbyshire DR, Elling AE, Smith G: Comparison of oral slow release morphine (MST) with intramuscular morphine for premedication. Anaesthesia 40:1082, 1985
144. Banning AM, Schmidt JF, Chraemmer-Jorgensen B, Risbo A: Comparison of oral controlled release morphine and epidural morphine in the management of postoperative pain. Anesth Analg 65:385, 1986
145. Brescia FJ, Walsh M, Savarese JJ, Kaiko RF: A study of controlled-release oral morphine (MS Contin) in an advanced cancer hospital. J Pain Sympt Manag 2:193, 1987
146. Vater M, Smith G, Aherne GW, Aitkenhead AR: Pharmacokinetics and analgesic effect of slow-release oral morphine sulphate in volunteers. Br J Anaesth 56:821, 1984
147. Pinnock CA, Derbyshire DR, Achola KJ, Smith G: The absorption of controlled release morphine sulfate in the immediate postoperative period. Br J Anaesth 58:868, 1986
148. Clyburn PA, Rosen M: Oral controlled-release morphine and gut function: a study in volunteers. Eur J Anaesthesiol 6:347, 1989
149. Hanning CD, Vickers AP, Smith G, et al: The morphine hydrogel suppository. A new sustained release rectal preparation. Br J Anaesth 61:221, 1988
150. Pandit UA, Kothary SP, Pandit SK: Intravenous dezocine for postoperative pain: a double-blind, placebo-controlled comparison with morphine. J Clin Pharmacol 26:275, 1986
151. Warren MM, Boyce WH, Evans JW, Peters PC: A double-blind comparison of dezocine and morphine in patients with acute renal and ureteral colic. J Urol 134:457, 1985
152. Glass PS, Camporesi EM, Shafron D, et al: Evaluation of pentamorphone in humans: a new potent opiate. Anesth Analg 68:302, 1989
153. Kaiko RF, Wallenstein SL, Rogers AG, et al: Intramuscular meptazinol and morphine in postoperative pain. Clin Pharmacol Ther 37:589, 1985
154. Moores MA, Frater R, Parry P, Hanning CD: Double-blind comparison of the efficacy and safety of single doses of meptazinol as a suppository and morphine by i.m. injection. Br J Anaesth 60:542, 1988
155. Brunelle RL, George RE, Sunshine A, Hammonds WD: Analgesic effect of picenadol, codeine, and placebo in patients with postoperative pain. Clin Pharmacol Ther 43:663, 1988
156. Sherline DM: Picenadol (LY 150720) compared with meperidine and placebo for relief of post-cesarean section pain: a randomized double-blind study. Am J Obstet Gynecol 147:404, 1983
157. Freye E, Hartung E, Schenk GK: Bremazocine: an opiate that induces sedation and analgesia without respiratory depression. Anesth Analg 62:483, 1983
158. Owen H, Reekie RM, Clements JA, et al: Analgesia from morphine and ketamine—a comparison of infusions of morphine and

ketamine for postoperative analgesia. Anaesthesia 42:1051, 1987

159. Hannington-Kiff JG: The need for analgesic cover after ENT surgery—comparison of nefopam and papaveretum. Anaesthesia 40:76, 1985
160. Rezvani A, Stokes KB, Rhoads DL, Way EL: Proglumide exhibits delta opioid agonist properties. Alcohol Drug Res 7:135, 1987
161. Lehmann KA, Schlusener M, Arabatsis P: Failure of proglumide, a cholecystokinin antagonist, to potentiate clinical morphine analgesia. A randomized double-blind postoperative study using patient-controlled analgesia (PCA). Anesth Analg 68:51, 1989
162. Lavigne GJ, Hargreaves KM, Schmidt EA, Dionne RA: Proglumide potentiates morphine analgesia for acute postsurgical pain. Clin Pharmacol Ther 45:666, 1989
163. Puig MM, Laorden ML, Miralles FS, et al: Endorphin levels in cerebrospinal fluid of patients with post-operative and chronic pain. Anesthesiology 57:1, 1982
164. Owen H, Galloway DJ, Mitchell KG: Analgesia by wound infiltration after surgical excision of benign breast lumps. Ann R Coll Surg Engl 67:114, 1985
165. Abdu RA: Ambulatory herniorrhaphy under local anesthesia in a community hospital. Am J Surg 145:353, 1983
166. Ryan JA, Jr., Adye BA, Jolly PC, Mulroy MF II: Outpatient inguinal herniorrhaphy with both regional and local anesthesia. Am J Surg 148:313, 1984
167. Hashemi K, Middleton MD: Subcutaneous bupivacaine for postoperative analgesia after herniorrhaphy. Ann Royal Coll Surg Engl 65:38, 1983
168. Bourne MH, Johnson KA: Postoperative pain relief using local anesthetic instillation. Foot Ankle 8:350, 1988
169. Moss G, Regal ME, Lichtig L: Reducing postoperative pain, narcotics, and length of hospitalization. Surgery 99:206, 1986
170. Hughes DG: Intra-articular bupivacaine for pain relief in athroscopic surgery. Anaesthesia 40:821, 1985
171. Gibbs P, Purushotham A, Auld C, Cuschieri RJ: Continuous wound perfusion with bupivacaine for postoperative wound pain. Br J Surg 75:923, 1988
172. Thomas DFM, Lambert WG, Lloyd-Williams K: The direct perfusion of surgical wounds with local anaesthetic solution: an approach to postoperative pain? Ann R Coll Surg Engl 65:226, 1983
173. Levack ID, Robertson GS: The direct perfusion of surgical wounds with local anaesthetic solution. Ann R Coll Surg Engl 66:146, 1984
174. Levack ID, Holmes JD, Robertson GS: Abdominal wound perfusion for the relief of postoperative pain. Br J Anaesth 58:615, 1986
175. Sinclair R, Cassuto J, Hogstrom S, et al: Topical anesthesia with lidocaine aerosol in the control of postoperative pain. Anesthesiology 68:895, 1988
176. Tree-Trakarn T, Pirayavaraporn S: Postoperative pain relief for circumcision in children: comparison among morphine, nerve block, and topical analgesia. Anesthesiology 62:519, 1985
177. Tree-Trakarn T, Pirayavaraporn S, Lertakyamanee J: Topical analgesia for relief of post-circumcision pain. Anesthesiology 67:395, 1987
178. McQuay H, Weir L, Porter B, et al: A model for comparison of local anesthetics in man. Anesth Analg 61:418, 1982
179. McQuay HJ, Carroll D, Moore RA: Postoperative orthopaedic pain—the effect of opiate premedication and local anaesthetic blocks. Pain 33:291, 1988
180. Wall PD: The prevention of postoperative pain. Pain 33:289, 1988 (editorial)
181. D'Athis F, Macheboeuf M, Thomas H, et al: Epidural analgesia with a bupivicaine-fentanyl mixture in obstetrics: comparison of repeated injections and continuous infusion. Can J Anaesth 35:116, 1988
182. Phillips G: Continuous infusion epidural analgesia in labor: the effect of adding sufentanil to 0.125% bupivacaine. Anesth Analg 67:462, 1988
183. Fischer RL, Lubenow TR, Liceaga A, et al: Comparison of continuous epidural infusion of fentanyl-bupivacaine and morphine-bupivacaine in management of postoperative pain. Anesth Analg 67:559, 1988

184. Lee A, Simpson D, Whitfield A, Scott DB: Postoperative analgesia by continuous extradural infusion of bupivacaine and diamorphine. Br J Anaesth 60:845, 1988
185. Anonymous: Analgesia in children after day-case surgery. Lancet 1:1084, 1988
186. Armitage EN: Caudal block in children. Anaesthesia 34:396, 1979
187. Kay B: Caudal block for post-operative pain relief in children. Anaesthesia 29:610, 1974
188. White J, Harrison B, Richmond P, et al: Postoperative analgesia for circumcision. Br Med J [Clin Res] 286:1934, 1983
189. Hinkle AJ: Percutaneous inguinal block for the outpatient management of post-herniorrhaphy pain in children. Anesthesiology 67:411, 1987
190. Markham SJ, Tomlinson J, Hain WR: Ilioinguinal nerve block in children. A comparison with caudal block for intra and postoperative analgesia. Anaesthesia 41:1098, 1986
191. Langer JC, Shandling B, Rosenberg M: Intraoperative bupivacaine during outpatient hernia repair in children: a randomized double blind trial. J Pediatr Surg 22:267, 1987
192. Fell D, Derrington MC, Taylor E, Wandless JG: Paediatric postoperative analgesia. A comparison between caudal block and wound infiltration of local anaesthetic. Anaesthesia 43:107, 1988
193. Reid MF, Harris R, Phillips PD, et al: Day-case herniotomy in children. A comparison of ilio inguinal nerve block and wound infiltration for postoperative analgesia. Anaesthesia 42:658, 1987
194. Cross GD, Barrett RF: Comparison of two regional techniques for postoperative analgesia in children following herniotomy and orchidopexy. Anaesthesia 42:845, 1987
195. Hannallah RS, Broadman LM, Belman AB, et al: Comparison of caudal and ilioinguinal/iliohypogastric nerve blocks for control of post-orchiopexy pain in pediatric ambulatory surgery. Anesthesiology 66:832, 1987
196. Tozbikian HG: Iliac crest nerve block (ICNB) for orchidopexy and herniorraphy in children. Reg Anaesth 11:53, 1986 (abstr)
197. Bacon AK: An alternative block for post circumcision analgesia. Anaesth Intensive Care 5:63, 1977
198. Broadman LM, Hannallah RS, Belman AB, et al: Post-circumcision analgesia—a prospective evaluation of subcutaneous ring block of the penis. Anesthesiology 67:399, 1987
199. Soliman MG, Tremblay NA: Nerve block of the penis for postoperative pain relief in children. Anesth Analg 57:495, 1978
200. Yeoman PM, Cooke R, Hain WR: Penile block for circumcision. Anaesthesia 38:862, 1983
201. Weiss GN: Local anesthesia for neonatal circumcision. JAMA 260:637, 1988 (letter)
202. Bramwell RGB, Bullen C, Radford P: Caudal block for postoperative analgesia in children. Anaesthesia 37:1024, 1982
203. Attwood AI, Evans DM: Correction of prominent ears using Mustarde's technique: an out-patient procedure under local anaesthetic in children and adults. Br J Plast Surg 38:252, 1985
204. Mather L, Mackie J: The incidence of postoperative pain in children. Pain 15:271, 1983
205. Cooper CM, Gerrish SP, Hardwick M, Kay R: EMLA cream reduces the pain of venepuncture in children. Eur J Anaesthesiol 4:441, 1987
206. Manner T, Kanto J, Iisalo E, et al: Reduction of pain at venous cannulation in children with a eutectic mixture of lidocaine and prilocaine (EMLA cream): comparison with placebo cream and no local premedication. Acta Anaesthesiol Scand 31:735, 1987
207. White PF: Use of patient-controlled analgesia for management of acute pain. JAMA 259:243, 1988
208. Gourlay GK, Kowalski SR, Plummer JL, et al: Fentanyl blood concentration—analgesic response relationship in the treatment of postoperative pain. Anesth Analg 67:329, 1988
209. Finley RJ, Keeri-Szanto M, Boyd D: New analgesic agents and techniques shorten postoperative hospital stay. Pain 2:S397, 1984 (abstr)
210. Bennett RL, Batenhorst RL, Graves D, et

al: Patient-controlled analgesia—a new concept of postoperative relief. Ann Surg 195:700, 1982

211. Graves DA, Foster TS, Batenhorst RL, et al: Patient-controlled analgesia. Ann Intern Med 99:360, 1983
212. Dahl JB, Daugaard JJ, Larsen HV, et al: Patient-controlled analgesia: a controlled trial. Acta Anaesthesiol Scand 31:744, 1987
213. Gambling DR, Uy P, Cole C, et al: A comparative study of patient controlled epidural analgesia (PCEA) and continuous infusion epidural analgesia (CIEA) during labour. Can J Anaesth 35:249, 1988
214. Harrison DM, Sinatra R, Morgese L, Chung JH: Epidural narcotic and patient-controlled analgesia for post-cesarean section pain relief. Anesthesiology 68:454, 1988
215. Rosenberg PH, Heino A, Scheinin B: Comparison of intramuscular analgesia, intercostal block, epidural morphine, and on-demand iv fentanyl in the control of pain after upper abdominal surgery. Acta Anaesthesiol Scand 28:603, 1984
216. Møller IW, Dinesen K, Søndergard S, et al: Effect of patient-controlled analgesia on plasma catecholamine, cortisol and glucose concentrations after cholecystectomy. Br J Anaesth 61:160, 1988
217. Fell D, Chielewski A, Smith G: Postoperative analgesia with controlled release morphine sulphate: comparison with intramuscular morphine. Br Med J 285:92, 1982
218. Bell MDD, Mishra P, Weldon BD, et al: Buccal morphine—a new route for analgesia? Lancet 1:71, 1985
219. Shah MV, Jones DI, Rosen M: "Patient demand" postoperative analgesia with buprenorphine: comparison between sublingual and i.m. administration. Br J Anaesth 58:508, 1986
220. Abboud TK, Zhu J, Gangolly J, et al: Transnasal analgesics: a new method for pain relief in post-cesarean section patients. Anesthesiology 69:A657, 1988
221. Wetchler BV, Alexander CD, Davis A, Uhll MA: Transnasal butorphanol for pain control following ambulatory surgical procedures: a pilot study. (in press)
222. Urquhart ML, Klapp K, White PF: Patient-controlled analgesia: a comparison of intravenous versus subcutaneous hydromorphone. Anesthesiology 69:428, 1988
223. Weinberg DS, Inturrisi CE, Reidenberg B, et al: Sublingual absorption of selected opioid analgesics. Clin Pharmacol Ther 44:335, 1988
224. Taylor E, White PF, Urquhart ML: Postoperative analgesia: SQ-PCA vs. IV-PCA. Anesthesiology 71:A685, 1989 (abstr)
225. Cohen SE, Tan S, White PF: Sufentanil analgesia following cesarean section: epidural versus intravenous administration. Anesthesiology 68:129, 1988
226. Risbo A, Chraemmer-Jørgensen BC, Kolby P, et al: Sublingual buprenorphine for premedication and postoperative pain relief in orthopedic surgery. Acta Anaesthesiol Scand 29:180, 1985
227. Ellis R, Haines D, Shah R, et al: Pain relief after abdominal surgery—comparison of i.m. morphine, sublingual buprenorphine, and self-administered i.v. pethidine. Br J Anaesth 54:421, 1982
228. Feld LH, Champeau MW, van Steenis CA, Scott JC: Preanesthetic medication in children: a comparison of oral transmucosal fentanyl citrate versus placebo. Anesthesiology 71:374, 1989
229. Sebel PS, Barrett CW, Kirk CJ, Heykants J: Transdermal absorption of fentanyl and sufentanil in man. Eur J Clin Pharmacol 32:529, 1987
230. Caplan RA, Ready LB, Olsson GL, Nessly ML: Transdermal delivery of fentanyl for postoperative pain control. Anesthesiology 65:A196, 1986
231. Varvel JR, Shafer SL, Hwang S, et al: Bioavailability and absorption of transdermal fentanyl. Anesthesiology 69:A593, 1988
232. Duthie DJR, Rowbotham DJ, Wyld R, et al: Plasma fentanyl concentrations during transdermal delivery of fentanyl to surgical patients. Br J Anaesth 60:614, 1988
233. Holley FO, Van Steenis C: Postoperative analgesia with fentanyl: pharmacokinetics and pharmacodynamics of constant-rate i.v. and transdermal delivery. Br J Anaesth 60:608, 1988
234. Bone ME, Fell D: A comparison of rectal

diclofenac with intramuscular papaveretum or placebo for pain relief following tonsillectomy. Anaesthesia 43:277, 1988

235. Bourke DL, Smith BAC, Erickson J, et al: TENS reduces halothane requirements during hand surgery. Anesthesiology 61:769, 1984
236. Tyler E, Caldwell C, Ghia JN: Transcutaneous electrical nerve stimulation: an alternative approach to the management of postoperative pain. Anesth Analg 61:449, 1982
237. Ali J, Yaffe C, Serrette C: The effect of transcutaneous nerve stimulation on postoperative pain and pulmonary function. Surgery 89:507, 1981
238. Jensen JE, Conn RR, Hazelrigg G, Hewett JE: The use of transcutaneous neural stimulation and isokinetic testing in arthroscopic knee surgery. Am J Sports Med 13:27, 1985
239. Thorsteinsson G, Stonnington HH, Stillwell GK, Elveback LR: The placebo effect of transcutaneous electrical stimulation. Pain 5:31, 1978
240. Cusheri RJ, Morran CG, McArdle CS: Assessment of transcutaneous electrical nerve stimulation (TENS) for postoperative analgesia following abdominal surgery. Br J Anaesth 55:1162P, 1983
241. McCallum MI, Glynn CJ, Moore RA, et al: Transcutaneous electrical nerve stimulation in the management of acute postoperative pain. Br J Anaesth 61:308, 1988
242. Smedley F, Taube M, Wastell C: Transcutaneous electrical nerve stimulation for pain relief following inguinal hernia repair: a controlled trial. Eur Surg Res 20:233, 1988
243. Smith CM, Guralnick MS, Gelfand MM, Jeans ME: The effects of transcutaneous electrical nerve stimulation on post-caesarian pain. Pain 27:181, 1986
244. Cooperman AM, Hall B, Mikalacki K, et al: Use of transcutaneous electrical stimulation in the control of postoperative pain. Am J Surg 133:185, 1977
245. Khiroya RC, Davenport HT, Jones JG: Cryoanalgesia for pain after herniorrhaphy. Anaesthesia 41:73, 1986
246. Jones MJT, Murrin KR: Intercostal block with cryotherapy. Ann R Coll Surg Engl 69:261, 1987
247. Wood GJ, Lloyd JW, Bullingham RES, et al: Postoperative analgesia for day-case herniorrhaphy patients: a comparison of cryoanalgesia, paravertebral blockade and oral analgesia. Anaesthesia 36:603, 1981
248. Sjölund B, Eriksson M: Electro-acupuncture and endogenous morphines. Lancet 2:1085, 1976
249. Hashish I, Hai HK, Harvey W, et al: Reduction of postoperative pain and swelling by ultrasound treatment: a placebo effect. Pain 33:303, 1988
250. Houle M, McGrath PA, Moran G, Garrett OJ: The efficacy of hypnosis- and relaxation-induced analgesia on two dimensions of pain for cold pressor and electrical tooth pulp stimulation. Pain 33:241, 1988
251. Postuma R, Fergusson CC, Stanwick RS, Howe JM: Paediatric day-care surgery: a 30-year hospital experience. J Pediatr Surg 22:304, 1987
252. Schulze S, Roikjaer O, Hasselstrøm L, et al: Epidural bupivacaine and morphine plus systemic indomethacin eliminates pain but not systemic response and convalescence after cholecystectomy. Surgery 103:321, 1988
253. Houde RW, Wallenstein SL, Beaver WT: Clinical measurement of pain. p. 75. In deStevens G (ed): Analgetics. Academic Press, Orlando, FL, 1965
254. Tierney E, Lewis G, Hurtig JB, Johnson D: Femoral nerve block with bupivicaine 0.25 per cent for post-operative analgesia after open knee surgery. Can J Anaesth 34:455, 1987
255. Nelson PS, Streisand JB, Mulder SM, et al: Comparison of oral transmucosal fentanyl citrate and an oral solution of meperidine, diazepam and atropine for premedication in children. Anesthesiology 70:616, 1989

20

Legal Considerations in Anesthesia for Outpatient Surgery

James B. Wieland
Laura L. Katz

Anesthesia was used in outpatient surgery as early as 1842, but it is only in recent years that its use in outpatient (ambulatory) surgical procedures has burgeoned into a major area of responsibility for many anesthesiologists. While this has been facilitated by advances in medical science in general, and in the medical specialty of anesthesia in particular, many of the pressures leading to the growth of ambulatory surgery are societal, such as the decreased cost of ambulatory care, its increased convenience to the patient, and changes in the American health care system's ability to effectively use inpatient bed space and other resources. The essential stages of anesthesia management for ambulatory surgery are no different than for inpatient procedures: patient selection and screening, prescription of the anesthesia plan and any premedication, provision of a safe and effective course of anesthesia, postoperative evaluation of the patient, discharge, and necessary post-discharge follow-up. The differences in ambulatory care are the degree of legal responsibility that is vested in the anesthesiologist and the environmental pressures to compromise a risk-management approach to anesthesia. External pressure for a speedy patient emergence and discharge may compete with the degree of vigilance that must be exercised at the time the patient is discharged directly to his or her home.

Ambulatory surgical procedures take place in hospital-based or hospital-affiliated units, often located in hospital outpatient departments or on medical center campuses, and in freestanding units that may be investor owned. The phrase "ambulatory surgery center" is used throughout this chapter to refer to all delivery sites, except in those instances in which distinctions are legally significant. This chapter focuses on the legal responsibilities of the anesthesiologist as a practicing physician, reviews the standards of the American legal system by which the anesthesiologist's actions will be judged, and suggests practices to manage the risks of liability for failure to meet those standards.

LEGAL DECISIONS AND THE ANESTHESIOLOGIST

In the American legal system, when a physician's professional conduct is called into question in a court of law, he or she will be held to an abstract standard, compliance with which is determined by the nonphysicians comprising the court or the jury. The physician's conduct is measured against what a hypothetical "reasonable physician" would have done in the same circumstances. Lacking medical training, courts turn to testimony from physicians or other expert witnesses who were not present when the events took place, and to legal precedent in judicial determinations based on analogous facts. This is a sobering realization for many physicians and, in our opinion, it should be. Whereas a physician's judgment may once have been seen by patients and the legal system as virtually unassailable, patients are increasingly inclined to question that judgment and, when there is a bad outcome, to seek redress in the courts. The American health care system's increased emphasis on quality assurance has meant increased scrutiny of complaints received concerning medical practitioners by state disciplinary boards and peer review organizations. There has also been heightened scrutiny of complaints under the federal Medicare program, including closer evaluation of care that is not deemed to meet standards established by the program itself. Subjective aspects of the physician-patient relationship make the potential for liability difficult to measure and prevent. For instance, many experienced malpractice attorneys feel that a patient may be more inclined to sue if the physician exhibits callousness or an apparent lack of empathy for the patient than if the physician-patient relationship is one that is built on a sense of caring and trust. Establishing a good rapport with the patient and providing necessary reassurance to allay the patient's fears or apprehensions may be more than an incidental part of a good work-up; it may be considered important in avoiding the risk of being named a defendant in a malpractice action.[1]

In a study of 104 claims randomly drawn from an insurance company's files, more than 25 percent involved cardiac arrest during or immediately after anesthesia. Closer evaluation showed that the anesthesia care was deemed below the legal standard in all of these cases.[2] In another study examining 27 deaths from cardiac arrest during anesthesia, it was determined that 20 deaths could have been avoided.[3] Next to obstetrics and gynecology, a leading source of medical malpractice claims has been anesthesia.[4] The practice of "good medicine" and the skills of a consummate technician are not always enough to protect against hostile patients or their lawyers.[1] While bad outcomes in an ambulatory surgery center should not be as high as in an inpatient setting by virtue of patient selection, procedure selection, and, at least historically, a less frequent use of general anesthesia, anesthetic morbidity remains a known risk. These morbidities may result from a variety of causes that are not always the result of poor training, bad judgment, or substandard care by the anesthesiologist.[5]

A review of reported decisions in which a court has found that an anesthesiologist failed to comply with the legal standard of care is a useful orientation to the principals that follow. Due to the recent emergence of outpatient surgery, there are as yet few reported decisions that involve anesthesiology in outpatient procedures. The majority of reported cases arose in the inpatient context. Discussion of the facts and findings of these cases is nevertheless instructive. Among other things, it should be noted that descriptions and medical terminology quoted in this chapter are those of the courts and may not be as precise or complete as would be demanded among physicians. This, in and of itself, is significant for the physician whose conduct may someday be scrutinized in a courtroom. An ambiguous, illegible, or hastily written anesthesia plan or chart note, for example, may seem an unavoidable byproduct of the pressure to get on to the next patient; however, 3 or 4 years later, in the very different environment of a courtroom, the physician may dearly wish that he or she could better document the care with which the patient's anesthesia was selected and delivered. Certainly, the courts have neither the ability nor the training to come to the physician's aid when the physician has made himself or herself vulnerable. This is demonstrated by a case decided by the Illinois courts in which failure to monitor a patient's adequate supply of oxygen during surgery rendered the anesthesiologist legally responsible for a bad outcome. The plaintiff received corrective eye surgery and suffered partial paralysis of his right side postoperatively. The allegation was that "asphyxial (characterized by suffocation) brain damage" occurred during the operation. Suit was brought against the anesthesiologist alleging that he was negligent in failing to "watch and record" the patient's respirations during the administration of anesthesia. Another anesthesiologist testified that the defendant anesthesiologist's failure to chart the plaintiff's respirations during the procedure "suggested that he may have been casual in his observation of the breathing." The anesthesiologist concluded by saying, "had the defendant placed his hand on the plaintiff's chest to monitor respiration, the 'parties wouldn't be here today.'"[6]

In the American legal system, injured patients typically exercise their right to select a trial before a jury. In a civil jury trial, the judge determines applicable legal principals and instructs the jury accordingly. Based on these instructions, and in the light of factual testimony and the testimony of expert witnesses in medicine or other relevant fields, the jury determines the "facts of the case." Experienced trial lawyers will invariably point out that there are two sides to every case. Partisan versions of what "really" happened, often diametrically opposed, are more the rule than the exception. This is not meant to impugn the judicial system or the integrity of counsel and witnesses who appear before it. It is meant, however, to recognize that there may be a lag of years between the events in question and the parties' day in court. Over and above that, "interested memory" is acknowledged by many judges and attorneys to affect the testimony of even the most scrupulous and honest of witnesses. Interested memory refers to a phenomenon by which, under the pressures of the courtroom environment, witnesses, unconsciously and without intent to deceive, color their testimony in a way that is perceived by them as helpful to the party advancing their testimony.

One of the best protections that an anesthesiologist can devise against undeserved legal liability is an accurate, complete, and legible medical record. Experienced trial lawyers often state that "if you haven't written it down, you haven't done it." This approach gives due recognition to the lapse of time between a bad outcome and a trial and to the partisan nature of our legal system. For adequate documentation, the patient's record should comply with recognized standards of medical practice existing at the time, and, when possible, the printed form should be supplemented with notations by the physician. Contemporaneous medical notations in the record are important components of the fact-determining process in any malpractice lawsuit, as they trace the specifics of the medical care provided. Care must be taken to restrict entries in the record to appropriate medical observations and to avoid legal conclusions or self-serving statements. The respect with which the patient's medical record must be treated extends to alteration or amendment of mistaken entries as well. While lawyers are generally reluctant to give absolute advice, experienced trial lawyers will invariably say that never, under any circumstances, should an entry in a medical record be erased, covered up, or otherwise rendered illegible. Such actions are invariably discovered in the course of litigation, and the very worst presumptions are raised against the party who made the alteration. If it is necessary to correct an entry, existing text should simply be lined through in a way that permits the entry to be read, and a corrective note should be appended immediately thereafter, with an explanation as to why correction was required.

While specific legal advice and guidance can only be given by a qualified attorney who is familiar with the facts of the situation, a general awareness and sensitivity to the way in which the legal system analyzes the conduct of physicians is the foundation for a practical, risk-management approach to the practice of outpatient anesthesia. This is the emphasis of the section that follows.

THE LEGAL BASIS OF LIABILITY FOR MALPRACTICE

Historically, civil litigation in the United States has been based on the legal theory on which the plaintiff relied to support the demand for judicial relief. Some theories that have been used against physicians may seem odd, at least when viewed in the abstract. For example, battery is a civil cause of action that protects an individual's right to freedom from harmful or offensive contact to his or her person. When a physician lays hands on a patient in the course of treatment without that patient's legally sufficient consent, some court's have found that the physician committed a battery. Other legal theories have been advanced to support a patient's monetary recovery against a physician for a bad result. The law of bilateral contracts deals with bargained-for exchanges of valuable consideration. Patients have successfully recovered against physicians who were found to have contracted to competently undertake a course of treatment, perhaps even to deliver a certain result, and subsequently failed to do so. Courts have found such contracts were implied, based on the conduct of the parties. Courts have also found that physicians guaranteed the patient that a certain result would be obtained. Failing to achieve that result, liability resulted for the physician based on a breach of warranty.

With respect to contract liability, two features of the American health care system have particular importance to anesthesiologists involved in outpatient care. In today's competitive, marketing-oriented milieu, brochures, pamphlets, or other materials designed by nonphysicians to attract patients to an ambulatory surgery center may be found by a court to have given a patient legal grounds to expect a specific result or to have guaranteed the patient a desirable outcome through incautious or overly optimistic wording. In a similar vein, many anesthesiologists provide their services at ambulatory surgery centers, especially investor-owned freestanding centers, by virtue of a written contractual agreement. Such contracts may properly specify a standard of anesthesia care that is reasonable and in accordance with accepted practice in the specialty, but when they obligate the anesthesiologist to "the highest and best" or to a "strict" standard of anesthesia care, they too can impose an inordinately high standard of care, and one that would not have been otherwise required. To guard against such consequences, anesthesiologists need to be aware of what is said about their care in seemingly tangential contexts and to maintain an active role in monitoring materials disseminated to the public.

Perhaps the legal maxim that "tough cases make bad law" explains those decisions relying on theories such as battery, contract, or warranty to support an injured patient's recovery. In any event, the prevalent legal theory on which physicians are brought to court to account for their care of patients is negligence, and it is that legal theory to which our attention will now turn.

Medical Malpractice: Care Negligently Given Causing Foreseeable Injury

In its most basic sense, the American legal system imposes a general duty of care on all human activity. In the conduct of daily affairs, whatever they are, each individual is charged with a legal duty to act as an ordinary, prudent, and reasonable person. This hypothetical reasonable person is expected to take precautions against creating an unreasonable risk of harm to others. A breach of this duty resulting in foreseeable harm to another is referred to as negligence and will confer on the breaching party financial responsibility for the injured party's damages.

Physicians, by virtue of their special training, skills, and licensure, are expected by our legal system to conform to a higher standard of care. This standard is an objective one predicated on a judicially created "reasonable physician" rather than a subjective standard that reflects the individual training, work environment, and other factors unique to the physician whose conduct is under scrutiny. In determining whether an anesthesiologist is liable for a bad patient outcome, a court will address the following four questions:

1. What was the applicable standard of care?
2. Did the anesthesiologist fail to comply with that standard; that is, did he or she fail to act as a reasonable physician would in similar circumstances?
3. If so, was it foreseeable that the patient could be injured as a result of the failure to meet the standard of care?
4. Was the patient's injury caused by the anesthesiologist's failure to comply with the standard of care?

The Legal Standard of Care for Physicians

Traditionally, the standard of care to which a physician was held was determined by reference to the locale in which he or she practiced. Under this so-called "strict locality" rule, the legal standard was that degree of care that would be exercised by a physician of ordinary skill in the same locale as the defendant physician. The idea was that it would be unfair to hold a small-town practitioner to the same standard as a physician practicing in a large city or in a teaching hospital; however, this rule proved to be harsh in its application. Since only physicians from the same locale could testify as medical experts, it was perceived to be difficult for injured patients to obtain expert testimony. The "strict locality" rule was eventually modified and, in a majority of jurisdictions, a physician was expected to exercise the skill and care of an ordinary physician in the "same or similar locality."

The modern trend, however, is to abandon any formula governed strictly by geographic considerations and to treat the size and character of the relevant medical community as only one factor to be considered in determining the standard of care. Particularly in cases involving board-certified physicians, a national standard of care has gained increasing judicial acceptance. Under this standard, the physician must exercise the degree of care and skill which is expected of a reasonably prudent practitioner of the same medical specialty, acting in the same or similar circumstances. Reasons for the erosion of the locality rule and the move toward uniform, national legal standards of medical care were aptly described in one court's opinion:

> Whatever may have justified the strict locality rule fifty or a hundred years ago, it cannot be reconciled with the medical realities today. 'New techniques and discoveries are available to all doctors within a short period of time through medical journals, closed-circuit television presentations, special radio networks for doctors, tape recorded digests of medical literature and current correspondence courses.' More importantly, the quality of medical school training itself has improved. . . . There now exists a national accrediting system which has contributed to the standardization of medical schools throughout the country.[7]

Expert testimony from physician witnesses is by no means the only basis for a judicial determination of the relevant standard of care. Standards established by national or state medical societies can be invoked in a courtroom to aid a jury in determining an individual physician's legal duty to his or her patient. The relationship between standards held by specialty societies and the legal standard of care imposed on physicians, especially under the emerging national standard just discussed, is brought into sharp focus by the lack of consensus regarding the use of new technologies. Intraoperative patient monitoring with pulse oximetry equipment is a good example. As a matter of legal precedent, there is not yet a judicially recognized consensus among "reasonably prudent anesthesiologists" that pulse oximetry must be used in all cases of general anesthesia, although the issue is a close one, and in some jurisdictions it might be required. The Standards for Intra-operative Monitoring of Patients, promulgated by the American Society of Anesthesiologists (ASA), provide that "during all anesthetics, the patient's oxygenation, ventilation, circulation, and temperature shall be continually evaluated." Continual is defined as "repeated regularly and frequently in steady rapid succession."[8] The use of pulse oximetry is encouraged by the ASA but is not required. As the availability and use of pulse oximetry equipment continue to grow, one may expect such benchmarks as the ASA standards to change and courts to begin to take the view that reasonable and prudent anesthesiologists should make use of the device in all appropriate cases. Adoption of such a requirement by the ASA will likely have a powerful effect in the courts. In the meantime, however, the issue will be determined by the testimony of expert witnesses as to local practice or custom, wherever it is alleged that failure to promptly detect deficient oxygenation contributed to an injury.

Standards for ambulatory surgery centers themselves have been established by the Joint Commission on Accreditation of Healthcare Organizations (JCAHO) and the Accreditation Association for Ambulatory Health Care (AAAHC). These organizations also set benchmarks for physician conduct in ambulatory surgery centers by specifying protocols or procedures that must be followed in an accredited center. The JCAHO standards were originally intended as a yardstick for hospitals to receive accreditation. With the development of alternative delivery systems, JCAHO has sought to foster comparable levels of outpatient care, regardless of the setting, and to make them consistent with the highest standards of ambulatory care organizations.[9] While there are differences between individual requirements, both JCAHO and AAAHC standards are comprehensive and authoritative. For the sake of simplicity, AAAHC standards are referred to in this chapter as the standard of care in an ambulatory surgery center. This decision on the part of the authors is not meant to imply a preference. In malpractice litigation, either JCAHO or AAAHC standards are admitted as evidence relevant to a determination of the legal standard of care; whichever standard is relied on is recognized as authoritative by physicians and others involved in outpatient care. If a center is accredited by either organization, even this relatively light burden is lessened. Assuming that an appropriate factual basis is established, either accreditation system gives the same evidentiary weight.

Failure to Comply With the Standard of Care

Typically, a physician's breach of his or her duty to comply with the applicable standard of care will be demonstrated in court by direct evidence consisting of medical records, testimony of the defendant physician and other individuals with factual knowledge of relevant events, and testimony of disinterested expert medical witnesses. In appropriate cases, however, the plaintiff may rely on circumstantial evidence, involving the existence of one fact from which other facts may be inferred. One form of such evidence particularly pertinent to medical malpractice is *res ipsa loquitur*, a Latin phrase literally meaning "the thing speaks for itself." This legal doctrine allows the jury to draw an inference that a physician breached the duty of care if the plaintiff proves the following:

1. The injury is of a nature that would not ordinarily occur in the absence of breach of the duty of care.
2. The defendant had exclusive control of the "instrumentality" which caused the injury.
3. The plaintiff did not contribute to the injury through his or her own conduct.[10]

This doctrine only applies when common knowledge or experience is sufficient to infer that the injury would not have existed but for negligence.[10] Although expert testimony is usually used by plaintiffs to build their case, it is not strictly required for a finding of liability based on this doctrine.

An anesthesiologist would seldom think of himself or herself as being in exclusive control of an ambulatory surgical procedure. However, many courts construe the requirement of control broadly. In a Colorado case, for example, the plaintiff was unable to prove whether his injury was caused by the hospital, the surgeon, the anesthesiologist, the nurse anesthetist, or the surgical nurse. The plaintiff was under general anesthesia for a cataract operation and "became inadequately anesthetized and coughed causing the expulsive loss of the eye." Testimony showed that the anesthesia machine had become disconnected, causing the cough. The court stated: "Because he was anesthetized [the plaintiff] had no knowledge as to the cause of the disconnection. His wife was not present in the operating room and the only conscious persons there were defendants or employees of the defendants. Thus, in the absence of voluntary disclosure by the participants as to the precise cause of the disconnection [the plaintiff] remained at an evidentiary disadvantage in this respect." The court stressed the fact that as an "insensible passive recipient of treatment administered by other parties" the plaintiff could not be expected to demonstrate each defendant's control. In adopting the rule of the majority of jurisdictions, the court found that the entire surgical team could be liable under the doctrine and that the jury should have been instructed accordingly.[11]

Violation of a statute governing medical practice may constitute negligence in and of itself, usually referred to as negligence per se, or may be presented by the plaintiff as evidence of negligence. In a Georgia case, the court found that a hospital, a student nurse anesthetist, an anesthesiology group practice, and an anesthesia assistant in the employ of the group, were all negligent per se under a state statute that established minimum qualifications for certified registered nurse anesthetists.[12] There, a senior student nurse anesthetist in the defendant hospital's training program had administered anesthesia, supervised only by a physician assistant specializing in anesthesia who was employed by the anesthesiology group. This was in violation of a Georgia statute limiting the administration of anesthesia to physicians and certified registered nurse anesthetists under the direction of a qualified physician. Even without a factual showing of what caused the injury, the court found that the breach of the statute was sufficient in and of itself to prove a breach of duty owed to the patient, who had suffered cardiac arrest and severe brain damage during a tubal ligation.

Other Legal Bases for Anesthesiologist Liability

The Georgia case discussed above raises a related point. In cases involving bad surgical outcomes, it is not unusual for a medical malpractice plaintiff to name the facility, the surgeon, the anesthesiologist, the nurse anesthetist, and even the operating room nurses as defendants. In many cases, a question arises as to which of these parties owe a duty to protect the patient from injury. Under a legal theory called vicarious liability, also known as *respondeat superior*, an employer will be responsible for the acts of employees within the scope of their employment. The legal basis for this liability is the right or authority of the employer to control the exact manner and means of the employee's performance, not simply to dictate the end result to be achieved. The ambulatory surgery center may be held vicariously liable for the negligence of its employees. Likewise, the anesthesiologist, besides being liable for his or her own direct acts, may also be vicariously liable for the performance of others acting under his or her direction and control. It is important for the anesthesiologist to realize that this form of vicarious liability is not limited to the acts of his or her employees.

There are many examples of nursing or other nonphysician personnel performing delegated medical responsibilities under direct or indirect physician supervision. Each situation carries its own legal risk of liability for the supervising physician and must be analyzed based on its individual facts. Typically, however, courts use the legal doctrine of agency to impute liability for a supervised nonemployee's actions to a physician. As the "principal," the supervising physician is legally responsible for the acts of his or her nurse or other nonphysician "agent" within the scope of the delegated medical task, the "agency relationship." Anesthesiologists who "medically direct" residents, interns, nurse anesthetists, or anesthesia assistants, in particular, have a unique legal responsibility. Medical direction is a term of art created largely by the federal Medicare program. Medical direction can best be thought of as a kind of focused, direct supervision. Under the Medicare law and administrative regulations, in order to medically direct a case, the anesthesiologist must personally perform a pre-anesthesia examination, prescribe the anesthesia plan, participate in the most demanding parts of the plan including induction and emergence, monitor the course of anesthesia at frequent intervals, and remain physically present and available in the event of an emergency.[13] The medically directing anesthesiologist need not be in the operating room at all times and may, in fact, be simultaneously directing several procedures. Medical direction is recognized as a physician service for which the Medicare program and a number of insurance companies or other so-called "third-party payers" will make payment. Even when he or she does not employ the nurse anesthetist or other medically directed individual, it seems clear that the "medically directing" anesthesiologist will be legally responsible for a bad outcome, either as a direct breach of his or her own duty or on a theory of vicarious liability, such as agency.

There are, in fact, more subtle issues regarding an anesthesiologist's responsibility for the acts of others involved in the provision of anesthesia, particularly those of nurse anesthetists. The legal system's concept of a nurse anesthetist's responsibility is in a state of flux. Each state has its own licensure law and regulations dictating the scope of such practice. In addition, most facilities that utilize nurse or other nonphysician anesthetists have their own means of determining the credentialing mechanism and medical responsibilities. Independent of reimbursement-oriented considerations, such as medical direction, state licensure or center accreditation may require the nurse anesthetist to be "supervised" by a physician or may permit some greater degree of independent practice. In this context, supervision can take a variety of forms. From a legal risk-management perspective, however it is defined, supervision carries with it legal responsibility and risk of liability. An anesthesiologist must be particularly alert to those situations in which his or her supervisory responsibility could be inferred in the event of a bad outcome, without the anesthesiologist ever having consciously formed a physician-patient relationship or otherwise clearly and knowingly assumed that responsibility. Depending on the laws of the particular state and the requirements of the individual center, the basis for such responsibility can be as subtle as past practice and custom, a general agreement to be the sponsoring or consulting physician, or the like. For the sake of the patient, as well as for the management of legal risk, all lines of legal responsibility and liability must be clearly understood by all concerned parties. In any doubtful situation, competent legal advice should be obtained, and the situation should be submitted to the anesthesiologist's malpractice carrier for a determination of coverage.

The law draws a distinction between employees and independent contractors, the latter being subject to control only as to the end result they provide and not as to the manner and means by which they provide it. Because courts do not normally impute an independent contractor's conduct to his or her "principal," anesthesiologists are often retained as independent contractors at the ambulatory surgical centers at which they practice. Consequently, responsibility for a poor patient outcome will remain with the anesthesiologist alone rather than also being imputed to the center. Patients, however, typically exercise little opportunity to obtain information about the anesthesiologist who will be caring for them, in contrast to their selection of surgeons. Thus, an ambulatory surgical center is often viewed by the courts as presenting anesthesia (implicitly if not explicitly) as part of its own patient care service. When an anesthesiologist is an employee of the center, there is no question that the center can be held vicariously liable for the anesthesiologist's negligent acts. As stated above, the anesthesiologist is frequently an independent contractor, not under the legal direction and control of the ambulatory surgery center. Nevertheless, if he or she is presented to patients and the public as an employee of the center, or is in fact controlled by the center in the manner and means by which anesthesia care is provided, the center may nonetheless be liable for a bad patient outcome. Curiously, in today's medical environment, in which administrators and other nonphysicians seek to exert more and more control over how physicians deliver anesthesia care, this possibility of vicarious liability for the center can be raised to support a proper degree of physician autonomy.

An exception to the general rule that the negligence of an employee is imputed to the employer is the so-called "borrowed servant" doctrine. This doctrine is important when the center employs nurse anesthetists but actually "loans them out" to nonemployed anesthesiologists for procedures performed in the center. When an employee is loaned for performance of a service, the individual who has direction and control over the employee will generally be the one held liable for the employee's negligent acts. The borrowed servant, in effect, becomes an employee of the party to whom he or she is loaned, with the resulting transfer of legal responsibility. As well as the overriding question of who had the right to control the actions of the borrowed servant, facts such as who was responsible for hiring and firing, the payment of wages, fringe benefits and liability insurance, and the establishment of professional guidelines will be considered by a court in determining vicarious liability of the center or the anesthesiologist.[14]

The so-called "captain of the ship" doctrine, a similar principle, has been adapted to the operating room and is at least nominally the law in several jurisdictions. The doctrine imposes vicarious liability on the surgeon in charge of an operation for the negligence of other practitioners during the period in which they were under the surgeon's control, even though the other practitioners may be independent professionals or employees of another, such as the ambulatory surgery center. Most courts recognize that as physicians anesthesiologists have special expertise and independent authority from that of the surgeon, and have determined that the surgeon should not be held legally responsible as an "insured" for their negligence.[15] There are still a few cases to be found that hold that the surgeon, as "captain of the ship," legally responsible for the care provided by the anesthesiologist. Those cases focus on the judicially perceived obligation of the surgeon to control the manner in which the anesthesiologist's duties are performed.[16] As with the theory of vicarious liability, the element of control becomes central to the analysis of any case employing the "captain of the ship" doctrine.

Legal Concepts of Causation

The judicial determination of causation requires a two-part analysis. First, an anesthesiologist's negligence will be deemed the legal cause of a patient's injury only when, without that negligence, the injury would not have occurred. This is known as "causation in fact." The plaintiff must therefore show that had the anesthesiologist adhered to the standard of care, the injury would not have occurred. Second, the plaintiff must show that the injury to the patient was a sufficiently direct and foreseeable result of the anesthesiologist's negligence to justify, as a matter of public policy, the imposition of legal liability, regardless of causation in fact. This is the issue of "proximate cause" and is ordinarily a question of fact for the jury to consider as part of its determination.[17]

Failure to anticipate and protect against a foreseeable but statistically remote risk of complication was the gravamen of the malpractice claim that was the underlying issue in a New York case. The plaintiff's husband suffered a rare fatal reaction to anesthesia diagnosed as malignant hyperthermia. The plaintiff asserted that conducting the surgery without an available supply of dantrolene, a widely accepted pharmacologic treatment for malignant hyperthermia, constituted negligence that proximately caused her husband's death.[18] That case and others have demonstrated the need to predict complications, to plan for dealing with foreseeable emergencies, and to ensure that necessary drugs and resuscitative equipment are made available to the surgical team at all ambulatory surgery centers.

Damages

In negligence litigation, monetary damages are awarded to compensate the plaintiff for actual harm or injury. Common elements of damages in medical malpractice litigation are reimbursement for medical expenses and lost earnings, monetary compensation for pain and suffering, and compensation for impairment of the patient's future earning capacity. The latter element of damages is discounted to its so-called "present value"; that is, the plaintiff is awarded the amount which, if prudently invested, will provide the sum of money that the court or jury believes appropriate to make up for the future loss of earnings. The principal of awarding money damages to compensate a patient for intangible injuries, such as pain and suffering, is not without its detractors, particularly in the current legal environment of seemingly upward spiraling monetary awards. The principal is grounded in a long-standing perception of the American legal system that pain and suffering are tangible injuries that may be redressed by the courts and that the only available form of appropriate redress is through monetary award.

It is not necessary for the malpractice plaintiff to prove that the precise harm suffered was foreseeable by the defendant physician. If a patient suffers greater harm than might reasonably be anticipated from a breach of the standard of care, however idiosyncratic the reason, the breaching physician will still be fully responsible, as long as some harm was reasonably foreseeable. As is frequently stated by the courts, a tortfeasor, that is, anyone who commits a tort such as negligence, "takes the victim as he finds him." Lawyers sometimes refer to this as the "easily bruised plaintiff" doctrine.

In extreme cases, punitive or exemplary damages may be awarded to supplement compensatory damages. This is one of the few instances in which the American legal system will award money in a civil proceeding, not to compensate the plaintiff for injuries but to punish the defendant for his or her conduct. Generally, punitive damages will not be allowed unless the defendant's conduct was grossly negligent, reckless, or willful.[19] A court in South Carolina found that punitive damages were available when, among other things, an anesthesiologist attempted to insert a central venous pressure line three times without success and did not have the patient x-rayed to determine if she had been harmed by the earlier attempts before proceeding further. The patient had in fact developed a hemomediastinum, spent 4 days of postoperative recovery in an intensive care unit, and thereafter suffered "painful breathing problems."[17]

Negligence in a Medico-administrative Capacity

Discussion has thus far focused on the legal responsibility of the anesthesiologist for the provision of individual patient care. In an ambulatory surgery center, an anesthesiologist may also hold the role of an administrator charged with development or enforcement of policies, protocols, and procedures. In today's legal environment, it must be remembered that negligent performance of these undertakings can lead to liability as well. Under principles of vicarious liability, the center itself may bear ultimate responsibility, but this does not relieve the anesthesiologist from being called to account, legally and financially, on an individual basis. One court, for example, found that when the chief anesthesiologist of a hospital had the responsibility to ensure that safe and adequate practices were followed, as well as the right and duty to direct the anesthesia staff to correct improper procedures, he was personally liable for negligent acts of a staff anesthesiologist that should have been corrected.[16] Anesthesiologists functioning in medico-administrative capacities should make certain that those activities are covered under their policies of malpractice insurance, which tend to be more patient-care oriented, or that specific additional coverage is obtained.

LEGAL CONSIDERATIONS IN OUTPATIENT ANESTHESIA

The stages of anesthetic management are essentially the same for inpatient and outpatient procedures. The overriding considerations and legal standards for both are identical: at each stage, what would a reasonable and prudent anesthesiologist do in the particular circumstances in order to ensure the safest possible course of anesthesia? While the witticism that "an anesthesiologist charges a dollar to put the patient to sleep and the balance of his or her fee to wake the patient up" isn't scientifically based, it does illustrate the fact that the anesthesiologist's patient care and legal responsibility are significantly broader than many realize. Although careful procedure selection and patient screening should result in a low risk of outpatients requiring unexpected hospital admission, patients with complex medical problems are being scheduled more frequently for elective outpatient surgical procedures. Irrespective of the outpatients' ASA physical status, there is absolutely no lowering of the legal standards by which an anesthesiologist's conduct will be judged as to foreseeable risks.

Extensive analysis is not necessary to demonstrate that a careless mistake or lapse in judgment that causes harm to a patient will lead to legal liability. What follows is an analysis of the less obvious risks of liability for the anesthesiologist practicing in an outpatient setting, focusing on a risk-management approach to anesthesia care.

Selection of Procedures

The selection of procedures to be performed in an ambulatory surgery center must be guided by considerations of the center's design and equipment, the qualifications of its staff, and its proximity to emergency services and inpatient facilities. The relative availability of consulting services or diagnostic testing is also a factor to be considered. The baseline standard is subjective: the ability of that particular center to respond in a timely and medically appropriate manner to the routine aspects as well as the complications or emergencies that are the reasonably foreseeable consequence of the type of procedures to be performed. Thus, what is or is not done at other centers is relevant only insofar as the other centers are demonstrably similar in all material respects. Obviously, this standard is not a fixed one. Because of ready access to the full resources of an acute general care institution, an ambulatory surgery center that is located within a hospital or on a medical center campus may undertake higher-risk procedures than a similarly equipped and staffed freestanding center located some distance from any inpatient center. On the other hand, a well-equipped freestanding center could perform procedures that a poorly equipped hospital-based center could not.

The general selection of procedures will typically not devolve to the anesthesiologist in his or her individual patient care capacity, but as a practitioner on the staff of the center or as a medico-administrative officer, the anesthesiologist will have an important role in procedure selection. The adoption of AAAHC standards limits the surgical procedures that can be offered by a medical facility to those that are approved by the governing body on the recommendation of qualified medical personnel.[20] Any list of approved procedures should not be static but should be reviewed periodically by the same multidisciplinary team of qualified medical personnel that established it in the first place, and the review should be conducted with equal care. The review should take cognizance not only of advances in medical science but of outcomes both in the center and as reported in the medical literature. Dropping a procedure from an approved list because of a bad outcome highlights a point of tension between our legal system and our health care system. Taking a remedial step in response to a bad outcome could be argued in a judicial context to constitute an admission of fault. However, most jurisdictions in the United States, if not all, recognize that such a result would inhibit the very sort of quality assurance analysis that ongoing review of approved procedures is designed to foster. Most courts therefore recognize that as a matter of public policy, such subsequent remedial steps are not admissible evidence in civil litigation based on medical malpractice.

Once a list of approved procedures is established, it should be adhered to despite pressures to make exceptions. Those responsible for permitting an unapproved procedure would be very vulnerable, should a bad outcome result, to the argument that the harm occurred because the procedure should not have been performed in that particular ambulatory surgical center in the first place.

Patient Selection and Screening

The same standards that apply to procedure selection form the basis of the patient selection process. No patient is an acceptable candidate for ambulatory surgery at a center unless the center has resources sufficient to properly handle any emergency that may foreseeably develop, given not only the nature of the procedure but also the medical history and health status of the individual patient. We believe that patient selection should be thought of as a two-stage process. At stage 1, when the patient first presents as a candidate for outpatient surgery, more general standards apply. When patients are young and healthy and the procedure is quick and straightforward, the overall risk of complication is low. However, when patients of ASA physical status III or IV are scheduled for an outpatient procedure, foreseeable risks obviously increase. When the patient presents a degree of risk that a reasonable and prudent anesthesiologist would consider unreasonable in the light of the capabilities of the center, that patient should be referred to another setting.

To satisfy possible judicial scrutiny, patient selection at this first stage requires careful, in-depth evaluation of every patient, including a thorough medical history. For example, the AAAHC requires that in an approved center "an appropriate and current history, physical examination, and pertinent preoperative diagnostic studies are incorporated into the patient's medical record prior to surgery."[20] However, abstract medical criteria alone should not govern. Although a certain amount of apprehension is common, patients voicing strong objections to undergoing a procedure in an ambulatory surgery center would be considered poor candidates.

As stated by the AAAHC, in an accredited center, "either the operating surgeon or an anesthesiologist must evaluate the patient immediately prior to surgery to assess the risk of the anesthesia relative to the surgical procedure to be performed."[20] Responsibility for this immediate preoperative evaluation will often fall to the anesthesiologist, because the operating surgeon may be engaged in completion of a preceding procedure or in scrubbing up for the next case. In our opinion, this immediate preoperative evaluation should be thought of as the second, discreet stage in the patient selection process. There may be great psychological pressures on the anesthesiologist performing this stage 2 evaluation not to disrupt the smooth operation of the center, the expectations and psychological preparedness of the patient, or even the schedule of the surgical room. Pressures such as these may be brought to bear in a subtle fashion. However, if it is borne in mind that this immediate preoperative evaluation is nonetheless an integral part of the patient selection process (as opposed to an "11th hour" last look), patients who passed the first stage of patient selection screening but who should not pass the second will be spared the risk of unsafe procedures, and the anesthesiologist will be spared the risk of legal liability for a bad outcome.

To ensure that presurgery instructions were followed, all patients should be routinely asked about food or liquid ingestion on arriving at the center and about the availability of an appropriate escort to take the patient home.

Surgeon Selection and Professional Relationships

Surgeon selection is, at least at its primary level, not the responsibility of the anesthesiologist, except when he or she is functioning as a medical staff member or medico-administrator for an ambulatory center. The AAAHC standards, for example, provide that "adequate supervision of surgery conducted in the organization is a responsibility of the governing body, is recommended by an anesthesiologist or another physician, and is provided by appropriate personnel."[20]

When there are serious questions about a surgeon's competence, reliability in surgical judgment, or lack of ability to work with the surgical team, that surgeon should not be selected to work in the ambulatory surgery center. In the event of denial of a surgeon's application, careful documentation of the justifications for exclusion can guard against any possibility of a suit alleging illegal boycott or unlawful restraint of trade. More to the immediate point, throughout the operation of an ambulatory surgery center, the relationship of the surgeon and the anesthesiologist is important to the patient's welfare. Since surgeons and anesthesiologists work as part of a medical team, they must be able to work in a cooperative and collaborative manner for the team to operate effectively. Lack of communication can contribute to a bad outcome. That may have been the situation in a Kansas case in which a husband brought a wrongful death action against an anesthesiology group practice, alleging medical malpractice because of improper administration of a spinal anesthetic to his wife. The plaintiff's wife was in labor, and an epidural anesthetic (Marcaine [bupivacaine], 0.25 percent) was administered. When it was discovered later that the baby was emerging brow first, a decision to perform a cesarean section was made. The patient was taken to the operating room and a spinal anesthetic was administered using bupivacaine, 0.75 percent, without a physician's presence or orders, by a nurse anesthetist employed by the anesthesiology group. Shortly after the administration of the spinal anesthetic, the patient vomited, suffered seizures, cardiac arrest, and a loss of consciousness. The patient died 4 days later. Since the anesthesiology group practice admitted 100 percent liability, the trial proceeded on the issue of damages alone.[21]

In the high-pressure environment of an ambulatory surgery center, where adherence to scheduling and rapid, efficient care of patients are required, the need for communication becomes at once more difficult and more important. The situation should call forth not only the best medical skills but also the best interpersonal communication skills. The anesthesiologist should take every opportunity, both in the context of specific surgical procedures and ongoing professional functions of the center, to establish mutual communication and to foster an understanding of the role and responsibilities of the anesthesiologist in the minds of all other members of the surgical team.

The Patient Interview

The patient interview, often called the preanesthetic visit, is likely to be the first face-to-face encounter between the anesthesiologist and the patient. In terms of legal requirements, the patient interview has two separate functions. The first is to gather information so the anesthesia plan can be formulated based on full knowledge of the patient's history and physical condition. The second, and equally important, function is to disseminate information sufficient to ensure that the anesthesiologist obtains an informed consent (see the following section) and psychologically prepares the patient for anesthesia. A not insignificant purpose of the information dissemination process is to foster the patient's understanding of the role of anesthesia in his or her care and to form a physician-patient relationship based on trust and confidence. The information gathering and dissemination functions interrelate. The anesthesiologist must convey information to the patient about the anesthetic modalities being considered and the risks of each and must elicit from the patient all relevant information as to personal and family history.

The timing of the patient interview is a critical element in its success, and nowhere is the contrast between ambulatory surgical procedures and inpatient surgery more apparent. In an inpatient setting, the interview is typically conducted the evening before surgery. By its very nature, ambulatory surgery does not require the patient's presence at the center until shortly before the procedure. Since the ambulatory surgical patient is not admitted to a designated bed, an appropriate physical location for the interview may also be more difficult to obtain. These differences must not be permitted to undermine the vital purpose of the patient interview. While there is no hard and fast rule about when or where this interview must take place, in all cases it should be conducted at a time and in a place designed to facilitate the meaningful exchange of information between the anesthesiologist and patient. It is virtually impossible for a meaningful exchange to take place as the patient is about to be wheeled into the operating room. Even in the absence of premedication, patient anxiety and the pressure to "get surgery over with" will be seen by a jury to have substantially impaired the patient's ability to understand and communicate. Furthermore, at that time, there is no opportunity to obtain consultation or diagnostic testing that may be indicated by the patient's history or condition.

In some centers, preprinted forms or questionnaires are provided to the patient, and there may be a telephone interview between anesthesiologist and patient prior to the day of surgery. While the ideal situation would involve a face-to-face meeting in an office, conference room, or at some other location conducive to the meaningful exchange of information, the realities of ambulatory surgical practice may make this impossible. In our view, a properly designed printed questionnaire and a telephone interview are acceptable as long as there is a personal meeting between the anesthesiologist and the patient prior to the procedure. At that time, the anesthesiologist must review with the patient the information contained on the form. The anesthesiologist must have had opportunity to analyze this form in advance of the actual meeting. While economic pressures increasingly discourage the routine administration of presurgical tests, the anesthesiologist must never lose sight of the obligation to obtain sufficient information far enough in advance of the surgical procedure to permit the ordering of tests that are medically necessary and to allow the retrieval and review of the patient's prior medical records, if those appear relevant.

INFORMED CONSENT

It is well-established that before commencing any course of treatment the physician has a duty to obtain the patient's informed consent. The touchstone of this requirement is the patient's right of self-determination—to decide what happens to his or her own body. The case law focuses attention on the physician's duty to disclose and on the nature and content of that disclosure. Although modified in emergency situations, when medical care is rendered without the physician first obtaining the patient's informed consent, the physician may be subject to an action for negligence or for technical battery, which is a tort consisting of intentionally causing a "harmful or offensive contact with the person of another."

The legal standard focuses on the scope of information that must be conveyed to the patient and the procedure for conveying that information. The extent of disclosure depends on the medical problem as well as on the patient.[22] We believe that a fertile breeding ground for claims alleging the lack of informed consent is the use of a "combined" consent form primarily directed to the surgery. The patient will allege that the surgery but not the anesthesia was discussed, and there will be little contradictory evidence in the medical record. For this reason there should be a separate process for, and record of, the patient's informed consent to anesthesia.

The preoperative visit clearly provides the best opportunity for the anesthesiologist to discuss with the patient the risks and alternatives of anesthesia. It is more difficult to demonstrate in court that valid consent was obtained by a meeting with the patient immediately prior to surgery, since the patient, even if not premedicated, is likely to have been preoccupied with fears or anxiety about surgery. Therefore, the safest cause from a legal perspective is to conduct the informed consent interview as far in advance of surgery as possible. When the patient grants permission for the procedure to be performed, he or she should be asked to sign an informed consent record that specifically describes the matters discussed. Entering a separate note in the patient's chart will provide further protection against any questions concerning the content of the discussion.

Of equal importance to disclosing the required information to the patient is the maintenance of a clear record of the disclosure and of the patient's response. Here, the anesthesiologist should remember that a consent record, however well-designed, is not the required consent itself, but is merely evidence of that consent. As evidence, the consent record must be able to demonstrate, often years after the fact, what was said on that particular occasion. For this reason, the use of consent forms that are simply a series of conclusory statements to be checked off are of considerably less legal value than forms that use, to the maximum practical extent, notations actually prepared by the anesthesiologist at the time the consent was obtained. Experienced trial lawyers often refer to a "13th juror called common sense." Common sense dictates that a contemporaneous writing is not only more persuasive than a check mark alongside a preprinted statement, but is also a better indication that appropriate time and care were invested by the anesthesiologist in the informed consent process.

The scope of the physician's legal duty to disclose is not subject to any uniform standard. "Indeed, the cases speaking in terms of 'full' disclosure appear to envision something less than total disclosure, leaving unanswered the question of just how much."[22] The patient must be informed of "material risks." However, the extent of disclosure as to other risks can be carried to extremes. The anesthesiologist is therefore faced with the difficult problem of discerning which risks should be made known to the patient. If he or she discloses risks that, for example, may occur in 1 of 200,000 cases, the patient may well become alarmed and refuse surgery. Precisely that issue was addressed in a case before the Texas courts. There, the patient signed a standard consent form granting the surgeon authorization to operate and to perform surgery "under any anesthetic deemed advisable." During surgery, the anesthesiologist administered halothane to the patient. One week after the patient's discharge she was readmitted to the hospital, where she died. The autopsy revealed an idiosyncratic reaction that was possibly related to the anesthesia (e.g., "massive hepatic necrosis"). The anesthesiologist admitted that she did not advise the patient of the risk of liver damage from halothane. Expert testimony estimated the risk to be an incidence between 1 in 3,000 and 1 in 40,000 and indicated that it was not standard practice to advise the patient of an adverse reaction occurring less than 1 percent of the time. Testimony also indicated that halothane was the "preferred anesthetic" at the time. Accordingly, the jury declined to find that the anesthesiologist failed to obtain the patient's informed consent.[23]

The traditional legal standard by which a jury determines whether a physician breached the duty of disclosure is to consider "what information would a reasonable physician of the same school disclose under the same or similar circumstances."[23] Referred to as the "professional community" standard, this test is accepted and applied in a number of states. States adhering to the traditional rule require the plaintiff to come forward with expert medical testimony to establish a standard of practice by which the physician's conduct at issue can be measured.

More recently, however, there has been an important shift from the professional community standard to a "prudent patient" standard, which is based on what a hypothetical reasonable patient would consider material to his or her decision-making process. Reasons for abandoning the traditional standard in favor of this more subjective one include concern (1) that professional custom should not furnish the legal test to measure the obligation to disclose, (2) that the focus should be on the patient's right to self-determination, and (3) that the requirement for expert testimony as to accepted practice in the physician community presents practical problems for patients. The prudent patient standard does not require expert testimony in addressing the question of whether a prudent person in the patient's position would have consented to surgery after full disclosure of material information.[23]

The two principal exceptions to the obligation of the physician to disclose relate to circumstances that apply infrequently in the ambulatory surgery setting. The first involves a genuine emergency in which the patient is incapacitated and incapable of giving consent. A physician faced with an immediate life-threatening situation and an unconscious patient will not be held liable for failure to obtain informed consent to appropriate emergency treatment. However, if the situation is not an emergency and the patient is unable to consent due to physical condition, age, disability, or the like, the courts require that the physician obtain consent from the patient's immediate next of kin or, if there is no next of kin available, from a court of appropriate jurisdiction. Many state or local judicial systems have an expeditious procedure by which physicians and legal counsel can approach the court, by telephone if necessary, to obtain judicial consent on behalf of an incapacitated patient. Each anesthesiologist should be aware of what the procedure is in the jurisdiction in which he or she practices.

The other exception to a duty to disclose is the withholding of information that could injure a patient's emotional state. The legal issue will be whether the decision to withhold information representing a sound medical judgment that the information would be injurious to the patient's well-being. Since the legal parameters of this exception have not been clearly defined, an anesthesiologist is at risk in relying on personal judgment alone. Even if this exception seems clearly applicable, the anesthesiologist should nevertheless seek the informed consent of next of kin, as a safeguard. If that is unavailable, we strongly recommend that a consultation from another physician be obtained, and his or her concurrence noted in the chart.

In summary, a general checklist of the elements of an informed consent for anesthesia appears below.

DISCHARGE POLICY

A significant hazard encountered almost exclusively in ambulatory surgery is premature discharge of the patient from the facility. The AAAHC standards provide that in an accredited center, "patients who have received anesthesia are evaluated by the operating surgeon or anesthesiologist

Elements of Informed Consent for Anesthesia

Identification of anesthesia as a medical specialty, and a statement of the anesthesiologist's planned role in the surgical procedure, particularly including any use of supervised, nonphysician anesthetists.

A concise explanation of the anesthesia modality chosen, the agents to be administered, the manner of their administration, and the way in which they induce anesthesia.

An explanation of alternative modalities or agents that were considered and the reasons why the chosen modality and agent is deemed to be best.

Identification and explanation of material risks associated with the particular modality or agent to be used.

Identification of material risks disclosed from the patient's history, symptoms, test results, and the like, as obtained in the patient interview.

Discussion of the special considerations particular to ambulatory surgery, such as the need to have another responsible adult take the patient home, the need to avoid operating dangerous equipment in the immediate postdischarge period, and the need to observe and report any postdischarge problems promptly.

A solicitation of questions and an offer to provide further information, particularly as to more remote risks not discussed.

after recovery from anesthesia, prior to discharge."[20] Responsibility for this evaluation is likely to fall on the anesthesiologist, since the surgeon may be involved in another procedure or may otherwise be unavailable. Accreditation standards reflect the reality of modern anesthesia practice by requiring that, in a qualified center, "an anesthesiologist or another physician qualified in resuscitative techniques is present or immediately available until all patients operated on that day have been discharged."[20]

A written policy establishing specific discharge criteria is a sound basis for a legally sufficient discharge decision. However, the patient must be individually evaluated at or just prior to actual discharge, not only to ensure that all discharge criteria are met, but also to ensure that there are no symptoms or complaints not specifically covered in pre-established criteria that would justify detaining the patient for further observation. Most physicians recognize that diagnosis is an art as well as a science, and if a patient simply does not "look right," even though his or her physical symptoms match established discharge criteria, that patient should remain in the center until the condition can be resolved. Other subjective criteria, such as the patient's degree of medical sophistication, overall intelligence, and relationship to the individual into whose custody he or she will be discharged, are appropriate factors to be considered, as well as the proximity of the postdischarge location to appropriate emergency facilities.

However strict the discharge criteria and however clearly those criteria are followed, a physician must be responsible for the discharge decision. In our opinion, granting permission to discharge by telephone should be discouraged, since it can contribute to liability exposure. In a courtroom, it could be argued that the contacting of the discharging physician shows the need for his or her assessment of the patient, but that this was done over the telephone, with no opportunity to observe the patient directly, indicates a substandard level of care. A back-up arrangement to ensure the availability of a qualified physician for this purpose should be in place in the event that neither the operating surgeon nor the anesthesiologist is available.

It is clear that the patient must be discharged into the hands of a "responsible adult." Even the accreditation standards are unambiguous and subject to no interpretation: "patients who have received anesthesia, except unsupplemented local anesthesia, are discharged in the company of a responsible adult."[20] There is no preestablished definition of a responsible adult, although a useful rule of thumb is an individual of legal driving age. In unusual circumstances, someone younger may be sufficiently responsible to meet the applicable legal standard, while someone older may fail to meet the criteria, particularly if that person is physically or psychologically impaired, either voluntarily or involuntarily. The judicial system will likely impose on the physician responsible for the discharge decision some responsibility for determining that the individual into whose custody the patient is discharged conforms to the standard. This responsibility is likely to increase as the likelihood or potential severity of postoperative complications increases or as the general mental state, sophistication, or level of comprehension of the patient decreases.

Written instructions should be given to the patient and to the patient's escort as to the time, place, and date of any follow-up appointment and as to whom the patient should contact in the event that complications arise. This duplication of instructions is a reasonable and prudent measure, since many sedative-anesthetic agents currently used in ambulatory settings can cause short-term postoperative amnesia (e.g., midazolam), even after appropriate discharge criteria are met. The patient and escort should also be warned of common complaints and possible complications that may arise after surgery. Equipped with this information, the patient is less likely to become alarmed if known complications occur and far more likely to recognize the need to seek follow-up care promptly.

As part of discharge planning, the patient's access to emergency facilities should be discussed. When the patient is referred to a hospital emergency room or other location outside the center for emergency treatment, the referral location should have access to basic information about the patient and the surgical procedure. A patient, even one not suffering complications, cannot be expected to describe his or her surgery and anesthesia in a medically appropriate manner.

Many centers have a telephone follow-up policy. A follow-up phone call the day after surgery not only communicates concern but also ensures that if unexpected complications do arise, arrangements can be made for the patient's continuing care. That call need not come from a physician. However, in the event that the follow-up call reveals problems, a physician must be available to promptly provide appropriate direction. Even if a duty is not imposed by law, whenever a duty is assumed, it must be performed competently, or liability may result.

SUMMARY

Although ambulatory surgery centers are still a relatively new development in the American health care system, many factors suggest their continued growth. As with inpatient care, a concern for the quality of outpatient care will have to be balanced with cost considerations. However, cost considerations should never be the sole guiding factor, nor should they outweigh concern for patient welfare.

In reducing exposure to liability, the same legal principles pertinent to an inpatient setting apply to the ambulatory surgical center. Thus, anesthesiologists practicing in the outpatient setting need to comply with standards of care, to anticipate and plan for complications, to obtain informed consent prior to any procedure, to properly discharge their patients, and to provide ample documentation of their care in the patient's chart. Anesthesia for ambulatory surgery also has its own distinct considerations. Additional risks related in part to the limited time for preanesthetic assessment and to the fact that patients are discharged to their home must be thoroughly considered so that adequate safeguards can be developed. Recognition of the legal hazards and pitfalls associated with anesthesia for ambulatory surgery can both advance the benefits of patient treatment and reduce the legal perils of patient care.

REFERENCES

1. Paxton, Why Doctors Get Sued, MED. ECON., April 18, 1980, at 50
2. Fuchsberg, Anesthesia Medical Malpractice, 17 TRIAL LAW. Q. 47 (1985)
3. Gavzer, What This Medical Battle Could Cost You, PARADE MAG., July 17, 1988, at 11
4. Kramer, *Anesthesia Complications*, 183 N.Y.L.J. 3 (1980)
5. Keats AS: p. 3. Complications in Anesthesiology. In Orkin F, Cooperman L (eds): Role of Anesthesia in Surgical Morbidity. JB Lippincott, Philadelphia, 1983
6. Vuletich v. Bolgla, 85 Ill App.3d 810, 407 N.E.2d 566 (1980)
7. Shilkret v. Annapolis Emergency Hosp. Ass'n, 276 Md. 187, 349 A.2d 245, (1975) (citation omitted)
8. American Society of Anesthesiologists Standards for Basic Intraoperative Monitoring. Approved by the House of Delegates October 21, 1986
9. JCAHO.7 Perspective 1 (September-October, 1987)
10. W. Prosser & W. Keeton, THE LAW OF TORTS, at 242. 5th Ed. 1984
11. Kitlo v. Gilbert, 39 Colo. App. 374, 570 P. 2d 544 (1977)
12. Central Anesthesia Associates P.C. v. Worthy, 173 Ga. App. 150, 325 S.E.2d 819 (1984), *aff'd* 254 Ga 728, 333 S.E. 2d 829 (1985)
13. 42 Code of Federal Regulations, Part 400, § 405.552(a) (1988)
14. Sanders v. Mt. Sinai Hospital, 21 Ohio app.3d 249, 487 N.E.2d. 588 (1985)
15. Thompson v. Presbyterian Hospital, Inc., 652 P.2d 260 (Okl. 1982)
16. Schneider v. Albert Einstein Medical Center, 390 A.2d 1271 (Pa. Super. 1978)
17. Cash v. Kim, 288 S.C. 292, 342 S.E. 2d 61, 63 (Ct. App. 1986)
18. King v. Retz, 115 Misc. 2d 836, 454 N.Y.S.2d 594 (Sup. Ct. 1982)
19. Restatement (Second) of Torts § 908(1) (1979)
20. ACCREDITATION HANDBOOK FOR AMBULATORY HEALTH CARE (1987–1988 Ed.). Standard 9 Anesthesia Surgical Services
21. Wentling v. Medical Anesthesia Services, P.A., 237 Kan. 503, 701 P. 2d 939 (1985)
22. Canterbury v. Spence, 464 F.2d 772 (D.C. Cir. 1972), cert. denied, 409 U.S. 1064 (1972)
23. Granado v. Madsen, 729 S.W.2d 866 (Tex. Ct. App. 1987)

21

Controversies in Outpatient Anesthesia

Burton S. Epstein

In a 1987 article, entitled "The Future of Ambulatory Surgery,"[1] I wrote, "it appears that 20 years after the opening of our in-and-out unit at George Washington University in Washington, DC, many unanswered questions remain as to the best management of anesthesia for the outpatient child and adult." In this chapter, Paul White requested that I respond to several questions that are frequently asked at meetings of individuals who have spent much of their professional careers involved in the management of anesthesia for outpatient surgery. Whenever possible, I have tried to support preferences with data from the medical literature. At other times, I have merely reflected or philosophized about the nature of the controversy and the current status of its resolution.

Many of my ideas will be considered controversial. How else can one address a subject that, by its own definition, remains unresolved? It is my hope that many of the topics discussed in this section will stimulate future clinical research activities. The results of carefully controlled studies will eventually lead to a resolution of some of the topics on the current list of controversies. In future years, we shall undoubtedly be faced with new challenges and controversies.

HOW DO WE IDENTIFY THE PATIENT WHO MAY NOT BE AN APPROPRIATE CANDIDATE FOR AMBULATORY SURGERY?

As anesthesiologists have become more experienced with the anesthetic management of the outpatient and insurance companies have insisted on justification for hospitalization prior to surgery, the list of procedures appropriate for elective surgery on an inpatient basis has dwindled. The usual indications are (1) unstable/uncontrolled medical condition requiring inpatient therapy, (2) prolonged intravenous antibiotic therapy, and (3) bowel preparation. Although hard data are not always available, it is most convenient to describe the "inappropriate" outpatient under two general headings: pre-existing medical diseases and inadequate social environment. Many of the patients with these medical and/or social conditions have been discussed in previous chapters. However, it is useful to consolidate these higher risk patient populations into one brief section.

Infants at Increased Risk

Infants at increased risk include (1) healthy full-term neonates less than 2 weeks of age, (2) expremature infants, (3) infants with bronchopulmonary dysplasia, and (4) infants at risk for sudden infant death syndrome (SIDS) (e.g., sibling with SIDS or history of apneic episodes).

It is sound medical practice to be cautious with the expremature infant *regardless* of the magnitude of the planned surgical procedure. Administration of an anesthetic is unwise before a postconceptual age of 50 weeks, or even later if the infant has not outgrown pulmonary or other systemic problems. It seems prudent to admit these infants so they may be monitored for possible apnea, bradycardia, and decreased oxygen saturation. Table 21-1 is a useful checklist of risk factors that must be identified and considered before determining the risk of the infant presenting for elective surgery on an outpatient basis.[2]

Adults at Increased Risk

Pre-existing Medical Conditions

Patients with an unstable American Society of Anesthiologists (ASA) physical status III or IV who require medical attention in an acute care facility as well as patients with an ASA physical status III who are morbidly obese are at increased risk. Although there are a few studies involving adults that relate the pre-existing medical condition to morbidity or mortality, the patient with coronary artery disease appears most likely to have an unplanned hospitalization.[3]

Inadequate Social Environment

Because outpatients are discharged home within hours after surgery, follow-up care relies largely on the patient's level of cooperation and the support of his or her social environment. Consequently, patients are at increased risk if they (1) are uncooperative, (2) are unwilling or unable to follow postoperative instructions, and (3) have no responsible adult available to care for them after discharge.

Selection of the geriatric-aged patient depends on the magnitude of the planned surgical procedure and the anesthetic requirements. Other important considerations include (1) overall physical and mental status, (2) physiologic (biologic) age, and (3) availability of competent home care.

The requirement that outpatients who have received any form of anesthesia be discharged in the company of a responsible adult has been in effect for decades. A responsible adult has been defined as a mature individual who is mentally and physically able to assist the patient with his or her healthcare needs. With the rapid increase in outpatient surgery among the geriatric population, many facilities are now requiring that a responsible adult also remain with the patient for a few days after surgery. What if the patient lives alone? How do we assess the physical and intellectual capabilities of the spouse/friend? How do we assess the mental status and capabilities of the patient? Should a test like the Folstein mini-mental status examination be administered before and after outpatient anesthesia? If dementia or delirium are identified preoperatively, how can we expect to improve the condition after anesthesia? The social issues surrounding the administration of anesthesia to geriatric outpatients need further study. However, concerns regard-

Table 21-1. Factors Affecting Risk of Infant for Outpatient Surgery

During perinatal period	Following perinatal period
Presence of respiratory difficulty	History of apnea monitor at home
Need for tracheal intubation	History of feeding difficulty or aspiration
Need for mechanical ventilation	Frequent "chest infections" or wheezing
Need for supplemental oxygen	

(From Epstein and Hannallah,[2] with permission.)

ing these healthcare issues are leading to innovative methods (e.g., the "23-hour clock" and "motel" arrangements) of intermediate care during the early postoperative period.

High-Risk Medical Conditions

Controversy exists over whether it is categorically inadvisable to perform outpatient surgery on patients susceptible to malignant hyperthermia or sickle cell disease.[4] The preoperative assessment and preparation, the magnitude of the procedure, and the intraoperative and postoperative course will ultimately determine the advisability of discharging these patients to their home on the day of surgery. In addition, for the patient who is susceptible to or has a previous history of malignant hyperthermia, the availability of support systems in the ambulatory facility is critically important. For example, how quickly can arterial blood gases be obtained? Is capnography in routine use?

WHAT ARE THE RISKS IN ANESTHETIZING THE GERIATRIC PATIENT?

I was somewhat amused in reading about the advantages of outpatient surgery for the geriatric patient (see Ch. 16). McLeskey and Nibel emphasize such things as the limited separation from family, friends, and familiar home environment, as well as less disruption in their daily routine, diet, and sleep pattern. Having worked 9 years in a pediatric hospital, I thought he was talking about pediatric outpatients, not their grandparents! One of the advantages of outpatient anesthesia for a child is the reduction in "separation anxiety." It appears that at least in this respect individuals at the extremes of age are similar.

The geriatric outpatient differs from most other candidates for ambulatory surgery in that the former frequently suffers from deterioration of major organ systems that may lead to increased perioperative morbidity and mortality. McLeskey and Nibel concentrated on a number of issues that deserve further comment: (1) the distinction between the age-related risk of complications and risk related to the patient's ASA physical status, (2) the influence of anesthetic techniques on the incidence of unanticipated hospital admissions, and (3) the influence of the type of surgery on the frequency of perioperative complications. I would agree that age per se does not necessarily relate to the risk of anesthesia and surgery in the otherwise healthy outpatient. One would predict, however, that there would be a correlation between the frequency of complications and pre-existing medical problems in the elderly outpatient population.

Interestingly, studies that have attempted to correlate ASA physical status and postoperative complications are not totally satisfactory and/or must be subject to interpretation. For example, Natof[5] reported that there was no statistical difference in the incidence of either major or minor complications in 15,984 outpatients without significant pre-existing diseases, compared with 1,984 outpatients with pre-existing diseases. The incidence of major complications was 1.12 and 1.16 percent in the two groups, respectively. Furthermore, there was a direct cause and effect relationship between the medical problem and the complication in only three cases. There were only four complications in the 642 ASA class III patients, and there was no clear evidence that the presence of serious disease increased the gravity of complications. Furthermore, Natof concluded that major complications associated with the ambulatory setting were much more likely to be related to the type of surgical procedure performed, rather than the physical state of the outpatient or the presence of pre-existing medical problems.

It is fascinating to note that Meridy[6] reported that "aside from patients undergoing dental surgery, neither the surgical procedure nor the extremes of age affected the duration of recovery or the rate of postoperative complications." It should be noted in interpreting these data that "in the older age group, local anesthesia was most frequently selected." Unfortunately, Meridy does not identify the specific types of surgical procedures performed and only lists them by categories. It would appear from both Natof's and Meridy's observations that in patients with pre-existing disease and/or at the extremes of age, less complex surgical procedures that can be performed under local anesthetic conditions are less likely to be associated with prolonged recovery times and postoperative complications. I would like to emphasize that it is imperative to match the patient, as well as his or her physiologic age and physical status, with the surgical procedure. To my knowledge, no one has yet conducted a randomized, controlled prospective study comparing the complication rate in patients with the above potential problems (i.e., pre-existing disease and/or increased age) undergoing superficial surgical procedures on either an ambulatory or inpatient basis.

Furthermore, generalizations are being made about the safety of geriatric ambulatory surgery in the United States under the Medicare Program and the new peer review organizations. The latter have established lists of surgical procedures that must be performed in an ambulatory unit on otherwise healthy patients over 65 years of age; otherwise, no payment is made to the facility. Data are being obtained on major complications during and immediately after outpatient surgery, particularly those complications necessitating overnight observation in a hospital. Unfortunately, there is no careful study of complications at home after discharge from the outpatient facility. Confusional states, bone fractures, and the inability to perform daily activities (e.g., bathing, cooking, and going to the bathroom) are common problems in the elderly surgical population. Yet, these elderly patients are only "acceptably" admitted overnight because of pre-existing disease and/or perioperative complications noted during or immediately after surgery. Should more studies be directed at the first few days at home? Should more emphasis be placed on developing less costly after-care facilities as an alternative to hospitalization and home care? At this time, a system to address these public health issues is probably more suitably established in Great Britain than in the United States. Although these comments were abstracted from an article entitled "The Future of Ambulatory Surgery," which was published several years ago,[7] they still appear to be accurate and timely today.

McLeskey and Nibel also discuss the issue of physical status, and cite a study by Cohen et al., who noted that the relative risk predicted by increased age was less dramatic than the relative risk predicted by poor physical status.[8] The ASA physical status classification system appears to predict intraoperative and major postoperative complications independently, but alone it is insufficient to predict anesthesia morbidity in the immediate postoperative period.[9] The major shortcomings of many articles that attempt to relate complications of ambulatory surgery to the type of surgery (without being specific about the nature of the procedure) and the patient's ASA physical status have been mentioned previously. In the special study conducted by the Federated Ambulatory Surgery Association involving 87,492 patients from 40 freestanding surgery centers, it was found that over 28,000 of the patients studied had no physical status value on their patient data collection form.[10] Obviously, accurate and complete data must be obtained before we generalize about which factors do or do not influence outcome.

SHOULD THE PATIENT BE SCREENED PRIOR TO THE DAY OF SURGERY? IF SO, WHAT FORMS SHOULD THIS EVALUATION TAKE?

There are many reasons justifying a visit to an outpatient facility, or at least telephone contact, prior to the day of surgery. Wieland and Katz (Ch. 20) comment that from a legal standpoint, an interview should be conducted at a time and in a place designed to facilitate the meaningful exchange of information between the anesthesiologist and his or her patient. The authors state, "it is virtually impossible for a meaningful exchange to take place as the patient is about to be wheeled into the operating room," adding that "patient anxiety and the pressure to 'get surgery over with' will be seen by a jury to have substantially impaired the patients' ability to understand and communicate." Likewise, from a medical viewpoint, if patient evaluation is conducted immediately prior to surgery, "there is no opportunity to obtain consultation or diagnostic testing that may be indicated by the patient's history or condition." Certainly, Roizen and Rupani (Ch. 9) have no quarrel with the role of the timely taking of a history. They consider this the best clinical indicator for detecting disease and the basis for ordering only necessary and appropriate laboratory tests.

In my opinion, much of the concern surrounding the anesthetizing of ambulatory surgical patients relates to the original and somewhat biased "ground rule" that limited ambulatory surgical procedures to those identified as ASA physical status I and II patients whose procedures were considered "superficial" operations. Initially, surgeons and referring physicians correctly associated ambulatory care with healthy patients and "minor" surgery. As a result, the preanesthetic evaluation was frequently short, cursory, and inadequate. Since the patients were largely young and healthy, and the procedures short and uncomplicated, little harm was done. When complications from anesthesia occurred, they were usually minor and not associated with inadequate preoperative evaluation and preparation of the patient. Although more extensive lists of operative procedures are now judged to be suitable for ambulatory surgery, many surgeons have not altered their original practice of neglecting to properly characterize the medical condition of outpatients. The patient's visit to the surgeon's office is frequently the only consistent point in the preanesthesia process where identification of potential problems can be made uniformly in a time frame suitable to allow medical consultation and alert the anesthesiologist. Unfortunately, when the surgeon believes he or she is acting in the role of technician, the patient appears in the ambulatory unit on the day of surgery improperly evaluated and poorly prepared for the operation. Delays, confrontations, and expedited evaluations continue to occur and may be even more frequent today than in the early days of ambulatory surggery.

Anesthesiologists who have not anticipated these problems or altered their practice will continue to be faced with the problem of what can be done safely and effectively to optimally prepare a patient on the day of the surgery. As a result of poor preparation, the operative schedule often has to be rearranged, and untimely delays then compound the frustrations of the operating team and the patient. In Chapter 9, Roizen and Rupani briefly survey various methods for preoperative evaluation in outpatient surgical units. They note that in some instances, no established practices are used to evaluate a patient prior to induction of anesthesia. It is my opinion that anesthesiologists must participate in the evaluation and management of the patient before the day of surgery. This can be done effectively by preinterviewing the patient by telephone and/or arranging a personal evaluation at the facility.

Whether a telephone or personal interview is preferred, the list of questions asked of the patient must be directed and focused on identifying risk factors that may influence the management and outcome of the surgical and anesthetic procedure. At Children's Hospital National Medical Center in Washington, D.C., a screening clinic is staffed by a pediatric nurse practitioner who is responsible to and remains in close contact with the Department of Anesthesiology. One of the functions of the clinic is to telephone all parents. The parents of each child are contacted initially by telephone after the operation has been posted and a second time within 48 hours of the scheduled surgery. The initial telephone "interview," in which a preoperative screening form (see Appendix 21-1) is completed, is highly specific and directed at identifying any past or present risk factors. For example, specific questions pertain to (1) breath-holding spells, (2) cardiac and respiratory problems, (3) history of prematurity, (4) muscular problems, (5) development delays, and (6) a detailed medical history. During a subsequent phone call, NPO orders are clarified, the patient's present health condition is reassessed, and instructions regarding the operational aspects of the short stay recovery unit are described. In a study performed at the Children's Hospital National Medical Center, significant problems were identified (Table 21-2). The cancellation rate of those outpatients who were not screened was almost twice that of those who were screened.[12]

Table 21-2. Results of Preoperative Screening Study of 5,031 Patients at Children's Hospital Medical Center

Outcome	Screened	Unscreened
Surgery completed as scheduled	79%	71%
Surgery postponed	5.4%	6.5%
Surgery cancelled	4.3%	8.2%[a]
Not on final schedule	5.9%	5.3%
Changed to PM admission	0.3%	1.3%[a]

[a] Significantly different from screened patients, $P < .05$.

(From Patel et al.,[11] with permission.)

At our adult outpatient facility at the George Washington University Hospital, approximately 25 percent of the outpatients are 65 years of age or older and 10 percent are ASA physical status III or IV. Ninety-five percent of these outpatients are evaluated in our screening unit at intervals up to 2 weeks prior to the day of surgery. A screening history is obtained, appropriate laboratory tests are ordered, consents are obtained, and, if appropriate, speciality consultations are requested. It has been apparent to us that many internists to whom we refer patients with complex medical problems are not aware of the appropriate form for a preoperative risk assessment evaluation when it is requested by an anesthesiologist. To standardize the assessment and make it more uniformly useful, we designed a Physician's Preoperative Assessment Summary (Appendix 21-2) in conjunction with the Department of Medicine. This and other endeavors applied before the day of surgery lead to a more uniform, comprehensive evaluation and preparation of the patient, as well as reduced delays, cancellations, and confrontations associated with unanticipated last-minute problems.

ARE ANY LABORATORY TESTS REQUIRED PREOPERATIVELY IN THE YOUNG HEALTHY PATIENT?

Anesthesiologists throughout the world are familiar with the approach used by Roizen and Rupani (Ch. 9) to deal with this question. The basic issue is whether the test and its results will affect the anesthetic management of the patient and the outcome of the surgical procedure. I recall hearing Fred Orkin state his philosophy as, "what do you do if the result of the test is positive? What do you do if it is negative? If the answer is the same, don't order the test."

Whether there is a requirement to order

a minimum set of data on every patient may depend on institutional, local, and regional policies, procedures, and legal statutes. The ASA has published a Statement on Routine Preoperative Laboratory and Diagnostic Screening[13] that states:

> Preanesthetic laboratory and diagnostic testing is often essential; however, no routine* laboratory or diagnostic screening† test is necessary for the preanesthetic evaluation of patients. Appropriate indications for ordering tests include the identification of specific clinical indicators or risk factors (e.g., age, pre-existing disease, magnitude of the surgical procedure). Anesthesiologists, anesthesiology departments, and/or health care facilities should develop appropriate guidelines for preanesthetic screening tests in selected populations after considering the probable contribution of each test to patient outcome. Individual anesthesiologists should order test(s) when, in their judgement, the results may influence decisions regarding risks and management of the anesthesia and surgery. Legal requirements for laboratory testing where they exist should be observed.

This is a "statement," not a guideline or standard. In my opinion, it displays the issue and outlines the options in a concise and authoritative manner. When used in conjunction with Tables 9-6 and 9-7, an objective approach for a department or institution is easily developed.

As far as the subject of preanesthetic testing is concerned, however, I believe there are even more controversial issues. These relate to the question of whether to test "routinely" for pregnancy, sickle cell disease, and the acquired immunodefiency syndrome (AIDS). Even if a policy is not adopted for routine testing, are there any risks involved in ordering tests on an individual in whom you suspect any of these conditions may exist? Furthermore, is it advisable for an anesthesiologist to order a test without considering what he or she may be getting involved in? This question involves issues of informed consent, determination of who has access to the information, provision of follow-up counseling, and protection of the patient's right to privacy.[14]

Roizen and Rupani touched on the issue of pregnancy in Table 9-7, which presents a simplified strategy for preoperative testing. "Possible pregnancy" is considered an indication for screening. Philip describes the position of the American College of Obstetricians and Gynecologists (ACOG) as stated in the sixth edition of its Standards.[15] She suggests, "a serum pregnancy test is *not* a specific requirement, but could be used if the history and physical examination are uncertain. The ACOG standard also identifies the need for a definite policy regarding pregnancy determination in each facility." I agree with this position because it identifies the role of the anesthesiologist as acting within the scope of the institution's framework. This is beneficial when controversies occur, such as who authorized the testing of an unmarried, adolescent patient who the parents did not know was sexually active.

Since many diagnostic and therapeutic modalities may pose a direct or indirect risk to an embryo, hospitals should establish specific procedures, applicable to all services, for identifying unsuspected pregnancies in hospitalized women of reproductive age. A menstrual history and physical examination can be helpful in this determination. If there is *any* reason to suspect pregnancy, a pregnancy evaluation should be performed.

The problem with "routine screening" for sickle cell hemoglobinopathies is more

---

* *Routine* refers to a policy of performing a test or tests without regard to clinical indications in an individual patient.

† *Screening* means efforts to detect disease in unselected populations of asymptomatic patients.

complex. The key question is who should be screened? Blacks? Patients of Middle Eastern or Mediterranean descent? Patients from India or Africa? What happens if a patient is identified as having sickle cell trait? Does the anesthesiologist have a responsibility to provide marriage counseling? What happens if the patient is applying for a position as an airline pilot or has applied for life or health insurance? Will the label of sickle cell trait modify their risk category? Again, I believe that the institution should generate a statement of policy on this issue so that the practicing anesthesiologist is not caught in the middle. In the absence of this, the attending physician should be consulted and made aware of the need to identify the presence of a hemoglobinopathy. Obviously, the anesthetic management and outcome of ambulatory surgery may be affected if the disease is identified. Whether a patient with the sickle cell trait is at increased risk for complications during the perioperative period remains controversial and is beyond the scope of this discussion.

Screening for AIDS is another dilemma with many of the same problems. Certainly, some institutions have chosen to adopt "universal precautions" to protect the health care worker from the potential consequences of contamination from blood, saliva, and so forth without ever needing to conclusively identify the patient "at risk." This, however, does not consider issues related to other patients who may be at risk because of a common dressing room, holding area, step-down recovery room, and bathroom. The need for isolation of the human immunodeficiency virus (HIV)-positive patient also remains controversial.

Additional issues that may be confronted when testing for HIV are (1) How do we identify at-risk patients (e.g., homosexuals, bisexuals, those who frequent prostitutes, intravenous drug users, adults with multiple sexual partners)? (2) Which health care workers should be informed if a patient tests positive? (3) If an anesthesiologist is stuck with a needle or splashed with blood from a high-risk patient, does the anesthesiologist have the right to order an HIV test? Should the anesthesiologist inform the patient if the test result is positive? A more comprehensive view of risk from exposure to the patient who is HIV-positive and the issue of confidentiality are described in two recent articles.[16,17] Some of the potential causes for malpractice suits related to these and other similar issues were described in a recent issue of *Medical Economics* (July 3, 1989). A recent survey of 33 doctor-owned liability insurers revealed that 13 have yet to see their first AIDS-related malpractice suite. The other 20 insurance carriers have received a total of only 52 claims against physicians (Table 21-3). These carriers believe that the number of claims could increase dramatically if doctors find a cure for AIDS because victims could sue physicians on the basis of their failure to diagnose or promptly treat the disease.

Obviously, I believe the anesthesiologist should act as a member of the health care team rather than as an independent operator. It is more appropriate to develop en-

Table 21-3. Reasons for Malpractice Suits by AIDS Patients

	Incidence[a]
Failure to inform about blood transfusions	33
Breach of confidentiality	11
Failure to inform or obtain informed consent	11
Negligent or unnecessary transfusions	10
Failure to warn third parties	7
Misdiagnosis or failure to diagnose	5
Testing without consent	5
Failure to provide counseling before or after testing	3
Failure to protect other patients, hospital personnel, or attending physicians	3
Miscellaneous reasons	11

[a] Percentage values were rounded to the nearest percent.

(Adapted from Kleven J, Midwest Medical Insurance Company, Physicians Insurers Association of America, 1989, with permission.)

compassing guidelines that allow input from administrators, surgeons, attorneys, and experts in control of communicable diseases than to leave such critical decisions to individual judgment. Institutional policies are essential when management of the anesthetic may affect outcome.

IS PREMEDICATION CONTRAINDICATED?

Steward (Ch. 8) considers it preferable to psychologically prepare the child scheduled for an outpatient surgical (or diagnostic) experience rather than use premedication. Pharmacologic preparation is used if considered necessary, although situations that might fit under this category are not described. Certainly, the child who is old enough to appreciate psychological preparation should benefit from it. Conversely, pharmacologic premedication without psychological preparation is unfair, unreasonable, and potentially harmful to children. The tactic of telling a child he or she is going to the grocery store to buy cookies and ice cream rather than honestly addressing the proposed surgical procedure should be a thing of the past.

In my opinion, the majority of children do not need preoperative sedation. Those children who may benefit from premedication include pediatric outpatients undergoing repeated painful procedures, those who are apprehensive, and those too young to benefit from verbal reassurance. Preoperative sedation should not be confused with various techniques that are used in the anxious or uncooperative child for induction of anesthesia (e.g., intramuscular ketamine or rectal methohexital).

Lichtor (Ch. 10) described his approach to treating the anxious adult patient scheduled for an elective outpatient procedure. If the lead time is sufficient, oral diazepam is administered. If the desired effect is not achieved and/or time does not permit the administration of an oral benzodiazepine, intravenous medication (e.g., midazolam) is administered in a holding area. I have no criticism of this approach. In my opinion, adults need to be psychologically prepared as much or more than children. Unfortunately, the primary emphasis in outpatient surgery is on processing, speed, and efficiency. The human element is often lacking. The patient, scantily garbed, is hustled through common corridors with little or no regard to privacy. It can be a humiliating experience for the patient.

Although it might be considered judicious to premedicate the patient in order to separate him or her psychologically from the environment, most anesthesiologists are reluctant to run the risk of delayed recovery secondary to sedation, dizziness, or vomiting. Although this is not necessarily the case,[18] many facilities do not have a designated holding area that enables premedication to be administered to a patient under observation. In my experience, the logistics of administering premedication to the outpatient is more of a problem than the potentially deleterious effects. I believe we should continue to investigate the efficacy of oral premedicants that reduce anxiety, allow the patient to remain seated without hypotension, and do not prolong recovery. Although not required by all patients, the availability of these drugs would certainly lead to the more widespread use of premedication in the outpatient setting.

SHOULD OUTPATIENTS RECEIVE ASPIRATION PROPHYLAXIS?

Lichtor (Ch. 10) and Kallar and Jones (Ch. 18) have addressed this question thoroughly. They conclude that routine aspiration prophylaxis is not essential in all situations but is indicated in outpatients with increased risk factors. (Their standards for patients at risk vary slightly.) Kallar and Jones identify increased risk in patients with hiatal hernia and obesity, and in pediatric patients, geriatric patients, and pregnant patients in late mid-trimester; Lichtor identifies increased risk in patients with hiatal hernia, morbid obesity, and pregnant patients in general. As has been noted, the incidence of aspiration is considered by many to be too low to justify the routine use of prophylactic drugs on all outpatients regardless of their perceived risk.

In my opinion, there are a few additional situations that may justify prophylaxis for aspiration. For patients in whom maintenance of the airway and/or intubation of the trachea may be difficult, it is virtually impossible to prevent inflation of the stomach with air. As intragastric pressure rises, regurgitation may be more likely to occur. In an editorial appearing in a leading anesthesia journal, Coombs stated that "patients receiving anesthesia by facemask without an endotracheal tube can and should be protected against the acid component of pulmonary aspiration injury with preoperative cimetidine or ranitidine."[19] Although not universally accepted, there are many anesthesiologists who routinely attempt to neutralize the acid secretions when general anesthesia without endotracheal intubation is planned. This is particularly true if the procedure is to be performed with the patient in the lithotomy or Trendelenburg position.

It should be noted, however, that neither cimetidine, ranitidine, nor metoclopramide has been approved for use as a prophylactic agent against acid aspiration in the patient undergoing general anesthesia. Although these drugs have been studied extensively with respect to their ability to reduce gastric acidity and residual gastric volume (i.e., factors that *may* modify outcome from aspiration), no study has been performed that demonstrates a beneficial effect of the H_2-antagonists on outcome per se.

SHOULD OUTPATIENTS RECEIVE PROPHYLAXIS AGAINST VOMITING?

Most anesthesiologists have become selective in the use of antiemetic agents prior to the onset of vomiting. As described by Kallar and Jones in Chapter 18 (Table 18-1), many factors must be considered as possible etiologies of nausea and vomiting in outpatients. It is common to use small doses of an agent such as droperidol when confronted with the outpatient at risk of developing postoperative emetic symptoms. Obviously, other factors that lead to nausea and vomiting (e.g., pain and hypovolemia) are best treated by alleviation of the causative factor.

I would like to take issue with one concept in the chapter by Kallar and Jones. These authors accept the findings of a study by Abramowitz et al. that says that when droperidol is used in doses up to 75 μg/kg for pediatric patients, the incidence of emetic symptoms is reduced "if it is given 30 minutes before the end of surgery."[20] Lerman et al. demonstrated that a further reduction would be obtained if droperidol (75 μg/kg) was given during induction of anesthesia.[21] In comparing these results with those of Abramowitz et al., it is important to realize that factors other than the time at which the drug was administered may have influenced the differing results obtained (Table 21-4). Lerman et al. have focused on the importance of timing the ad-

Table 21-4. Comparison of Two Studies Designed to Evaluate the Effect of Droperidol on the Incidence of Postoperative Nausea and Vomiting

	Thiopental	Atropine	Succinylcholine	Gastric contents emptied
Lerman et al.[21]	yes	yes	yes	no
Abramowitz et al.[20]	no	no	no	yes

ministration of droperidol so it precedes manipulation of the extraocular muscles. They may be correct, and there is no reason not to administer a long-acting agent like droperidol prior to the stimulus; however, in my opinion, a better-designed study is still needed to validate this theory.

Korttila (Ch. 17) reminds us that "the total dose of droperidol should not exceed 1.25 mg because larger doses are likely to cause excessive postoperative drowsiness and disorientation, thereby jeopardizing early discharge from the outpatient unit." This guideline is certainly supported by reasonable data in the anesthesia literature. However, in the study by Abramowitz et al.,[20] if 75 μg/kg droperidol (versus placebo) was administered, patients who vomited did not take longer to meet discharge criteria. In the study by Lerman et al., this was also true of the patients who received droperidol when compared with those who received acetaminophen or codeine. Nevertheless, I agree with Korttila that whenever possible, the dose of droperidol should not exceed 1.25 mg. For procedures associated with a high frequency of postoperative vomiting (e.g., strabismus and orchiopexy) or in a patient in whom protracted vomiting remains after the usual low-dose treatment (e.g., 0.6 to 1.25 mg droperidol), it is preferable to run the risk of having a patient sleep comfortably for a few hours than for he or she to be awake, vomiting, and hypovolemic.

It is somewhat amusing that at the 1989 annual meeting of the ASA, some 6 years following the publication of our study,[20] two abstracts were published in which the use of droperidol, 75 μg/kg, was advocated in outpatient pediatric strabismus surgery.[22,23] Average discharge times were 170 minutes and 208 minutes, respectively. This was considerably shorter than the times reported by Abramowitz et al. (300 minutes) and Lerman et al. (384 minutes). How is it possible to use the same drug in an identical dose and route of administration in the same group of patients for a given procedure with widely divergent times to discharge? The earlier studies required tolerating oral fluids as a criterion for discharge. I suspect in the two most recent studies, this criterion was not required. This is not intended to be a criticism, merely an observation. Whether one should require that patients tolerate oral fluids prior to discharge is still controversial.

IS OXYGEN SATURATION AND CARBON DIOXIDE MONITORING THE STANDARD OF CARE?

One of the most misunderstood concepts in the field of anesthesiology today is the question of what constitutes the "standard of care." In an enlightening article, Rubsamen[24] states that the standard of constant monitoring of the pulse "did not evolve from some textbook, from how the judge instructed the jury, or from a board of experts. It depended on the jury hearing conflicting expert testimony on what the standard was and then deciding whom to believe." He further describes the process of how, for example, continuous oximetry monitoring could become a standard in the near future. In summary, the instruments will first have to be widely used throughout a given jurisdiction. In a particular case, an expert witness will have to testify that the instrument is safe, noninvasive, reliable, and the due care standard. If the instrument was not used and there was an adverse event, the jury will not be especially sympathetic, which will convince hospitals that they cannot be without continuous oximetry monitoring. Finally, a defense attorney will not be able to find expert witnesses who will deny that this is the standard of care for every anesthetic.

Blitt (Ch. 11), an acknowledged expert in the field of monitoring, believes that a pulse oximeter should be used on every anesthetized patient and that capnography should be used on all patients receiving general anesthesia. This is not a universally-accepted practice. The most important message in his chapter, however, may be the statement that monitoring the patient undergoing surgery and anesthesia on an ambulatory basis should be essentially the same as monitoring similar patients who have been admitted to the hospital. The philosophy on monitoring in our department in the outpatient surgical setting is based on two fundamental considerations: (1) that neither the point of entry to or exit from the facility, nor (2) the type of anesthesia, should modify the extent of the patient's evaluation and management.[25] Hornbein[26] adds that "the assumption is that more attentive monitoring will diminish the frequency and severity of adverse outcomes, particularly those occurring in low risk (healthy) patients, where the incidence of an untoward event should ideally be zero." This implies that even in an outpatient facility in which only healthy, ASA physical status I or II patients are managed, vigilance is the byword!

Currently, we conform to the Standards for Basic Intraoperative Monitoring of the ASA, which are described in detail by Zelcer and White in Chapter 12, and in which pulse oximetry is required and capnography is strongly encouraged. Since an overwhelming majority of anesthesiologists currently use pulse oximetry for all anesthetics and are "tooling up" to use capnography for general anesthesia when endotracheal intubation is employed, experts will probably testify to this practice in the future. This latter point is particularly important since, as Rubsamen[24] emphasizes, this is how the standard of care is derived. However, an individual physician has the opportunity to show that the care he or she rendered to a patient, even if departing from the alleged "standard of care" in some respects, satisfies the physician's duty to the patient under all the facts and circumstances. It would have to be demonstrated conclusively that failure to use the instrument(s) contributed to the mishap.

DO PEDIATRIC OUTPATIENTS NEED AN INTRAVENOUS CATHETER?

In Chapter 8, Steward notes that "many infants and children who have had fluids up to 3 or 4 hours preoperatively, who are having minor surgery, and who are predicted to resume fluid intake soon after the operation do not require intravenous fluids." Although not specifically stated, it is implied that an intravenous catheter is not required, at least under the above conditions or if the use of intravenous medications is not planned. In 1985, the Committee on Drugs (Section on Anesthesiology) of the American Academy of Pediatrics (AAP) addressed the issue of the need for an intravenous catheter for use in ambulatory ASA physical status I or II pediatric dental patients receiving conscious sedation, deep sedation, or general anesthesia.[27] It was recommended that an intravenous line be placed during deep sedation and that an intravenous line be required during general anesthesia. One year later, the Committee agreed that under some circumstances (e.g., very brief procedures, availability of persons skilled in establishing intravenous lines in children), it may not be necessary for an intravenous line to be in place during surgery.[28]

The AAP guidelines were modified as follows:

> *Deep Sedation*—Patients receiving deep sedation should have an intravenous line in place or have immediately available a person skilled in establishing intravenous infusions in pediatric patients.
> *General Anesthesia*—Patients receiving ambulatory general anesthesia shall have an intravenous line in place or have immediately available a person skilled in establishing intravenous infusions in pediatric patients.

Although the above guidelines were aimed at the healthy dental outpatient, no mention is made of this fact in the title of the article or in the text. As a result, it represents an authoritative statement by the AAP on this controversial issue. I would agree that many pediatric anesthesiologists do not feel compelled to have intravenous access in all patients undergoing general anesthesia. Obviously, factors such as the child's age, weight, physical status, state of hydration, and length (or severity) of the surgical procedure will influence the anesthesiologist's decision-making process.

As mentioned previously by Hannallah and myself,[29] "it is reassuring to remember that the two emergency drugs that are most likely to be needed in the healthy day-surgery child are succinylcholine and atropine. In the absence of an intravenous infusion or visible veins, these two drugs are rapidly effective when administered intramuscularly (in a dose twice that used for intravenous administration)."

IS AN ENDOTRACHEAL TUBE REQUIRED FOR LAPAROSCOPIC PROCEDURES?

When I began training in anesthesia 30 years ago, the first 3 months were spent administering general anesthesia without an endotracheal tube. Although most anesthetics consisted of combinations of ether, cyclopropane, and nitrous oxide, some used thiopental, nitrous oxide, and a muscle relaxant drug. Operative procedures included cholecystectomy and gastrectomy; patients were frequently obese; and the position during surgery could be lithotomy, Trendelenburg, or even prone. Ether and cyclopropane have disappeared from our anesthetic armamentarium and so has the art of administering anesthesia by facemask. The question posed relates to the requirement for endotracheal intubation in a specific procedure. I believe that if this question is pertinent, it more properly applies to experienced, "mature" anesthesiologists trained in an era when the use of mask anesthetic techniques was more prevalent.

In this context, whether endotracheal intubation is selected depends on the size of the patient, the ability to establish a patent airway without difficulty, and the experience of the laparoscopist and anesthesiologist. Certainly, the surgical conditions under mask anesthesia are suboptimal. Abdominal distension with a patient in steep Trendelenburg position can only be made more complicated by gastric distention secondary to a partially obstructed airway. Insertion of the trocar into the distended stomach has been reported and is a well-known complication. Surgical conditions during a laparoscopy might predispose the patient to hypoventilation, regurgitation, and even aspiration of gastric contents. In the presence of an obstructed airway, administration of a skeletal muscle relaxant is a double-edged sword.

Certainly, there are patients in whom an endotracheal tube represents a specific risk (e.g., asthmatic), and the combination of variables may allow for administration of a reasonably uneventful anesthetic without an endotracheal tube. There is also the proverbial professional vocalist whose livelihood depends on intact, properly functioning vocal cords. However, these types of patients can often be managed successfully with regional anesthetic techniques. We have seen a few cases of postobstructive, noncardiogenic pulmonary edema following extubation. This usually occurs after a paroxysm of coughing results in laryngospasm in a patient with a previously irritable airway secondary to smoking or a recent upper respiratory tract infection. Administration of anesthesia by mask to this type of patient is also hazardous. Production of secretions, laryngospasm, and bronchospasm can occur with the patient prepared and draped, and even while the procedure is being performed if the patient is inadequately anesthetized.

At the last several meetings of the Society for Ambulatory Anesthesia "straw polls" usually have shown an overwhelming preponderance of anesthesiologists electing to routinely intubate the trachea for laparoscopy. If an anesthesiologist decided to use a facemask technique, most would not quickly come to his or her defense. Although rare, one of our outpatients experienced a carbon dioxide embolism during a routine laparoscopy.[30] The trachea had been intubated, and the decrease in end-tidal CO_2 concentration was promptly diagnosed, leading to a successful resuscitation. Diagnosis and therapy in this case were aided tremendously by elective tracheal intubation.

WHEN DOES "CONSCIOUS SEDATION" BECOME GENERAL ANESTHESIA?

In Chapter 12, Zelcer and White list in tabular form the specific differences between conscious sedation and deep (unconscious) sedation. As suggested by these authors, the problem with taking these definitions literally is that "conscious sedation clearly lies on a dose-dependent continuum leading from minimal sedation to general anesthesia." Cardiac, respiratory, and reflex functions are altered accordingly. In many aspects, the adverse effects of deep sedation can be equated with those of general anesthesia. This is often a difficult concept to understand for those who administer sedation/analgesia in more than a calming dose. The results of "slipping over the edge" from conscious sedation to an unconscious state can be a dramatic and life-threatening experience. The Joint Commission on Accreditation of Health Care Organizations (JCAHO) Standards for Anesthesia Services apply to all patients who receive general, spinal, or other major regional anesthesia and/or intravenous, intramuscular, or inhalation sedation/analgesia that may result in the loss of the patient's protective reflexes.[31] The word "may" has the same connotation that is described above by Zelcer and White as a dose-dependent continuum.

Why the uproar with respect to combination local anesthesia-sedation techniques? In a recent report of an anesthesia follow-up program involving approximately 100,000 anesthetics, monitored anesthesia care (MAC) was associated with the highest rate of mortality (209 deaths per 10,000 anesthetics).[32] The ASA has recognized the potential dangers of MAC by equating the requirements of standards for basic intraoperative monitoring[33] for the patient undergoing MAC to be equivalent to those for patients undergoing either general or regional anesthesia. No attempt was made to define the state of central nervous system depression produced by adjunctive drugs. It is the "potential" for organ depression that is most important. In this situation, the major risk factor contributing to morbidity and mortality is respiratory depression. The reader is referred to the sections in Chapter 12 that describe the use of sedative-analgesic drugs during MAC and the effects of these agents on patient outcome.

Anesthesiologists and members of the anesthesia care team, as well as practitioners of other disciplines (e.g., gastroenterology, cardiology, pulmonary medicine) who administer sedation/analgesia to the point at which it may result in the loss of protective reflexes should adhere to the same procedures for evaluating and monitoring the patient, as well as drug management during and after the procedure. This is particularly relevant during a diagnostic procedure like an endoscopy, in which it is possible for the endoscopist to be responsible for prescribing the medication(s) for sedation and analgesia while at the same time performing the procedure. The responsible physician may not even be observing the patient at a time when these depressant drugs are producing their peak effects. Alternatively, he or she delegate this responsibility to someone who has no formal training in recognizing signs of cardiorespiratory depression (e.g., hypoxia, airway obstruction, hypotension). This unacceptable practice, coupled with the tendency of some physicians to continue to prescribe fixed drug combinations in which the dose is determined in advance based on body weight (e.g., meperidine 1 mg/kg and midazolam 0.07 mg/kg IM), is more likely to result in organ depression when compared with slower, careful titration methods for administering these intravenous medications (e.g., 1-mg incremental bolus doses of midazolam). Knowledge of the pharmacokinetic and pharmacodynamic effects of the sedative and analgesic drugs will further decrease the incidence of adverse complications in those patients at increased risk (e.g., geriatric patients, those with respiratory disease, and morbidly obese patients).

The question is how to optimally provide analgesia, alleviate anxiety (anxiolysis), and produce amnesia without compromising respiratory or circulatory function. I have no real answer on how to avoid converting a planned conscious sedation technique into deep sedation or general anesthesia other than to adhere to the principals advocated in the chapters on MAC and sedation techniques. As a result, it becomes essential to anticipate the potential catastrophic events and to plan ahead with respect to the management of these potentially life-threatening problems.

CRITERIA FOR DISCHARGE—SHOULD ALL PATIENTS BE REQUIRED TO TOLERATE FLUIDS BY MOUTH AND VOID PRIOR TO DISCHARGE?

As noted by Korttila in Chapter 17, the abilities to void and maintain orally administered fluids have yet to be established as criteria for discharge. Certainly, it is unacceptable to discharge a patient home when he or she is vomiting or retching. It is also undesirable to continue to administer oral fluids when they produce vomiting. The determination to discharge the outpatient should be based on the state of hydration, medical condition, age, size (infants), distance between the home and the ambulatory facility, availability of a responsible adult, and anticipation of whether the patient is likely to suffer any serious complications if little or no fluids are taken on the day of surgery (e.g., diabetics).

The requirement to void prior to discharge is one of the most complex and unresolved issues faced during recovery of the adult outpatient. It is rarely, if ever, a consideration in the pediatric patient. Inability to void, urinary retention, and the need for subsequent catheterization have been related to reflex urethral spasm or reflex inhibition of normal bladder detrusor muscle activity by pain, distention of the anal canal, and prolonged block of bladder autonomic innervation (e.g., epidural or subarachnoid blockade). The following factors have been mentioned by at least one author to be related or unrelated to overdistention of the bladder:

1. Site of surgery: rectal, pelvic-related operations
2. Age: in elderly males (secondary to prostatic hypertrophy) and young adults (secondary to anxiety or embarrassment)
3. Fluid administration: reduced incidence of catheterization after fluid restriction or deprivation, while an increased incidence has been reported after vigorous fluid therapy[34–36]
4. Pain and anxiety: both pain and anxiety are increased when focus is placed on the requirement to void during the discharge process
5. Anesthesia: related to sympathetic denervation (e.g., spinal or epidural anesthesia) following the use of long-acting local anesthetic agents in the subarachnoid (e.g., tetracaine) or epidural space (e.g., bupivacaine), and less likely to occur when shorter-acting drugs are used (e.g., lidocaine)[37]

Emphasis should be placed on anticipation and prevention of an overdistended bladder, as well as the recognition that normal or vigorous fluid therapy during sympathetic block may lead to an overdistended bladder and a reduction in detrusor activity (which is necessary to open the bladder neck at the beginning of micturition, as well as for complete emptying of the bladder). If voiding is not a criterion for discharge, patients must be fully informed as to their responsibility to contact the physician or to return to the facility if the problem persists after discharge. As noted by Mulroy (Ch. 14), further studies are needed to determine whether simple drainage of the bladder with "in-and-out" catheterization prior to discharge home would decrease recovery times in outpatients receiving spinal or epidural anesthesia without increasing postoperative morbidity.

HOW IMPORTANT IS THE TREATMENT OF PAIN POSTOPERATIVELY?

Poler et al. (Ch. 19) have provided a comprehensive overview of the current concepts in the evaluation and treatment of pain in the outpatient setting. Why is it that the issue of pain has taken on such an important role today compared with 10 or 20 years ago?

In the 1960s, one of the considerations in the selection of a procedure suitable for outpatient surgery was that an opioid (narcotic) analgesic not be required for treatment at home. The presumption was that a procedure associated with pain requiring opioid therapy exceeded the allowable or acceptable extent (or magnitude) of surgery. In the 1990s, the issue of whether a procedure is associated with severe or intense pain is a social problem that in itself is not an indication for overnight hospitalization. Yet, home health care and/or reimbursement for the treatment of pain in an intermediate care facility are concepts that are not yet universally approved.

In addition, when I entered the field of pediatric anesthesia in the early 1970s, it was widely taught that most children (particularly younger ones), really did not experience pain. In retrospect, many health care providers looked the other way, assuming that there would be no long-term damage from a "good cry." Furthermore, the hazards of administering potent opioid analgesics or using regional anesthetic techniques like caudal analgesia were considered to be "overkill." At that time, the risk-to-benefit ratio was considered to be too high. What has changed?

Obviously, it is now the exception to the rule that a patient undergoing a potentially painful procedure, like arthroscopy, orchiopexy, hemiorrhaphy, or circumcision, is scheduled on an inpatient basis. In addition, since the mid-1970s, we have gained more experience in the use of rapid and short-acting narcotics like fentanyl to treat severe postoperative pain. Our ability to anticipate the type of patient and procedure that are more frequently associated with the need for intense analgesic treatment allows us to more effectively select the proper drug or combination of drugs. In addition, we are now almost routinely using local anesthetics both prophylactically and therapeutically.

One of the problems that our group at Children's Hospital National Medical Center experienced was how to evaluate the need and success of a given therapy in an infant or child unable to communicate verbally. At the Children's Hospital, designing a pain/discomfort scale was an invaluable aid in assessing the response to different analgesic regimens[38] (Table 21-5). In randomized studies in which either a caudal or an ilioinguinal-iliohypogastric nerve block was used, patients had a dressing applied over the groin and the sacrum was painted with poviodide-iodide and covered with a

Table 21-5. Pain/Discomfort Scale Used to Assess Postoperative Pain in Children[38]

Observation	Criteria	Points
Blood pressure	± 10% of preoperative value	0
	> 20% preoperative value	1
	> 30% preoperative value	2
Crying	Not crying	0
	Crying but responds to tender loving care (TLC)	1
	Crying and does not respond to TLC	2
Movement	None	0
	Restless	1
	Thrashing	2
Agitation	Patient asleep or calm	0
	Mild	1
	Hysterical/crying	2
Posture	No special posture	0
	Flexing legs and thighs	1
	Holding scrotum or groin	2
Complaints of pain (where appropriate by age)	Asleep or states no pain	0
	Cannot localize pain	1
	Can localize pain	2

"band-aid" type strip to conceal possible block markings and prevent observer bias. In these clinical studies, the anesthetic records were sealed, the observer was prohibited from entering the operating room, and the use of well-defined stringent discharge criteria were required.

Use of this rigorous investigative protocol allowed us to advocate the use of uncomplicated techniques, such as subcutaneous ring block of the penis for circumcision,[37] and to evaluate the efficacy of caudal and ilioinguinal-iliohypogastric nerve blocks for control of postorchiopexy pain.[36] It was also possible to verify that children do, in fact, experience severe pain and discomfort. These studies also demonstrate the effectiveness of small doses of the potent opioid analgesics (e.g., fentanyl, 1 to 2 μg/kg IV) as alternatives to regional block techniques.[38] Studies by our group did not always demonstrate effective control of pain by local or regional block (e.g., use of local anesthetics following tonsillectomy).[40] Likewise, Poler et al. note that the use of intraarticular bupivacaine following knee arthroscopy may not be efficacious, although it is a widely practiced technique.

The approach to the treatment of postoperative pain in the outpatient setting has improved dramatically over the last few years. The availability of drugs, drug combinations, and the applicability of regional anesthetic techniques (using long-acting local anesthetics) allows for patients to leave the facility with little or no discomfort. We must, however, broaden our horizons and attempt to spread the use of these newer techniques to the home environment. Although pain and discomfort begin at the surgery facility, they do not end there! Follow-up phone calls are extremely valuable in assessing the physical well-being of ambulatory surgery patients (Ch. 5).

The use of patient-controlled analgesia, nonsteroidal anti-inflammatory drugs, and other methods for pain control, such as transcutaneous electrical nerve stimulation, need to be investigated scientifically, and, if found to be efficacious, they should be more widely applied during the postdischarge period. As stated by Poler et al., "safer and simpler delivery systems are needed to improve our ability to provide cost-effective pain relief after surgery in the outpatient setting."

WHO IS RESPONSIBLE FOR DETERMINING WHEN IT IS SAFE TO DISCHARGE A PATIENT HOME AND HOW CAN THIS BE PERFORMED?

Korttila (Ch. 17) refers to the fact that the "major accreditation body in the United States (the Joint Commission of Accreditation of Health Care Organizations) requires that policies and procedures be implemented for safe recovery after anesthesia." The guidelines for safe discharge (outlined in Table 17-2), with the exception of ability to void and tolerate fluids by mouth, are well-accepted and not controversial. Korttila further states that the "patient must be discharged by the person who gave anesthesia, performed surgery, or their designees." I would like to take issue with this guideline since it is ambiguous and does not state who is responsible for discharge or whether or not that individual must be present at the time of discharge. Furthermore, Korttila does not define the role of the "designee."

The JCAHO guidelines states, "a licensed independent practitioner* who has appropriate clinical privileges and who is familiar with the patient is responsible for the decision to discharge the patient." They further stipulate, "when the responsible licensed independent practitioner is not personally present to make the decision to discharge or does not sign the discharge order, the name of the licensed independent practitioner responsible for the discharge is recorded in the patient's medical record, and relevant discharge criteria are vigorously applied to determine the readiness of the patient for discharge. The discharge criteria must be approved by the licensed independent practitioner's staff."[41]

How did this policy evolve? Certainly, the preferable medical practice would be for a physician familiar with the patient to be personally present to evaluate the patient at the time of discharge. Unfortunately, it is not always possible for the physician to "drop everything" and run to the recovery room when an ambulatory surgical patient is ready to go home. This is particularly true after normal working hours in a small hospital where there may only be one anesthesiologist who is administering an anesthetic or is otherwise occupied (e.g., in the intensive care unit). In addition, there are some anesthesiologists or physicians who are satisfied with one look at the patient and who will sign a discharge order without regard to the use of any uniform discharge criteria.

More recently, the emphasis has been shifted to assessing the condition of the patient rather than mandating that a physician be present at the time of discharge. The option to delegate the release of the patient, for example, to a nurse when specific discharge criteria (approved by the medical staff) have been satisfied implies that a nurse is acting as an observer, much as he or she would in assigning points in the determination of an Apgar score. If formal discharge criteria are adhered to by the recovery room nurses, patients will be allowed to go home when ready, while the physician still assumes the responsibility for setting the conditions for discharge. I believe this is a reasonable mechanism for providing uniform safe care of the ambulatory surgery patient. Appendix 21-3 provides an example of discharge criteria.

In its standards for postanesthesia care,[42] the ASA encourages the use of an appropriate recovery room scoring system for each patient on admission, at appropriate intervals prior to discharge, and at the time of discharge. As stated in Standard V, "a physician is responsible for the discharge of

* Licensed independent practitioner: any individual who is permitted by law and who is also permitted by the health care organization to provide patient care services without direction or supervision within the scope of his/her license and in accordance with individually granted clinical privileges.

the patient from the postanesthesia care unit.'' The ASA obviously recognized that an anesthesiologist may not be available when it uses the term ''physician'' as the responsible individual. The standard further states that ''in the absence of the physician responsible for the discharge, the recovery room nurse shall determine that the patient meets the discharge criteria. The name of the physician accepting responsibility for the discharge shall be noted on the record.''

Both the JCAHO and ASA documents are intended to allow the patient safe passage home when he or she is ready for discharge. They also encourage the use of discharge criteria and mandate them when a physician is not personally present.

REFERENCES

1. Epstein BS: The future of ambulatory surgery. Anesthesiol Clin N Am 5:217, 1987
2. Epstein BS, Hannallah RS: Anesthetic considerations for pediatric ambulatory surgery. Cur Rev Clin Anesth 8:146, 1988
3. Gold BS, Katz DS, Lecky JH: Clinical characteristics of ambulatory surgery patients requiring hospital admission. Presented at annual meeting of SAMBA. Washington DC, April 1987
4. Bender K, Spear R, Pasternak LR: The role and delivery of pediatric outpatient anesthesia. Anesthesiol Rep 1:21, 1988
5. Natof HE: Complications. p. 321. In Wetchler BV (ed): Anesthesia for Ambulatory Surgery. Philadelphia, JB Lippincott, 1985
6. Meridy HW: Criteria for selection of ambulatory surgical patients and guidelines for anesthetic management. A retrospective study of 1553 cases. Anesth Analg 62:921, 1982
7. Epstein BS: The future of ambulatory surgery. Anesthesiol Clin N Am 5:217, 1987
8. Cohen MM, Duncan PG, Tate RB: Does anesthesia contribute to operative mortality? JAMA 260:2859, 1988
9. Cohen MM, Duncan PG: Physical status score and trends in anesthetic complications. J Clin Epidemiol 41:83, 1988
10. Federated Ambulatory Surgery Association Special Study I. FASA, Alexandria, VA, 1985 (unpublished data)
11. Patel RI, Kasprazak S, Hannallah RS: Effectiveness of preoperative comprehensive telephone screening in pediatric ambulatory surgery. Soc Amb Anesth Annual Meeting, Scottsdale, AZ, April 1988
12. Patel RI, Hannallah RS: Effectiveness of preoperative comprehensive telephone screening in pediatric ambulatory surgery. Part II. Soc Amb Anesth Annual Meeting, San Antonio, TX, April 1989
13. Statement on the routine operative laboratory and diagnostic screening, American Society of Anesthesiologists (approved by House of Delegates), October 14, 1987
14. Luban LC, Epstein BS, Watson SP: Sickle cell disease and anesthesia. p. 289. In Gallagher TJ (ed): Sickle Cell Disease and Anesthesia in Advances in Anesthesia. Vol. 1. Year Book Medical Publishers, Chicago, 1984
15. Philip B: In Ambulatory Anesthesia Newsletter, Society for Ambulatory Anesthesia, Vol 2, June 1987
16. Hagan MD, Meyer KB, Parker SG: Routine preoperative screening for HIV—does the risk to the surgeon outweigh the risk to the patient? JAMA 259:1357, 1988
17. Dickens BM: Legal limits of AIDS confidentiality. JAMA 259:3449, 1988
18. Shafer A, White PF, Urquhart ML, Doze VA: Outpatient premedications: use of midazolam and opioid analgesics. Anesthesiology 71:495, 1989
19. Coombs DW: Aspiration pneumonia prophylaxis. Anesth Analg 62:1055, 1983
20. Abramowitz MD, Oh TH, Epstein BS, et al: The antiemetic effect of droperidol following outpatient strabismus surgery in children. Anesthesiology 59:583, 1983
21. Lerman J, Eustis S, Smith DR: Effect of droperidol pretreatment on postanesthetic vomiting in children undergoing strabismus surgery. Anesthesiology 65:322, 1986
22. Grunwald Z, Nicolson SC, Browne PM, et al: Comparison of the effects of oral versus intravenous droperidol in children having outpatient strabismus surgery. Anesthesiology 71:A1044, 1989
23. Lin DM, Rodarte A: Metroclopramide pro-

phylaxis against postoperative vomiting in pediatric strabismus patients. Anesthesiology 71:A1064, 1989

24. Rubsamen DS: The standard of care and where it comes from. Semin Anesth 5:237, 1986
25. March MG, Shaffer MJ, Epstein BS: Monitoring for outpatient surgery. Semin Anesth 8:130, 1989
26. Hornbein TF: The setting of standards of care. JAMA 256:1040, 1986
27. Committee on Drugs, Section on Anesthesiology, American Academy of Pediatrics: Guidelines for the elective use of conscious sedation, deep sedation, and general anesthesia in pediatric patients. Pediatrics 76:317, 1985
28. Committee on Drugs, Section on Anesthesiology, American Academy of Pediatrics: Clarification. Guidelines for the elective use of conscious sedation, deep sedation, and general anesthesia in pediatric patients. Pediatrics 77:754, 1986
29. Epstein BS, Hannallah R: The pediatric patient. p. 141. In Wetchler BV (ed): Anesthesia for Ambulatory Surgery. JB Lippincott, Philadelphia, 1985
30. McGrath B, Zimmerman J, Williams JF, Parmet J: Carbon dioxide embolism treated with hyperbaric oxygen. Can J Anaesth 36:586, 1989
31. Accreditation Manual for Hospitals. Joint Commission on Accreditation of Healthcare Organizations, 1988
32. Cohen MM, Duncan PG, Tate RB: Does anesthesia contribute to operative mortality? JAMA 260:2859, 1988
33. Standards for basic intraoperative monitoring. Approved by the House of Delegates, American Society of Anesthesiologists, October 21, 1989
34. Axelsson K, Mollefors K, Olsson JO, et al: Bladder function in spinal anesthesia. Acta Anaesthesiol Scand 29:315, 1985
35. Bailey HR, Ferguson JA: Prevention of urinary retention by fluid restriction following anorectal operations. Dis Colon Rectum 19:240, 1976
36. Campbell ED: Prevention of urinary retention after anorectal operations. Dis Colon Rectum 15:69, 1972
37. Ryan JA, Adya BA, Jolly PC, Mulroy MF: Outpatient inguinal hemiorrhaphy with both regional and local anesthesia. Am J Surg 148:313, 1984
38. Hannallah RS, Broadman LM, Belman AB, et al: Comparison of caudal and ilioinguinal/iliohypogastric nerve blocks for control of post-orchiopexy pain in pediatric ambulatory surgery. Anesthesiology 622:832, 1987
39. Broadman LM, Hannallah RS, Belman AB, et al: Postcircumcision analgesia—a prospective evaluation of subcutaneous ring block of the penis. Anesthesiology 67:399, 1987
40. Broadman LM, Patel R, Feldman B, et al: The effects of peritonsilar infiltration on the reduction of intraoperative blood loss and post-tonsillectomy pain in children. Laryngoscope 99:578, 1989
41. Ambulatory Health Care Standards Manual. Joint Commission on Accreditation of Health Care Organizations, 1988
42. Standards for Post Anesthesia Care. American Society of Anesthesiologists. Approved by the House of Delegates, October 12, 1988

Appendix 21-1

Preoperative Telephone Screening*

* Courtesy of Children's Hospital National Medical Center, Washington, DC

CHILDREN'S HOSPITAL NATIONAL MEDICAL CENTER

AMSAC

PRE-OPERATIVE TELEPHONE SCREENING

Patient's Name: ______

DATE SCHEDULED FOR SURGERY:	HOME PHONE:	WORK PHONE:
SURGEON/DENTIST:	DATE AND TIME OF CALL:	DISPOSITION:
CHIEF COMPLAINT: *(TYPE OF SURGERY):*		AGE:
RESPONDANT:	RELATIONSHIP	

SUBJECTIVE FINDINGS:

Does your child have or ever had:	CHECK (✓) BOX YES	NO	COMMENTS
Asthma	☐	☐	
Breath-holding spells *(apnea)*	☐	☐	
Croup/Bronchitis/Pneumonia	☐	☐	
Heart problems, heart murmurs *(Rheumatic)*	☐	☐	
Hepatitis (*Hepatitis B Carrier/liver disease)*	☐	☐	
Kidney Disease	☐	☐	
Bleeding disorders (*bruises easily)*	☐	☐	
Diabetes	☐	☐	
Sickle Cell Disease or Trait	☐	☐	
Seizures or convulsions	☐	☐	
Allergies to medicines, food, environmental factors	☐	☐	
Prematurity	☐	☐	
Was O_2 or ventilator required	☐	☐	
History of Apnea/Bradycardia	☐	☐	
Is your child currently on any medications	☐	☐	
Has your child ever had:			
Previous hospitalization/surgery	☐	☐	
If the child had previous surgery:			
Problems with anesthesia	☐	☐	
(delayed awakening, unexplained fever, MH, jaundice/vomiting/difficult intubation)	☐	☐	
Does anyone in your family have a history of			
Bleeding disorders	☐	☐	
Muscle disease	☐	☐	
Trouble with anesthesia/M.H.	☐	☐	
Does your child wear any prosthesis	☐	☐	
Glasses/Braces/Bridges/Hearing aid/Trach/ Wheelchair/Crutches	☐	☐	
Does your child have:			
Any developmental delays/learning disabilities	☐	☐	
Is your child prepared for surgery	☐	☐	
Will you bring your child in on the day of surgery? If NO, who will?	☐	☐	
Does your child have any problems I have not mentioned?	☐	☐	
Adolescents:			
History of smoking	☐	☐	
Drug/alcohol use	☐	☐	
Chance of being pregnant	☐	☐	

PAGE 1 OF FOUR

CHILDREN'S HOSPITAL NATIONAL MEDICAL CENTER

PLANS: (1) Counsel:

	CHECK (✓) BOX YES	NO	COMMENTS
Phone call from Admissions Counselor, RN will call day before with food instructions, time of surgery, time to arrive	☐	☐	
Puppet show and why prepare	☐	☐	
Explain NPO and why	☐	☐	
Any questions parent has	☐	☐	
Rules of SSRU/Surgical Unit	☐	☐	

AMSAC/SSRU
DAY BEFORE SURGERY TELEPHONE CALL

Signature: ______________________

DATE AND TIME OF CALL:	DISPOSITION:	RESPONDANT:	RELATIONSHIP:
DATE OF SURGERY:		ARRIVAL TIME TO AMSAC:	
TIME OF SURGERY:	NPO TIME:FULL	CLEAR:	

SUBJECTIVE FINDINGS:

Does your child now have:	CHECK (✓) BOX YES	NO	COMMENTS
Cold symptoms/sore throat/cough	☐	☐	
GI symptoms *(diarrhea)*	☐	☐	
Fever	☐	☐	
Rashes/cold sores	☐	☐	
Loose teeth, tooth aches, dental problems	☐	☐	
Has your child been exposed to: Chicken pox, German measles, measles, mumps in the past 3 weeks	☐	☐	
Is your child now taking any medications?	☐	☐	
Did you and your child attend the Puppet Show or Is your child prepared for surgery?	☐	☐	
Are there any other medical problems not discussed?	☐	☐	
Does your child have any nicknames	☐	☐	

ASSESSMENT: ______________________

PLANS: (1) Counsel:

	CHECK (✓) BOX YES	NO	COMMENTS
Times as above	☐	☐	
Reinforce What and Why NPO *(No tooth-brushing, gum)*	☐	☐	
Review rules of SSRU/Surgical Unit	☐	☐	
Other *(Trach protocol, crutches, etc.)*	☐	☐	
Any questions parents have?	☐	☐	

Signature: ______________________

ASSESSMENT: ______________________

PAGE 2 OF FOUR

CHNMC 144.1/144.2

CHILDREN'S HOSPITAL NATIONAL MEDICAL CENTER
111 Michigan Avenue, N.W. Washington, D.C. 20010

PEDIATRIC FLOW SHEET

DATE: ____________ HEIGHT: ____________ WEIGHT: ____________

MASK: ____________ CAUDAL: ____________

ETT: ____________ LOCAL: ____________

ALLERGIES: ________________________

NPO TIME: ________________________

ADDRESSOGRAPH

____________ ( ) Signature/Initials ____________ ( ) Signature/Initials ____________ ( ) Signature/Initials

ASSESSMENT											DISCHARGE CRITERIA							INTERVENTIONS					CROUP					
TIME	TEMP./MODE	HEART RATE	RESPIRATIONS	BLOOD PRESSURE	COLOR/ACTIVITY	BREATH SOUNDS	SURGICAL SITE				VITAL SIGNS STABLE	SWALLOW/ COUGH/GAG	ABLE TO AMBULATE	NAUSEA/VOMITING/ DIZZINESS (min)	ABSENCE OF RESPIRATORY DISTRESS	ALERT AND ORIENTED		D/C TEACHING/ NSG. CONSULT	P.R.N. MED (✓)				INSPIRATORY SOUNDS	STRIDOR	COUGH	RETRACTIONS/FLARING	CYANOSIS	TOTAL SCORE
COMMENTS																												

INTAKE				OUTPUT			
TIME	DIET/AMOUNT	P.O. FLUID	AMOUNT	URINE	STOOL/AMOUNT	EMESIS	SHIFT TOTALS FOR INTAKE & OUTPUT
							(I.V.) T-
							(P.O.) T-
							(T.F.) T-
							T INTAKE-
							URINE T OUTPUT-

	1					2					COMMENTS FOR INTRAVENOUS MEDICATIONS ONLY
SOLUTION A											
SOLUTION B											
SITE											
TIME	RATE / CHANGE	PUMP VOLUME	VOLUME INFUSED	MED ADDED/SITE	TIME	RATE / CHANGE	PUMP VOLUME	VOLUME INFUSED	MED ADDED/SITE		

PAGE 3 OF FOUR

CHNMC 688.1

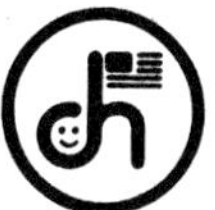

CHILDREN'S HOSPITAL NATIONAL MEDICAL CENTER
SHORT STAY UNIT
POST-OPERATIVE PHONE CALL

Date Call Made: ______________________ Informant: ______________________

Procedure: ______________________ Home Phone: (   ) ______________

CHECK (✓) APPROPRIATE ANSWER and COMMENT IF NECESSARY

Call not Completed: ☐ N/A ☐ Busy ☐ Wrong No. ☐ Not in Service ☐ Disconnected ☐ Unlisted

☐ Message Left with No Response From Parents Comment: ______________________

Any Vomiting? ☐ None ☐ 1 Time ☐ 2 Times ☐ 3 Times ☐ 4 Times ☐ > 4 Times

Comment: ______________________

If any item below is checked ☑ Yes, describe in COMMENT Section.

Sleep Extra Hours? ☐ No ☐ Yes When was child back to normal, alert self? ______________

Oozing from Suture Line/Dressing? ☐ Normal ☐ Excessive

Elevation of Temperature? ☐ If yes ______ °F

☐ Sore Throat (If Adenoidectomy, please state "Adenoids" in COMMENT Section) ☐ Croupiness

☐ Cough Post-op ☐ Cough pre-op

Loss of Appetite? ☐ Yes ☐ No

For children over the age of 2 years ☐ Bad Dreams ☐ Muscle Pain ☐ Dizziness ☐ Headache ☐ Upset Stomach

Comments: ______________________

CHNMC 144.3

PAGE 4 OF FOUR

Appendix 21-2

Preoperative Assessment Summary*

* Courtesy of the George Washington University Medical Center, Department of Medicine, Division of Internal Medicine, Washington, DC

THE GEORGE WASHINGTON UNIVERSITY MEDICAL CENTER
DEPARTMENT OF MEDICINE
DIVISION OF GENERAL INTERNAL MEDICINE

PHYSICIAN'S PREOPERATIVE ASSESSMENT SUMMARY

Patient
name ______________________ Age _____ Sex _____ Ht _____ Wt _____
Date of surgery ______________________ Surgical procedure ______________________
Vital signs: Pulse ________ BP ________ Resp ________ Temp(degrees C) ________

RISK ASSESSMENT - Please explain all positive responses. (Note: The following is just a partial list of some of the known risk factors for surgery. Further description of medical problems is appropriate below.)

1. *Cardiovascular* – Does the patient currently have

Yes	No	
( )	( )	Valvular heart disease
( )	( )	Abnormal cardiovascular examination? If yes, which of the following are present? ( ) rales ( ) jugular venous distention ( ) S3 gallop ( ) murmur ( ) edema ( ) other ________
( )	( )	Hypertensive CV disease
( )	( )	Coronary artery disease
( )	( )	Arrhythmia
( )	( )	Congestive heart failure
( )	( )	Hx of pulmonary edema
( )	( )	A hx of MI? If yes, when was it? ( )<3 months ago ( )3-6 months ago ( )>6 months ago ( )Unknown
( )	( )	History of CABG, if yes, give date ________
( )	( )	Pacemaker
( )	( )	Is endocarditis prophylaxis indicated?
( )	( )	Other cardiovascular problems ________

2. *Pulmonary* – Does the patient currently have

Yes	No	
( )	( )	URI/Productive cough? If yes, what is the status? ( ) active ( ) resolving
( )	( )	Wheezing?
( )	( )	A Hx of asthma? If yes, what is the status? ( ) active ( ) inactive
( )	( )	Chronic obstructive pulmonary disease?
( )	( )	Chronic bronchitis?
( )	( )	Kyphoscoliosis?
( )	( )	Smoking history? If yes, quantify in pack years ________
( )	( )	Other pulmonary problems ________

3. *Endocrine* – Does the patient currently have

Yes	No	
( )	( )	Diabetes? If yes, what therapy is patient receiving? ( ) diet alone ( ) diet and oral agent ( ) diet and insulin: insulin type and dose ________ What is the degree of control? ( ) glucoses <120 ( ) glucoses 180-240 ( ) glucoses 120-180 ( ) glucoses >240

4. Renal – Does the patient have

Yes No

( ) ( ) Renal failure?

( ) ( ) Current urinary infection?

5. Hematology – Does the patient have

Yes No

( ) ( ) Hemoglobinopathy?

( ) ( ) Bleeding diathesis?

6. Rheumatology – Is there

Yes No

( ) ( ) Cervical spine disease?

7. Neurology – Does the patient have

Yes No

( ) ( ) Hx of CVA? If yes, when?

( ) <6 weeks ago

( ) >6 weeks ago

( ) ( ) Hx of Seizures?

( ) ( ) Hx of TIAs?

( ) ( ) Myopathy/Neuropathy?

( ) ( ) Carotid bruit?

8. Gastroenterology – Does the patient have

Yes No

( ) ( ) Gatroesophageal reflux?

( ) ( ) Peptic ulcer disease?

( ) ( ) Liver dysfunction?

What is the patient's exercise tolerance?

( ) Sedentary only

( ) Normal activities

( ) Able to walk 2-3 flights without difficulty

( ) Participates in aerobic activities

Please elaborate on any positive responses above and describe any other medical problems which may be important:

Laboratory – Which tests have been ordered? (Only some of these tests may be required. You may wish to consult with outpatient anesthesiology regarding specific cases.)

( ) CBC ( ) SMA-6 ( ) SMA-12 ( ) UA ( ) CXR ( ) ECG ( ) PFTs ( ) ABG

( ) Protime ( ) PIT ( ) Bleeding time ( ) Pregnancy test

Other____

Note: The following tests are the minimal requirements of the hospital:

All patients: CBC, UA

Age ≥50: CXR & SMA-12

Males ≥40 and females ≥50: ECG

Results: Copies of lab reports are appreciated. Please check any of the following abnormalities that are present:

( ) $K < 3.5$ ( ) $pCO_2 > 50$ ( ) Hct < 30 ( ) SGOT > 40
( ) $K > 5.5$ ( ) $pO_2 < 70$ ( ) BUN > 50 ( ) Creat > 3.0

( ) Abnormal ECG. If ECG abnormal, check appropriate boxes:
( ) Premature atrial contractions ( ) >5 PVCs/minute
( ) Heart block ( ) Myocardial Infarction
( ) Rhythm other than sinus, specify ____________
( ) Other abnormality, specify

( ) Abnormal pulmonary function tests. Specify.

( ) Abnormal Chest X-ray. If CXR abnormal, check appropriate boxes below:
( ) Cardiomegaly ( ) Congestive heart failure ( ) Atelectasis
( ) Effusion ( ) Infiltrates
( ) Other, Specify ____________

( ) Other lab abnormalities (specify): ____________

Current medications/treatment (Include all OTC preparations)

1. ____________ 4. ____________

2. ____________ 5. ____________

3. ____________ 6. ____________

Allergies: ____________ ____________

____________ ____________

Anesthesia history: (Problems in patient or family)

____

____

Assessment of medical risk:

( ) Low risk ( ) Somewhat increased risk ( ) Moderate risk ( ) High risk

Discussion/Recommendations for perioperative medical care: ____________

____

____

____

Physician
(Print) ____________ Signature ____________ Date ____________

Should any questions or problems arise, please contact the GWUMC Preoperative Clinic.

Appendix 21-3

Guidelines for the Use of the Discharge Criteria*

Ideally, a physician should be available to personally discharge all surgical patients. However, short stay surgical patients may be released by a nurse when the patient meets discharge criteria as established by the hospital. (Physicians may discharge patients who do not meet criteria only after a personal evaluation and by a discharge order.) The physician indicates those patients who may be discharged, utilizing the discharge criteria stamp by writing the following provisional discharge order at the time of the surgical procedure: "(patient's name) may be discharged when discharge criteria are met." However, two circumstances require special consideration.

1. Patients whose anesthesia management has included endotracheal intubation must remain in the hospital a minimum of 3 hours (time in recovery room plus time on ward) even in the absence of respiratory distress. A patient who meets the discharge criteria but has had less than 3 hours of combined recovery time may be discharged by the anesthesiologist after a personal evaluation.

2. Patients who receive depressant medication for relief of pain, vomiting, dizziness, and so forth must be observed in the hospital at least 2 hours following its administration.

When the patient meets each of the discharge criteria, it is noted in the nurse's notes. When the criteria are all met, the discharge stamp is entered on the progress note, along with the current time. The nurse then signs the discharge stamp and the patient may be discharged at that time. To avoid confusion over the interpretation of some portions of the discharge criteria, the following guidelines have been proposed:

1. Vital signs: These include temperature, pulse, respiration, and blood pressure. Postoperative vital signs are taken every 15 minutes in the recovery room, then twice at 30-minute intervals, once at 60 minutes until stable, and then at 4-hour intervals in the unit. Vital signs are stable if over the period of 1 hour following transfer from the recovery room they are appropriate for age and consistent with the patient's preanesthesia vital signs and those in the recovery room.

2. Ability to swallow, cough, and gag: The patient must demonstrate the ability to swallow oral fluids and to cough or to demonstrate a gag reflex.

* Courtesy of the George Washington University Medical Center, Department of Anesthesiology, Washington, DC

3. Ability to ambulate: The patient must demonstrate the ability to perform movement consistent with his or her developmental age level and usual movement patterns (as determined during the nursing admission history).

4. Minimal nausea, vomiting, and dizziness: The patient must demonstrate the ability to swallow and maintain sips of fluids for 1 hour. (Because maintenance fluids are provided by intravenous fluids during the surgical procedure, the patient need not retain more than sips of fluid.) If vomiting is persistent (more than 3 times in 1 hour) notify the appropriate personnel. If dizziness is present the patient must still be able to perform movements consistent with age. Parents of pediatric patients should be taught to manage their child's fluid intake the remainder of the day following discharge. Initial fluids offered should be water, cola, or ginger ale at room temperature. Small amounts of fluids should be offered in an amount the child accepts.

5. Absence of respiratory distress: The patient may not present any of the signs of respiratory distress—snoring, cyanosis, or dyspnea. If these signs are present, notify the department of anesthesia immediately, so the patient may be evaluated and treated if necessary.

6. State of consciousness: The patient must be alert and oriented to person, place, and/or time as appropriate to his or her developmental level. Consult parents when evaluating state of consciousness in pediatric patients.

The discharge criterion policy does not require that a patient voids prior to discharge, unless specifically noted in doctor's orders. If voiding is required but has not occurred, the attending physician or resident should be consulted by phone before the patient is discharged.

Index

Page numbers followed by **f** denote figures; those followed by **t** denote tables.